AF443154

MEDICINE MEETS VIRTUAL REALITY 02/10

Studies in Health Technology and Informatics

Editors

Jens Pihlkjaer Christensen (EC, Luxembourg); Arie Hasman (The Netherlands);
Larry Hunter (USA); Ilias Iakovidis (EC, Belgium); Zoi Kolitsi (Greece);
Olivier Le Dour (EC, Belgium); Antonio Pedotti (Italy); Otto Rienhoff (Germany);
Francis H. Roger France (Belgium); Niels Rossing (Denmark); Niilo Saranummi (Finland);
Elliot R. Siegel (USA); Petra Wilson (EC, Belgium)

Volume 85

Earlier published in this series

ISSN: 0926-9630

Medicine Meets Virtual Reality 02/10

Digital Upgrades: Applying Moore's Law to Health

Edited by

James D. Westwood

Program Coordinator, MMVR02/10
Aligned Management Associates, Inc., New London, CT, USA

Helene Miller Hoffman, PhD

Assistant Dean, Curriculum & Educational Computing
Associate Adjunct Professor of Medicine
Director, Learning Resources Center
University of California, San Diego, School of Medicine, La Jolla, CA, USA

Richard A. Robb, PhD

Scheller Professor in Medical Research
Professor of Biophysics & Computer Science
Director, Mayo Biomedical Imaging Resource
Mayo Clinic & Foundation, Rochester, MN, USA

and

Don Stredney

Director, Interface Laboratory
Research Scientist, Biomedical Applications
OSC, Columbus, OH, USA

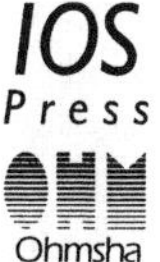

IOS
Press

Ohmsha

Amsterdam • Berlin • Oxford • Tokyo • Washington, DC

ISBN 1 58603 203 8 (IOS Press)
ISBN 4 274 90491 1 C3047 (Ohmsha)
Library of Congress Control Number: 2001098682

Publisher
IOS Press
Nieuwe Hemweg 6B
1013 BG Amsterdam
The Netherlands
fax: +31 20 620 3419
e-mail: order@iospress.nl

Distributor in the UK and Ireland
IOS Press/Lavis Marketing
73 Lime Walk
Headington
Oxford OX3 7AD
England
fax: +44 1865 75 0079

Distributor in the USA and Canada
IOS Press, Inc.
5795-G Burke Centre Parkway
Burke, VA 22015
USA
fax: +1 703 323 3668
e-mail: iosbooks@iospress.com

Distributor in Germany, Austria and Switzerland
IOS Press/LSL.de
Gerichtsweg 28
D-04103 Leipzig
Germany
fax: +49 341 995 4255

Distributor in Japan
Ohmsha, Ltd.
3-1 Kanda Nishiki-cho
Chiyoda-ku, Tokyo 101
Japan
fax: +81 3 3233 2426

LEGAL NOTICE
The publisher is not responsible for the use which might be made of the following information.

PRINTED IN THE NETHERLANDS

Preface

James D. Westwood and Karen S. Morgan
Aligned Management Associates, Inc.

Digital Upgrades: Applying Moore's Law to Health. We chose this year's theme to acknowledge that virtual reality, as an aid to medical diagnosis and therapy, is now being validated by clinical experience. No longer merely conjectural or start-up, it's well on its way to becoming routine.

In a half-humorous way, "Digital Upgrades" refers to upgrading our bodies the way we now upgrade software. Now the stuff of science fiction, personal health augmentation devices and programs will become, we predict, commonplace tools in the future. Already, networks connecting physicians, patients, and data are upgrading our methods of care. Sensors and microdevices, constantly improving, will become eyes, ears, fingers, noses, and tongues for these networks.

The doubling of efficiency and capability that Moore's Law describes does not directly apply to healthcare, as Richard Robb explains in his paper. However, we can expect accelerating progress as the utility of imaging, robotics, and informatics is demonstrated in the doctor's office and hospital. Kirby Vosburgh and Ronald Newbower examine how information technology already assists clinical care, and they address the barriers that discourage physicians and the healthcare industry from adopting novel tools and methods. What's noteworthy to us is that ordinary patients now benefit from the research shared at *MMVR* over the past ten years. Inevitably, continuing technological leaps and refinements will merge electronic tools with our bodies in ways we can now only imagine.

MMVR02/10 takes place in the wake of September 11, 2001, and we believe there is a relationship between that day's events and what this conference is for. On that morning, it became clear *why* healthcare should be transformed along the lines of Moore's Law. September 11 taught us that data has become the most critical political and economic resource, that which determines the power of nations. To address some particular fears, the United States and other wealthy nations are confronting the urgent need for improved data-intensive biomedical tools. For all its agonies, war does stimulate medical progress. We're sure to see increased government and private investment in electronic aids to medical training, surgery, telemedicine, data networks, and sensors — what *MMVR* is all about. Our ability to defend ourselves depends upon this investment.

On the preventive side of conflict, if medical excellence were to proliferate the way cellular phones, personal computers, and the internet have, then the inequality — generally, as well as in healthcare — between rich and poor nations would diminish. (And inequality will increasingly deter peace because global communications are making disparities between nations more obvious.) Although we can't replicate healthcare workers like we can computer chips, the ever cheaper production of health-supporting technology — per Moore's Law — would make medical care better and more available in the developing world. Healthier, more valuable individual lives will add up to a more peaceful world.

This volume is the product of the tenth annual *Medicine Meets Virtual Reality* conference. Noting this special anniversary, we wish to thank the hundreds of researchers who, during the past decade, have shared their knowledge and vision and made *MMVR* a tool for giving better health to all.

Contents

Medicine Meets Virtual Reality 02/10
J.D. Westwood et al. (Eds.)
IOS Press, 2002

1

The Virtualization of Medicine: A Decade of Pitfalls and Progress

Richard A. Robb, Ph.D.
Scheller Professor in Medical Research
Professor of Biophysics and Computer Science
Director, Biomedical Imaging Resource
Mayo Clinic/Foundation

Abstract. This paper is a personal perspective on VR in medicine over the last decade.

This brief review is not intended to be comprehensive nor inclusive of all developments or viewpoints regarding the role and impact of Virtual Reality (VR) in medicine in the past 10 years. It is primarily based on the author's experience and opinion. Although such a review begs for many references to confirming published works, that too is eschewed in order to remind the reader that the text herein is largely the author's perspective and views, for better or for worse. However, six references [1-6] are included which themselves contain many references to much of the material touched upon in this essay. Facts are in evidence that in the past decade there has been remarkable intrusion by advanced technology into the world of medicine and healthcare, including virtual reality technology. To the extent that one hopes to learn from such history, this synopsis may be helpful but may not fully meet expectations, primarily because VR in medicine has been a roller coaster ride of failures and successes that has squandered some time and resources but has also made some useful contributions. This treatise will summarize a few of these more obvious and egregious pitfalls and some of the generally acclaimed progress of VR in medicine during the past decade. These are listed in relational order in Table 1.

Table 1
Some Pitfalls and Progress of VR In Medicine

Pitfalls	Progress
wire frame models	surface and volume rendering
primitive geometry-"cartoons"	true anatomic volume scanning
rigid models only	deformable models
artificial surfaces	photo-realistic texture mapping
high latency	rapid computing-interactivity
2D display only	hi-resolution 3D display
no tactile or other senses	haptic and aural devices
difficult image segmentation	image registration/fusion
artificial intelligence	augmented/mixed reality
no "Killer App"	virtual endoscopy, surgery planning
crude robots	high precision robots
magnetic trackers, tethered	untethered optical trackers
poor communication	education/training, telemedicine
no software toolkits	comprehensive software
lack of standards	emerging standards
lack of validation	improving validation

VR has a relatively short history [1]. One reasonable starting point coincides in the early 1960s with the development of the *"Sensorama Simulator"*. This device placed the user in a surrounding visual and audio field to provoke a sense of immersion in the scene. The device was marginally successful as an oddity in the entertainment industry. More significant and useful developments followed this nascent stage. To mention a few, the development of the first head-mounted display in 1966, and in the early 1970s the development of high resolution screens for generating realistic scenes in flight simulation. The military rapidly adapted this technology in flight simulators, developing flight helmets and other interactive simulators to train pilots and other military personnel. A great amount of this work was unpublished. Other contributions to VR came in the early 1980s with the development of LCD-based head-mounted displays and in 1982 the first VR system, called VIVED or *"Virtual Visualization Environmental Display"*. This system consisted of a mini-computer, a graphics system, and a magnetic non-contact tracker. Feedback devices also began to appear in the 1980s, including the first sensory gloves. In the late 1980s another system called VIEW for *"Virtual Interface Environment Workstation"* was developed incorporating 3D virtual sound and some of the very first surface renderings instead of wire frame graphics.

Medical VR began in the very late 1980s [1,2]. In 1989 the first simulated surgery procedure for doing tendon transplants was published and in 1991 an abdominal surgery simulator was reported [3]. In 1993 detailed graphics of highly realistic images of the human torso, including deformable models, began to be published. The advent of the Visible Human Dataset from the National Library of Medicine in 1994 generated a large number of efforts to produce more realistic simulations of a variety of medical procedures. A hysteroscopy simulator using haptics was developed and published in 1995. Virtual endoscopy had its beginnings in the middle 1990s with simultaneous developments by several groups. By the late 1990s, a wide array of imaging, advanced visualization, and VR devices and systems were being developed for and used in medicine [4]. One remarkable system was developed in Tokyo which consisted of two 16-degree of freedom haptic input-output navigation devices, one for each hand, and a high resolution head-mounted display which permitted trainers and surgeons to perform two-handed 3-dimensional surgical simulations and rehearsals with sensitive tactile feedback. More recently, incorporation of realistic physical properties into deformable models, ultra-high resolution displays, more sensitive haptic devices and intelligent mapping of physiological properties onto anatomy have moved virtual reality into the mainstream of medical technology research, and useful clinical applications have begun to appear [5]. One successful paradigm for use of VR in medicine has emerged involving virtualization of volume image scans of the body (Figure 1). The ultimate value of VR in medicine may derive more from the sensory enhancement or augmentation of real experience than from the simulation of normally-sensed reality. This variant of VR is often referred to as AR (Augmented Reality) or sometimes MR (Mixed Reality).

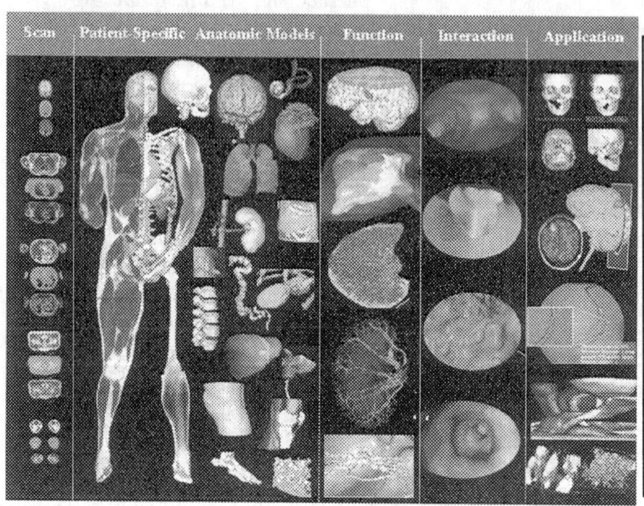

Figure 1. Paradigm for Virtual Reality in Medicine. Involves virtualization (modeling) of advanced high spatial and temporal resolution volume images of the body for clinical applications. Scanning systems provide 3D image data for patient-specific models in every region of the body, ranging in size from cells to organs. Functional and physical properties are fused with the anatomic models, and visual interaction with models provides detailed exploration and regional measurement and analysis directed at specific clinical applications. Evolution of capabilities holds promise for synchronous detection, differentiation and treatment of disease that will become the future successor of current image-guided diagnosis and therapy methods.

The first generation of VR in medicine actually started in the 1960s and 70s with attempts to analytically represent anatomic shapes. This generation contributed to an early major pitfall in VR, at least in medicine. Wire frame drawings and rigid modules were "neat", but not really useful. Oversimplified geometries were used to represent even complex body shapes. To compound the problem, the models were displayed on low-resolution 2D displays. The hype surrounding artificial intelligence and expert systems in the 1960s and 70s also mislead many who looked to this "new science" to make up for the shortcomings of simplistic anatomic and biologic models. It was the wrong solution to the wrong problem. The second generation added more sophistication to these models, providing elastic properties, which permitted tissue deformations and kinematics. Initially this was too crude for medical applications, but these capabilities became sufficiently realistic to be useful in the late 1980s and early 1990s. This was progress. Then physiology and even more complex physical properties were added to the simulations and anatomic models to more accurately depict structure and function, providing realistic and useful simulations of fluid flows and muscle dynamics, for example. High resolution, high performance graphic displays, along with true volume rendering, stereoscopic and immersive display formats, significantly advanced the usefulness of these higher order models. More recently, micro-anatomy models and cellular mechanics simulations have been possible with the advent of 3D microscopic imaging systems (e.g., confocal microscopy and optical coherence tomography. More exciting progress. The next generation of virtual anatomy and function will incorporate biochemistry and metabolic functions at the molecular level. Such capabilities will permit study and understanding of fundamental biologic processes and systems, such as the endocrine and immune systems. We have not yet reached this stage of sophistication.

In spite of numerous "fits and starts", progress has been sufficient to deploy VR technology in the operating or procedure room to provide the physician or surgeon with on-line, intra-operative access to and viewing of 5-D volume images of the anatomic regions of interest, along with associated physiological functions, all translated faithfully to the patient on the procedure table. Pre-operative volume image data and models can be fused with real-time data in the procedure room to provide enhanced visualizations of dynamic functional processes as well as anatomy, to make on-line measurements and generally to manipulate, control and guide interventional procedures [6]. Accurate tracking devices for reliable interactive navigation in such procedures have only recently become available. In the past, magnetic trackers were seriously compromised by the "unfriendly" metallic environment in the procedure room, and often required the physician to be tethered to the device. Free-standing optical and very recent metal-immune magnetic tracking/navigation systems are now providing working solutions. And, not withstanding the pitfalls, the quality of current VR-based capabilities have largely dispelled the notion that participants must "suspend disbelief" to make VR useful. Immersion and interaction are still needed, but advanced technology now renders the simulations and environments so realistic and responsive as to minimize or negate the need for imagination or conscious effort to suspend disbelief. VR techniques have also evolved to a three-fold stratification of types. First, *simulated reality* which involves an imitation or a model of real objects and procedures. Examples of simulated reality in medicine are virtual endoscopy or virtual surgery planning. The second stratification is *augmented reality*, which is a fusion of simulated and real time data. Image guided surgery and computer-aided interventions are examples of augmented reality. Fully *synthetic reality* refers to an optimized, totally artificial, yet absolutely faithful, environment and procedures and tools that replace or significantly augment actual procedures. Examples of optimized synthetic reality are telepresence surgery and robot manipulator performers.

Arguably one of the greatest pitfalls experienced by researchers and practitioners in medical VR early in the past decade has been the relative isolation of workers in the field, and lack of communication among them. Another pitfall was the false notion, at least originally, that sufficiently realistic simulations without validation could augment medical procedures in ways that would be acceptable to physicians. Much work was done in the early days of medical VR with unrealistic models based on analytical geometry rather than true anatomical geometry, and with artificial textures applied and no physical properties included. Even though such primitive efforts could be expected at the beginning, they were often promoted as useful without validation for way too long, to the detriment of the field. Because of such fallacious efforts, VR in medicine became unfairly stereotyped as "science fiction" – a waste of time in terms of making any positive contribution to the practice of medicine.

The Medicine Meets Virtual Reality (MMVR) Conference series has done a lot to minimize and overcome such pitfalls. Since its inception in 1992, the goal and theme of this conference series has been to bring engineers and physicians together to communicate and share and explore the cutting edges of VR technology and its potential applications in medicine. Initially, MMVR was never intended to be a forum to communicate or evaluate practical, routine use of VR technology in medicine, but rather to be forward looking and provide a venue for commercially promising new developments, ranging from novel ideas to innovative technology. To a large extent, the thread of this mission has continued throughout the ten MMVR conferences. However, as the decade has marched on, more and more reports on practical applications and careful evaluations of VR methods and devices in medicine have penetrated the series. This author believes this has been a good thing, rendering MMVR more inclusive of clinicians – an important original goal that had become marginalized. Scientists and engineers can occupy hours and days sharing their theories and gadgets, but dialogue with physicians is eventually essential if these are ever to be useful. Innovative technology and clever ideas are still an important part of the MMVR series, but the applications "promised" for several years are now being delivered – a welcome trend for this unique conference. As the decade milestone of conferences approached, the theme in 2001 of *Outer Space, Inner Space and Virtual Space* again solicited contributions that were leading edge developments in VR. Papers on multidimensional approaches, biointelligence, advanced deformations of models, data fusion, realistic mapping of structure and function established the meeting again as a forum for exposition of state-of-the-art technology and its promise in medicine. The theme for 2002, *Digital Upgrade: Applying Moore's Law to Health,* continues in this vane, but with a somewhat tongue-in-cheek inference that Moore's Law might be applicable to health and/or healthcare in a way similar to computer technology – that is, a doubling of capabilities and/or improvements about every 18 months. However, looking back over the past decade, it is evident that this law does not apply to the rate and magnitude of improvements in healthcare. It is problematical to apply such a formula to health or the healthcare system where there is such a high degree of variability, uncertainty and inertia, due to conservatism. Nonetheless, the theme provokes a retrospective analysis of where we've been and how far we have come, as well as tempts a prospective look at the future of virtual reality in medicine. The present overview finds itself in the saddle of these perspectives.

A significant contributor to pitfalls <u>and</u> progress in medical VR over the last decade has been developments (or not) in medical imaging. The field of medical imaging enjoyed continued improvements in resolution, speed and differential clinical applications in the past ten years. However, issues of image latency, interactivity, and validation have proven challenging. The speed of image acquisition and computation has almost followed Moores Law over the last decade. The amount of detail that can now be presented at interactive rates, even near real-time rates, is several-fold higher than available in 1990. There has been similar improvement in the photo-realistic quality of the images used in simulations and augmented reality scenarios and in the sensory responsiveness and interactivity of the systems. Even so, this increase does not obey Moore's formula. Improvement has often been slow and fraught with difficulties. Similarly, although there has been great progress in data processing, e.g., multimodality registration, image classification, volume rendering, and quantitative measurement, image segmentation is still the Achilles heel in achieving practical routine use of medical images. Even though medical images have improved significantly in quality, they are still relatively "noisy" in terms of absolute and reproducible quantitative representation of bodily tissue properties, making methods for automatic, rapid and reproducible segmentation of desired features from medical image scans very difficult. There are some niche successes for certain algorithms, modalities and tissue types, but the *"Killer App"* in image segmentation has yet to be developed. When it is, Moore's Law may well be applicable to the rate of progress that will ensue.

What is needed to avoid some of the pitfalls and blind alleys that have occurred in the past is a concerted effort on due diligence. Proposed new methods should be based on real clinical needs and align with the expectations of physicians. The method(s) should be relevant to problems without satisfactory current solutions and that have distinct promise to improve outcomes. Safety of the equipment and procedures needs to be documented and demonstrated. Reliability, accuracy, ease of use, modularity, and versatility of the method or procedure are all important factors to consider and document. Lack of comprehensive software toolkits for rapid prototyping and testing of VR methods, procedures and devices has impeded progress. Conversely, recent availability of such resources has significantly empowered the field and moved it forward. One must consider several practical issues commonly associated with new methodology, including the training of new users and the maintenance of new systems and/or devices. Conformance to existing standards or development of new standards is often crucial to success. Standards in VR have been slow to develop, but emerging conventions (e.g., VRML) are promising. Validation and evaluation are critical, as is careful assessment of cost versus benefit. Without question, one of the greatest pitfalls and inhibitors to reduction to practice and routine use of new methods and technologies involving imaging and virtual reality in medicine has been the lack of adequate scientific and clinical validation. The general approach to validation that scientists routinely take is a necessary but not sufficient first step, involving a sequence of mathematical simulations, phantom studies and testing on synthetic data derived from real data. Such evaluation can quantitatively characterize the performance and error margins of a new method. Such results should then be compared to ground truth or gold standards, if available, and multiple trials and comparisons conducted with existing standard methods targeted for replacement. In addition to this objective validation, scientists must interact with physicians who are expert in the specific clinical application and evaluate together subjective factors associated with the new method (e.g., clinical relevance, procedure safety, ease of use, training, etc.) Such interaction insures that when an absolutely unique feature(s) of a new method is determined to have compelling merit, i.e., no other method can produce the useful measure or effect, efforts must be accelerated to get the method accepted and implemented into routine practice.

Current and future VR medical research will continue to focus in four main areas: 1) devices and instrumentation, 2) algorithm development, 3) modeling and simulation and 4) application prototyping. Important ongoing needs and developments include 1) increased multidimensional resolution through space and time of images, procedures and devices, 2) automatic accurate anatomic and functional segmentation from image data produced by medical volume scanners of the human body, 3) fast and robust multi-dimensional registration and data fusion, 4) faithful tissue feature and property classification, and 5) realistic, real-time volume rendering and visualization. Many projects that have been initiated in the last decade will continue into the next decade, including virtual surgery, virtual endoscopy, image-guided diagnosis and treatment, virtual histology and pathology, robotics, manipulations, telepresence, performance assessment, etc. These are predicted to have an ever-increasing positive impact on medicine and healthcare. We will move toward the future successfully the same as we have done in the past, through a synergistic combination of ideas and tools. Ideas alone are not worth much. Tools that have not been based on good ideas are not worth much. But good ideas and good tools together are the key to future success, and what a bright future it is. Table 2 indicates some of the developments that can be expected in the next decade or two – progress toward fully non-invasive real-time diagnosis and treatment made possible through VR-related technologies.

Table 2
Future Medical VR : Non-Invasive Real-Time Diagnosis and Treatment

- **Multidimensional Dynamic Displays**
  Ultrahigh resolution, real-time holograms, dynamic immersion
- **Image Gloves**
  Bare hand control, unconstrained gesturing
- **Voice Control**
  Voice pick-up, tracking, recognition, synthesis
- **Smart Rooms**
  Whole body location sensing/tracking
- **Smart Clothes**
  Neural interfaces, bio-signal monitoring (EMG, EEG)
- **High Performance Medical Robots**
  Intelligent, remotely programmable, micro-precision, teletherapy
- **Smart Micro-Probes**
  Miniature devices inserted into body, controllable outside
- **Dick Tracy Computers**
  Wristwatch super-computers, voice programming, real-time models
- **Hospital Palmtops**
  Hand-held device for synchronous diagnosis and therapy

Multidimensional dynamic displays, image gloves for hands-free navigation in virtual space, and voice control will epitomize next generation Mixed Reality and greatly enhance medical procedures. Intelligent rooms and clothing that perform real-time tracking and monitoring will provide comprehensive and instantaneous input for informed, even automated, decision making. Special high precision robots remotely contollable will establish routine practical use of telemedicine and teletherapy. Moore's law will continue to apply to computers through the next decade, although an asymptote in computational performance may be eventually approached (not within the next decade - DNA computers will maintain the slope!). Real-time model generation capabilities and programming computers in natural language will be possible, and super computers will, in fact, be micro or even nano computers, and used both outside and inside the body. Intelligent diagnostic and/or therapeutic probes will be introduced into the body and either pre-programmed or externally controlled to proceed to the anatomic site of interest – "seek and destroy" nanobots!). Real-time model generation capabilities and programming computers in natural language will be possible, and super computers will, in fact, be micro or even nano computers, and used both outside and inside the body. Intelligent diagnostic and/or therapeutic probes will be introduced into the body and either pre-programmed or externally controlled to proceed to the anatomic site of interest – "seek and destroy" nanobots!). Eventually we will have the kind of totally non-invasive real-time technology that we only see in Star Wars and Star Trek movies – devices that simultaneously perform diagnosis and treatment – sort of *"one-stop shopping"*. Satava's *"Door to the Future"* may be such a device, but this author believes it will be much smaller than a door – more like a flashlight.

One of the pitfalls that any technology age suffers is that there are more false prophets than true pioneers (I firmly assert to be neither). We have to more expediently discern those really useful tasks from those that are destined to be useless, and not give heed to those voices that are *"full of sound and fury, signifying nothing"* (Shakespeare's Macbeth). At any given moment in history, it may be challenging to discern the false prophet from the true pioneer. John Lawton said *"The irony of the information age is that it has given new responsibility to uninformed opinion."* I agree with this. We indeed are in the Age of Information, for better <u>and</u> for worse! One might even refer to it as the Age of Information Glut, so enormous is the magnitude and ready accessibility of the information. We are not well poised to take maximum advantage of the available information. To compensate, some short cuts are taken by the false prophets, resulting in deductions that are not substantiated by good, hard facts and experimentation. Again, that **"V"** word, validation. Be wary!

The cost of new technology should not be the driving nor limiting factor to future progress. It is important, but if the cost of developing and proving a new technology can be demonstrated with high probability to improve and impact positively healthcare and eventually reduce costs, then fortitude and foresight must prevail to make the required capital investment. There is ample room in the field for true pioneers and visionaries, indeed they are always needed, but there is also need for rationale practitioners who exercise common sense and are committed to reduction to practice. As Carl Popper said *"I hold it to be morally wrong not to believe in reality"*. The degree to which virtual reality will ultimately be successful in improving healthcare and advancing the state-of-the-art in medicine will surely be commensurate with the degree to which we understand reality and are sensitive to it. The reason for this is simple: the object of medicine is the patient, and the patient is real.

<u>References</u>

1. Burdea G, Coiffet P: Virtual Reality Technology. New York: Wiley, 1994

2. Akay M, Marsh A: Information Technologies in Medicine, vol. 1. New York: Wiley, 2001

3. Satava R: Cybersurgery: Advanced Technologies for Surgical Practice. New York: Wiley, 1998

4. Robb RA. Biomedical Imaging, Visualization, and Analysis. New York: Wiley, 2000

5. IEEE Computer Graphics and Applications: Issue On Virtual Reality. November/December 2001

6. Robb RA. The Biomedical Imaging Resource at Mayo Clinic. IEEE TMI 2001; 20(9):854-867

Medicine Meets Virtual Reality 02/10
J.D. Westwood et al. (Eds.)
IOS Press, 2002

Moore's Law, Disruptive Technologies, and the Clinician

Kirby G. Vosburgh, Ph.D.
CIMIT/MGH/Harvard Medical School
65 Landsdowne Street, Suite 200, Cambridge, MA 02139
kvosburgh@partners.org

Ronald S. Newbower, Ph.D.
Partners HealthCare System/Harvard Medical School
11th Floor, 50 Staniford St, Boston, MA 02114

Abstract. The advancement of technical power described by Moore's Law offers great potential for enabling more cost-effective medical devices and systems. However, progress has been slow. Many factors for this failure have been cited, including the anti-rational economic structure of healthcare and the complexity and long time scale of medical development. Christensen et al. suggest that "disruptive technologies" may circumvent some of these difficulties. "Disruptive Technologies" are defined as those that are established in one market, but then penetrate and overwhelm another market. These incursions are accelerated by economic factors, and capitalize on functionality, reliability, and advancements supported by the original market. Christensen has cited many examples from industrial and service businesses, but few examples can be found yet in healthcare.

We argue that positive technology impacts in medicine occur most readily when innovators augment the skills of and collaborate with caregivers, rather than seeking to displace them. In the short term, a new approach may improve efficiency or quality. In the longer term, such approaches may obviate human tasks at lower-skill levels, and even permit task automation. One successful example has been the introduction of flexible monitoring for physiologic information. Systems for computer-aided diagnosis, which have failed to impact complex decision making, have succeeded in simpler specialty areas such as the interpretation of EKG's and mammograms, and may do the same with analysis of some pathology images. The next frontier may the operating room, and the adoption of such systemic technologies by caregivers in emergency medicine and general care may then have an even wider "disruptive" effect. Responding to time and cost pressures, and the desire to move care to the patient, other workers, such as radiologists, will drive the trend away from isolated, complex, large-scale devices, and toward integrated, modular, and simpler networked technologies.

In summary, technological "push" will continue in the demanding cutting-edge application areas as always, but the "disruption" will occur through wider application of lower-cost technologies, pulled by the users. The capabilities described by Moore's Law will allow the advancements necessary to facilitate this dissemination of capability and its ultimate benefit, so long sought.

1.   High Technology in Healthcare

The advancement of technical power, exemplified by Moore's Law predicting the doubling rate of semiconductor system capability, ought to have great potential for creating more cost-effective medical devices and systems. Over the past decade, it has been postulated that the improvements in communications and the development of standards [1] would simultaneously create a richer and more extensive pattern of relationships, leading directly to better care. However, frustration with the difficulties of applying high technology to meaningful use in clinical care is common.

Gladfelter [2] has listed some of the factors that have constrained the implementation of the "Holy Grail" of high tech medicine: the Electronic Patient Record. We have rewritten and expanded the list to include other factors which are often evident in the development of new devices and systems for patient care. These are drawn from our own experience and diverse sources, including the work of Kuttner [3] on the applicability of the market model:

Skills Barriers
- The range of capabilities required to successfully create, demonstrate, validate and commercialize new medical technology is very broad, and few individuals, or even organizations, have the full set.
- Medical care problems are highly complex; extensive knowledge and a sophisticated approach are required to partition the work so that commodity technology may be used effectively.

Market Barriers
- Medical product channels are often structured by medical specialty; new technologies often bridge or merge specialties.
- Different types of product compete to serve the same need, thus complicating market analysis: a surgical device may compete with a drug.
- The market is geographically (and socially) dispersed.

Technology Barriers
- Demonstrated reliability and robustness are required in the medical environment.
- Information systems must supply complex information reliably at the point of care, while preserving confidentiality, maintaining data security, and enabling authentication.
- New technologies must work easily with disparate systems, standards, and islands of automation.
- Systems must accommodate images and multimedia data.

Organizational Barriers
- Traditions of professional autonomy and extensive departmentalization
- Failure to understand the changing environment in healthcare
- Uniqueness of each organization, so solutions are not transportable

Physician Barriers
- Physicians are conservative and reluctant to abandon working systems.
- New technology often compromises the physician's unique access to and management of information.
- Physicians are not willing to constrain dialog to accommodate technical interfaces.
- Physicians fear displacement by MDs with other specialties, less qualified workers, or machines.

Structural/Financial Barriers
- Healthcare demand drivers are frequently non-rational.
- The volume of medical products is often small, so economies of scale may not be realized.
- The market model is not well adapted to medicine, so the benefits of new technology can often not be justified through a simple cost model.
- The prevailing economic incentives are often not aligned with general societal needs or even the patient's best interests.
- Many aspects of the current financial system perpetuate, or even reward, inefficiency.
- It is hard to assign value to individual process steps in clinical care.

Regulatory Barriers
- Clinical trials are the only practical way (today) of validating new approaches, but they are very expensive and time consuming, particularly when long-term benefits must be quantified.
- The regulatory process is unpredictable.
- The regulatory landscape is evolving: Current examples: HIPAA, Patient's Bill of Rights.

Despite these challenges, there is an overwhelming belief, which can easily be supported by macro-economic analysis [4], that high-tech medicine is cost-effective. The challenge is then to find ways to accelerate these changes, which may include stimulating and supporting "disruptive innovation."

2. The Potential of Disruptive Technologies.

Christensen and colleagues [5] have argued that "disruptive technologies" may offer a successful path to faster clinical use. "Disruptive Technologies" are defined by Christensen [6] as those with capabilities that are developed and validated in one market, and then penetrate and overwhelm another market. Christensen has cited many examples from conventional markets where penetration occurs in low-end applications, the needs of which are met by commoditized technologies originally developed for other purposes. They disrupt the overly complex and vulnerable products previously filling the market needs. These disruptions are accelerated by economic factors, but also by the availability of rapid technological advances and related attributes of improved functionality, reliability, etc. There are many such examples in industry and commerce (such as the evolution of banking), yet few examples can be found in healthcare.

We argue that positive technology impacts in medicine occur most readily when innovators and designers seek to augment the skills of and collaborate with caregivers, rather than seeking to displace them. In the short term, a new approach can improve efficiency or quality. In the longer term, such approaches can obviate human tasks at lower-skill levels, and even permit some level of task automation.

Our approach does not conflict with that of Christensen; rather, it supports it. In Christensen's analysis of manufacturing and service industries, the disruptive changes are generally initiated by the customer, rather than the supplier, of the product. The customer makes an informed choice to replace a high priced, over-featured product with one that is adequate to the task, but less costly. Once the new technology is in place, it may provide additional disruptive opportunities. The classic example of this is the substitution of a PC for a special purpose processor. Once the PC is inserted, the primary application may simply run adequately, but manifold additional advantages may be derived from the other attributes of the PC (software, communication, display, peripherals, etc.). These are almost "free" from the beginning, but position the user to tap into a universe of commoditized hardware technology and software applications, thus providing significant downstream benefits.

This may be so logical that its subversive nature is not apparent, but it does invert conventional models of driving technical innovation into medicine. Consider the use of information system technology: The traditional approach often involves setting standards, providing interfaces and connections to all possible sources, capturing all the information, and assuming that the power of the system will enable good things to happen. Examples of such approaches are the first several generations of Picture Archival Communications Systems (PACS) and thirty years of effort on the electronic patient record. Conversely, a more effective approach is to insert computers to do the jobs they can do successfully, keep a weather eye on compatibility and standards, and let the users grow into the capabilities, while providing better service along the way. The leaders of this revolution are then the physician, the biomedical engineer, the nurse, and their peers, and the job of the technologist is to support them at their working level.

3.　Successful Disruptive Technologies in Medicine

3.1　Automated EKG Reading

Systems for computer-aided diagnosis have failed to impact complex decision making, but have penetrated more routine specialty areas such as the interpretation of EKG's and diagnostic mammography, and may do the same with analysis of some pathology images. The interpretation of electrocardiograms (EKGs) was formerly a challenging task, particularly for non-specialists. The development of automated systems for this analysis was then pursued by the academic, government, and industrial communities. Initial results were poor: after many years of work, in 1972 the US Regional Medical Programs service concluded, in a report written by a committed of leading clinicians, [7] that available EKG analysis software showed "a significant incidence of disagreement" between the computer and trained cardiologists. Development continued, and by 1988, half of the EKG readings in the US were assisted by a computer [8]. By the early 90's, a review published in the New England Journal [9] concluded that some of the nine programs tested in a multi-site blinded study "perform almost as well as cardiologists in identifying several major cardiac disorders." Today, physicians routinely place high confidence in computer automated readings; a leading cardiologist remarked that "it's uncommon that he disagrees with the machine." Thus, computer–automated EKG reading fully fits Christensen's definition of disruptiveness: the computer has slowly and steadily displaced a specialist in doing a demanding task, allowing much less trained individuals to use the results of EKG examinations correctly. Of course, there are still situations in which the specialist's skills are called for, but as Christensen has predicted, these are an increasingly small segment of the total market, at the highest and costliest end.

3.2　Computer-Aided Diagnosis for Mammography

The interpretation of screening mammograms is an important, but difficult task. Early disease is often nearly occult and the anatomy is complex. Most examinations are normal, so reader fatigue is a factor. Yet, radiographic mammography has been shown, particularly in older women, to be a highly cost-effective screening procedure. [10] Thus attempts have been made for over thirty years to apply computers to assist the diagnosis. Originally, these built on work to pre-screen normal examinations from radiographs of coal miners with the potential for pneumoconiosis, which was successful by the early 1970s. However, mammography proved much more difficult, and it was only in 2000 that convincing data were presented showing the ability of a computer system to improve the effectiveness of radiologists in reading screening mammograms. [11] The way in which this technology has been marketed bears examination. The successful strategy used by the commercial supplier [12] has emphasized the ability of the system to "check" the reading of the radiologist; the analogy used is with a "spell checker" in word processing software. The documented advantage is to improve the likelihood that suspicious lesions will not be missed, while keeping constant the rate of "False Positives." Thus the radiologist feels that the system is supporting him, and avoiding the feared problem of missing an easy "True Positive" diagnosis, while at the same time practicing in a cost-effective fashion.

3.3　System Level Success: Flexible Monitoring for Physiologic Information

Another successful example has been the introduction of flexible monitoring for physiologic information. The low cost and high power of computational chips (Moore's law!) has finally allowed engineers to liberate physiologic monitoring from the bolt-to-the-wall "main-frame" ICU monitoring boxes. It has now been implemented in small portable wirelessly networked devices, which can then follow the patient from place to place. Thus

ICU-level technology moves to and with the patient, rather than requiring the patient to be transferred to an ICU for high-acuity episodes of monitoring needs.

4. Impact in the Operating Room, and Beyond

The operating room (OR), where equipment and information integration should lead to better care and lower costs, has long seemed ripe for disruption. Yet the variability of the procedures conducted in that venue and the personal preferences of surgeons have frustrated technologists. Rampant development at the sub-system level, without standardization, driven by performance criteria set by different user constituencies (surgeons, anesthesiologists, nurses), has led to inefficient and crowded conditions. However, now, with the evolution of standardized setups for minimally invasive surgical techniques, we see a fresh opportunity now for re-thinking the OR as a truly integrated system. These issues may be attacked systemically with technology that is (or is soon to be) commercially available. The physical architecture can be made more flexible, to permit setups for different procedures to be grouped together and stored out of the operating field when not in use. Equipment can be consolidated, with computers, displays, and power supplies becoming more integrated, with only the "end effectors" being different. Acuators, such as the ubiquitous foot pedals, may be combined. These trends may lead to the physical partitioning of the non-essential pieces of equipment into non-sterile control rooms, simplifying operation and cleaning, and accelerating the implementation of "plug and play" standards. Systems for the tracking, management, and storage of supplies and instruments may be adapted from technologies already in place in other industries. With greater automation and effective remote monitoring, the staffing may be reduced without reducing (or perhaps even improving) patient safety, and more effective space and time utilization will result. The use of smart objects, intelligent devices, and wireless communication will drive further improvements, and their insertion will be facilitated by the standardized systems already in place.

The subsequent flow of systemic technologies from the OR into emergency medicine and general care may then have an even wider "disruptive" effect. Other fields such as radiology may see a similar trend away from isolated, complex, large-scale devices, and toward integrated, modular, and simpler networked technologies. In all the areas, we expect the increasing time-pressure on procedures to favor the development of technologies that move to the patient, rather than technologies that require movement of the patient from venue to venue.

5. Summary

In summary, technological "push" will continue in the demanding cutting-edge application areas as always, but the "disruption" will occur through wider application of lower-cost technologies, pulled by the users when the improvements in capability become so large as to overwhelm the barriers unique to healthcare. The capabilities described by Moore's Law will allow the advancements necessary to facilitate this dissemination of capability and its ultimate benefit, so long sought, and will encourage innovators to undertake fresh assaults on long-standing systems problems in healthcare.

References

[1]   Evans, Philip and Thomas S. Wurster "Blown to Bits: How the New Economics of Information Transforms Strategy", HBS Press, Boston, MA 1999.

[2]	Gladfelter, Thomas, "Barriers to the Implementation of the Computerized Patient Record",
	http://www.uic. edu/~gladfelt/barriers.html
[3]	"Markets and Medicine" Chapter 4 of "Everything for Sale" by Robert Kuttner, Knopf, New York,
	1997
[4]	Cutler, DM and M. McClellan, "Is Technological Change Worth it?" Health Affairs, September-
	October 2001: 11-29.
[5]	Christensen, Clayton M., Richard M.J. Bohmer, and John Kenagy. "Will Disruptive Innovations
	Cure Health Care?" Harvard Business Review (September-October 2000): 102-117.
[6]	Christensen, Clayton, "The Innovator's Dilemma: When New Technologies Cause Great Firms to
	Fail", Harvard Business School Press, Boston, MA 1997
[7]	"Regional Medical Programs Service and Computer Assisted EKG Analysis Systems," Draft Report,
	division of Professional and Technical Development, US Regional Medical Programs Service,
	(unpublished), 1972
[8]	Drazen, E., et al., "A Survey of Computer Assisted Electrocardiography in the United States," J.
	Electrocardiol 1998:2; Supl:S98-S104
[9]	Willems, Jos L. et al., "The Diagnostic Performance of Computer Programs for the Interpretation of
	Electrocardiograms," New Engl J.Med 1992:325;1767-1773
[10]	See, for example, "Breast Cancer Facts and Figures," published annually by the American Cancer
	Society, or reviews such as Saveane, G. et al., Editors, "Screening Mammography, Breast Cancer
	Diagnosis in Asymptomatic Women," Mosby, 1993.
[11]	Burhenne, LJ, et al., "Potential Contribution of Computer-aided Detection to the Sensitivity of
	Screening Mammography", Radiology 2000;215;554-562
[12]	R2 Technology, Inc, 325 Distel CircleLos Altos, CA 94022

Medicine Meets Virtual Reality 02/10
J.D. Westwood et al. (Eds.)
IOS Press, 2002

Heuristic Haptic Texture for Surgical Simulations

Eric Acosta, MS, Bharti Temkin, Ph.D.
Dept. of Computer Science, Texas Tech University
Lubbock, TX 79409,
(806) 742-3527, Bharti.Temkin@coe.ttu.edu

John A. Griswold MD[1], Sammy A. Deeb MD[1], Tom Krummel MD[2]
Randy S. Haluck, MD[3], Louis R. Kavoussi, MD[4],
[1] *Dept. of Surgery, Texas Tech University Health Science Center,*
[2] *Emile Holman Professor and Chair Department of*
Surgery, Stanford University School of Medicine
[3] *Penn State Geisinger Health System*
[4] *Johns Hopkins School of Medicine*

Abstract

Generation of credible force feedback renderings adds the sense of touch crucial for the development of a realistic virtual surgical environment. However, a number of difficulties must be overcome before this can be achieved. One of the problems is the paucity of data on the in-vivo tissue compliance properties needed to generate acceptable output forces. Without this "haptic texture," the sense of touch component remains relatively primitive and unrealistic. Current research in the quantitative analysis of biomechanics of living tissue, including collection of in-vivo tissue compliance data using specialized sensors, has made tremendous progress. However, integration of all facets of biomechanical data in order to transfer them into haptic texture remains a very difficult problem. For this reason, we are attempting to create a library of heuristic haptic textures of anatomical structures. The library of heuristic haptic textures will capture the expert's sense of feel for selected anatomical structures and will be used to convey the sense of touch for surgical training simulations. Once the techniques for converting biomechanical data into haptic texture become more robust, this library can be used as a benchmark to verify theoretical computational models used for generating output forces in haptic devices.

1. Introduction

In order to develop a realistic surgical simulator, one must be able to develop a force feedback rendering mechanism that will produce credible forces via a haptic device. In turn, extensive knowledge of the characteristics of the tissues being simulated must be known. Basic research in quantitative analysis of biomechanics of living tissue has made tremendous progress, especially in topics such as new methods of testing of mechanical properties of soft tissues [1]. However, the integration of all facets of this field has yet to become a reality and it is an extremely difficult task to convert this knowledge into a form useable for haptic simulations. In addition to biomechanical factors, the perception of feeling objects by touch is subjective and dependent on a number of physiological and psychological factors. Despite such difficulties, the sense of touch is an integral part of medical practice, and simulating it, even at an imperfect level, is an essential step towards the development of comprehensive medical training simulators.

The capability of simulating palpation of different tissue types is an enormous hurdle for developers of computer haptics. Even though haptic rendering of soft bodies in a simple volumetric situation has been achieved [5], the general problem of haptic rendering, including dynamic tissue manipulations, remains unsolved. This is due to the intricacy and unpredictability involved in tissue structure representation as well as the visualization and deformation processes. In order to achieve realistic tissue simulation, a library of *in-vivo* tissue compliance properties is essential. If the sense of touch is not authentic enough to convince the user that the object being touched is real, it may only serve as a distraction rather than an aid.

Collection of biomechanical sensor data is currently the prevalent approach for generating *in-vivo* tissue compliance properties [2,3,4]. This is an important approach, but it does not take into account human perception. This is an important issue since even a perfect mathematical representation of a tissue is insufficient if the end result does not feel correct to the user. The fundamental solution to this problem will be very difficult to obtain and it will take a long time to produce reliable data for a variety of tissues. We thus believe that the collection of heuristic data is imperative. Such a heuristic database can play a critical role in testing of theoretical and computational models and can be used until sensor data can be converted into a form useful for haptics. Eventually, the quality of haptic textures will be improved by a combination of heuristic data reflecting human perceptual factors with biomechanical models.

2. Haptic textures

Haptic textures define how objects feel as they are palpated with a haptic device. Each texture has a unique combination of stiffness, damping, and static and dynamic friction components needed for haptic rendering of different body structures. The initial set of heuristic data will be collected by asking anatomy and surgery experts to generate haptic textures for geometrical models of anatomical structures. The expert's sense of perception will be taken into account when compiling a library of heuristic textures for three-dimensional haptic anatomical structures (3D-HAS). Each expert user will tweak and individual settings of haptic textures of anatomical structures and save them into a database. This will result in a baseline database containing the average (default) textures and a range of acceptable values. The resulting textures can then be analyzed and incorporated into future haptic surgical training and research simulations. Once the computational infrastructure is completed, more refined values of the existing parameters, as well as additional parameters needed to represent living tissues, can be easily incorporated into the heuristic database.

Haptic textures will be generated with our "touch&tell" system, Figure 1, which gives the user the ability to manipulate the tissue compliant properties. The system queries the database for a preferred haptic texture and, unless a previously saved haptic texture exists, the default value is assigned to the 3D-HAS. Users can modify haptic texture properties using the material's editor. Changes made to a haptic texture are updated on the fly to allow users to teak the haptic texture as they palpate the 3D-HAS. The user can then record satisfactory settings in the database. Users can also load haptic textures defined by other users, or the average haptic texture of all expert users who saved their settings for a particular 3D-HAS. The "touch&tell" system provides an option of turning off the visualization component to fine tune and to capture the texture data, thus collecting truer sense of the touch data.

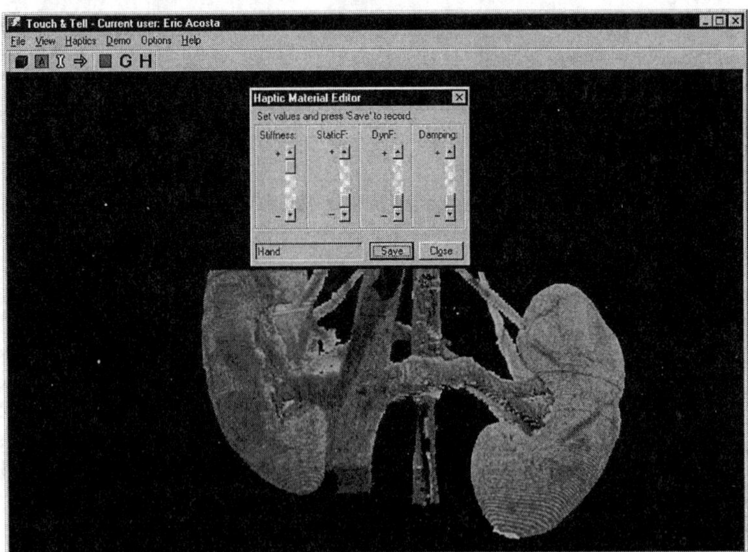

Figure 1. User interface with haptic material editor.

3. Conclusion

Our "touch&tell" system generates haptic textures using geometrical models of anatomical structures. The textures are compiled into a library of three-dimensional haptic anatomical structures (3D-HAS). In creating 3D-HAS we will be able to capture the expert's sense of touch. The data collection feature of the system can also be used to formulate various experiments in order to analyze and understand other factors related to human sense of touch, e.g. psychological and physiological factors.

4. Acknowledgements

Our work is supported by State of Texas Advanced Research Project, Grant # 003644-0117 and the Surgery Department of Texas Tech University Health Science Center.

5. References

1. Fung YC. Biomechanics, mechanical properties of living tissues, 2nd Ed, Springer-Verlag, New York, 1993.
2. Ottensmeyer, Mark P., Ben-Ur, Ela, Salisbury, Dr. J. Kenneth. "Input and Output for Surgical Simulation: Devices to Measure Tissue Properties in vivo and a Haptic Interface for Laparoscopy Simulators." Proceedings of Medicine Meets Virtual Reality 2000, Newport Beach, CA. IOS Press. 236-242. 27-30 Jan 2000.
3. Maab H, Kuhnapfel U. Noninvasive Measurement of Elastic Properties of Living Tissue, CARS '99: Computer Assisted Radiology and Surgery: proceedings of the 13th international congress and exhibition, 865-870, Paris, 23-26 June 1999.
4. Scilingo EP, DeRossi D, Bicchi A, Iacconi P. Haptic display for replication of rheological behavior of surgical tissues: modeling, control, and experiments, Proceedings of the ASME Dynamics, Systems and Control Division, 173-176, Dallas, TX, 16-21 Nov 1997.
5. Jon Burgin, Bryan Stephens, Farida Vahora, Bharti Temkin, William Marcy, Paul Gorman, Thomas Krummel, "Haptic Rendering of Volumetric Soft-Bodies Objects", The third PHANToM User Workshop (PUG 98), Oct 3-6, MIT Endicott House, Dedham, MA.

Medicine Meets Virtual Reality 02/10
J.D. Westwood et al. (Eds.)
IOS Press, 2002

Mastoidectomy Simulation with Combined Visual and Haptic Feedback

Marco Agus, EE[1], Andrea Giachetti, Ph.D. [1], Enrico Gobbetti, Ph.D. [1],
Gianluigi Zanetti, Ph.D. [1], Antonio Zorcolo, Dipl.-Inform[1]
Nigel W. John, Ph.D. [2], Robert J. Stone, Prof[3].

[1]CRS4, Uta (CA) Italy – http://www.crs4.it
[2]Manchester Visualization Centre, University of Manchester, Manchester, UK,
[3]Virtual Presence Ltd., Manchester, UK

Abstract. Mastoidectomy is one of the most common surgical procedures relating to
the petrous bone. In this paper we describe our preliminary results in the realization
of a virtual reality mastoidectomy simulator. Our system is designed to work on
patient-specific volumetric object models directly derived from 3D CT and MRI
images. The paper summarizes the detailed task analysis performed in order to
define the system requirements, introduces the architecture of the prototype
simulator, and discusses the initial feedback received from selected end users.

Introduction

Mastoidectomy is one of the most common surgical procedures relating to the petrous
bone. It consists of removal of the air cavities just under the skin behind the ear itself, and
it is performed for chronic infection of the mastoid air cells (mastoiditis). It is a surgical
procedure undertaken by a wide range of surgeons in everyday practice. The site anatomy
is widely variant. The main risks are related to the detection and avoidance of the facial
nerve and of aberrant jugular veins (or branches) and to the resection of adequate amounts
of the mastoid air cells. The ability to rehearse the procedure using patient-specific data is
extremely rare. A VR simulator realistically mimicking a patient-specific operating
environment addresses this shortcoming. A number of groups are working toward this goal
[4][5][6][7].

In this paper we describe our preliminary results in the realization of a virtual reality
mastoidectomy simulator designed to work on patient-specific volumetric object models
directly derived from 3D CT and MRI images. The simulator runs on a multiprocessing PC
platform and provides realistic visual and haptic feedback, including secondary effects
such as the obscuring of the operational site due to the accumulation of bone dust and
other burring debris.

The rest of the paper is organized as follows: first, we describe the detailed task analysis
performed to define the system requirements; we then provide a brief description of the
architecture of the prototype simulator, and we conclude with a discussion of the first
results obtained and a view of our future work.

1. Human-Centered Design

A detailed task analysis, following ISO 13407 [3], has been carried out in order to
identify the essential ergonomic components [9]. The analysis involved a review of

existing documentation, training aids, and video recordings, interviews with experienced operators, as well as direct observation of the procedure being performed in theater.

In the typical mastoidectomy surgical setup, Fig. 1, the ENT surgeon looks at the region of interest through a stereoscopic microscope and holds in his hands a high speed burr and a sucker. These tools are used, respectively, to cut the bone and to remove water (used to cool the burr bit) and bone paste produced by the mixing of bone dust with water.

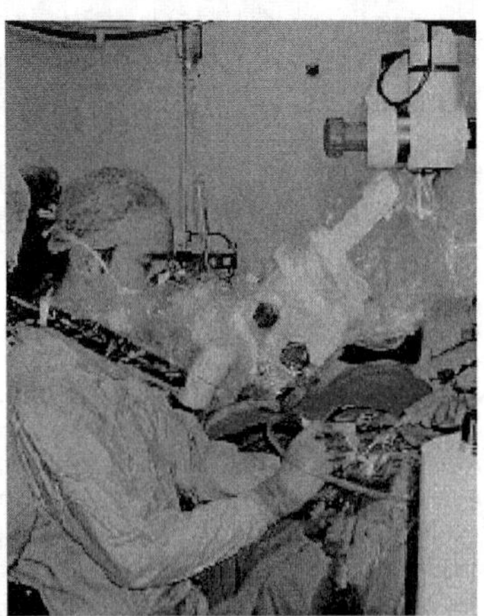

Figure 1: The typical mastoidectomy surgical setup: the ENT surgeon looks at the region interested by the procedure via a stereoscopic microscope and holds in his hands a high speed burr and a sucker, that he uses, respectively, to cut the bone and to remove bone paste produced by the mixing of bone dust with water.

Subjective analysis of video records, together with *in-situ* observations highlighted a correlation between drilling behaviours and type and depth of bone. In the case of initial cortex burring and recess preparation for, e.g., a cochlea implant receiver/stimulator, drill tip/burr motions of around 0.8 cm together with sweeps over 2-4 cm were evident, as were fine flexion and extension movements of the forefinger and thumb around the drill. Shorter (1-2 cm) motions with rapid lateral strokes characterized the post-cortex mastoidectomy. For deeper drilling, ~1 cm,- strokes down to 1 or 2 mm were evident with more of a "polishing" motion quality, guided using the contours from prior drill procedures. "Static" drill handling was also noted, eroding bone tissue whilst maintaining minimal surface pressure.

As for the visual effect of the drill on the surface of the bone, the task analysis hilighted that the graphical process must simulate drill site obscuration by bone dust paste, because its absence would reduce the importance placed by a trainee on the need for regular irrigation and suction. Realistic and meaningful bleeding is a perennial problem for VR researchers. We have concluded that, visually, the actual drill representation needs only be quite simple, and it is felt that representing the spinning of the cutter or diamond burr is unnecessary. What is considered necessary, from a functional standpoint, is an effective collision detection mechanism which not only copes with increased resolution as the virtual drill proceeds deeper into the temporal bone, but is also capable of generating error states when (for example) a large burr is inserted into a narrow drill site.

As for the nature of the technology required for displaying drill, drill site, bone, and so on, there is no conclusive evidence or support for the premise that the use of a stereoscopic system will aid performance in this case. Binocular viewing systems are deployed in the operating theatre and used by surgeons, and so binocular imaging should be available to the simulator. However, the wearing of any form of stereoscopic display, such as a head-mounted display or liquid crystal shutter glasses should be avoided. The surgeon or trainee does not want to use cumbersome eyewear that is not necessary for carrying on the real procedure. We make the hypothesis that, if the simulation achieves a reasonable level of fidelity, then the combination of high-resolution images and haptic feedback will, more than likely, suffice.

As well as the visual and 6-DOF input/3-DOF haptic feedback for drill simulation (including high frequency vibration), the training system might also be enhanced by the inclusion of audio effects. Some surgeons suggest that they are able to detect subtle changes in sound depending on the nature of the bone they are working with (eg. cortex *vs.* petrous). However, this quality is considered to be "overkill" in a training system such as that being considered here.

2. Prototype System Architecture

We have built a prototype system, simulating the effects identified by the task analysis. The system is running on a dual PC platform (Fig. 2). It exploits both message passing and shared-memory parallelism to meet the performance constraints imposed by the human

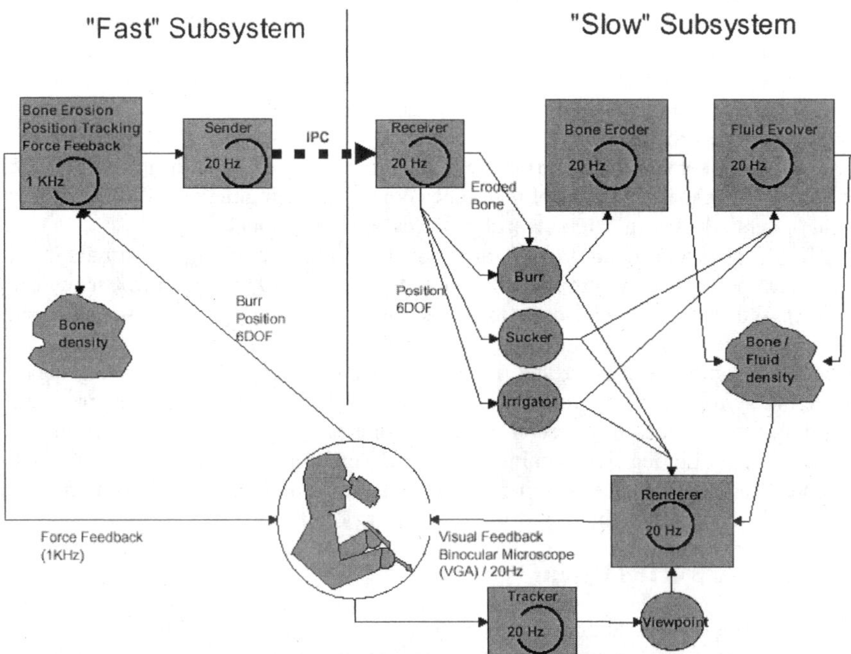

Figure 2: Decoupled simulation architecture. The system uses a volumetric approach, with the initial configuration of the model directly derived from patient CT data. The data is initially replicated on the two machines. The first machine is dedicated to the high-frequency tasks: haptic device handling and bone removal simulation. The second machine concurrently runs at 10-20 Hz the low-frequency tasks: bone removal, fluid evolution and visual eedback. The two machines are synchronized using one-way message passing with a dead reckoning protocol.

perceptual system. The system uses a volumetric approach, with the initial configuration of the model directly derived from patient CT data. The final version will use volumetric tissue probability maps derived from CT, MRI and MRA data using a multi-dimensional classification technique [8]. The data is initially replicated on the two machines. The first machine is dedicated to the high-frequency tasks: haptic device handling, one for the dominant hand controlling the burr and the irrigator, and the other controlling the sucker, as well as bone removal simulation. These tasks require at least 1 kHz update frequency because of the need of simulating hard contacts. The second PC concurrently runs at 10-20 Hz the low-frequency tasks: bone dust evolution and visual feedback. The two machines are synchronized using one-way message passing with a dead reckoning protocol.

In our volumetric description of the scene, voxels labeled as bone must bone must react to the manipulators through the haptic feedback devices, but they do not evolve unless they are removed by burring. In the data replicated in the machine dedicated to low frequency tasks, further values are introduced in the volume labelling voxels occupied by dust, blood and water. These values are used directly by the volume rendering thread.

The "fast" subsystem performs the burring simulation, i.e. the force feedback calculation and the bone removal from the dataset, sending the force value to the haptic devices, and sending information on manipulator positions and bone removed to the "slow" subsystem.

This task is extremely difficult to perform at over 1 Khz. We have thus organized our simulation so that each time step is divided into two sub-steps. The first sub-step estimates the bone material deformation and the resulting elastic forces, given the relative position of the burr with respect to the bone. The second sub-step estimates the local rate of cutting of the bone by using a postulated energy balance between the mechanical work performed by the burr motor and the energy needed to cut the bone, which is assumed to be proportional to the bone mass removed.

The "flow" subsystem performs the visual simulation of bone dust and fluid dynamics as well as the visual rendering of the scene. We are modeling the dust/fluid dynamics using what essentially amounts to a hybrid particles/sand pile model.

The visual rendering subsystem must operate within the timing constraints imposed by the human perceptual system (i.e. a latency of less than 300 ms, and a frequency above 10-15 Hz). We reach this goal by using a parallel processing approach, which exploits the capabilities of current graphics PC architectures. In our system, the renderer is totally decoupled from the simulator and the tracking system, and runs at its own frequency. The rendering system is based on a volumetric approach. We use texture mapping and alpha blending for a back to front reconstruction of the scene. Shading effects are implemented by exploiting the register combiner OpenGL extension on most modern commodity graphic boards. Surgical instruments are rendered as polygons, and combined with the volumetric rendering of the rest of the scene using Z-buffering.

3. Implementation and Results

Our current configuration is the following:

- a single-processor PIII/600 MHz with 256 MB PC100 RAM for the high-frequency tasks; two threads run in parallel: one for the haptic loop (1 KHz), and one for sending volume and instruments position updates to the other machine;
- a dual-processor PIII/800 MHz with 512 MB PC800 RAM and a NVIDIA GeForce 2 GTS and running a 2.4 linux kernel, for the low frequency tasks. Three threads are continuously running on this machine: one to receive volume and position updates, one to simulate bone removal and fluid evolution, and one for visual rendering;
- a Phantom Desktop haptic device for the dominant hand; the device is connected to the single processor PC. It provides 6DOF tracking and 3DOF force feedback for the burr/irrigator;

- a Phantom 1.0 haptic device for the non-dominant hand; the device is connected to the single processor PC. It provides 6DOF tracking and 3DOF force feedback for the sucker;
- a N-vision VB30 binocular display for presenting images to the user. The VB-30 contains a small high resolution LCD display and is connected to the S-VGA output of the dual processor PC.

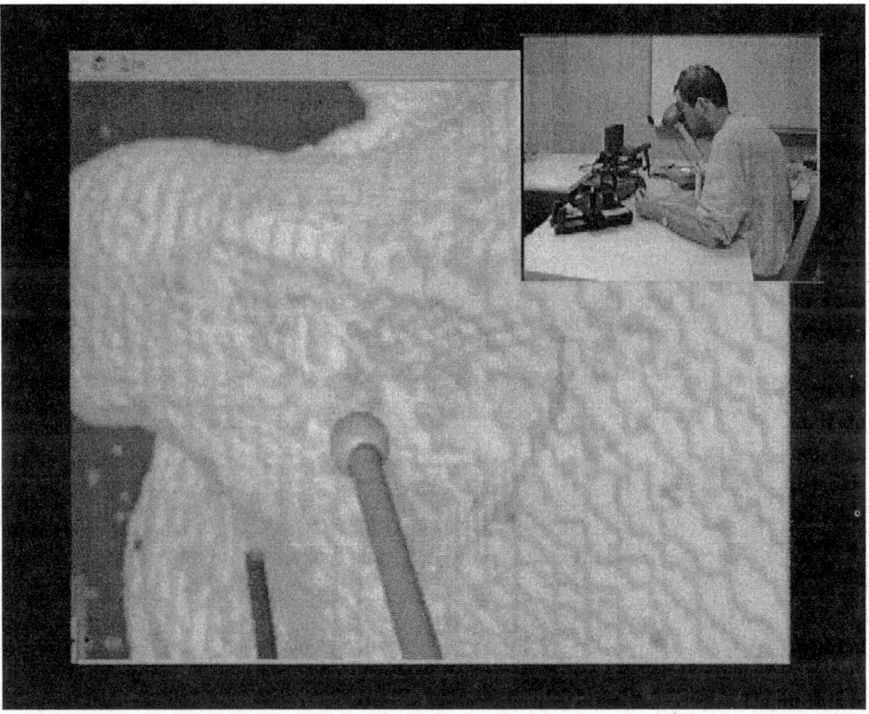

Figure 3: Snapshot from a video demonstration of a simulated mastoidectomy. The central image show the image viewed by the training surgeon with bone, water, blood and manipulators. In the top right corner it is possible to see the corresponding external view with the training surgeon feeling the haptic feedback through the Phantoms while observing the scene in the binocular display

We have gathered initial feedback about the prototype system from the Otolaryngology surgeons that are collaborating with this project.

The performance of the prototype is sufficient to meet the timing constraints for display and force-feedback effects, even though the computational and visualization platform is made only of affordable and widely accessible components. We are currently using a volume of 256x256x128 8-bit cubical voxels (0.3 mm side) to represent the region where the operation takes place. The force–feedback loop is running at 1 KHz using a 5x5x5 grid round the tip of the instruments for force computations. The computation needed for force evaluation and bone erosion takes typically 20 µsec, and less than 200 µsec in the worst case configuration. Shaded volume rendering of dynamic volumes currently takes 70 ms per frame (i.e. over 14 frames per second) using 256 depth slices on an 800x600 window with 16 bit color and 2X zoom rendering.

The overall realism of the simulation is considered sufficient for training purposes. As required by the task analysis, the haptic sub system is able to provide a reasonable force feedback effect, bone removal and noise simulation. The visual system is able to provide bone dust and water bleeding effects, blood simulation, and manipulators displayed at the required frame rate.

Subjective input is currently being used to tune the parameters that control force feedback. The speed of the water flow simulation has been identified as a principal area for improvement.

Fig. 3 shows a snapshot of the current system in use. The surgeon is looking at the scene with the binocular display and manipulates the burr and sucker through the two PHANToM devices. Fig. 4 shows selected frames of the initial phase of a virtual mastoidectomy, where debris formation and suction effects are clearly visible.

4. Conclusions and Future Work

We have described our preliminary results in the realization of a virtual reality mastoidectomy simulator designed to work on patient-specific volumetric object models directly derived from 3D CT and MRI images.

We carried out an in-depth task analysis, that highlighted key human interface features, including visual and haptic feedback requirements, as well as burring primary and secondary effects. Our simulator prototype demonstrates the possibility of building, exploiting parallelism on a PC platform, and a VR simulator mimicking a realistic patient-specific operating environment, including key secondary effects such as debris formation and the related visual masking effects.

The results obtained thus far were judged of good quality by the Otolaryngology surgeons collaborating to the project. The prototype is currently running directly using patient specific data as input, opening, therefore, the road towards the use of the simulator for pre-operation planning and rehearsal. This would make it possible to plan surgery directly on a model of the individual patient, rather than by referring to a model surgical procedure on a standard anatomy.

While subjective input from selected end users is encouraging, it has been realized that it would be of extreme interest to have available direct forces measurements obtained by drilling actual samples, since there are, to our knowledge, no available data on the subject in the literature. In the near future we plan to start an activity aimed at defining an experimental setup and measurement procedures.

Our current work is also concentrating on improving the quality and speed of fluid flow simulation.

Acknowledgments

These results were obtained within the framework of the European Union IERAPSI project (EU-IST-1999-12175). The authors would like to acknowledge the contributions from members of the University of Pisa's Department of Otolaryngology, University of Pisa's Department of Radiology, Manchester Royal Infirmary's Department of Otolaryngology, Head & Neck Surgery, and of the Department of Surgery and North of England Wolfson Centre for Minimally Invasive Therapy.

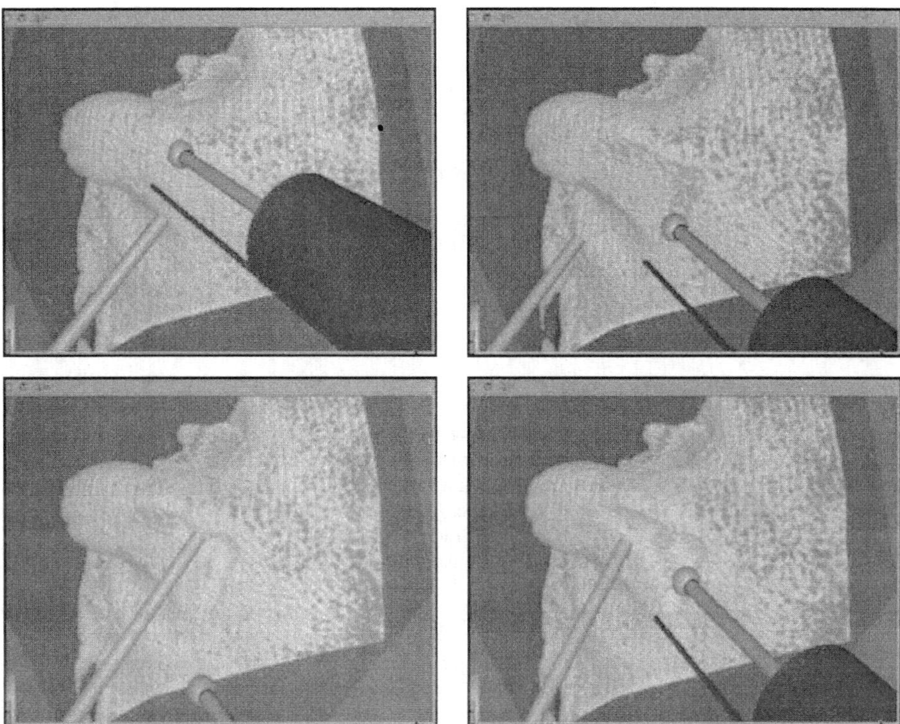

Figure 4: From top left to bottom right, selected frames of the initial phase of a virtual mastoidectomy. Debris formation and suction effects are clearly visible.

References

[1]   A. Jackson, N. W. John, N. A. Thacker, E. Gobbetti, G. Zanetti, R. J. Stone, A. D. Linney, G. H. Alusi, and A. Schwerdtner, Developing a virtual reality environment for petrous bone surgery: a "state-of-the-art" review. *Journal of Otology & Neurology*, To appear.

[2]   N. W. John, N. Thacker, M. Pokric, A. Jackson, G. Zanetti, E. Gobbetti, A. Giachetti, R. J. Stone, J. Campos, A. Emmen, A. Schwerdtner, E. Neri, S. Sellari Franceschini, and F. Rubio. An integrated simulator for surgery of the petrous bone, In J. D. Westwood, editor, *Medicine Meets Virtual Reality 2001*, Amsterdam, The Netherlands, January 2001. IOS.

[3]   ISO. *Human-Centered Design Processes for Interactive Systems*. International Standard ISO 13407, ISO, 1999.

[4]   G. Wiet, J. Bryan, D. Sessanna, D. Streadney, P. Schmalbrock, and B. Welling. Virtual Temporal Bone Dissection Simulation. *Proc. Medicine Meets Virtual Reality*, Newport Beach, CA. 2000.

[5]   C.V. Edmond, et al. Simulation for ENT Endoscopic Surgical Training. *Proc. Medicine Meets Virtual Reality 5*, San Diego, CA, January 1997.

[6]   S. Weghorst, et al. Validation of the Madigan ESS Simulator. *Proc. Medicine Meets Virtual Reality*, San Diego, CA. 1998.

[7]   J. Bryan, D. Stredney, G. Wiet and D. Sessanna. Virtual Temporal Bone Dissection: a Case Study, *Proc. IEEE Visualization*, San Diego, CA, 2001.

[8]   M. Pokric et al. Multi-dimensional Medical Image Segmentation with Partial Voluming. Proceedings of Medical Image Understanding and Analysis, July 2001

[9]   R. J. Stone, A Human-Centered Definition of Surgical Procedures, IERAPSI (IST-1999-12715) Work Package 2, Deliverable D2 (Part 1), July 2000

Medicine Meets Virtual Reality 02/10
J.D. Westwood et al. (Eds.)
IOS Press, 2002

Tele-Immersive Medical Educational Environment

Zhuming Ai, Fred Dech, Jonathan Silverstein and Mary Rasmussen
University of Illinois at Chicago
VRMedLab, School of Biomedical and Health Information Sciences
1919 W. Taylor St. (MC 530), Chicago, IL 60612-7249
Email: zai@uic.edu

Abstract. By combining teleconferencing, tele-presence, and Virtual Reality, the Tele-Immersive environment enables master surgeons to teach residents in remote locations. The design and implementation of a Tele-Immersive medical educational environment, Teledu, is presented in this paper. Teledu defines a set of Tele-Immersive user interfaces for medical education. In addition, an Application Programming Interface (API) is provided so that developers can easily develop different applications with different requirements in this environment. With the help of this API, programmers only need to design a plug-in to load their application specific data set. The plug-in is an object-oriented data set loader. Methods for rendering, handling, and interacting with the data set for each application can be programmed in the plug-in. The environment has a teacher mode and a student mode. The teacher and the students can interact with the same medical models, point, gesture, converse, and see each other.

1 Introduction

There are many complex regions of the human anatomy which are difficult to understand using traditional educational methods. Text books, 2D illustrations and movies have limited ways of showing complex 3D information. Cadaver dissection has always been important to the study of anatomy, however the availability of cadavers has declined, and sometimes meaningful dissection is made difficult by poorly delineated anatomic structures. A clear understanding of the intricate spatial relationships between anatomic structures is essential for the diagnosis and the treatment of disease. Immersive Virtual Reality (VR) provides a powerful tool to address these problems. Some medical educational applications have been developed in VR environments. An earlier version of Virtual Temporal Bone application developed here is one of them.[1] An eye diseases simulation program, which could be used for resident education as well as patient education, has also been developed by us.[2]

While teacher-student interaction is very important in education, expert medical educators are few in numbers for increasingly specialized procedures. By combining teleconferencing, tele-presence, and Virtual Reality, the Tele-Immersive environment enables master surgeons to teach residents in remote locations.[3] Tele-Immersion is Virtual Reality combined with high speed networks. With Tele-Immersion, surgeons can use superior 3-dimensional (3D) visualization of VR, and share networked, interactive anatomic models and radiological imaging. With high quality networked 2-way audio and video integrated in the VR environment, gestural communication and body language are also represented.

The Electronic Visualization Lab at the University of Illinois at Chicago has developed a general purpose Tele-Immersive framework, Limbo[4]. Although many educational applications share the same identical basic functionality, a general purpose environment can not provide all the features necessary for specific applications. To address this problem, we have designed and developed a Tele-Immersive medical educational environment which has many common VR functions as well as a Application Programming Interface (API), and a plug-in structure for loading different data sets. This allows us to quickly get medical educational applications running in VR.

2 Design of Tele-Immersive Medical Educational Environment

Tele-education is the use of telecommunications technology to deliver education from a distance. Most current Internet-based tele-education applications are distributing multimedia text books on the Internet. State-of-the-art network and visualization technology has made it possible to go one step further - distributing classrooms on the next generation networks.

2.1 Immersive VR

The sense of presence in a virtual world elicited by immersive VR technology indicates that VR applications differ fundamentally from those commonly associated with interactive computer graphics or multimedia systems. Immersive Virtual Reality can be a very powerful tool for providing realistic 3D anatomic information. It even provides information which is difficult to obtain from cadaver dissection due to poorly delineated anatomic structures in anatomic dissection and lack of capability for transparency.

The CAVE[5], the ImmersaDesk[6], and the head-mounted display are some of the most commonly used Immersive display devices nowadays. The CAVE and the ImmersaDesk can present a virtual world to a group of people at the same time, which make it promising for medical education. The ImmersaDesk has an appropriate scale for anatomic models, as well as being more economic and portable than the CAVE, we are using the ImmersaDesk to do VR medical education.

2.2 Real-Time Networking

The Network is an essential part of Tele-Immersive educational environment. The data transmitted on the network includes video, audio, models, model manipulation matrix, and control data. All this data needs to be transmitted in real time. Jitter and latency control is crucial for the quality. Quality of Service (QoS) and multicasting techniques in the Next Generation Internet (NGI) and Internet2 projects are helpful for establishing distributed classrooms.

2.3 Tele-Immersive Classroom

A Tele-Immersive classroom gives the teacher and the students the sense of presence in an environment where they can talk to one another, see each other and manipulate the same model. The Tele-Immersive classroom mimics a real classroom in such a way that the teacher and the students do not feel the distance between them. They can interact with each other and they can interact with the medical models.

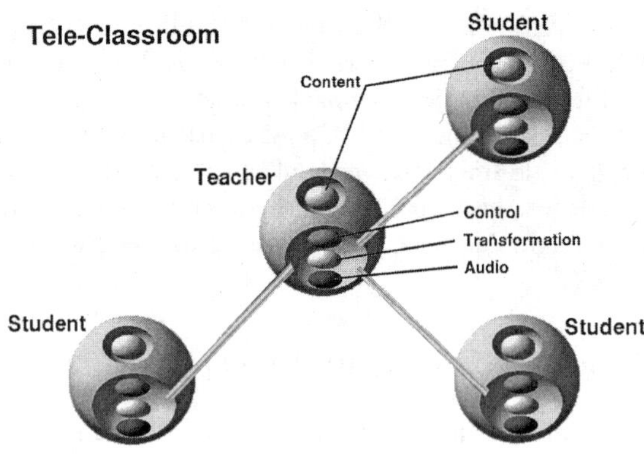

Figure 1: Tele-Immersive classroom for medical education.

Real-time streaming audio is enabled in the Tele-Immersive classroom so that people can hear each other; avatars are used so that people can see each other. Electronic control methods are provided for the teacher to control the classroom discipline, and to organize discussions.

2.4   Reusability

The development of Tele-Immersive educational applications is time consuming. It involves the use of many different libraries and APIs. Networking, visualization, VR, modeling, content and educational expertise need to be well organized.

In the real world, a classroom can is used by different teachers to teach different courses. In Tele-Immersive education, each course is usually a set of computer programs and associated data. Some parts of the program code are common among different courses, some are unique. From an application developer's perspective, it will save considerable effort if the virtual classroom is reusable, and different courses can be put into one virtual classroom.

3   Implementation

A Tele-Immersive medical educational environment, Teledu, has been development for Silicon Graphics, Inc. (SGI) machines based on Limbo. Limbo is designed as a programming framework or template that can be used as a start point of Tele-Immersive programming. One problem in the development of the Tele-Immersive educational environment is that a general purpose environment can not provide all the features for different applications, although many applications share the same basic functionality. Teledu defines basic functionality for Tele-Immersive medical education.(Figure 1) It provides a user interface for Tele-Immersion. In addition, an API is provided so that developers can develop different applications with different requirements. With the help of this API, a programmer only needs to implement a plug-in in order to load their application-specific data set. The plug-in is an object-oriented data set loader. Methods for rendering, handling, and interacting with the data set are programmed in the plug-in for each application.

3.1 User Interface

Teledu has two basic modes, teacher mode and student mode. The teacher controls the environment: he/she can run demos and manipulate the models. He/She can also control a student's viewpoint and can pass control to a student. The students can watch the models and demos, ask questions, and control the models when permitted by the teacher. The teacher and the students can interact with the same medical models, point, gesture, converse, and see each other. Teledu supports one teacher and a virtually unlimited number of students. In practice, each ImmersaDesk can have 4 or 5 people working together. If 4 or 5 ImmersaDesks are linked at a time, a teacher can teach a class with about 20 students.

Teledu has all the basic functions a VR application needs. These include picking, moving, and rotating the objects. In the case of our ImmersaDesk, the only tool used for interaction is a device called a wand. It has only 3 buttons and a joystick. With a tracker mounted on it, its position and orientation information in 3D space are also available. It is common in VR setups that tools for interaction are very simple and people do not have access to the keyboard or mouse. So the user interface needs to be designed differently compared to monitor/keyboard/mouse based applications.

A menu is useful in VR, but it is not as efficient as it is in 2D applications. The font needs to be much larger, showing fewer menu items on the available screen space. Also it is much more difficult to select menu items in 3D space. In Teledu, the menu interface is different for teacher and students. The teacher has a programmer-defined menu system. The students' names are listed on the menu so the teacher can pass control to a particular student by clicking his/her name. Students are allowed to select the menu only when they are given control, so that the commands from the teacher and the students do not conflict.

Voice control is much more important in VR applications then it was in 2D applications. We have set up a voice recognition server developed with IBM's ViaVoice library on a PC running the Linux operating system. The user's voice is transmitted from the SGI machine's microphone to the Linux PC over the network. CAVERNsoft is used here to handle the real time transmission. The recognition engine on the Linux PC processes the voice and transfers the recognized text back to the SGI machine. Then the application on the SGI machine takes actions based on the text sent back. For simple command phrases voice recognition is very accurate.

Instead of showing text on the ImmersaDesk, voice feedback is used in Teledu to let the user hear error messages and other information the application wants the user to know. IBM's ViaVoiceTTS library is used here to set up a server to do the text to speech conversion. This server is also on the Linux PC. The application on the SGI machine sends the text to the Linux PC over the network, and the server sends back the synthesized voice so it can be played back on the SGI's speakers.

Sometimes the teacher wants to show the medical model to the students from a particular view point. What the teacher can do in the normal VR environment is to move his/her own head to that position and ask the student with the head tracker at the remote location to do the same thing. In practice, the student at the remote site, who may have little experience with VR, may not know what to do. And when the teacher is talking about what they should see from this view position, the student may have no idea what the teacher is talking about. To solve this problem, the teacher needs to have the ability to control the students' view points. So in teacher control mode we send the data from the tracker mounted on the teacher's head to the student sites, and use this data, instead of the local tracker data, to control the students' view points. In this way all the students at all the networked VR setups have the same perspective as the teacher.

3.2 Application Programming Interface

Teledu is a tele-classroom. It also has an Application Programming Interface (API) with which programmers can develop object-oriented data set loaders as plug-ins.

The API contains a set of C++ classes. A C++ menu class is provided with which a programmer can build a customized menu system. A voice processing class is also implemented in this system. The developer can make use of voice recognition and speech synthesis functions. The functions communicate with a server running on a Linux PC. This server does the actual speech related work. A communication channel between teacher and students is embedded within the API. The developer can send application specific data among connected VR sites.

Teledu is based on IRIS Performer, which provides a programming interface for creating real-time graphics applications and offers high-performance rendering in a 3D graphics toolkit. Teledu can load all the database formats Performer supports.

It is very difficult, if not impossible, to define the contents of an educational course in a standard file format. In medical education, the contents of a course could include a set of 3D models, the manipulation of the models, and the animation of the models. Such a course, if defined in a computer, includes not only the data, but also the functions handling the data. In Teledu, we designed the course as a plug-in which contains the collection of data (usually 3D models) and the code to handle the data. We put the models into a data file, and the code into a Dynamically Linked Library. The data file and the library have a one-to-one correspondence. When the application is directed to load the data, the code in the library is also loaded automatically.

4 Applications

Using this environment, we have developed the Virtual Pelvic Floor application, the Virtual Temporal Bone application, and an application to view radiological volumetric data sets. Other applications are also under development in this environment.

4.1 Virtual Pelvic Floor

The pelvic floor and its associated structures is an anatomic region which is complex and difficult to understand from traditional educational resource material such as two-dimensional drawings in textbooks and cadaver dissections. Tele-Immersion allows us to not only view and manipulate these structures in stereo from an infinite number of perspectives, but also to simultaneously transmit this information over high-speed networks to any other properly equipped location in the world.

The Virtual Pelvic Floor application (Figure 2) has been used at the University of Illinois at Chicago (UIC) to train medical students and residents. Initial training and testing of medical students and residents suggests improved understanding of the complex anatomic structures of the pelvic floor.[7]

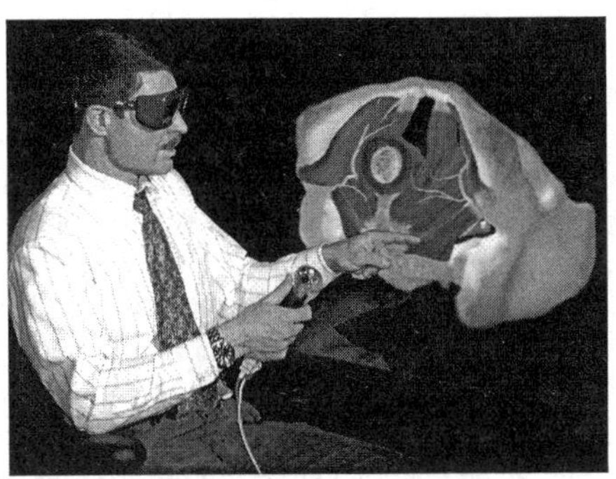

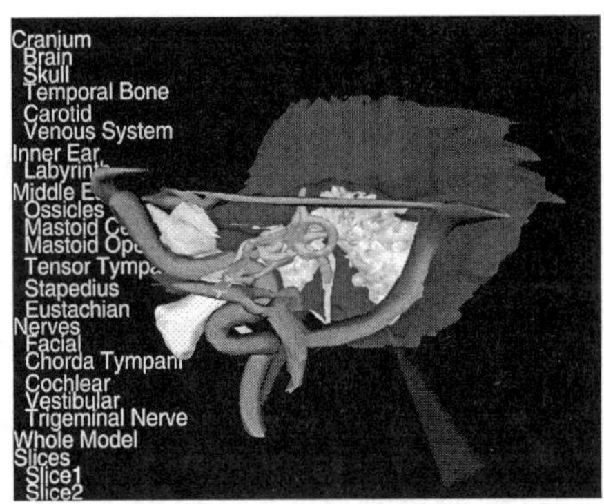

Figure 2: Virtual Pelvic Floor application.   Figure 3: Virtual Temporal Bone application.

4.2 Virtual Temporal Bone

The temporal bone of the skull contains the delicate organs of hearing and balance, the nerve that controls the muscles of facial expression, as well as blood vessels, nerves, and muscles that are essential for normal sensory and motor function. The anatomic structures within the temporal bone are in a complex 3-dimensional arrangement that is very difficult to conceptualize, and the complex interrelationships of these structures are hidden from normal view because they are embedded within dense bone. Because of the minute size and compact nature of the structures within the temporal bone, visual inspection of these structures is extremely difficult by dissection or by imaging techniques.

The Virtual Temple Bone (Figure 3) is a Tele-Immersive educational application which is a new method of teaching the complex anatomy of the middle and inner ear utilizing Virtual Reality and current networking technology.[1]

4.3 Radiological Volumetric Image

We have developed plug-ins that automatically combine 3D medical data with the methods for handling the data. The most commonly used radiological data format is DICOM. We have developed plug-ins which can read DICOM and 3D TIFF format data sets.[8]

Collaborative, interactive methods currently implemented in the plug-ins include cutting planes and windowing. A 3D windowing bar is used to represent the position and the width of the window, which determines the gray scale range displayed in the radiological data. A user can press a button on the wand to activate the windowing bar, and move the wand up and down to change the width of the window, or left and right to change the position of the center of the window. A cutting box is also implemented which encloses the radiological data model. A user can press a button to activate the movement of the box. Then the user can move or rotate the cutting box by moving or rotating the wand. The part of the model of interest remains in the cutting box, and the remaining external data is not visible.

The changes of windowing and cutting planes are distributed through a TCP channel to other participants who are involved in the Tele-Immersive environment. With the support of streaming audio, participants, who are at the different ends of the world, can see each other, work on the same data set, and talk to each other in real-time.

5   Conclusions

Tele-Immersive medial education has many advantages. Master surgeons can teach residents in remote locations. Surgeons can use superior 3D visualization of VR. We can benefit from shared, networked, interactive anatomic models and radiological imaging. High quality networked 2-way audio, video, and avatars integrated into VR environment can support oral as well as gestural communication and body language.

Using the method presented in this paper, different kinds of models can be loaded in Teledu together with the functions handling the models. With this environment, the coding of a general purpose Tele-Immersive educational environment is separated from different applications. Teledu and its plug-in structure can significantly reduce the time and efforts needed to put more medical models into Tele-Immersive educational environments. Different courses can be easily loaded into this tele-classroom.

Tele-Immersion allows educators to overcome some of the barriers of teaching surgical principles based upon understanding of highly complex 3D anatomy. Tele-Immersion also supports widespread dissemination of anatomic expertise.

6   Acknowledgments

This project has been funded in part with federal funds from the National Library of Medicine/ National Institutes of Health, under contract No. N01-LM-9-3543.

References

[1] Mary Rasmussen, Theodore P. Mason, Alan Millman, Ray Evenhouse, and Daniel Sandin. The virtual temporal bone, a tele-immersive educational environment. *Future Generation Computer Systems*, (14):125–130, 1998.

[2] Zhuming Ai, Balaji K. Gupta, Mary Rasmussen, Ya Ju Lin, Fred Dech, Walter Panko, and Jonathan C. Silverstein. Simulation of eye diseases in a virtual environment. In *Hawaii International Conference on System Sciences (HICSS-33)*, Jan 2000.

[3] J. Leigh, A. Johnson, T. DeFanti, S. Bailey, and R. Grossman. A tele-immersive environment for collaborative exploratory analysis of massive data sets. In *Proceedings of ASCI 99*, Heijen, the Netherlands, June 1999.

[4] J. Leigh, P. Rajlich, R. Stein, A. E. Johnson, and DeFanti T. A. Limbo/vtk: A tool for rapid tele-immersive visualization. In *Proceedings of IEEE Visualization'98*, Research Triangle Park, NC, October 1998.

[5] C. Cruz-Neira, D. J. Sandin, and T. A. DeFanti. Surround-screen projection-based virtual reality: The design and implementation of the CAVE. In *Proc. Siggraph 93*, pages 135–142, New York, 1993. ACM Press.

[6] M. Czernuszenko, D. Pape, D. Sandin, T. DeFanti, G. Dawe, and M. Brown. The ImmersaDesk and infinity wall projection-based virtual reality displays. *Computer Graphics*, 31(2):46, MAY 1997.

[7] Howard D. Dobson, Russell K. Pearl, P. Orsay, Charles, Mary Rasmussen, Ray Evenhouse, Zhuming Ai, Gregory Blew, Fred Dech, Jonathan C. Silverstein, and Herand Abcarian. Virtual reality: New method of teaching anorectal and pelvic floor anatomy, pathology, and surgery. In *The American Society of Colon and Rectal Surgeons*, Boston, MA, June 24-29 2000.

[8] Zhuming Ai, Fred Dech, Mary Rasmussen, and Jonathan C. Silverstein. Radiological tele-immersion for next generation networks. In James D. Westwood et al., editors, *Medicine Meets Virtual Reality 2000*, pages 4–9. IOS Press, 2000.

Medicine Meets Virtual Reality 02/10
J.D. Westwood et al. (Eds.)
IOS Press, 2002

An Immersive Simulation System for Provoking and Analyzing Cataplexy

Kurt Augustine, Bruce Cameron, Jon Camp, Lois Krahn, M.D., Richard Robb, Ph.D.
Mayo Clinic/Foundation, Rochester Minnesota 55905

Abstract. Cataplexy, a sudden loss of voluntary muscle control, is one of the hallmark symptoms of narcolepsy, a sleep disorder characterized by excessive daytime sleepiness. Cataplexy is usually triggered by strong, spontaneous emotions, such as laughter, surprise, fear or anger, and is more common in times of stress. The Sleep Disorders Unit and the Biomedical Imaging Resource at Mayo Clinic are developing interactive display technology for reliably inducing cataplexy during clinical monitoring. The use of immersive displays may help bypass patient defenses, and game-like "unreality" allows introduction of surprising, threatening, or humorous elements, with little risk of offending patients. The project is referred to as the "Cataplexy/Narcolepsy Activation Program", or CatNAP. We have developed an automobile driving simulation to allow the introduction of humorous, surprising, or stress-inducing events and objects as the patient attempts to navigate a simulated vehicle through a virtual town. The patient wears a stereoscopic head-mounted display, by which he views the virtual town through the windows of his simulated vehicle. The vehicle is controlled via a driving simulator steering wheel and pedal cluster. The patient is instructed to drive his vehicle to another location in town, given initial directions and street signs. As he attempts to accomplish the task, various objects, sounds or conditions occur which may distract, startle, frustrate or cause laughter; responses which may trigger a cataplectic episode. The patient can be monitored by reflex tests and EMG recordings during the driving experience. An evaluation phase with volunteer patients previously diagnosed with cataplexy has been completed. The goal of these trials was to gain insight from the volunteers as to improvements that could be made to the simulation. All patients that participated in the evaluation phase have been under a physician's care for a number of years and control their cataplexy with medication. We believe this is a novel and innovative approach to a difficult problem. CatNAP is a compelling example of the potentially effective application of virtual reality technology to an important clinical problem that has resisted previous approaches. Preliminary results suggest that an immersive simulation system like CatNAP will be able to reliably induce cataplexy in a controlled environment. The project is continuing through a final stage of refinement prior to conducting a full clinical study.

1. Introduction

Narcolepsy was first described in 1880 by Jean Baptiste E. Gelineau, [1] a neuropsychiatrist in France, who recognized a group of patients who had irresistible sleep triggered by strong emotions. His recognition of excessive daytime sleepiness and cataplexy helped clarify that these symptoms represented a distinct neurologic disease [1,2]. Sleep paralysis and hypnagogic hallucinations were added to excessive daytime sleepiness and cataplexy by Yoss and Daly [3] in 1957, resulting in a tetrad of core narcoleptic symptoms. In 1960, Vogel [4] observed REM sleep occurring at sleep onset in patients with narcolepsy. Several years earlier, REM sleep had been first observed and was known to typically occur 90 minutes after initially falling asleep. However, by 1963, Rechtschaffen et al [5] recognized that many patients with the classic symptoms of narcolepsy experienced REM sleep within minutes, instead of an hour, after sleep onset.

Most patients with narcolepsy are initially identified because of severe daytime sleepiness that interferes with their functioning. Essentially all patients with narcolepsy experience this potentially disabling symptom, which can lead to motor vehicle crashes, occupational difficulties, and social problems [6]. However, excessive daytime sleepiness is not unique to narcolepsy and can be caused by a number of other conditions.

Cataplexy is the symptom that is clearly most specific for narcolepsy. Cataplexy is often triggered when a patient experiences a strong emotion like laughter, anger, surprise, or excitement. Patients can have either partial or complete muscle weakness that can involve the face, neck, legs, or total body. During cataplexy, patients are aware of their surroundings but cannot move their body normally. They can recall information spoken to them and can repeat this after the event. They do not lose consciousness, although with prolonged cataplexy, they can fall asleep. The ability to observe and recall events occurring during the cataplectic event is a helpful feature that allows discrimination between cataplexy and other debilitating states like seizures and sleep. Typical cataplectic episodes can last from several seconds to several minutes.

Apart from the muscle atonia, which is characterized by a transient areflexia of the deep tendon reflexes, the patient is medically stable without cardiovascular or respiratory compromise. Several studies have indicated that because of the muscle atonia, electrophysiologic testing, such as H-reflex testing done with electromyography (EMG), yields abnormal results [7]. This occurs because the spinal alpha motor neurons are inhibited postsynaptically by activated cells in the medial medulla. The H-reflex is a monosynaptic spinal reflex induced by electrical stimulation of the tibial nerve. It is the electrophysiologic parallel of the deep tendon reflex induced by stimulation of the Achilles tendon. The H-reflex is reduced during sleep and absent during REM sleep. This abnormal EMG finding strongly suggests that cataplexy represents a partial REM state. The muscle paralysis seen as a typical feature of normal REM sleep inappropriately intrudes into wakefulness leaving a subject unable to move certain muscles for a period of time.

Why this partial REM state is typically triggered by strong emotions remains unexplained. However, this is a clear example of the mind-brain interface. A subject has a powerful emotional experience, and immediately, changes in the neurotransmitter levels, suspected to be related to excessive cholinergic stimulation and reduced noradrenergic activity, lead to muscle atonia [7-10].

Clear-cut cataplexy coexisting with excessive daytime sleepiness points directly to the diagnosis of narcolepsy. Although no community-based study of narcolepsy has been published, approximately 25% of patients with narcolepsy are thought not to have cataplexy. Controversy exists regarding the patients with narcolepsy, based on abnormal REM sleep observed during a multiple sleep latency test (MSLT), who do not have cataplexy. The debate centers on whether narcolepsy with and without cataplexy represents the same or different diseases. Future studies of hypocretin or other neurotransmitters may soon settle this controversy.

The other two classic symptoms found in narcolepsy are sleep paralysis and hypnagogic hallucinations. In sleep paralysis, a patient becomes transiently unable to move before sleep onset or just after awakening. Hypnagogic and hypnopompic hallucinations are vivid, frightening dreams, often with a sensation of flying, that similarly occur at the time of transition from sleep into wakefulness or the reverse. These symptoms may be very distressing to patients. Over time, these symptoms have been found to be less specific than cataplexy in helping to distinguish a patient with narcolepsy from those with other sleep disorders. Both of these conditions have been known to occur in people without sleep disorders. Nonetheless, a relatively large group of patients with narcolepsy have the classic tetrad of symptoms-excessive daytime sleepiness, cataplexy, sleep paralysis, and hypnagogic hallucinations. Sleep paralysis and hypnagogic hallucinations, like cataplexy, represent partial intrusion of REM phenomena into wakefulness. Both of these conditions occur at the time of sleep onset or awakening.

Since cataplexy is the most specific sign of narcolepsy, there has been interest in developing a cataplexy test that could be used to diagnose narcolepsy. Unlike excessive daytime sleepiness, cataplexy occurs only rarely in the absence of narcolepsy. Attempts have been made to provoke cataplexy by telling jokes to a patient [7, 11]. More recently, an attempt has been made to standardize the cataplexy test by having susceptible patients view humorous videotapes while undergoing polysomnographic monitoring. Assessing deep tendon reflexes before, during and after a possible cataplectic episode is very helpful in verifying that cataplexy has indeed occurred. The PSG can show reduced tone on the EMG [12].

2. Purpose

One of the challenges in studying cataplexy is the difficulty in reliably inducing the condition in a clinical setting. There are several reasons for this. Induction of a cataplectic episode requires the purposeful evocation of strong emotions in the patient. The social and ethical concerns surrounding such an experiment create a dilemma for sleep disorder researchers. Any number of negative social stimuli can reliably evoke strong negative emotions, particularly in situations where escape is not possible. This requires deception in order to provoke the desired response, may involve feigned behaviors that practitioners find repugnant, and risks loss of patient confidence. Evoking a more positive emotional response requires a level of familiarity and spontaneity seldom found in a clinical setting. Even humor is such an individualized response that material that reliably produces laughter in the majority of cases will leave some unmoved and others offended. The disorder itself can make it difficult to induce a state of cataplexy in patients. Episodes of daytime sleepiness may distract the patient from any presented stimuli, or mute their emotional response. This limits the time available for reliable testing, and may confound the detection of cataplexy. Finally, cataplexy provocation can be very difficult in patients who have had to deal with the disorder for a long time. They learn to develop strong defense mechanisms that aid in resisting any of the emotions that might trigger an episode. They often keep their emotions under tight control, become somewhat humorless, avoid conflicts, and can be difficult to draw into conversation.

The Sleep Disorders Center (SDC) and the Biomedical Imaging Resource (BIR) at Mayo Clinic have collaborated to develop a system that will provoke cataplexy in a predictable manner, which in turn will provide a reliable means for studying the disorder. The BIR has a well-equipped virtual reality laboratory and considerable experience in developing interactive simulations for clinical studies and education [13-18]. Using immersive display and interactive control technology, we have developed a simulation system for provoking and analyzing cataplexy. Through the use of immersive displays we expect that defenses-mechanisms will be bypassed without offending patients. The simulation is realistic enough to suspend disbelief while providing a game-like "unreality" that safely allows introduction of surprising, threatening or humorous events.

3. Methods

The project developed between the SDC and the BIR is referred to as the "Cataplexy/Narcolepsy Activation Program", or CatNAP. The goal of the CatNAP project is to create a system that immerses a cataplexy patient into a virtual environment designed to provoke strong emotions considered to be cataplexy triggers. The simulation needs to be sufficiently realistic to temporarily "fool" the patient into letting down their guard and bypassing their well-developed defense mechanisms. The primary component of the CatNAP project is the immersive simulation system, which consists of both "off-the-shelf" hardware and software, and custom developed software. It is based on an automobile driving simulation which introduces of humorous, surprising, frustrating or stress-inducing events. The patient wears a stereoscopic head-mounted display (HMD) while attempting to navigate a simulated vehicle through a virtual town. A tracking device is attached to the HMD to provide realistic views in any direction the patient's head is turned. The vehicle is controlled via a driving simulator steering wheel and pedal cluster. The patient is instructed to drive his vehicle to various locations throughout the town after being given an initial set of instructions. As he attempts to reach his destinations, various objects, sounds or conditions occur which may distract, startle, frustrate, or cause laughter. The emotional responses evoked during the driving experience, if strong enough, trigger a cataplectic episode. Because cataplexy can manifest itself with varying degrees of muscle atonia, the observer may not even be aware that a patient is experiencing an episode. For this reason, the patient is monitored throughout the experience by reflex tests and EMG recordings.

The hardware system is made up of several components. The workstation driving the entire system is a Silicon Graphic Onyx 2 with InfiniteReality graphics. Additional components include a Dexxa steering wheel and pedals along with an Unwinder multifunction adapter, a Proview head-mounted display, and a Motionstar electro-magnetic tracking system. The system is illustrated in Figure 1. There is no special purpose computing hardware included in the CatNAP project.

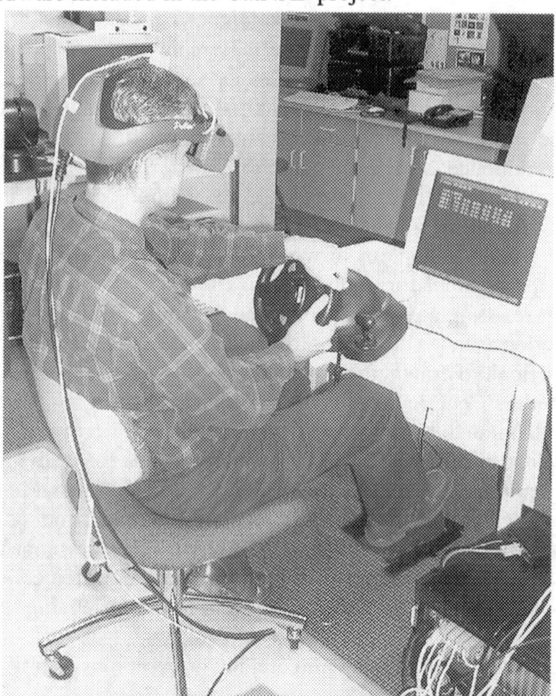

Figure 1: CatNAP immersive simulation display system

The software toolkit used for the project is Vega, which consists of a graphical user interface called LynX, Iris Performer and Vega libraries, and header files of C-callable functions. We started with the Vega supplied town as the basis for the driving simulation. To increase both the surprise factor and humor, we added numerous objects to the environment, which the driver comes across as he drives through the town. Among the new objects were animals darting across the highway (see Figure 2a), a space ship diving between tall downtown buildings, vehicles driving erratically, startling noises like loud car horns or screeching cats, fog that suddenly appears and disappears, a large toy train racing along the tracks (see Figure 2b), humorous "Burma Shave" signs (see Figure 2c), and a tall ship traversing a small river (See Figure 2d).

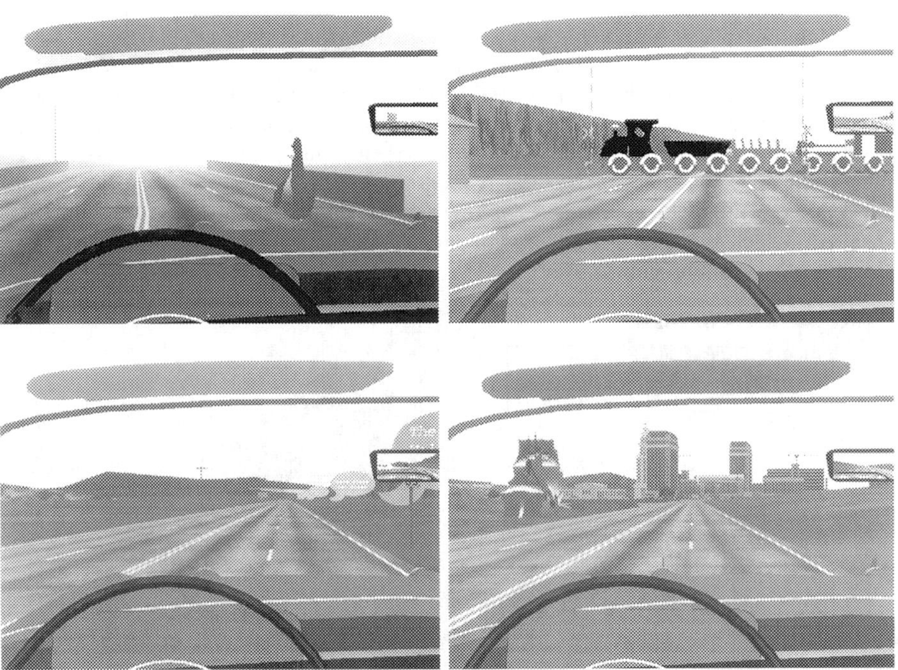

Figure 2: a) penguin crossing road in fog, b) toy train crossing road, c) "Burma Shave" signs on right side of road, d) tall ship sailing down river on left side of road

In addition to the objects that were added to the environment, actions were programmed into the simulation. While the patient waits for the program to begin, a set of simple instructions is printed on the screen. At this time, the patient is asked by the observer if he has any additional questions. Because the surprise factor is crucial to provoking a cataplectic episode, written and verbal instructions are kept to a minimum. At the beginning of the experience, the patient is provided a short period of time for practice driving. This gives him a chance to get accustomed to the simulated driving experience without the fear of penalty. It is important for the patient to become comfortable with steering wheel sensitivity, placement of the gas and brake pedals, rate of acceleration and braking speed and the changing field of view while moving his head. During the practice period (2 minutes by default) the patient does not know what the penalties are, only that they exist and are invoked when the vehicle leaves the road or hits certain objects. After the practice period has expired, the patient's vehicle must stay on the road. If he leaves the road for more than an instant, he hears a person scream or a cat screech, and then is set back to his starting location. If the patient is not careful, he is continually "reset" back to the beginning, which leads to a great deal of frustration, one of the emotions that triggers cataplexy. As the patient drives through the simulated town, perhaps the most startling and stressful events are those caused by a truck. A large military truck is programmed to follow the patient vehicle wherever it goes. At the beginning, the patient can barely see the trucks headlights in the rear view mirror but as time passes, the truck gets increasingly closer to the vehicle. No matter where the patient tries to turn, or how fast he tries to go, he cannot lose the truck (see Figure 3a). When all that can be seen in the rearview mirror is the front grill of the truck, a loud horn is blasted, which usually startles and flusters the driver. At that point, the truck backs off but continues to follow. Once again, the truck tries to close in on the patient's vehicle. After several close encounters, the truck eventually smashes into the rear of the patient vehicle with a very loud crashing sound. Instead of blowing up, however, the patient's vehicle suddenly starts to rise. As he continues his ascent, the patient may steer and accelerate, allowing him to maneuver above the town, flying around and between the tall buildings (see Figure 3b). What was a highly stressed environment a moment ago is now a serene and peaceful setting. After a flying above the town for a short period (2 minutes by default), the patient begins to see smoke coming from the engine. After several seconds of increasing smoke, a shrill alarm is sounded and the vehicle begins a nosedive towards the earth, spinning as it drops. At the moment of impact, the screen is filled with smoke and flames and a loud and prolonged crash is heard. The simulation is over.

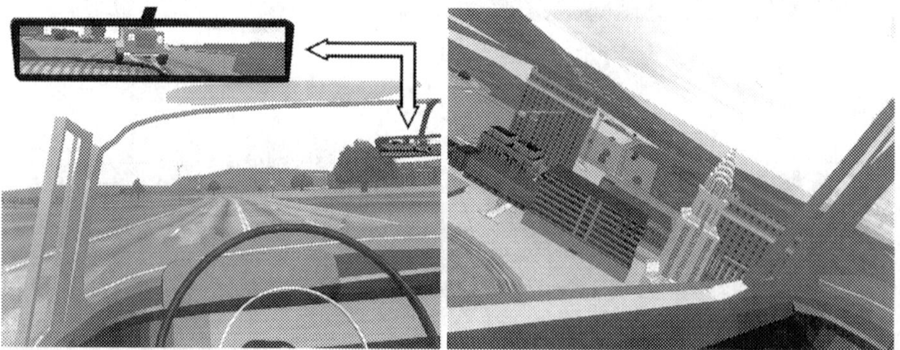

Figure 3: a) truck approaching in rearview mirror, b) view of city while flying

4. Results

During the development of the immersive simulation system, SDU patients helped evaluate the project and give suggestions on how to make it more effective. Six patients evaluated the system. One patient was a female age 24. The rest were men ranging in age from 18 to 75. All six patients had confirmed diagnoses of cataplexy and had been under a physician's care for at least four years. These patients were not ideal subjects for testing the true effectiveness of the CatNAP system. They had been controlling their condition through medication for a number of years. In addition, most of them are very good at defending against the emotions that might lead to a cataplectic episode. However, they provided valuable insight as evaluators, which was used to enhance the system. After each test, the patient was asked for suggestions on how to make the experience effective for recently diagnosed patients. Although none of the subjects had a cataplectic episode, they usually suggested practical ways to enhance the simulation. Several patients felt they would have had an episode during the test if they experienced it prior to therapy. One patient experienced slight nausea from the simulated movement. Most patients found the steering wheel sensitivity to be annoying, which ironically is an emotion that could actually trigger cataplexy. We did not monitor heart rate but some patients thought their heart rate might have increased during some of the more stressful parts of the simulation. We found the most difficult emotion to provoke through a simulation system is humor. Sense of humor is a very personal trait and one that cannot easily be provoked or predicted for a wide variety of test subjects. Most of the volunteers agreed that getting them to laugh would be the most difficult task for the simulator.

5. Conclusions

The CatNAP simulator is a novel and innovative approach to a difficult problem – clinical study of cataplexy. Virtual reality has been used to treat. patients with certain phobias, such as acrophobia, claustrophobia, and fear of flying, each with a modest amount of success [19-21], but CatNAP may be the first application of VR to studies in sleep disorders. Preliminary results suggest that an immersive simulation system like CatNAP will be able to reliably induce cataplexy in a controlled environment. After final refinements to the system, the next phase of the project is to conduct a full clinical study.

6. References

1. Gelineau JBE: De la Narcolepsie. Lancette Fr., 53: 626-628, 1880.
2. Culebras A., Sleep and narcolepsy. [published correction appears in Arch Neurol. 56(5): 632, 1999]. Archives of Neurology, 56(1): 117-118, 1999.
3. Yoss RE, Daly DD: Criteria for the diagnosis of the narcoleptic syndrome. Proc Staff Meet, Mayo Clin, 32: 320-328, 1957.
4. Vogel G: Studies in the psychophysiology of dreams, III: The dream of narcolepsy. Archives of General Psychiatry, 3: 421-428, 1960.
5. Rechtschaffen A, Wolpert EA, Dement WC, Mitchell SA, Fisher C: Nocturnal sleep of narcoleptics. Electroencephalography & Clinical Neurophysiology, 15: 599-609, 1963.
6. Broughton RJ, Guberman A, Roberts J: Comparison of the psychosocial effects of epilepsy and narcolepsy/cataplexy: a controlled study. Epilepsia, 25(4): 423-433, 1984.
7. Guilleminault C, Wilson RA, Dement WC: A study on cataplexy. Archives of Neurology, 31(4): 255-261, 1974.
8. Siegel JM, Nienhuis R, Fahringer HM, et al: Neuronal activity in narcolepsy: identification of cataplexy-related cells in the medial medulla. Science, 252(5010): 1315-1318, 1991.
9. Guilleminault C, Gelb M: Clinical aspects and features of cataplexy. Advances in Neurology, 67:65-77, 1995.
10. Hodes R: Effects of age, consciousness, and other factors on human electrically induced reflexes (EIRs). Electroencephalography & Clinical Neurophysiology, Suppl. 25: 80-91, 1967.
11. Dyken ME, Yamada T, Lin-Dyken DC, Seaba P, Yeh M: Diagnosing narcolepsy through the simultaneous clinical and electrophysiologic analysis of cataplexy. Archives of Neurology, 53(5): 456-460, 1996.
12. Krahn L, Boeve B, Olson E, Herold D, Silber M: A standardized test for cataplexy. Sleep Medicine, 1: 125-130, 2000.
13. Robb RA, Cameron BM: Virtual Reality Assisted Surgery Program. Book chapter in: <u>Interactive Technology and the New Paradigm for Healthcare</u>. Eds., R. Satava, et. al., IOS Press, vol. 18, pp. 309-321, 1995.
14. Robb RA: Virtual reality assisted surgery planning using patient specific anatomic models. IEEE Engineering in Medicine and Biology. Ed., Metin Akay, 15(2): 60-69, 1996.
15. Kay PA, Robb RA, Myers RP, King BF: Creation and validation of patient specific anatomical models for prostate surgery planning using virtual reality. Proceedings of the Fourth Conference on Visualization in Biomedical Computing, 1131: 547-552, September 22-25, 1996, Hamburg, Germany.
16. Blezek DJ, Robb RA: Evaluating virtual endoscopy for clinical use. Journal of Digital Imaging, 10(3)(Suppl. 1-August): 51-55, 1997.
17. Martin DP, Blezek DJ, Robb RA: Simulating lower extremity nerve blocks with virtual reality. Techniques in Regional Anesthesia and Pain Management, 3(1): 58-61, 1999.
18. Robb, RA: Virtual Reality in Medicine and Biology. Book chapter in: <u>Information Technologies in Medicine: Medical Simulation and Education</u>, ed. Metin Akay and Andy Marsh, John Wiley & Sons, Inc., New York, NY, vol. 1, chapter 1, pp. 3-31, 2001.
19. Rothbaum BO, Hodges LF, Kooper R, Opdyke D, Williford JS, North M: Effectiveness of computer-generated (virtual reality) graded exposure in the treatment of acrophobia. American Journal of Psychiatry, 152(4): 626-628, 1995.
20. Botella C, Banos RM, Villa H, Perpina C, Garcia-Palacios A: Virtual reality in the treatment of claustrophobic fear: A controlled, multiple-baseline design. Behavior Therapy, 31(3): 583-595, 2000.
21. Wiederhold BK, Gevirtz R, Wiederhold MD: Fear of flying: A case report using virtual reality therapy with physiological monitoring. Cyberpsychology & Behavior, 1(2): 97-103, 1998.

Medicine Meets Virtual Reality 02/10
J.D. Westwood et al. (Eds.)
IOS Press, 2002

Soft-tissue simulation using LEM - Long Elements Method

Remis Balaniuk
Department of Surgery, School of Medicine
Stanford University
Stanford, CA. USA 94305-5655
remis@stanford.edu

Abstract: This paper discusses the use of the Long Elements Method – LEM in soft tissue modeling and surgery simulation. The LEM is a new method for real time, physically based, dynamic simulation of deformable objects, based on a new meshing strategy, using long elements. The method uses a combination of static (state-less) and dynamic approaches to simulate deformations and dynamics, obtaining a higher degree of compliance per time step. Global deformations that conserve volume and are convincingly compliant are obtained. Models are defined using bulk material properties. Elastic and plastic deformations can be simulated. The real time performance of the method and its intrinsic properties of volume conservation, modeling based in material properties and simpler meshing make it particularly attractive for soft tissue modeling and surgery simulation.

1. Introduction

Physically based simulation of deformable objects is a key challenge in Virtual Reality (VR). Deformable object modeling has been studied in computer graphics and animation for three decades. As computational power increases deformable models start being used in VR as well. Researchers from new fields as human tissue modeling, interactive character animation and surgical simulation, are working to extend the simulation of deformable models to a virtual interactive reality. They essentially aim at physically based simulations of complex deformable objects, and enhanced multi-modal interactivity: graphic and haptic interfaces to manipulate and to change the topology of the objects in real time. A major application area for this research is the simulation of biomaterials. Physical modeling of biomaterials has a broad range of applications ranging from understanding how soft and hard tissue respond under loading, to patient-specific planning of reconstructive procedures, to the training of surgical skills, and much more. Real-time interaction with these models is necessary in order to impose conditions of interest, to examine results and alternative solutions, to learn surgical procedures by performing them in simulation.

Modeling the biomechanics of muscles, tissues, and organs is intrinsically a computationally difficult undertaking - doing so at haptically real-time rates requires significant computational resources and algorithmic finesse. The development of sufficiently real-time modeling of biomaterials is a topic of intense interest to a worldwide research community, and methods to simulate deformable materials are at the center of this research.

A number of methods have been proposed to simulate deformable objects ranging from non-physical methods, where individual or groups of control points or shape parameters are manually adjusted to shape editing and design, to methods based on continuum mechanics, which account for material properties and internal and external forces on object deformation. Simpler methods, as the mass-spring, are mainly non-physical and inaccurate. Accurate physically based methods, as the Finite Elements (FEM), are typically simulated off-line, and the changes on these methods to achieve real time performance normally compromise or their accuracy or their interactiveness.

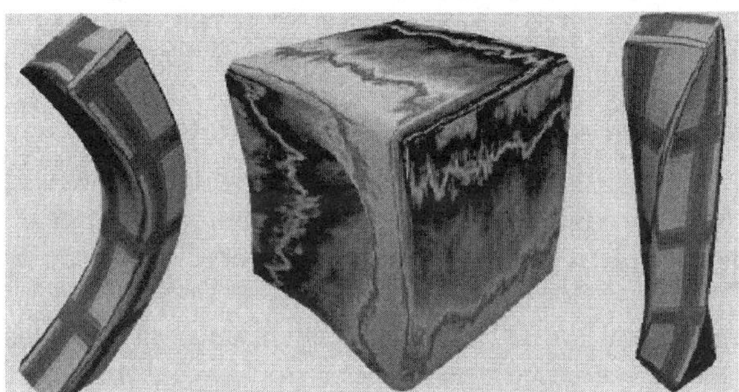

Figure 1: *Soft-tissue simulation: (a) bend (b) palpation (c) twist*

Simulation methods can be classified as *Dynamic* or *Static*. Dynamic methods simulate the time evolution of a physical system state. The bodies are assumed to have mass and energy distributed throughout. Differential equations and a finite state vector define each model. Numerical integration techniques approximate the system state (position and velocity) at discrete time steps. In static methods equilibrium equations or closed form expressions describe the system and these equations are solved to find a static solution at each time step. In static and quasi-static methods the time and the system state are usually not considered (e g spring-only models respond immediately to load change).

For a more comprehensive and accurate simulation of deformable objects a state-based approach should be used, given the significant internal dynamics of the deformable media, as well as the dynamics of the movements (translations and rotations) of the object in space. Nevertheless, static and quasi-static methods can be useful in applications where the objects deform but do not move, or move slowly, and the deformable media is highly damped. If the problem permits, a static solution seems more attractive than a dynamic one. Dynamic solutions usually pose various problems, which depend on the type of method used.

The LEM proposes a combination of dynamic and static approaches. A static state-less *Deformation Engine* solves the deformation problem for a given input of internal and external stresses calculating the respective strains while a *3D Integrator* performs the dynamic simulation integrating the forces generated by the strains to update the state of the system. The link between static and dynamic simulation is made using the duality between pressure (stress / strain) and force.

The method integrates the simplicity and compliance of the static method to a full 3D dynamic simulation of the deformable media. Highly deformable material can be simulated. Localized or global deformations can be simulated. Figure 1 illustrates some results, showing the bend of an elastic rod (a), a palpation of a soft object with a rigid haptic probe (b) and a twist of the rod (c).

This method was previously presented in [1] and [2]. For a survey of deformable modeling in computer graphics the reader is referred to [3]. Others recent methods proposed are the "Geometric Nonlinear finite element method" [5], the "Boundary Element Method" [4] and some medical simulators [6], [7], [8].

2. Method

The LEM is based on a combination of static solution for elastic deformations of objects filled with uncompressible fluid and dynamic simulation of movements. The volumes are discretised in a set of Long Elements (LE) (Fig. 2), and an equilibrium equation is defined for each element using bulk variables. The set of static equations plus the Pascal principle and the volume conservation are used to define a system that is solved to find the object deformations and forces. The forces obtained are integrated to simulate movement: translation and rotation, for each element.

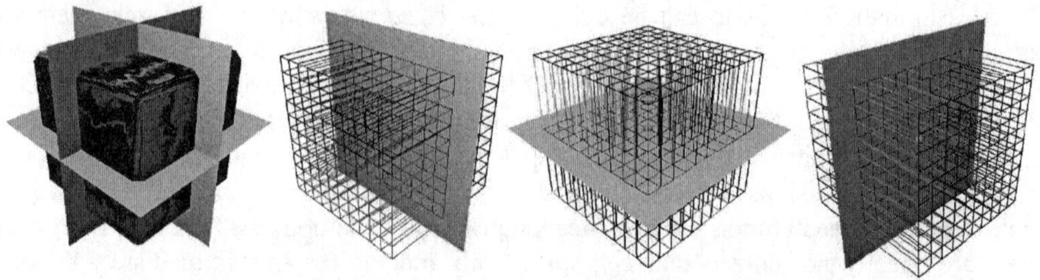

Figure 2: *Meshing an object in long elements*

The long elements define an original and efficient 3D meshing strategy that permits the approximation of the state and the strain at any point on a volume from a reduced number of explicitly updated points. An innovative 3D modeling approach is used, based on the decomposition of the object by projection of the object into three orthogonal spaces. This decomposition uses three mutually perpendicular reference planes that cross the object, and the relative positions of points inside the object with respect to these *reference planes* are simulated (Fig. 2). The objects are meshed in 3 superposed orthogonal sets of long strips that cross the object from face to face in a direction defined by a reference plane. The total number of elements used to mesh an object is about $O(6.n^2)$ where n is the average number of elements in one side of the grid.

The LE is an elastic spring. The state-less Deformation engine simulates a LE as a mass-less spring, defined by its length, area and elasticity (Fig. 3(a)). These values are defined for each element based on the material properties of the simulated media. An equilibrium equation is defined for each LE relating its stress (internal and external pressures) to its strain, or deformation (change in length). The static equilibrium condition states that the forces, or pressures, inside the element should be equal to the external forces, or pressures, applied externally. Using this equation we can estimate the change in length (the deformation) of the LE when a stress exists. The set of LEs used to fill an object define a set of equations. To correlate these equations 3 global conditions are considered: superficial tension, the Pascal principle and the incompressibility of the material.

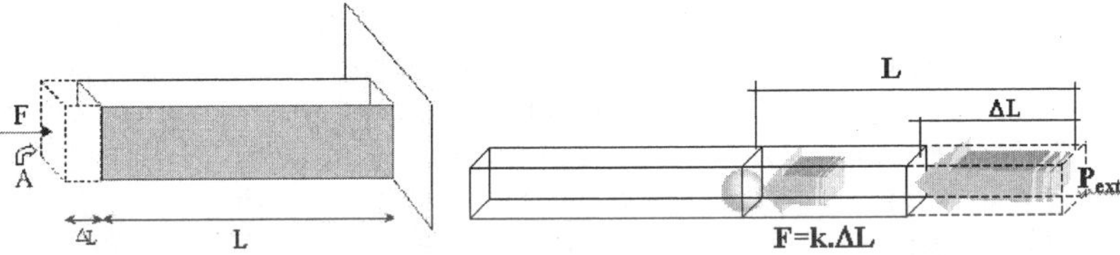

Figure 3: *(a) static LE (b) dynamic LE*

Superficial tension can be defined as a force field created by local changes on the surface area of a deforming object. We simulate superficial tension by means of elastic connections between neighbor elements, coupling their changes in length. Figure 4 illustrates the smoothing effect of the superficial tension.

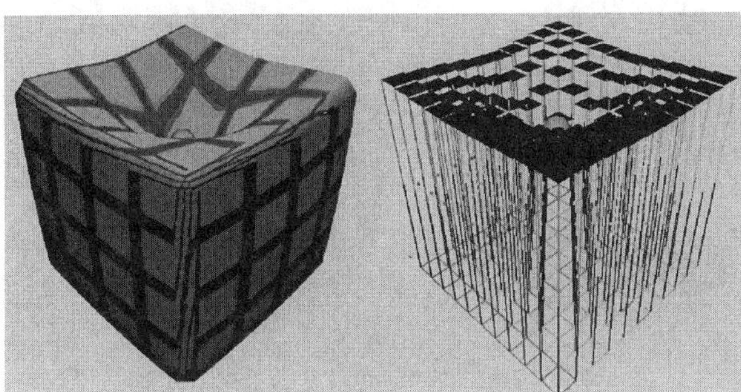

Figure 4: *Superficial tension*

We suppose that the simulated objects are filled with uncompressible fluid (what is a good approximation for biological tissues). The Pascal's principle states that *an external pressure applied to a fluid confined within a closed container is transmitted undiminished throughout the entire fluid.* It means that the equilibrium condition must be satisfied simultaneously at all elements to define an object in equilibrium. If the filling fluid is incompressible then the *volume conservation* must be guaranteed. One equation is added to the system to implement the volume conservation, stating that the sum of the deformations of all LEs (the changes in lengths) must be 0.

The equilibrium equations plus the volume conservation equation define a typical numerical problem of type $A.x=B$. A is a sparse matrix and the system is solved **once** using standard numerical methods to estimate the inverse matrix A^{-1}. Unless some topological change occurs during the simulation, the vector of deformations x can be estimated performing the multiplication of the pressures vector B by A^{-1}. Note that the number of equations is also strongly reduced if compared to other simulation methods where the number of elements is usually of order $O(n^3)$ of the granularity of the mesh.

To simulate a state based dynamic system the same mass-less LEs used by the deformation engine are simulated as energy-storing elements by the 3D Integrator. Elastic potential energy due to either compression or stretching is simulated to create forces and derive a state for each element. The LE is now modeled as a spring attached to a particle with a known mass. A combination of two LEs attached to the same particle is used as the basic element to mesh the volumes (Fig. 3(b)). These particles are the only points where forces are known inside the object. Each particle exists in a simplified one-dimensional space. The particles initially lie on the reference plane where its LE is defined. The reference planes remain static while the particles move. The state of a particle corresponds to the position and velocity of the particle with respect to its reference plane.

The 3D state of any point inside the object can be approximated based on the state of the particles. For a given configuration (state of the particles + vector of deformations estimated by the Deformation Engine) it is also possible to approximate the internal stress at any point inside the object. The internal stress, together with the external pressures are used as feedback to the Deformation Engine.

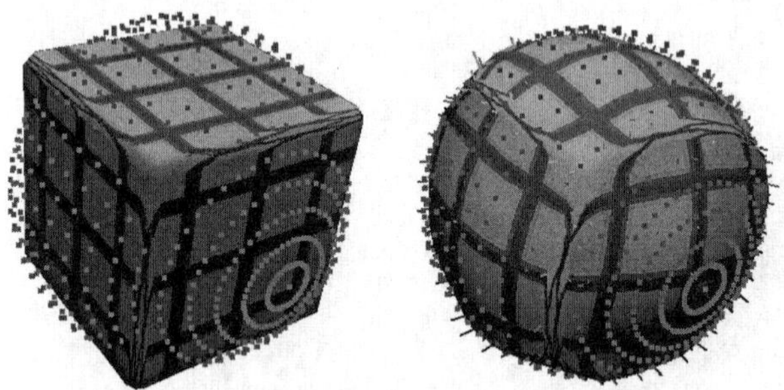

Figure 5: *Plastic deformation*

Both elastic and plastic deformations can be simulated using the LE method. However, in a plastic deformation the system of static equations change, requiring a new matrix inversion. Using plastic deformation is also possible to mesh new objects. A "modeling clay" can be implemented mapping points from an meshed object to a new one. The differences in distance between the two sets of points are used to create external forces applied on the original object, molding it to fit the new shape. Figure 5 shows the molding of a sphere starting from a cube.

The LEs can take arbitrary forms. They can be initially defined as straight lines, but the simulation continuously estimates the direction of the LE at each segment. This estimation is based on the relative positions of an LE and its neighbors. Non-homogeneous materials can be simulated as well. The material properties can be specifically defined at each segment of a LE.

3. Results

A prototype was implemented, and used to simulate various materials (homogeneous and non-homogeneous) and forms (Fig. 6). In a standard dual 700MHz desktop PC one iteration of the simulation loop takes about 0.05 seconds for a 600 elements mesh. A haptic interface was implemented, enabling touching, moving and palpation of the deformable objects with excellent results.

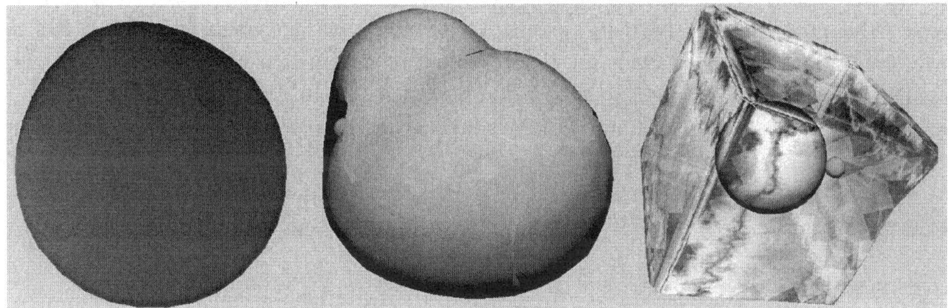

Figure 6: *Deformations with LEM*

Compared to existing methods the LEM seems to be better suited for soft tissue and surgery simulation. It is physically based, reproducing important global phenomena such as the simultaneous movement of all parts of the solid when it is touched. Preservation of volume is also very important when virtual organs are manipulated because they are usually highly deformable. The state-less Deformation Engine enables a more compliant and realistic simulation of the deformations at the surface of the object. This is because there is no inertia on the deformations, only on the movements, requiring less time steps to get to an equilibrium configuration when external forces are applied. Compliance is very important when the object is touched using the haptic interface. Models are defined based on material properties, strongly simplifying the definition and tuning of the virtual objects. Most methods require experimental data and empirical tuning to define the properties of the objects and the behavior of the simulation. Non-homogeneous biologic-like materials can be defined and simulated. The meshes are one order of magnitude smaller if compared to cubic or tetrahedral meshes used by most methods. The reduced number of elements and equations makes the simulation much less computationally expensive and also more stable. In normal use, when no real-time topologic changes are made, the simulation of deformations requires only a multiplication of a matrix by a vector, instead of inversion of matrices as in most other methods, making the computation much faster. Topologic changes are also possible. Real time remeshing of the objects, like in a cutting, suturing or removing of material, can be implemented, requiring new matrices inversions, but still faster then in most methods because of the reduced size of the matrices.

4. Conclusion

The LEM approach introduces two new concepts to the simulation of deformable objects: the meshing based on long elements and the combination of static and dynamic approaches to simulate the same object. Using the long elements we are able to model the 3D internal state at any point inside a deforming object from a reduced number of explicitly updated elements. The reduction in one order of magnitude of the number of elements enables the simulation of more complex objects with less computational effort. The combination of a state less and a dynamic approach improves the compliance of the simulation. Large deformations that rapidly change the entire shape of the object can be simulated in a reduced number of time steps. Much of the simulation occurs in the LE 1D space, where the complexity of all aspects of the simulation is strongly reduced. State-less deformations are estimated using only multiplications of matrices by vectors. The reduced number of elements minimizes instability problems. Automatic meshing of objects can be defined using plastic deformation. The method is particularly promising for soft tissue modeling and surgical simulation.

References

[1]	Balaniuk, Remis and Costa, Ivan Ferreira.
	"LEM - An approach for physically based soft tissue simulation suitable for haptic interaction".
	Conference Paper, *Fifth PHANTOM Users Group Workshop - PUG00*, Aspen, USA, October 2000.
[2]	Costa, Ivan Ferreira and Balaniuk, Remis.
	"LEM - An approach for real time physically based soft tissue simulation ". Proceedings of the IEEE International Conference on Robotics and Automation - ICRA2001, May 2001, Seoul, Korea.
[3]	Sarah F. F. Gibson and Brian Mirtich.
	"A survey of deformable models in computer graphics."
	Technical Report TR-97-19, Mitsubishi Electric research Laboratories, Cambridge, MA, November 1997. (http://www.merl.com/reports/TR97-19/index.html).
[4]	D. James and D. Pai,
	"Artdefo Accurate Real Time Deformable Objects",
	Computer Graphics, vol. 33, pp: 65--72, 1999.
[5]	Yan Zhuang and John Canny.
	"Haptic Interaction with Global Deformations". Proceedings of the IEEE International Conference on Robotics and Automation - ICRA 2000, 2428-2433, 2000.
[6]	M. C. Cavusoglu, F. Tendick, M. Cohn and S. Shankar Sastry.
	"A Lapraroscopic Telesurgical Workstation". IEEE Transactions on Robotics and Automation, 15(4), 728-739, 1999.
[7]	M. Downes, M. Cenk Cavusoglu, W. Gantert, L. W. Way and F. Tendick.
	"Virtual Environments for Training Critical Skills in Laparoscopic Surgery". Proc. Medicine Meets Virtual Reality, 6, 316-322, 1998.
[8]	Stephane Cotin, Herve Delingette and Nicholas Ayache.
	"Real-time Elastic Deformations of Soft Tissues for Surgery Simulation".
	IEEE Transaction on Visualization an Computer Graphics}, 5(1), 62-73, 1999.

SELF-ADMINISTERED DECISION SUPPORT TOOL FOR TRIAGE: RESULTS OF A RETROSPECTIVE STUDY

Afsaneh Barzi, MD, Sarmad Sadeghi, MD, Brent R. King, MD
Dynasty Technologies, Inc.
University of Texas at Houston
ABarzi@Dynasty.com

ABSTRACT

BACKGROUND: This study was designed to evaluate the safety of a self-administered triage tool. MATERIALS: Ninety-five patients older than 14 years who presented to Memorial Hermann Hospital emergency room (ER) with chief complaint of abdominal pain were included in the study. Their ER disposition and final diagnoses were logged into a database. The assigned disposition and top three diagnoses by the triage tool for each patient were also logged into the database. An emergency physician blinded to the actual disposition reviewed all cases and provided a disposition for each patient. RESULTS: The system disposed 51.1% of cases appropriately and under-disposed 4.4% of cases. Comparison between the system and the emergency physician shows that all cases under-disposed by the system are also under-disposed by the physician.

INTRODUCTION

Triage has become part of emergency medicine over time because the volume of patients using emergency room has been increasing [1]. The increase in the volume of emergency visits reflects the increase in the number of patients using the emergency department for primary, non-acute care. Indeed, in most surveys, the percentage of patients with non-acute illness is about 50 percent. In this situation it is of utmost importance to triage patients properly and consistently, for this purpose the emergency department nurse should be an experienced and efficient triage officer [2]. The more experienced the nurse, the better as he/she can use more of his/her previous experiences, collect less data and have a better judgments [3]. But unfortunately triage assessments (both inter-rater and intra-rater) by experienced personnel are inconsistent [4].

Delivering a system that can perform the task of triage consistently and with minimum training requirement can not only help decrease the load of emergency departments but also can empower and educate consumers to make a decision when faced with a medical problem.

We have developed a powerful self-administered triage tool [5] that enables individual consumers, with or without the help of a triage nurse, to determine the cause of the symptom(s) they are experiencing – self-diagnosis. This also helps the consumer to decide how quickly he/she needs to seek medical attention – triage.

We performed a retrospective study to assess the accuracy of the tool for self-diagnosis and triage; the results of which are reported here.

THE SELF-ADMINISTERED TRIAGE TOOL

The tool is composed of a number of modules – chief complaints – and will approach the patient based on the chief complaint. As abdominal pain is one of the most common chief complaints presented to emergency departments [1] in this study we evaluated the validity of the abdominal pain module,

The abdominal pain module has two divisions, adult abdominal pain and pediatric abdominal pain. Adult abdominal pain covers the patients 15 years or older and pediatric abdominal pain covers the rest of the patients.

Each module is has two main parts:

- Screening part: In one page the life threatening situations are ruled out. There are six questions on this page and at the end of the page a decision is provided to the patient. No diagnosis is given to the patient who is positive for a screening question. Examples are, overt bleeding or history of fainting.
- Diagnostic part: Patients can reach the diagnostic part only if they are negative for all of the screening questions. For adult abdominal pain a patient would have to answer 22 questions on average – the number of questions vary depending on the provided answers – and at the end he/she will receive a message as to what to do and a list of possible diagnoses for his/her problem. The questions are only about the history of the present illness and answering them doesn't need the interaction of a healthcare professional.
The diagnostic part utilizes Bayesian reasoning as inference mechanism. There are a number of diagnoses that are considered for abdominal pain algorithm; these diagnoses are sorted from the most common to the least common based on the demographic information of the patient. Then based on the provided answers by the patient the list will be resorted and at the end the top 3 diagnoses will be given to the patient as differential diagnoses. Based on the urgency of the diagnoses and their probability an advice will be rendered and offered to the patient.

There are four levels of decision in this system; in the rest of this paper we will use the term "disposition" to explain about these decisions. The dispositions are listed below:

1. Call 911
2. Go to the emergency room (ER)
3. Make an office appointment
4. Self-care

The last two dispositions are followed by a message that encourages the patient to recheck with the system if any change happens in their presentation.

MATERIALS AND METHODS

One hundred eighteen patients older than 15 years who presented to Hermann Hospital emergency room (ER) with chief complaint of stomach pain were included in the study. Each chart was reviewed and those patients who were positive for any of the screening questions were excluded from the study.

The symptoms of the patients at the time of presentation were extracted and stored in a database; their disposition in the ER – admission, referral and discharge – and their final diagnoses based on the hospital record were also logged into the database. The presenting symptoms for each patient was then entered into the triage tool by a person who was blind to the final diagnoses and ER disposition, and the disposition and the top three differential diagnoses were logged into the same database – the triage tool is capable of providing diagnoses and disposition even when there are some missing information but its accuracy will decrease. The presented symptoms were also presented to an emergency physician who was blind to the ER diagnoses and dispositions and was asked to provide a disposition.

To adapt for taxonomic differences in disposition, four levels of system disposition were mapped onto three levels of ER disposition. The first 2 levels – "call 911" and "go to ER" – mapped to "admission" in the ER at the time of the visit. The third level – "make an office appointment" – is mapped to "referral from ER to a clinic." And the forth level – "Self-care" – is mapped to "discharge" from ER. The dispositions of the ER and triage system were then compared and the following categories were used for analysis:

1. If the dispositions from ER and triage system were at the same level the disposition of the system was considered an *appropriate disposition*.
2. If the disposition of the triage system was higher than the ER disposition the disposition of the system was considered an *over-disposition*.
3. If the disposition of the triage system was lower than the ER disposition the system disposition was considered an *under-disposition*.

The same comparison was made between the physician's dispositions and those of the system and ER.

Considering the limited number of diagnoses available in the triage system we created four categories:

1. The ER diagnosis was in the triage system list of diagnoses and the triage system diagnosis matched the ER diagnosis. This condition was considered as *ER-Triage System diagnosis agreement*.
2. The ER diagnosis was in the triage system list of diagnoses and the triage system diagnosis didn't match the ER diagnosis. This condition was considered as *ER-Triage System diagnosis disagreement*.
3. The ER diagnosis was not in the triage system list of diagnoses but the triage system diagnosis, based on the judgment of the emergency physician, was reasonable compared to the ER diagnosis [6]. This condition was considered, as *ER diagnosis is not in Triage System ER-Triage System diagnosis agreement*.

4. The ER diagnosis was not in the triage system list of diagnoses and the triage system diagnosis, based on the judgment of the emergency physician, was not reasonable compared to the ER diagnosis [6]. This condition was considered, as *ER diagnosis is not in Triage System and ER-Triage System diagnosis disagreement.*

The SPSS software version 10.0 was used for analysis.

RESULTS

- The system disposed 51.1% of cases appropriately over-disposed 44.4% of cases and under-disposed 4.4% of cases (Fig-1).
- The ER specialist under-disposed 17.8% of cases (Fig-1).

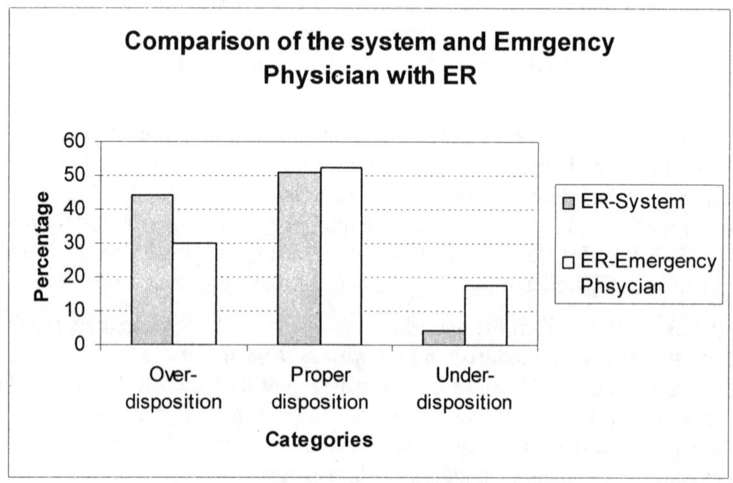

Fig-1. Comparing the performance of the system against ER and the physician against ER.

- Comparison between the system and the emergency physician against ER shows that all cases under-disposed by the system are also under-disposed by the emergency physician (Fig-2).

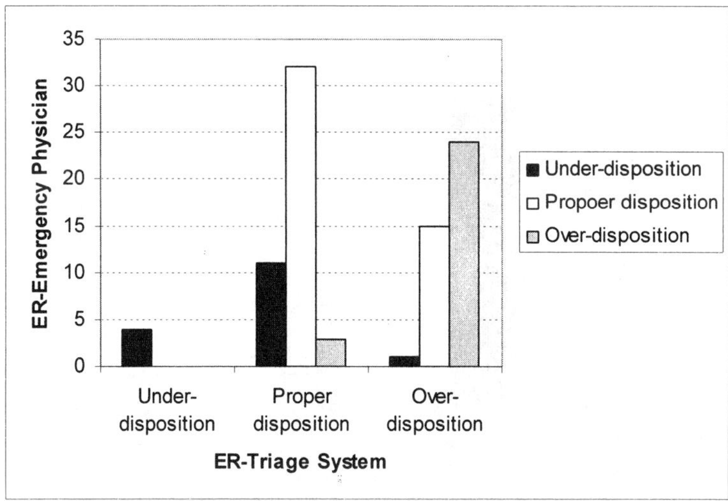

Fig-2. This chart shows the frequency of any of the 3 possible classifications (under, proper, and over-disposition) by the emergency physician among the cased that were classified into the same categories based on the performance of the ER-Triage System. For instance, the chart shows that all of the case that were under-disposed by the ER-Triage System, were also under-disposed by the emergency physician.

- 58.1% of cases had accurate diagnosis, *ER-Triage System diagnosis agreement*. The diagnoses that didn't exist in the triage system 16.1% of total assigned diagnoses were reasonable compared to the ER diagnosis; *ER diagnosis is not in Triage system ER-Triage System diagnosis agreement* (Fig-3).
- 19.4% of cases had inaccurate diagnosis, *ER-Triage System diagnosis disagreement* and 6.5% of cases were in the category of *ER diagnosis is not in Triage System and ER-Triage System diagnosis disagreement* (Fig-3).

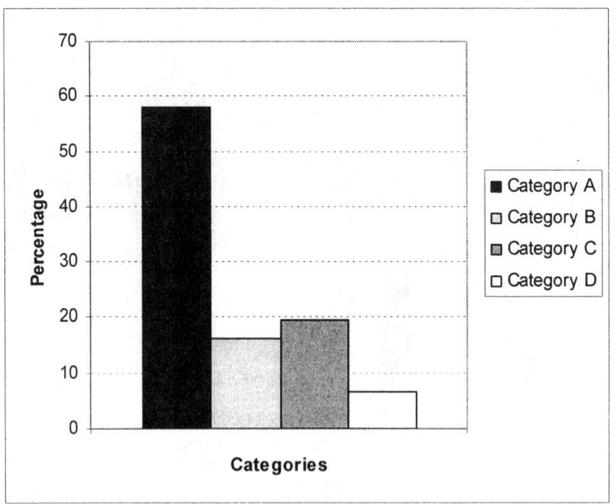

Fig-3. Accuracy of diagnosis of the System compared to ER diagnoses. Category A: *ER-Triage System diagnosis agreement.* Category B: *ER diagnosis is not in Triage system ER-Triage System diagnosis agreement.* Category C: *ER-Triage System diagnosis disagreement.* Category D: *ER diagnosis is not in Triage System and ER-Triage System diagnosis disagreement.*

DISCUSSION

As mentioned in the introduction one of the major problems of healthcare is emergency department over crowding [7]. Decreasing the load in the ER should be one of the main focuses of any triage tool but at the same time the tool should be safe for use.

Considering the fact that there is no real standard for triaging the patients, routinely a triage nurse makes the triage decision based on the protocols she has and based on her personal experience[3;8;9]. An emergency physician can make as good a decision as a triage nurse and comparing our tool with the emergency physician, our tool under-disposed 4.4% of patients while the emergency physician under-disposed about 17.8% of patients. So our triage tool is safer than a physician doing a telephone triage. Besides, the tool is not subject to fatigue or interpersonal relations and can make consistent diagnoses for two patients presenting with the same symptoms, while the physician or any triage nurse can have different judgments for a similar presentation based on the situation they are facing. The group of patients that the system under-disposed was all under-disposed by the physician which means that the visual, or physical exam information available in the ER had a larger impact on decision (Fig- 2).

The results of the study shows a tendency for over-disposing the patients but it is worth considering that many of the patients discharged from ER or referred to a clinic were observed in the ER for a few hours and then discharged. That observation period is not considered admission and so those patients are counted as over-disposition. In reality, that observation period is necessary to make a final decision and so those patients are false over-dispositions. Unfortunately, we didn't have accurate data for the length of observation for all of the patients to analyze the relation between observation period and over-disposition.

The diagnosis and decision in the ER are the gold standards for this study and our null hypotheses are

- "There is no difference between the system dispositions and those decisions made in ER".
- "There is no difference between system diagnoses and those made in the ER".

The statistical analyses failed to reject either of the null hypotheses. As the tool is safe compared to ER decisions and emergency physician's decisions, based on the descriptive data expanding the database could help increase statistical power of the study.

Although we analyzed the data from the patients who have already made a trip to ER the system would have advised 17.9% of them to make an office appointment. This number is very encouraging and shows that this triage tool has the capability of decreasing the ER load if used in the ER.

CONCLUSION

Current standard triage systems are run by a nurse practitioner providing advice to patients who call about their problem. An ER specialist, in our study, makes decisions under the same situation, but the system under-disposed only a small subset of the ER specialist's under-dispositions. Results, taken as a whole, support the conclusion that this system is safe within the current standards.

REFERENCE LIST

(1)　Schappert SM. National Hospital Ambulatory Medical Care Survey: 1992 Emergency Department Summary. Vital Health Stat 13 1997;(125):1-108.

(2)　Lowe RA, Bindman AB. Judging who needs emergency department care: a prerequisite for policy-making. Am J Emerg Med 1997; 15(2):133-136.

(3)　Gerdtz MF, Bucknall TK. Why we do the things we do: applying clinical decision-making frameworks to triage practice. Accid Emerg Nurs 1999; 7(1):50-57.

(4)　Wuerz R, Fernandes CM, Alarcon J. Inconsistency of emergency department triage. Emergency Department Operations Research Working Group. Ann Emerg Med 1998; 32(4):431-435.

(5)　Sadeghi S, Barzi A, Zarrin-Khameh N. Decision support system for medical triage. Stud Health Technol Inform 2001; 81:440-442.

(6)　Berner ES, Jackson JR, Algina J. Relationships among performance scores of four diagnostic decision support systems. J Am Med Inform Assoc 1996; 3(3):208-215.

(7)　McCabe JB. Emergency department overcrowding: a national crisis. Acad Med 2001; 76(7):672-674.

(8)　Gerdtz MF, Bucknall TK. Triage nurses' clinical decision making. An observational study of urgency assessment. J Adv Nurs 2001; 35(4):550-561.

(9)　Cioffi J. Triage decision making: educational strategies. Accid Emerg Nurs 1999; 7(2):106-111.

Medicine Meets Virtual Reality 02/10
J.D. Westwood et al. (Eds.)
IOS Press, 2002

Calibration and Accuracy Testing for Image-Enhanced Endoscopy

Michael R. Bax, Rasool Khadem, Jeremy A. Johnson, Eric P. Wilkinson
and Ramin Shahidi
Image Guidance Laboratories, Department of Neurosurgery,
300 Pasteur Drive #S-012, Stanford, CA 94305-5327, USA
http://igl.stanford.edu

Abstract. New surgical navigation techniques may combine the use of live video from a surgical endoscope with 3D volumetrically-reconstructed images of a patient's anatomy. This *image-enhanced endoscopy* requires calibration of the endoscope to ensure that the mapping of the real endoscope image to its virtual counterpart is properly performed. The application of a technique to calibrate an endoscope prior to use in a diagnostic or therapeutic procedure is described, as well as a simple yet effective linear method for lens-distortion compensation. The results of accuracy testing of the calibration technique using a dedicated testing apparatus are reported.

1. Background

Computer-assisted methods now provide real-time navigation during surgical procedures, including analysis and inspection of three-dimensional (3D) diagnostic images from magnetic resonance (MR) and computed tomography (CT) data [1]. Endoscopic technology has also undergone rapid development, providing lightweight endoscopes able to be used in small body cavities. Endoscopes are however able to display only visible surfaces, and are also limited by their inability to provide views of the interior of opaque tissue.

The combination of both endoscopic and computer-generated 3D images has the potential to provide the previously unavailable capability of overlaying volumetrically-reconstructed patient images onto the endoscopic view of the surgical field. This technique can permit surgeons to look beyond visible surfaces and provide "on-the-fly" 3D and two-dimensional (2D) information for planning and navigational purposes [2,3]. Due to the many parameters involved in the function of an endoscope, however, multiple small errors in the settings of the device may have relatively large and cumulative effects on the final discrepancy between the position of the overlaid endoscopic images and the patient's anatomy. For this reason, precise calibration of the endoscope and exhaustive accuracy testing of the calibrated endoscope is necessary to ensure surgical quality.

2. Theory

Calibration of an endoscope is more involved than calibration of a surgical probe, where only six extrinsic parameters must be estimated — three for translation and three for

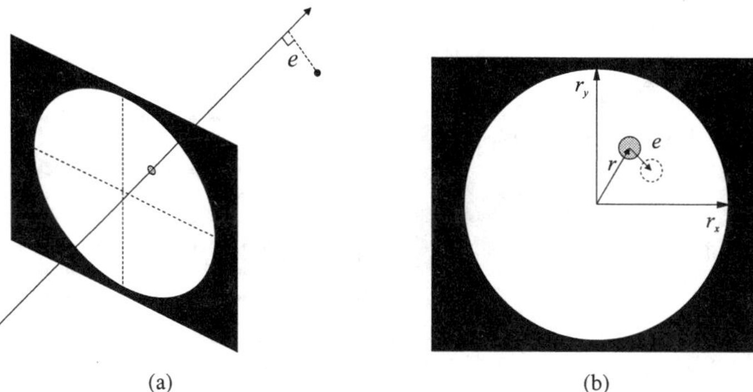

(a)   (b)

Figure 1. Endoscope view and errors in feature prediction. (a) Physical space error in which the projection of the image into physical space is the basis of the accuracy measurement. (b) Image space error in which the video image is used to determine accuracy. The grey dot represents the actual image of a point captured and the dashed circle shows the prediction based on the camera model.

rotation. Endoscopic calibration requires the estimation of five additional intrinsic parameters that model the operation of the camera itself [4].

The camera is modelled as a pinhole projection camera, described by its focal length (f), radial lens distortion (k_1), image coordinates of the center of radial distortion and piercing point of camera's z-axis with sensor plane (C_x, C_y), and a horizontal scale factor (s_x). Once all 11 parameters are known for a particular endoscope and the tracking sensor's position and orientation are measured, a virtual endoscopic image can be rendered from the preoperative volume dataset to match the endoscope video image.

It remains to be determined how closely the virtual endoscopic image matches the video image of the physical endoscope. Two types of errors can be characterized: physical space error and image space error.

In physical space error analysis, the question is how well the endoscope can be used as a targeting tool. In the camera model, a point seen in the video image corresponds to a ray from the center of projection (the camera model's optical origin) passing through the image projection plane (the model's equivalent to the camera CCD). If there is no tracking or modelling error this ray will also pass through the corresponding physical point, but if there is residual lens distortion, tracking error or other errors unaccounted for in the system model, the ray will miss the corresponding physical point by some distance, denoted e. This is defined as the shortest distance between the physical point and the ray, as shown in Figure 1(a).

In image space error analysis, the goal is to predict how closely locations of the features in the virtual image match the same features in the captured endoscope video image. In other words, the object of this analysis is to measure the closeness of the real image to the virtual image as shown in Figure 1(b). This is the approach taken here.

3. Materials and Methods

3.1. Endoscope Tracking

For testing purposes, the Polaris optical tracking system in a hybrid mode of passive/active (Northern Digital, Inc., Waterloo, Ontario, Canada) was used as the tracking system. In active mode, infrared emission from IR LEDs is captured by the camera. In passive mode,

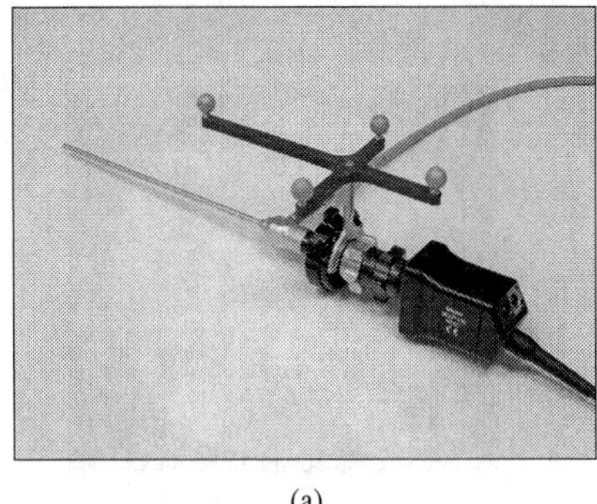
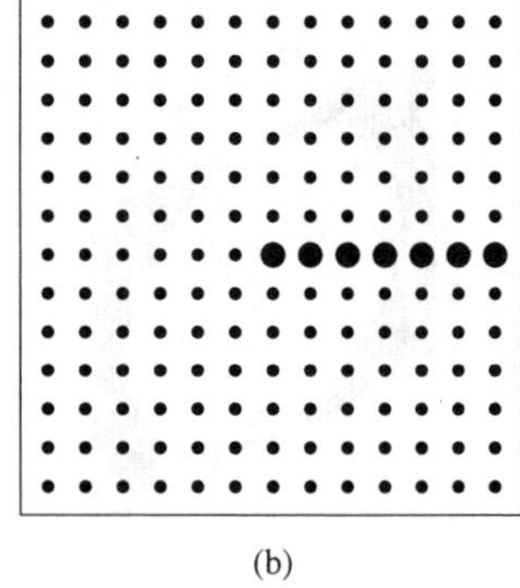

(a)   (b)

Figure 2. (a) Universal tracking tool attached to the endoscope. (b) Grid used for endoscope calibration.

infrared beams are emitted from the emitter/camera and reflected by balls on a tracking device attached to the endoscope.

An endoscope from STORZ (Karl Storz Endoscopy America, Inc., Culver City, CA) encoded with a passive reflector-ball tracking device was used as the principal endoscope. The following equipment was used during development: the Storz Tricam SL camera; the Storz Nova Light Source; and a Storz 50200A zero degree telescope. To track the surgical tools a universal tracker from Traxtal, Inc. was attached to the endoscope, as shown in Figure 2(a). This tracking device may be mounted on top of various surgical devices, such as a surgical probe (used for dissecting down to the surgical site) and the endoscope.

3.2. Endoscope Calibration

A common method used for obtaining both the extrinsic and intrinsic camera calibration parameters simultaneously is that developed by Tsai [4]. The input parameters to the algorithm are the world coordinates (x, y, z) of a set of known points and their corresponding coordinates (u, v) in the endoscope video image. The features are identified in the camera image and mapped to the reference pattern; in this way, the real-world coordinates of the features can be found. The best results are obtained when the collection of points are distributed across x, y, and z in world coordinates, and fill as much of the camera image as possible.

For the system described in this paper, a planar grid pattern of black dots 1 and 2 mm in diameter and with 3 mm spacing between the grid rows and columns was used, as shown in Figure 2(b). The world coordinates of the dots were defined with respect to a tracking tool rigidly attached to the calibration unit. The endoscope, equipped with the universal tracker, was then placed into the calibration unit with its lens roughly 15 mm away from the center of the pattern. In order to achieve a sufficient distribution of the points in the z-direction, the telescope lens view direction is constrained to an angle of $30°$ from the normal of the pattern plane.

One of the parameters determined by this algorithm is the lens distortion parameter k_1, a coefficient of the radial lens-distortion model polynomial. Incorporating this non-linear model into the 3D perspective rendering engine results in a drop in performance; if this lens distortion compensation is omitted, a choice has to be made about the "effective FOV" of the virtual endoscope. If this FOV is set to match that of the physical endoscope, the result is that the center part of the virtual image is smaller than that in the video image. This effect is undesirable because this is the primary region of interest for the surgeon. An alternative method, here named "constant-radius linear compensation", is to scale the virtual FOV such that the radii of the region of interest in each image are made equal.

3.3. Calibration Accuracy Testing

A planar grid of 1 and 2 mm black dots with 3 mm of spacing between grid rows and columns, large enough to fill the field of view of the endoscope at a distance of 65 mm, was used as a physical target. The grid was mounted on a moveable plate with a universal tracking device fixed on it. A tracked pointer was used to manually locate and register the positions of 8 crosshairs on the grid with reference to the tracking device on the plate; the positions of the grid dots were computed using the known positional relationship between the dots and the set of crosshairs.

The endoscope was calibrated and mounted facing this grid, and the grid was positioned at a set of distances from 5 to 65 mm from the tip of the endoscope's telescope. At each position the physical location and orientation of the endoscope, the grid plate tracking device, and the endoscope video image were stored. The dots in each image were detected and matched with the corresponding grid dots.

The virtual image was formed by projecting a ray from the camera's focal point through the virtual image plane to each physical dot identified in the endoscope video image. The error was determined as the distance between the image coordinates of the virtual dot and the corresponding dot in the endoscope video image. This procedure was repeated for 20 separate calibrations.

4. Results

Figure 3(a) shows the error as a function of distance from the center of the image normalized to the radius of FOV. The choice of distortion compensation method affects the error values at points far from the center of the image.

Figure 3(b) shows mean error between the location of the predicted dots in the virtual image and the corresponding dots in the endoscope video image as a function of the distance of the target plane from the endoscope tip. It can be seen that this is essentially independent of distance, since the error in the image plane is determined by the angle between the rays from the camera model's center of projection to each point pair.

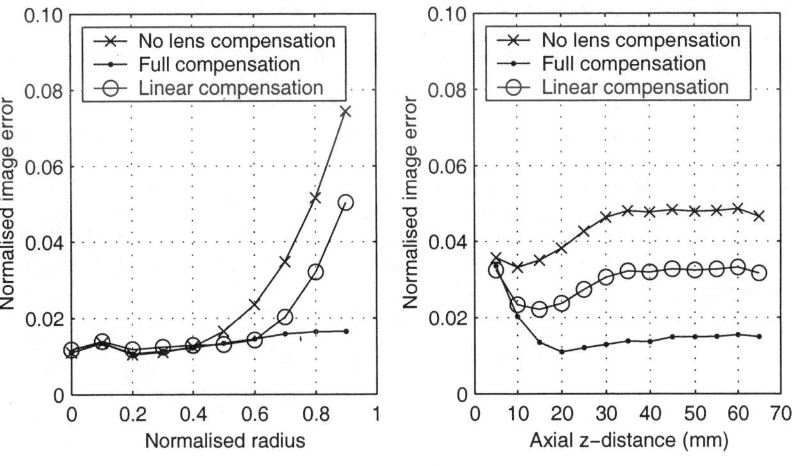

Figure 3. (a)   3. (b)

In each case the error is normalized to the diameter of the FOV: on a 512×512 pixel display where the endoscope video fills the screen, a normalized error of 0.01 corresponds to an error of approximately 5 pixels.

5. Discussion

Endoscope calibration is an essential part of an image-enhanced endoscopy system. Mismatches between virtual image and video output of the endoscope have a variety of sources. Sources of error in the overall system accuracy include errors in the calibration of the endoscope, errors in the tracking system and errors in the registration process. The main focus of this work was on errors associated with the calibration process.

The errors inherent to the calibration may be categorized into three groups: errors in the detection of dots, deficiencies of the camera model, and errors from tracking system. Accuracy of the detection of the dots is bound by the resolution of the camera. The Tsai algorithm is sensitive to errors in image space localization and therefore the best possible algorithm should be used for dot detection: sub-pixel accuracy should be obtained, with the lowest possible sensitivity to the lighting conditions and to image noise.

Although the camera model used by this algorithm is a simplification of optical geometry, it is sufficient for the purpose of image-guided surgery as other sources of error dominate in determining the overall accuracy of the system.

Tracking system errors are known to impact the accuracy of localization of the endoscope tip [6]. The image guidance system also suffers from tracking system error in determining the direction of the tool; this error is magnified, as objects in the virtual image may be a considerable distance from the endoscope itself.

Since image-plane error is constant with respect to target feature distance from the endoscope tip, it shows that the projected physical error is linearly proportional to this distance.

It can also be seen that constant-radius linear compensation is an effective scheme for overcoming lens distortion without an associated performance loss.

References

[1] M.Viergever (ed.), Special Issue on Image-Guidance of Therapy, *IEEE Trans on Medical Image* **17** (1998) 669–685.

[2] R. Shahidi, Applications of Virtual Reality in Stereotactic Procedures: Volumetric Image Navigation Via a Surgical Microscope, Ph.D. Dissertation, Rutgers University, Rutgers, NJ, 1995.

[3] D.J. Vining, Virtual Endoscopy: Is It Reality? *Radiology* **200** (1996) 30–31.

[4] R.Y. Tsai, An Efficient and Accurate Camera Calibration Technique for 3D Machine Vision. In Proceedings of the IEEE Conference on Computer Vision and Pattern Recognition, 1986, pp. 364–374.

[5] E. Krotkov, K. Henriksen, and R. Kories, Stereo Ranging with Verging Cameras, *IEEE Trans on Pattern Analysis and Machine Intelligence* **12** (1990) 1200–1205.

[6] R. Khadem, C. Yeh, M. Sadeghi-Tehrani, M.R. Bax, J.A. Johnson, J.N. Welch, E.P. Wilkinson, R. Shahidi. Comparative Tracking Error Analysis of Five Different Optical Tracking Systems, *Computer Aided Surgery* **5** (2000) 98–107.

Medicine Meets Virtual Reality 02/10
J.D. Westwood et al. (Eds.)
IOS Press, 2002

Open Surgery Simulation

Daniel Bielser and Markus H. Gross

Computer Science Department, ETH Zurich, Switzerland
email: {bielser, grossm}@inf.ethz.ch

Abstract The design of simulators for surgical training and planning poses a great number of technical challenges. Therefore the focus of systems and algorithms was mostly on the more restricted minimal invasive surgery. This paper tackles the more general problem of open surgery and presents efficient solutions to several of the main difficulties. In addition to an improved collision detection scheme for computing interactions with even heavily moving tissue, a hierarchical system for the haptic rendering has been realized in order to reach the best performance of haptic feedback. A flexible way of modeling complex surgical tools out of simple basic components is proposed. In order to achieve a realistic and at the same time fast relaxation of the tissue, the approach of explicit finite elements has been substantially improved. We are able to demonstrate realistic simulations of interactive open surgery scenarios.

1. Introduction and Previous Work

The design of surgical simulators poses a great number of technical challenges: appropriate soft tissue models have to be chosen and the underlying differential equations have to be solved efficiently. Very often, surgical tools such as scalpels and hooks are involved, featuring complex interactions with the soft tissue. High speed haptic rendering of these tools requires sophisticated mechanical models.

Systems and algorithms for surgical training and planning proposed over the past years have mostly focused on minimal invasive surgery [1]. The underlying datastructures are often restricted to surface meshes [13] or regular grids [18],[9]. Apart from a few approaches, open surgery and real time soft tissue cutting is still largely unexplored. First approaches calculating intersection surfaces in retrospect can be found in the algorithms of [16] and [15]. The removing of entire tetrahedra in [5] is real-time but generates very uneven surfaces. A dynamic subdivision algorithm using an operator framework is introduced by the authors of this paper in [3] and has then be refined in [2] and [14] as well as extended to multiresolution grids by [8].

In this paper we will present interactive open surgery scenarios in which surgical hooks and large scalpel intersections are applied simultaneously. Our real-time system is based on arbitrary tetrahedral meshes and shows capable of interactively modeling incisions with high accuracy and topological freedom (chapter 3).

Previous volume collision detection algorithms like the one described in [3] and [2] have had difficulties in reliably registering all intersections between a tool and the tissue structures while the tissue is being deformed. We show a solution that solves the consistency problems even when the tissue is moving heavily (chapter 4).

The computationally most accurate but also most expensive methods for the modeling of elastic soft tissue use Finite Element procedures to solve the governing equations (e.g [11] and [12]). Recently, Boundary Element Methods (BEM), like [4] or [10] were proposed, condensing the solution into the domain boundary. Condensation, however, is very problematic because the whole stiffness-matrix has to be recomputed when cutting some surface elements. The formulation of explicit finite elements of [5], [7] and [6] helps here to reduce the computational complexity and allows for iteratively solving of the system. Whereas these works still solve the resulting differential equations with explicit numerical methods, the work in hand improves the approach of explicit finite elements by using the fast and robust (implicit) Theta-schemes, by parallelization, and by supporting individual time-steps for each node (chapter 5).

In most approaches, force feedback devices are utilized to implement the interface to the user. While haptical surface rendering of complex rigid objects has been already introduced in [17] and applied in many other works (e.g. [19]), we have developed algorithms to render surfaces of deforming objects including static and dynamic surface friction as well as more tool specific forms of tool-object-interaction. (chapter 2)

2. Simulation Overview

All main modules of a surgery simulator, like *Collision Detection, Geometrical Updates, Relaxation, Rendering* and *Haptics*, are realized as individual components of the simulation. During simulation the different components work in parallel. This enables the relaxation of the model in parallel with geometrical modifications and it makes the frame rate dependent only on the graphics hardware. In the following we focus on the interaction between the haptic simulation and the tissue model, which may be located on different machines connected via a TCP/IP connection.

The difficulty of haptic rendering deforming tissue is the slow response of the underlying physical model. In order to achieve the high update rates required for qualitatively sufficient haptic rendering we implemented a three stage simulation hierarchy (Fig. 1). On a haptic client the surface is approximated by a tangent plane and rendered with static and dynamic friction at an update rate of several thousand Hertz (**Haptics Simulation**). This plane is updated from the server side at high speed taking into account the actual local curvature of the model (   ). In a first step the output force is roughly approximated through the client by a simple spring model. It is then overlaid by the real external tissue forces as being computed by the relaxation process at the server side (**Relaxation**).

Fig. 2 explains the interplay of the three components in more detail: As soon as a tool approaches the surface an estimation of the tangent plane through which the tool may enter the surface is sent to the client. Once the first interaction of the tool with the tissue occurs (a) only the haptic client is fast enough to calculate a responding force F_{spring} . A fraction of a second later (b), the reaction force from the tissue model F_{tissue} arrives together with an

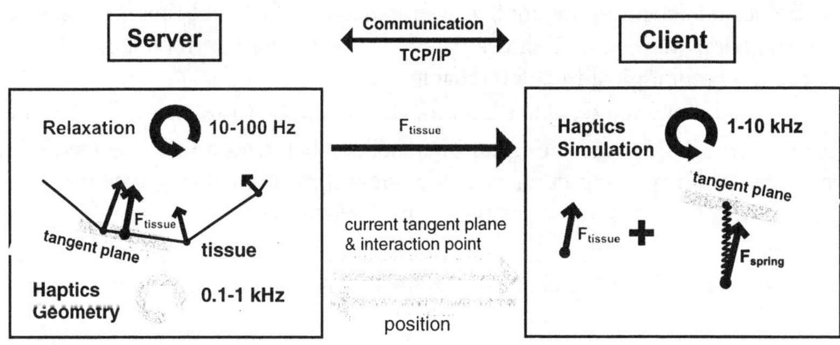

Figure 1: 3 stage simulation hierarchy

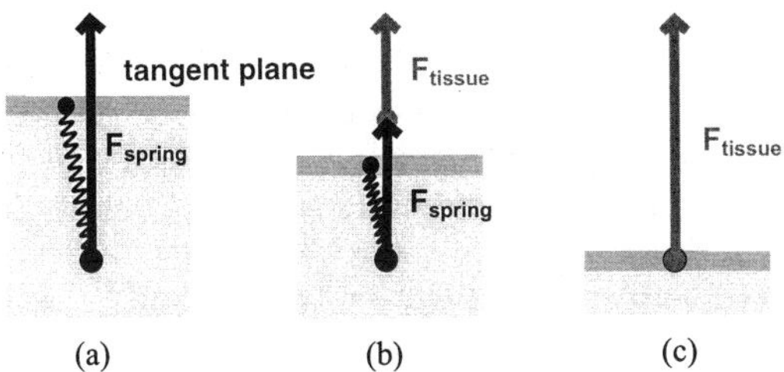

Figure 2: Interplay of the force components

update of the shifted tangent plane and is overlaid with $\mathbf{F_{spring}}$. If the tool does not move any further (c) $\mathbf{F_{spring}}$ nearly vanishes and the haptic output consists solely of $\mathbf{F_{tissue}}$. With this procedure we manage to keep the point of the haptic tool outside the tissue.

3. Tool Tissue Interaction

As depicted in Fig. 3 the tools contain three representations of different complexity. The first representation is the graphical surface model consisting of several thousands of triangles. The second one is a simple line model used for collision detection. Finally, the third one presents the current interaction point for the haptic simulation.

The collision detection model (b) can be made up of any number of two different types of lines. One line-type results in deformation when interacting with an object and the other type cuts the tissue. For each line of the model the penetration with the object's surface is calculated. Special algorithms have been developed to handle the case of lines that have shown two or more intersections with the object's surface.

The haptic model (c), responsible for the calculation of the haptic output, is the same for all tools and supports only one interaction point. This is necessary because the applied PHANToM® device only supports positional force feedback for the tip of the pin. Therefore a procedure to determine the interaction point in relation to the current collision detection state has to be defined for each tool. The interaction point can be chosen from the colliding lines or computed as their average.

As for surgical tools, a *virtual scalpel* and a *surgical hook* have been realized so far. During an operation several of these tools can be activated. Depending on their orientation the hooks either deform the tissue while sliding over the surface or hook in and transmit the applied forces directly. In case of the scalpel the tetrahedra are cut progressively, thus continuously providing a consistent representation of the cut surface up to the actual position of the scalpel. Immediate computation of the interactions with the mesh structures allows us to simulate deformations resulting both from cutting and friction.

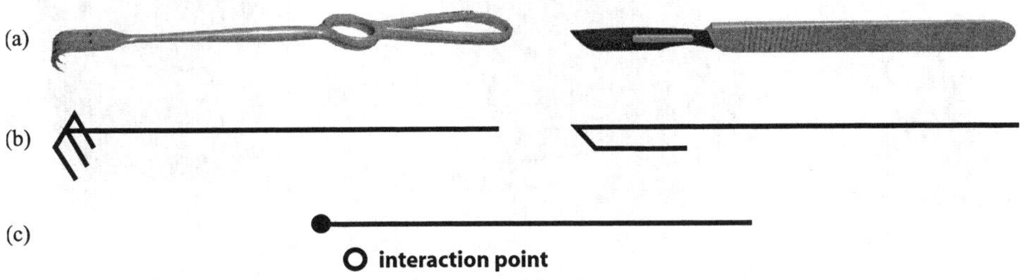

Figure 3: 3 tool representations for: (a) graphics, (b) collision detection, and (c) haptics

4. Local Collision Detection

Our system not only performs high performance surface proximity checks, but also supports local volume collision detection. Starting with some penetrated entry faces the algorithm iterates through the tetrahedra mesh along the current scalpel blade. With these penetrated tetrahedra as starting points, all tetrahedra affected by the preceded motion of the scalpel are retrieved by a recursive algorithm. In order to compute scalpel interactions even within heavily moving tissue structures, the local volume collision detection algorithms as described in [2] have been modified in the following way:

Each time the tetrahedra penetrated by the current scalpel blade are determined, the collision points between the tetrahedra faces and the blade line are calculated and stored locally inside the tetrahedra in form of barycentric coordinates (**ENPi** in Fig. 4 (a)). In contrast to storing a global scalpel position, the locally barycentric intersection points follow potential mesh transformations (Fig. 4 (b)). No matter how large the positional displacements of the mesh nodes are, each face intersection point **ENPi** stays relative to its face's nodes at the same position.

In order to actually mark the penetration between the scalpel trajectory and the tetrahedral edges a surface is spread between the previous marked collision points at time t_i and the current position of the scalpel blade at t_{i+1}. From each line segment between two face intersection points (e.g. **ENP1** and **ENP2**) a triangle is spanned to one of the current scalpel intersection points **currentSP** or **currentENP**. From a topological point of view this procedure guarantees that the same tetrahedra edges will be cut whatever the motion of the tetrahedra nodes is.

Whereas in Fig. 4 only one tissue intersection is depicted, in real simulation situations several distinct parts of a tool may intersect the tissue at the same time. Approximating the tool by a set of lines, the two types of intersections symbolized in Fig. 5 (**ENP1** to **EXP3** and **ENP4** to **SP**) and the spaces in between need to be treated. The corresponding algorithm constructs the swept surface by proceeding from tetrahedron to tetrahedron and always constructing triangles between its entry point and the entry point of the subsequent tetrahedron. In order to bridge the gaps between two line segments the exit point of the last tetrahedron of a segment is always linked with a triangle with the entry point of the first tetrahedron of the next segment. The intersection points between the trajectory of the tool tip and the tetrahedra faces have to be calculated separately. For that reason a line is drawn between the current tool tip **currentSP** and its previous position **SP**, which both are stored as 4D barycentric coordinates relative to the nodes of the surrounding tetrahedron.

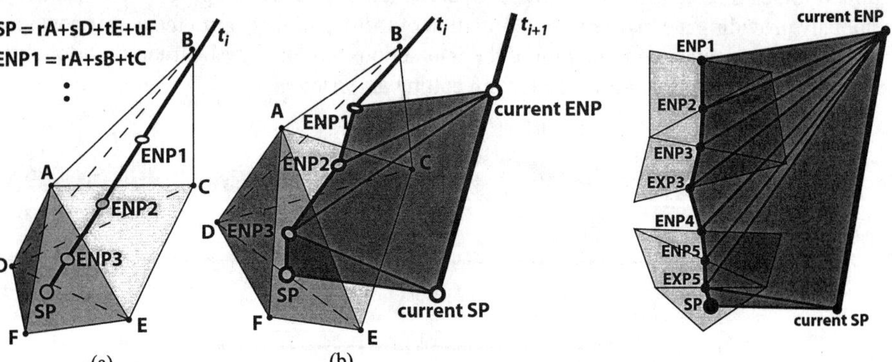

Figure 4: Benefit of local intersection points: (a) initial tetrahedra mesh (b) mesh after transformation   **Figure 5:** Collision algorithm

5. Relaxation

For the calculation of the underlying tissue structures two different physical models have been applied. On the one hand there exists already a very fast implicitly solved mass-spring system [2] and on the other hand we have developed an improved version of the more realistic tensor mass system introduced in [5]. This approach bases on continuum mechanics and describes the energy of elasticity in the tissue with linearized stresses as

$$E_{\text{elast}} = \int_V \left(\frac{\lambda}{2} \cdot (trE)^2 + \mu \cdot tr(E^2) \right) dV$$

whereas tr is the trace of the matrix and λ, μ are the two Lame-coefficients.

$$\lambda = \frac{\nu \cdot E_{\text{Young}}}{(1 + \nu) \cdot (1 - 2 \cdot \nu)} \qquad \mu = \frac{E_{\text{Young}}}{2 \cdot (1 + \nu)} \qquad \begin{array}{l} E_{\text{Young}}: \text{modulus of elasticity} \\ \\ \nu: \text{poisson ratio} \end{array}$$

The energy thereby is defined by the displacement vector $\vec{U}$ in relation to the restposition as

$$E = \frac{1}{2} \cdot (\nabla \vec{U} + (\nabla \vec{U})^T) \qquad \nabla: \text{laplacian}$$

In order to achieve a local calculation scheme the nodes are visited iteratively and their positional changes are calculated by applying Newtons equation. The external force is obtained by precalculation of the force parts of the participating elements in the direct adjacency. The influence of the tissue force onto a specific node is divided into a part for the incident edges (edge tensors) and into one for the neighboring nodes (node tensors).

The indicated explicit finite element approach adapts very well to our parallelized iterative solving strategy which has already been successfully used to speed up mass-spring systems [2]. In contrast to the explicit numerical methods of the initial approach [5] we propose implicit Theta-schemes. This class of stable numerical methods enables to perform the time integration of the actually stiff differential equations with large time steps.

The θ-scheme evaluates the partial derivation $dx/dt = f(x, t)$ two times, one time at the current position x_i and one time at the subsequent position x_{i+1}. This two values are then weighted with a parameter θ.

$$x_{i+1} = x_i + \Delta t \cdot ((1 - \theta) \cdot f(x_i) + \theta \cdot f(x_{i+1}))$$

Furthermore, we support adaptive time steps for each individual node in order to better cope with the stiff differential equation system. For an absolute stable convergence of the relaxation process the size of the time step of each single node is controlled by fixing the largest possible velocity of a node. Whenever a node exceeds this upper bound its time-step will be halved and the node's position will be recalculated as long as the bound is not met.

6. Results

A prototype of a surgery simulator supporting all the features described above has successfully been realized. The system allows high quality rendering at real-time frame rates and reacts interactively for substantial mesh sizes (up to 3000 tetrahedra). Due to the progressive subdivision of the tetrahedral mesh, the virtual scalpel can be guided with high precision. The haptic output of the tool–tissue interaction for both of the implemented tools is free of any vibrations and oscillations and is considered realistic according to various test persons. The figures 6 to 10 give some sequential screen shots from the simulation of a operation in the abdominal area. The processed model consists of initially 3800 tetrahedra. The simulation setup is depicted in figure 11. (Visit the project website *http://graphics.ethz.ch/artist* in order to see the figures in color.)

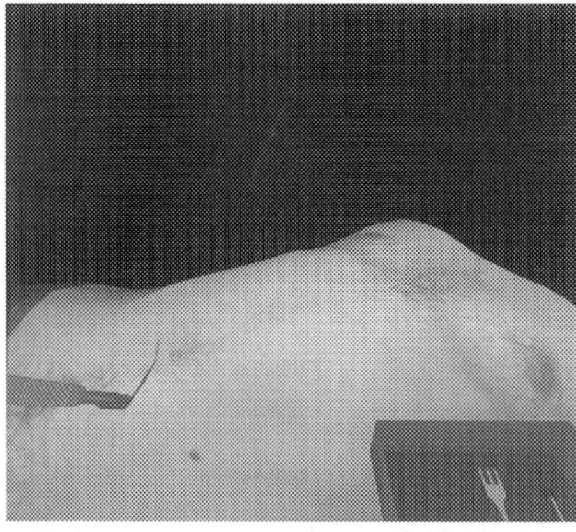

Figure 6: First scalpel cut in order to open the skin tissue

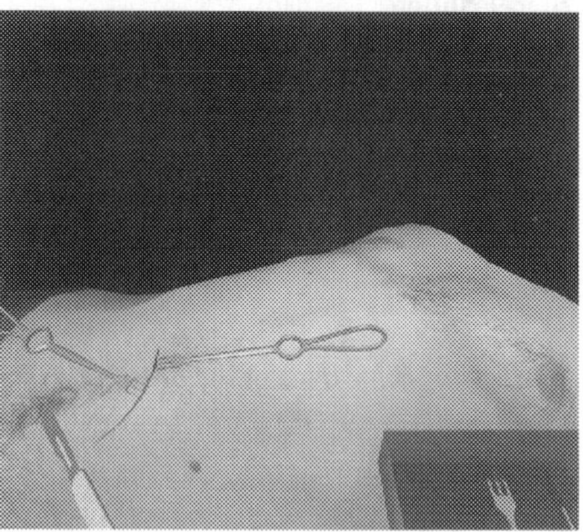

Figure 7: Insertion of the hooks

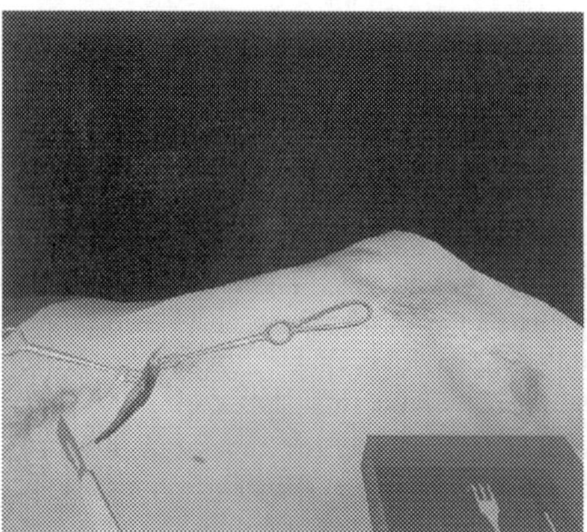

Figure 8: Opening the intersection

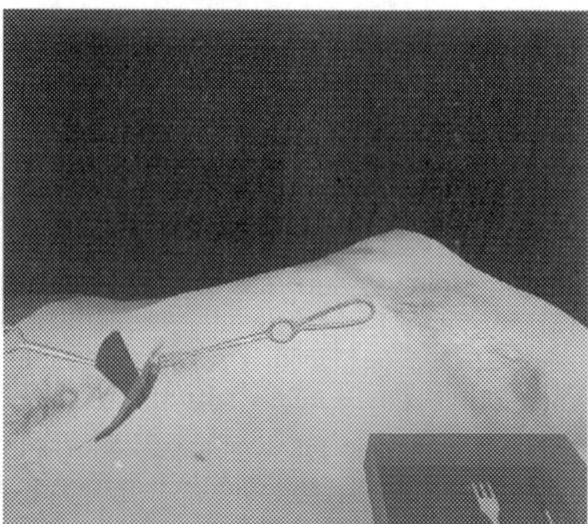

Figure 9: Fitting in the scalpel in order to perform a further cut

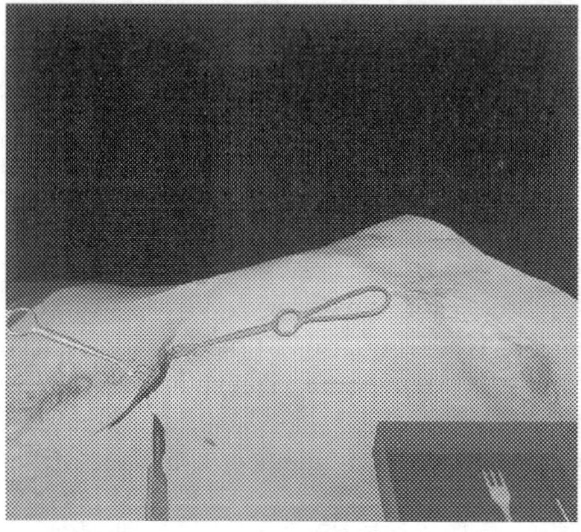

Figure 10: Carrying out a further cut

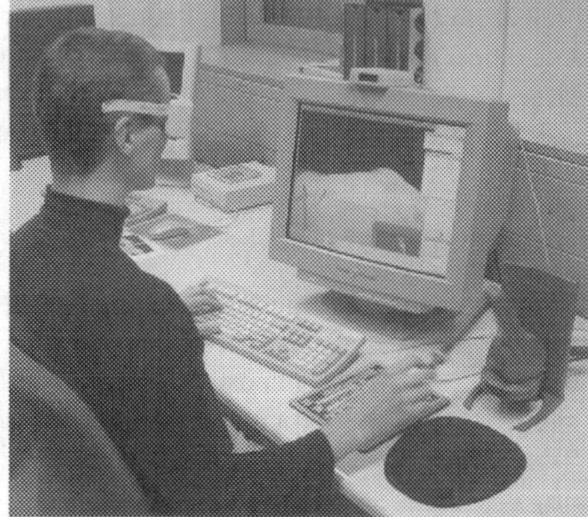

Figure 11: Simulation setup with PHANToM® force feedback device and stereo glasses

7. Conclusion and Future Work

We designed a realistic surgery trainer that features topological flexibility and accuracy for tool–tissue interactions occurring during open surgery procedures. The presented tools combined with an efficient and realistic tissue model allow us to simulate various surgical procedures with highly realistic force feedback.

Future work will expand the tool-tissue interaction approach of pure positional force feedback to the haptic rendering of torques by taking into account multiple interaction points with the tetrahedra mesh.

8. Acknowledgement

We would like to thank Remo Ziegler, Stefan Benkler, and Arno Jost for their contribution to the current implementation of our surgery training software.

9. References

[1] C. Basdogan, Chih-Hao, and M. A. Srinivasan. "Simulation of tissue cutting and bleeding for laparoscopic surgery using auxiliary surfaces." In *Medicine Meets Virtual Reality*, pages 38–44. IOS Press, 1999.

[2] D. Bielser and M. H. Gross. "Interactive simulation of surgical cut procedures." In *Proceedings of the Pacific Graphics 2000*, pages 116–125, 2000.

[3] D. Bielser, V. A. Maiwald, and M. H. Gross. "Interactive cuts through 3-dimensional soft tissue." In *Proceedings of the Eurographics '99*, volume 18, pages C31–C38, 1999.

[4] M. Bro-Nielsen and S. Cotin. "Real-time volumetric deformable models for surgery simulation using finite elements and condensation." *Computer Graphics Forum*, 15(3):C57–C66, C461, Sept. 1996.

[5] S. Cotin, H. Delingette, and N. Ayache. "A hybrid elastic model allowing real-time cutting, deformations and force-feedback for surgery training and simulation." *The Visual Computer*, 16(8):437–452, 2000.

[6] G. Debunne, M. Desbrun, M.-P. Cani, and A. H. Barr. "Dynamic real-time deformations using space & time adaptive sampling." In *SIGGRAPH'01 Proceedings*, pages 31–36, 2001.

[7] G. Picinbono and H. Delingette and N. Ayache. "Non-linear and anisotropic elastic soft tissue models for medical simulation." In *ICRA2001: IEEE International Conference Robotics and Automation*, Seoul Korea, May 2001.

[8] F. Ganovelli, P. Cignoni, C. Montani, and R. Scopigno. "A multiresolution model for soft objects supporting interactive cuts and lacerations." In *Proceedings of the Eurographics 2000*, volume 19, pages C271–C282, 2000.

[9] S. F. Gibson. "3d chainmail: a fast algorithm for deforming volumetric objects." In *Proceedings 1997 Symposium on Interactive 3D Graphics*, pages 149–154, Apr. 1997.

[10] D. L. James and D. K. Pai. "Accurate real time deformable objects." In *SIGGRAPH Proceedings*, pages 65–72. ACM Press, 1999.

[11] R. Koch, M. Gross, D. von Bueren, G. Frankhauser, Y. Parish, and F. Carls. "Simulating facial surgery using finite element models." In *Proceedings of SIGGRAPH 96*, pages 421–428, 1996.

[12] R. Koch, S. Roth, M. Gross, A. Zimmermann, and H. Sailer. "A framework for facial surgery simulation." *Technical Report No. 327, Computer Science Department, ETH Zurich*, 1999.

[13] U. Kuehnapfel, C. Kuhn, M. Huebner, H. Krumm, H. Maafl, and B. Neisius. "The karlsruhe endoscopic surgery trainer as an example for virtual reality in medical education." In *Minimally Invasive Therapy and Allied Technologies*, volume 6, pages 122–125. Blackwell Science Ltd., 1997.

[14] A. B. Mor and T. Kanade. "Modifying soft tissue models: Progressive cutting with minimal new element creation." In *CVRMed-Proceedings*, volume 19, pages 598–607, 2000.

[15] K. D. Reinig, H. L. Pelster, V. M. Spitzer, T. B. Johnson, and T. J. Mahalik. "More real-time visually and haptic interaction with anatomical data." In K. M. et al, editor, *Medicine Meets Virtual Reality*, pages 155–158. IOS Press, 1997.

[16] K. D. Reinig, C. G. Rush, H. L. Pelster, V. M. Spitzer, and J. A. Heath. "Real-time visually and haptically accurate surgical simulation." In S. H. H. Sieburg and K. Morgan, editors, *Health Care in the Information Age*, pages 542–546. IOS Press, 1996.

[17] D. Ruspini, K. Kolarov, and O. Khatib. "The haptic display of complex graphical environments." In *SIGGRAPH Proceedings*, pages 345–352, 1997.

[18] N. Suzuki, A. Hattori, S. Kai, T. Ezumi, and A. Takatsu. "Surgical planning system for soft tissues using virtual reality." *Medicine Meets Virtual Reality*, pages 159–163, 1997.

[19] T. V. Thompson and E. Cohen. "Direct haptic rendering of complex trimmed nurbs models." In *Proceedings of Symposium on Haptic Interfaces*, 1999.

Medicine Meets Virtual Reality 02/10
J.D. Westwood et al. (Eds.)
IOS Press, 2002

Virtual Reality-*Based* Post-Stroke Hand Rehabilitation

**R. Boian[1], A. Sharma[2], C. Han[2], A. Merians[3, 4], G. Burdea[1],
S. Adamovich[4], M. Recce[2], M. Tremaine[2] and H. Poizner[4]**

[1] Center for Advanced Information Processing, Rutgers University,
Piscataway, NJ, USA
[2] Department of Information Systems, New Jersey Institute of
Technology, Newark, NJ, USA
[3] University of Medicine and Dentistry of New Jersey, Newark, NJ,
USA
[4] Center for Molecular and Behavioral Neuroscience, Rutgers
University, Newark, NJ, USA

Abstract.
A VR-based system using a CyberGlove and a Rutgers Master II-ND haptic glove
was used to rehabilitate four post-stroke patients in the chronic phase. Each patient
had to perform a variety of VR exercises to reduce impairments in their finger range
of motion, speed, fractionation and strength. Patients exercised for about two hours
per day, five days a week for three weeks. Results showed that three of the patients
had gains in thumb range (50-140%) and finger speed (10-15%) over the three
weeks trial. All four patients had significant improvement in finger fractionation
(40-118%). Gains in finger strength were modest, due in part to an unexpected
hardware malfunction. Two of the patients were measured against one-month post
intervention and showed good retention. Evaluation using the Jebsen Test of Hand
Function showed a reduction of 23-28% in time completion for two of the patients
(the ones with the higher degrees of impairment). A prehension task was performed
9-40% faster for three of the patients after the intervention illustrating transfer of
their improvement to a functional task.

1   Introduction

The American Stroke Association states that stroke is the third leading cause of death in the
United States and a major cause for serious, long-term disabilities [1]. Statistics show that
there are about four million stroke survivors living today, with 500,000 new cases being
added each year. Impairments such as muscle weakness, loss of range of motion, decreased
reaction times and disordered movement organization create deficits in motor control,
which affect the patient's independent living. Recent studies have showed that intensive
and repetitive training may be necessary to modify neural organization [11,12,13,14] and
recover functional motor skills [17,18]. Several authors have reported significant
improvement in patients' daily activities due to higher training intensities, even in the
chronic phase of the disease.

The current health care system provides stroke rehabilitation in the acute care
hospital setting, in the rehabilitation setting and in the outpatient setting. The frequency of
training in the outpatient rehabilitation phase is usually once or twice a week. It is clear that

the limited amount of therapy offered by the current system makes it difficult to provide the training intensity needed for neural reorganization and functional changes.

Research is currently focused on various approaches to provide better rehabilitation means for post-stroke patients. Virtual environments are a technology suitable for rehabilitation therapy due to their inherent ability of simulating real-life tasks. Besides helping to engage the patient in life-like activities, virtual environments provide the means to better measure and evaluate the patient's performance. Sensors can be attached to the patient's body to measure the motions, and the sensor readings can be transparently stored and evaluated by the system. Virtual environments can also improve the motivation of the patient toward the therapy by providing an engaging interface to the exercises.

Virtual environments have been used by Holden et al. [6] to develop a hand-reaching task for patients with chronic hemiplegia. Popescu et al. [16,15] have developed a library of VR exercises for hand rehabilitation in orthopedic patients. Virtual reality has been used for children with cerebral palsy to enhance spatial awareness and the operation of motorized wheelchairs [3,7]. A Stewart platform robot coupled to a virtual environment has been used to rehabilitate orthopedic and neurological patients with ankle problems [4,2].

Jack et al. [8,9] used VR exercises and traditional non-VR manual task practice in interventions on post-stroke patients. Lessons learned from our earlier study lead to the research reported here, in an attempt to see if VR exercise *alone* can improve post-stroke patients in the chronic phase.

2　Rehabilitation System

The rehabilitation system is distributed over three sites connected to each other through the Internet, as illustrated in Figure 1. The *rehabilitation site* is the location where the patient is undergoing upper extremity therapy. The system components deployed at this site are a PC workstation, a CyberGlove and a Rutgers Master II (RMII) haptic glove [5]. The two sensing gloves are integrated with VR exercises running on the PC host. The patient interacts with the system using the sensing gloves. Feedback is given on the computer screen. The *data storage site* is the location of the main server of the system. The server hosts an Oracle database, a monitoring server and a web site for access to the data. *Data access sites* do not have a fixed location, being computers with Internet access. Using a web browser, a therapist or physician can access the web portal and view the patient data remotely. The three sites of the system are presented in more detail in the next sections.

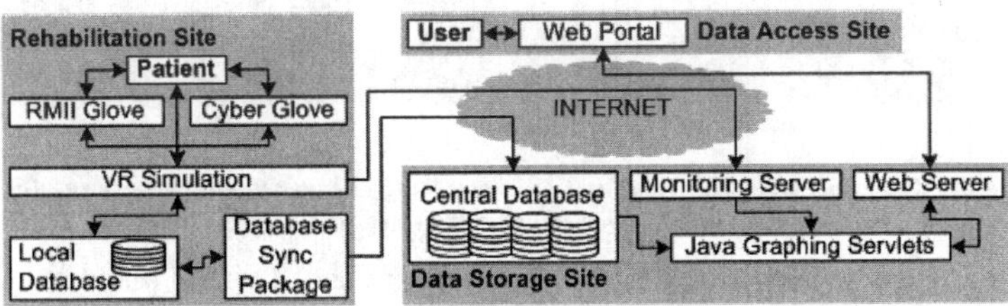

Figure 1- Rehabilitation system architecture. © Rutgers University 2001.

2.1　Rehabilitation Application

The rehabilitation exercises target four major hand impairments: finger range of motion, finger speed of motion, degree of independence of (finger fractionation), and finger strength. Each corresponds to a specific VR simulation [8,9]. The first three exercises use the CyberGlove, while the strength exercise uses the RMII haptic glove.

All the rehab exercises ask the patient to close one or more fingers, starting from a fully open position. The beginning of the range, speed and fractionation exercises has a transparent hand overlapped on the virtual hand controlled by the patient. The finger angles of the transparent hand are set to the desired degree of extension, and patients are required to match the transparent hand before starting each exercise. The beginning of the strength exercise uses the RMII glove to apply forces to help the patient open the hand before switching to the target of the exercise.

The range of motion exercise is executed in two phases: one for the thumb and one for the fingers. The exercise provides performance feedback for each finger. As shown in Figure 2(a) each finger motion "cleans up" a portion of the image. The higher the range of motion, the larger the portion of the image is revealed.

The speed of motion exercise consists of a virtual butterfly flying in circles just above the virtual hand controlled by the patient (see Figure 2-b). The goal is to scare the butterfly away by closing the hand fast enough. If the speed performance does not exceed the target the butterfly continues flying above the hand. Since this design has no "start" signal, the patient is free to initiate the motion at any time (unlike an earlier version of this exercise that combined reaction time and speed of motion [8,9]).

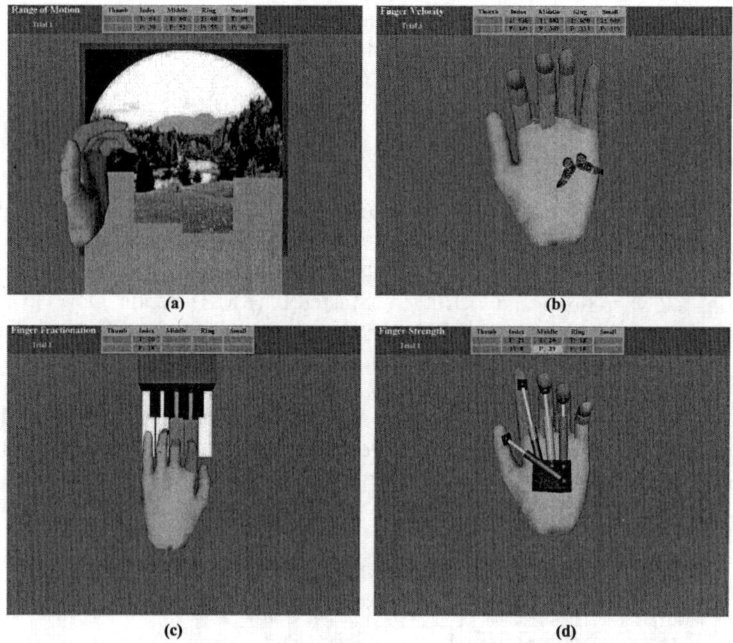

Figure 2 – VR exercises: (a) Range of motion exercise; (b) Finger velocity exercise; (c) Finger fractionation exercise; (d) Finger strength exercise. © Rutgers University 2001.

The finger fractionation exercise has the patient play a virtual piano with one finger (Figure 2(c)). The patient has to flex the active finger and press the corresponding key while the other fingers (passive) must be kept extended. The performance is measured as the difference between the active finger flexion and the maximum finger flexion of the passive fingers.

The finger strength exercise (Figure 2(d)) measures the piston displacement that the patient can achieve against a constant force applied to the fingers. The VR simulation consists of a virtual model of the RMII glove attached to a patient-controlled virtual hand. The virtual pistons fill with color proportional to the displacement of the real ones.

The top portion of the screen provides performance feedback in a numerical format. This feature was added based on feedback from our earlier trials. Patients felt that numerical scores were a better indication of their progress. The exercises also contain a feedback bar displaying the name of the exercise, the trial number and the targets and performances for each of the fingers involved in the current exercise. The displayed performance (a letter P followed by a number) changes in real-time as the patient's hand moves.

2.2   Target Calculation

The design of the rehabilitation procedure relies on a moving target approach. The exercises are executed in blocks, each block containing a number of trials. Each block is assigned an average target. The individual targets for each trial are chosen from a normal distribution around the assigned average target. The average block target is computed by first averaging the performances of the patient in the previous block. Then, the algorithm computes a new target by adding or subtracting a fraction to/from the current target. Thus, as the patient improves their performance they are pushed by higher target level to perform even better. The fraction change is positive if the current target was achieved and negative if it was not. The amount of target change is computed so that the day's trial success rate is kept close to 80%. This success rate was chosen to keep patients motivated.

2.3   Data Storage and Access

The current version of our system stores the recorded data and reads the rehabilitation session configuration from an Oracle database. When the system uses directly the central database, the data storage site is updated in real-time with records from the rehabilitation site. If the network connection is unreliable (or slow), then the necessary data is replicated in a local database, as illustrated in Figure 1. The central database is then synchronized with the local database with a customizable frequency.

To provide the therapist with the possibility of monitoring the patient's activity we developed a client-server architecture that brings the data from the rehabilitation site to the data storage site in real-time. The server stores only the last record data. Due to the small size of the data packets and the lack of atomic transactions, the communication works even over a slow connection.

Data access is provided through a web portal implemented as a Java applet that accesses the data through Java servlets running on the data storage site. The therapist can access stored data, or monitor active patients, through the use of a web browser. The portal provides a tree structure for intuitive browsing of the data displayed in graphs such as performance histories (day, session, trial), linear regressions, or low-level sensor readings. The graphs are generated in PDF format to allow easy printing.

The real-time monitoring of the patient activity is done through a Java3D applet displaying a simplified virtual hand model. The virtual hand's finger angles are updated with the data retrieved from the monitoring server at the data storage site. The therapist can easily open multiple browser windows for different patients.

3   Patient Trials

The system described above has been tested on patients during a three-week pilot study in Summer 2001. Four post-stroke hemiplegic subjects, three male and one female, ages 58 to 72, participated in this study. These patients sustained a right hemisphere stroke (left hand affected) one to four years prior to the study.

One week prior to the study, all patients went through a baseline procedure to measure their performance for each of the four exercises. Subsequently the patients completed a one-week pilot to fine-tune the system followed by a three-week study. Each patient exercised daily (five days per week) for approximately two hours. A rehabilitation session consisted of four blocks of each exercise. A block contained ten trials except for the fractionation exercise, which contained 20 trials because it exercised individual fingers. After the first week, the number of exercise blocks in a day was increased to five. After the second week the number of strength blocks was increased to six. Two of the subjects participated in post-therapy retention tests at one week, two weeks and one month after the intervention.

To evaluate the transfer from our rehab exercises to real life functions, the subjects were asked to pick up and move objects of various sizes, shapes and weight. The patients' motions during these tasks were recorded using a CyberGlove and four electromagnetic trackers (Flock of Birds, Ascension Technology). In addition to computerized tests and exercises, the patients' performance was evaluated using clinical tests such as the Jebsen Test of Hand Function [10].

4   Results

Figure 3 shows the percentage change in the patients' performance on each of the four movement tasks over the three-week intervention. Three subjects had substantial improvement in range of motion for the thumb (50-140%), while their gains in finger range were more modest (20%). One patient had an 18% increase in thumb speed and three had between 10-15% speed increases for their fingers. All patients improved their finger fractionation substantially (40-118%). Only one subject showed substantial gain in finger strength, in part due to unexpected hardware problems during the trial. This subject had the lowest levels of isometric flexion force prior to the therapy.

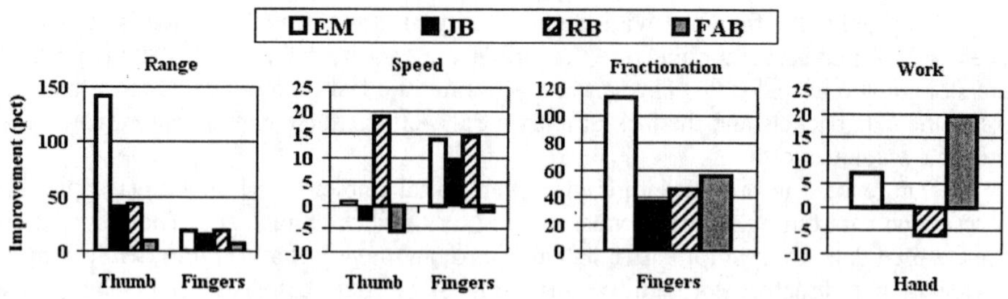

Figure 3 - Percentage increase between the first and the last day for each of the four VR exercises.
© Rutgers University 2001

Figure 4 shows the retention in the two patients that were measured, again for the four variables for which they trained. Their range and speed of motion either increased (patient RB) or decreased marginally (patient FAB) at one-month post intervention. Their finger strength increased significantly (about 80%) over the month following therapy, indicating they had reserve strength that was not challenged during the trials.

Figure 5 shows the results of the Jebsen evaluation, namely the total amount of time it took the patients to complete the seven component manual tasks. It can be seen that two of the patients (RB and EM) had a substantial reduction in the time from the measures taken prior to the intervention (23-28%, respectively). There was essentially no change in the Jebsen test for the other two patients (JB and FAB). Most of the gains occurred early in the intervention, with negative gains in the second half of the trials.

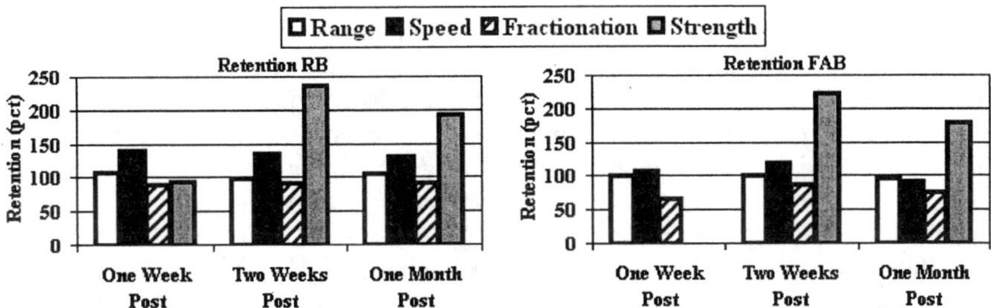

Figure 4 - Percentage of retention. © Rutgers University 2001.

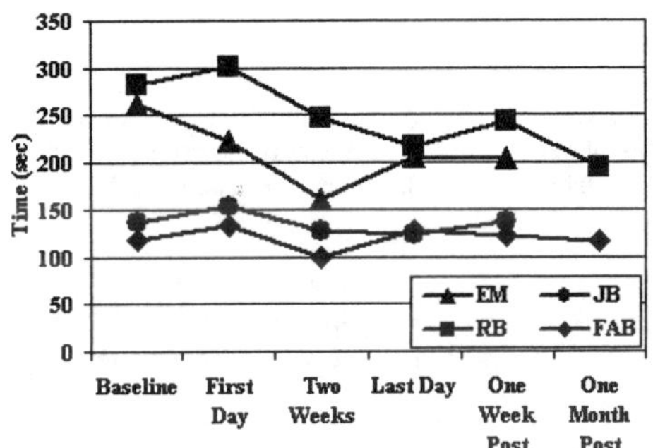

Figure 5 - Jebsen test results on the affected hand (sum of completion times for seven manual tasks).
© Rutgers University 2001.

The transfer-of-training results for a reach-to-grasp task are shown in Figure 6. There was no training of this particular task during the trials. However, results indicate improvements in impairments appeared to transfer to this functional activity, as measured by the reduction in task movement time. Three of the patients had improvements of between 15% and 38% for a round object and between 9% and 40% for a square object. There was no change for subject RB for picking up a square object while the time to pick up a round object increased by about 11%.

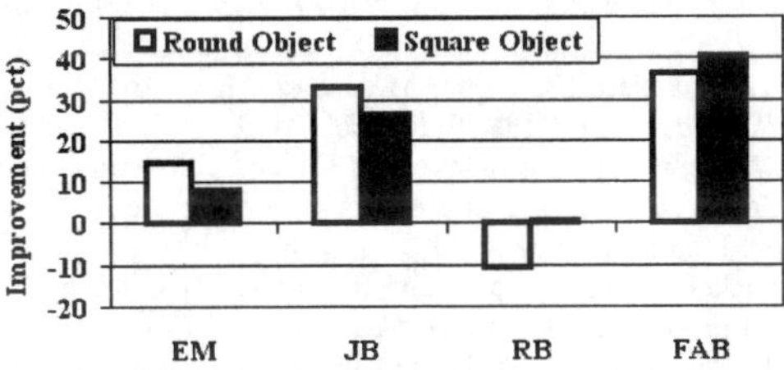

Figure 6 - Percentage improvement between the first and last day for the transfer-of-training test.
© Rutgers University 2001.

5　Conclusions

The study described here was performed to determine whether VR *alone* could be used as a therapeutic intervention modality to improve the hand of chronic post-stroke patients. A CyberGlove was used to train finger range, speed and fractionation. A prototype RMII-ND glove was used to train finger strength. A library of VR simulations was created, using

WorldToolKit for graphics and an adaptive targeting algorithm developed for setting performance levels. Oracle databases were used to transparently store data locally and remotely, and to allow remote physicians/therapists to follow patient progress. Results of a three-week pilot on four patients showed various degrees of improvement in hand impairment following this unconventional therapeutic intervention. There was good retention in gains and a positive subjective evaluation of the system by the patients and therapist that participated. The patients with a higher degree of impairment showed gains in manual ability as measured by a reduction in the cumulative time (of 23-28%) to perform the seven subtasks of the Jebsen Test of Hand function. Three of the four patients participating in the study showed transfer to function for a pickup task with a reduction in the completion time of up to 40%.

Acknowledgment

The research reported here was supported by an R&D Excellence Grant from the New Jersey Commission on Science and Technology. The authors wish to thank Karin Peterson and Anu Arora from the University of Medicine and Dentistry of New Jersey for their assistance in running the VR training trials.

References

[1] The American Stroke Association. http://www.strokeassociation.org/, 2001.

[2] J.E. Deutsch, J. Latonio, G. Burdea, and R. Boian. Post-Stroke rehabilitation wit the Rutgers Ankle System – A Case Study. In *Presence*, volume 10, pp. 416-430. MIT Press, August 2001.

[3] Foreman, N., P. Wilson, and D. Stanton, VR and Spatial Awareness in Disabled Children. *Communications of the ACM*, 1997. 40(8): pp. 76-77.

[4] M. Girone, G. Burdea, M. Bouzit, and V.G. Popescu. "A Stewart Platform-Based System for Ankle Telerehabilitation". *Autonomous Robots*, 10: pp. 203-212, 2001

[5] Gomez, D., G. Burdea, N. Langrana, "Integration of the Rutgers Master II in a Virtual Reality Simulation," *Proc. of IEEE VRAIS'95 Conference*, Research Triangle Park NC, pp. 198-202, March 1995

[6] Holden, M., et al., Virtual Environment Training Improves Motor Performance in Two Patients with Stroke: Case Report. *Neurology Report*, 1999. 23(2): pp. 57-67

[7] Inma, D., et al., Teaching Orthopedically Impaired Children to Drive Motorized Wheelchairs in Virtual Reality, in Center on Disabilities Virtual Reality Conference. 1994.

[8] D. Jack, et al.. A Virtual Reality-Based Exercise Program For Stroke Rehabilitation. In *Proceedings of ACM SIGCAPH ASSETS 2000*, Arlington Virginia, pp. 56-63, November 13-15, 2000.

[9] Jack D., R. Boian, A. Merians, M. Tremaine, G. Burdea, S. Adamovich, M. Recce, and H. Poizner, "Virtual Reality-Enhanced Stroke Rehabilitation," *IEEE Trans. Neurl Sys. Rehab. Eng.*, Vol. 9(3), pp. 308-318, 2001.

[10] Jebsen RH, Taylor N, Trieschman RB, Trotter MJ, Howard LA. An Objective and Standardized Test of Hand Function. *Arch Phys Med Rehabil* 1969; 50:pp. 311-19

[11] Jenkins, W. and M. Merzenich, Reorganization of Neocortical Representations After Brain Injury: A Neurophysiological Model of the Bases of Recovery From Stroke., in *Progress in Brain*, F. Seil, E. Herbert, and B. Carlson, Editors. 1987, Elsevier.

[12] Kopp, Kunkel, Muehlnickel, Villinger, Taub, and Flor Plasticity in the motor system related to therapy-induced improvement of movement after stroke. *Neuroreport*. 10(4) pp. 807-10, 1999 Mar 17

[13] Liepert, J., Bauder, Hl, Miltner, W., Taub, E., and Weiller, C. Treatment-induced cortical reorganization after stroke in humans. *Stroke*, 2000, 31:1210-1216

[14] Nudo, R.J., Neural Substrates for the Effects of Rehabilitative Training on Motor Recovery After Ischemic Infarction. *Science*, 1996. 272: pp. 1791-1794.

[15] V.G. Popescu, G. Burdea, M. Bouzit, M. Girone, and V. Hentz. A Virtual Reality-Based Telerehabilitation System with Force Feedback. *IEEE Trans. Inf. Tech. Biomed.*, 4(1):pp. 1-8, 2000

[16] V.G. Popescu. Design and Performance Analysis of a Virtual Reality-Based Telerehabilitation System. PhD thesis, Rutgers University, January 2001

[17] Taub, E., et al., Technique to Improve Chronic Motor Deficit After Stroke. *Arch Phys Med Rehab*, 1993. 74: pp. 347-354.

[18] Wolf, S., et al., Forced use of Hemiplegic Upper Extremities to Reverse the Effect of Learned Non-use Among Chronic Stroke and Head Injured Patients. *Experimental Neurology*. 1989. 104: pp. 125-132.

Computer-Controlled Motorized Endoscopic Grasper for *In Vivo* Measurement of Soft Tissue Biomechanical Characteristics

Jeffrey D. Brown[a]; Jacob Rosen Ph.D.[b]; Manuel Moreyra MSME[c];
Mika Sinanan M.D., Ph.D.[d]; Blake Hannaford Ph.D.[b]

[a] *Department of Bioengineering, University of Washington,*
email: jdbrown@u.washington.edu
[b] *Department of Electrical Engineering, University of Washington*
[c] *Haptic Technologies, Inc., Seattle, WA*
[d] *Department of Surgery, University of Washington*

ABSTRACT

Accurate biomechanical characteristics of tissues are essential for developing realistic virtual reality surgical simulators utilizing haptic devices. Surgical simulation technology has progressed rapidly but without a large database of soft tissue mechanical properties with which to incorporate. The device described here is a computer-controlled, motorized endoscopic grasper capable of applying surgically relevant levels of force to tissue *in vivo* and measuring the tissue's force-deformation properties.

1. Introduction

Accurate biomechanical characteristics of tissues are essential for developing realistic virtual reality surgical simulators utilizing haptic devices. Surgical simulation technology has progressed rapidly but without a large database of soft tissue mechanical properties with which to incorporate. In addition, the majority of the research done on measuring mechanical properties of abdominal soft tissues has been performed *in vitro* on animals and cadavers. As simulation technologies continue to be capable of modelling more complex behavior, an (*in vivo*) tissue property database needs to be developed to fill this gap.

2. Background

The biomechanics of soft tissues that are load-bearing during physiological activities have been well studied (muscles, tendons, intervertebral discs, cartilage, blood vessels). Most of that work, however, has been done *in vitro* and/or on animal specimens. Much less testing has been done on the abdominal organs relevant to laparoscopic surgery.

A seminal work presenting tests of a wide variety of organs and tissues was done by Yamada.[1] Mechanical properties of a large number of tissues were compiled by Yamada. Some of the surgically relevant soft tissues were lung, esophagus, stomach, small and large intestines, liver, and gallbladder. Much of the work was done on animals *in vitro*, and a few were done on human cadavers. Viscoelastic behavior was not described. Other work has been done in testing and modelling the kidney.[2,3] Melvin *et al.* conducted *in vivo* experiments on rhesus monkey kidney and liver by placing the whole live organ onto a load cell and performing uniaxial unconfined compressions.[2] Farshad *et al.* tested pig kidney *in vitro* under various (multi-axial) loading conditions.[3] Both of those studies were done with the application of high impact injury modelling in mind, not the slow loads and displacements typically performed in surgery. Perhaps more directly relevant to surgery, some recent work was done by Carter *et al.*, in which they measured *in vitro* the force required to puncture pig liver and spleen with a scalpel and the displacement of the tissue at puncture.[4]

It has only recently become a major thrust of researchers to obtain *in vivo* measurements of tissue mechanical properties. Brouwer *et al.* developed several instruments for measuring porcine tissue response to extension and indentation *in vivo*.[5] Ottensmeyer *et al.* have been developing a set of instruments for obtaining *in vivo* multi-axial tissue response to quasi-static and dynamic loading.[6] Their group has designed a 1-D indenter for applying small, time-varying displacements, and a 3-D indenter for applying larger but slower displacements. Our previous instrument was capable of applying compressive force via voice-coil actuators.[7,8] This instrument was used to test several porcine abdominal tissues *in vivo* to measure their force-deformation response, similar to the work done by Brouwer *et al.*[5]

3. Methods & Tools

To study and characterize the abdominal tissues relevant to laparoscopic surgery, a few objectives must be met in the design of the testing device. First, most soft tissue structures within the body demonstrate aspects of nonlinear, viscoelastic behavior, so the ability to induce time-varying loads is critical in characterizing the tissue's true mechanical behavior. Second, the device should be capable of applying levels of force and deformation consistent with those seen in laparoscopic procedures. The device should also be hand-held, lightweight, have interchangeable tool tips, and be capable of entering the body through an endoscopic port.

To achieve these goals, we have adapted our previous design for the force-reflecting endoscopic grasper (FREG) [7,8] to a motorized endoscopic grasper (MEG) that uses a brushed DC motor instead of a voice-coil actuator. The motor is attached to a capstan that drives a cable and partial pulley. The pulley is attached to a ball joint that converts the rotational motion of the motor and pulley to a linear translation. (The linear movement occurs in a standard laparoscopic grasper shaft, which then drives the opening and closing of the jaws.) The motor is capable of producing 29 mNm of continuous torque, but it is coupled with a 19:1 planetary gearhead and partial pulley that increase the torque to 3.98 Nm. This torque is equivalent to 52 N of grasping force applied by a surgeon on an endoscopic grasper's finger loops, close to the maximum value applied by surgeons in our previous work.[9] Standard laparoscopic instruments can be attached to the base plate mount and inserted into the ball joint, allowing tool type to be changed with relative ease. Two strain gage force sensors are embedded in the partial pulley to provide accurate grasping force measurement for robust and precise control. A digital encoder, attached to the motor, measures position. Computer control is provided real-time via a PC using a PD (position) controller implemented in Simulink and dSPACE user interface and hardware. The MEG is a hand-held device that weighs about 0.7 kg (including grasper and protective covers) and can be inserted into the body through regular endoscopic ports to perform computer-controlled dynamic and static uniaxial compressive displacements of soft tissues *in vivo*. Compressive loadings can be static or dynamic, allowing for ramp-and-hold, creep, and stress relaxation tests.

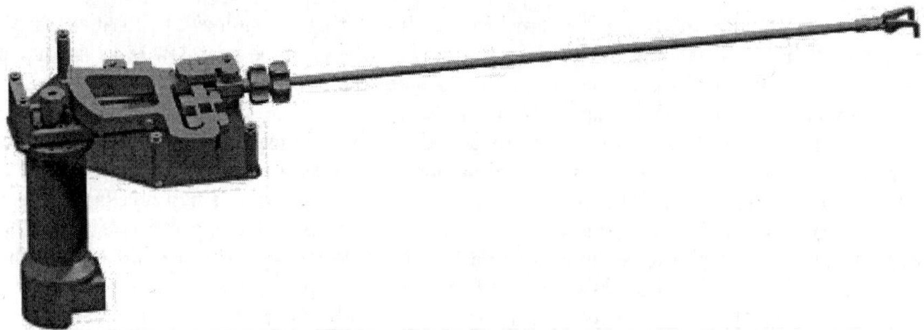

Figure 1. Motorized Endopscopic Grasper (MEG) (top cover not shown).

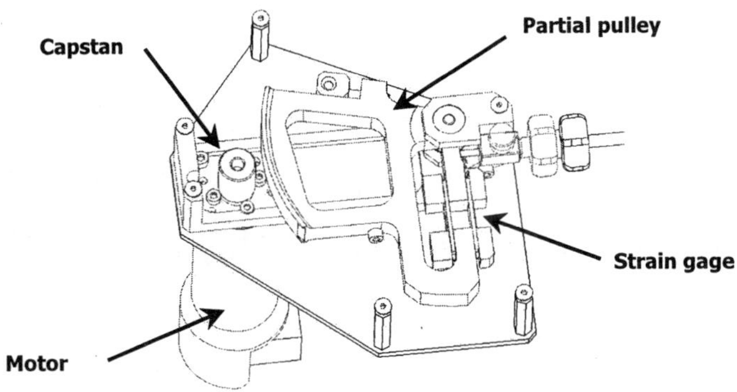

Figure 2. Close-up of the MEG drive system components.

4. Conclusion

The device reported here is a newly developed tool for taking measurements of soft tissues *in vivo* using a minimally invasive or open setup. The new device can control and measure grasping force and deformation of tissues, accept a wide variety of tool types, and can apply physiological and surgically realistic levels of force and deformation to the tissues. The MEG will help provide realistic data for surgical simulation and corroborate the results of other researchers.

The MEG is currently being used on latex rubber samples (tissue physical models) and porcine soft tissues. These tissues will have their stress-strain properties characterized under various loading types, including static and dynamic. Time-dependent properties such as creep and stress relaxation will also be studied. Other work will compare *in vivo* MEG data with *in vitro* MEG and universal testing machine data to observe changes in tissue mechanical properties postmortem. Determination of tissue response (damage) to various loadings and tool tips will also likely be performed.

5. References

[1]　H. Yamada, *Strength of Biological Materials*, ed: F.G. Evans, Robert E. Krieger Publishing Co., Inc.: Huntington, N.Y., 1973.

[2]　J.W. Melvin, R.L. Stalnaker, V.L. Roberts, M.L. Trollope, "Impact injury mechanisms in abdominal organs," *Proceedings of the 17th Stapp Car Crash Conference*: 115-126, 1973.

[3]　M. Farshad, M. Barbezat, P. Flueler, F. Schmidlin, P. Graber, P. Niedere, "Material characterization of the pig kidney in relation with the biomechanical analysis of renal trauma." *J Biomechanics*, 32(4): 417-25, 1999.

[4]　F.J. Carter, T.G. Frank, P.J. Davies, A. Cuschieri, "Puncture forces of solid organ surfaces," *Surg. Endosc.*, 14(9): 783-6, 2000.

[5]　I. Brouwer, J. Ustin, L. Bentley, A. Sherman, N. Dhruv, F. Tendick, "Measuring in vivo animal soft tissue properties for haptic modeling in surgical simulation," Proceedings, MMVR-2001:69-74, 2001.

[6]　M.P. Ottensmeyer, J.K. Salisbury, "In vivo mechanical tissue property measurement for improved simulations," Proceedings of the SPIE, 4037: 286-93, 2000.

[7]　B. Hannaford, J. Trujillo, M. Sinanan, M. Moreyra, J. Rosen, J. Brown, R. Lueschke, M. MacFarlane, "Computerized Endoscopic Surgical Grasper," Proceedings, MMVR-98, 1998.

[8]　J. Rosen, B. Hannaford, M. MacFarlane, M. Sinanan, "Force Controlled and Teleoperated Endoscopic Grasper for Minimally Invasive Surgery - Experimental Performance Evaluation," *IEEE Transactions on Biomedical Engineering*, 46(10): 1212-1221, 1999.

[9]　J. Rosen, M. Solazzo, B. Hannaford, M. Sinanan, "Objective Laparoscopic Skills Assessments of Surgical Residents Using Hidden Markov Models Based on Haptic Information and Tool/Tissue Interactions," Proceedings, MMVR-2001:417-23, 2001.

Medicine Meets Virtual Reality 02/10
J.D. Westwood et al. (Eds.)
IOS Press, 2002

Generalized Interactions Using Virtual Tools within the *Spring* Framework: *Probing, Piercing, Cauterizing and Ablating*

Cynthia D. Bruyns[1,2] Kevin Montgomery[2]
[1]*Center for Bioinformatics, NASA Ames Research Center, Moffett Field, CA 94035*
[2]*National Biocomputation Center, Stanford University, Stanford, CA 94305*

Abstract

We present schemes for real-time generalized interactions such as probing, piercing, cauterizing and ablating virtual tissues. These methods have been implemented in a robust, real-time (haptic rate) surgical simulation environment allowing us to model procedures including animal dissection, microsurgery, hysteroscopy, and cleft lip repair.

1. Introduction

When trying to create a simulation environment, whether for surgical training, clothing design or manufacturing, it inevitably becomes necessary to model object to object interactions [1-3]. We have developed generalized methods for allowing a user to interact with patient-specific models using detailed virtual tools in a real-time virtual environment. These methods strive to provide a general method for interactions that can then be realized by many different virtual instruments.

2. Methods

When implementing a simulation system, many tasks are required to be performed at each timestep. Within our simulator, the basic simulation engine loop is deformable object solution, collision detection, collision response, and user interface information. For a detailed description of the simulation environment, the reader is directed to [4] and for a description tool behavior [5]. The goal of this paper is to describe the implementation of several forms of interactions common to surgical simulations. These interactions are implemented within each object's collision response routine. The result of each collision is determined by the object's interaction type. This paper briefly describes four such interactions: probing, piercing, cauterizing, and ablating. In each case, the collision resolution algorithm processes each of the elements in a collision pair list, performs their interaction function, and computes the resulting haptic force of that interaction upon the virtual tool performing the manipulation. Once this process is completed, the interaction forces are combined to calculate the overall force vector that should be realized upon the virtual instrument. This resultant interaction force is then rendered upon a haptic interface device.

Collision Detection

Each object in the virtual environment is partitioned into a bounding sphere hierarchy [6]. Currently we are storing intersection information as collision pairs with pointers to the objects that were in collision, the point at which collision occurred, and the primitives that were intersected (node, edge, or triangle). This list of collision pairs is then passed to the collision response method of the tool and provides the necessary information to perform a probing, piercing, ablating or cauterizing interaction.

Collision Response

Probing

When a virtual probing tool (such as a hand, pick, dilator, etc) has penetrated a deformable object, the deformable surface displaces itself until force within the springs becomes larger than the yield force of the deformable material being simulated [7]. To handle this displacement we compute the intersection of the object and the tool then, based on the direction the tool followed, we can determine which direction the deformable object should be moved. We resolve the collision in real-time by displacing nodes of the deformable object until the objects are no longer in collision.

Currently we are storing pairs of intersecting primitives, which determine the *boundary* of the subset of the surface that is interpenetrating, but not all of the faces that are in that subset. In order to resolve the interpenetration as fast as possible, it may be advantageous to determine all of the faces that are interpenetrating [8] and start collision response on the face that is farthest into the other object. However, in order to avoid additional computation, we force the faces of the deformable object to walk down the contour of the other object in order to resolve the object-to-object interpenetration. Figure 1 demonstrates the real-time probing interaction being implemented by a virtual hand composed of 3,000 triangles and a piece of virtual tissue composed of 5,000 triangles.

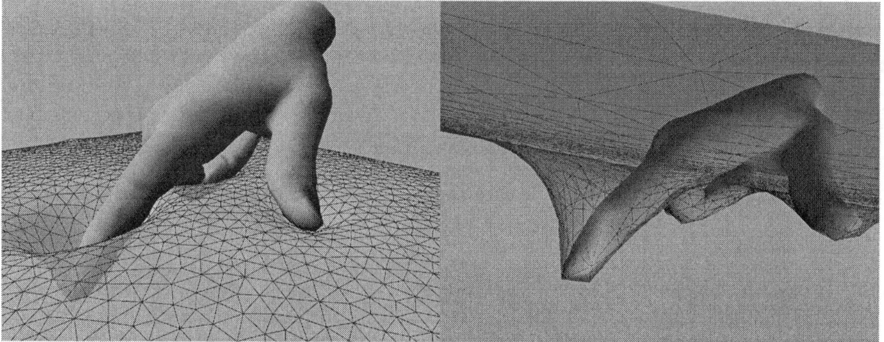

Figure 1. Pushing. [Left]: Top view. [Right]: Side view.

Piercing

For a piercing interaction (e.g., syringe, needle), the virtual instrument pierces through a surface, producing a local subdivision at the point of entry. The rest of the object merely has a probing interaction. In this way, the tip of the syringe is "sharp" and can pierce through tissue, while the rest of the syringe merely bumps the tissue upon interaction.

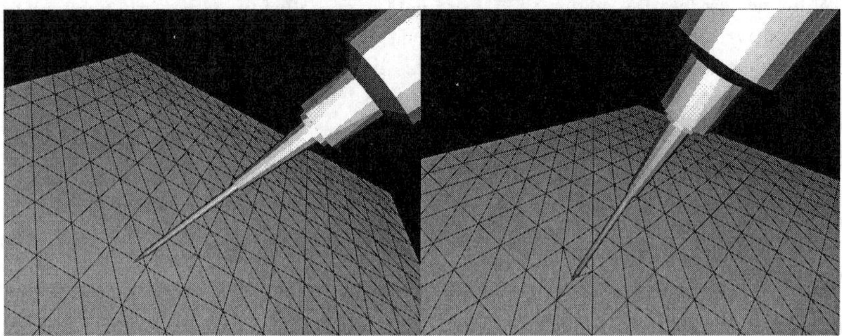

Figure 2. Piercing. [Left]: Before intersection. [Right]: After subdivision.

Ablation

An ablating instrument (roller ablator) when active and in contact with tissue, progressively yellows, browns, then blackens the area of contact. This interaction is performed by changing the color of the contacted faces and using blended textures to achieve the desired graphical result. Specifically, the underlying surface is originally set to completely white which, with an overlayed, blended texture, merely yields the original texture image. As the active cauterizing tool comes in contact with the surface, the triangles that are in collision with the "hot" part of the tool decrease their blue intensity (thereby leaving a more and more yellow color remaining). When the blue intensity is zero, then the red and green channels are also decreased, with the rate of decrease of the green channel being twice that of the red (thereby producing a brown color that fades toward black as both the red and green approach zero). By modifying the colors in this way, along with blended textures, the visual appearance of the texture is that of progressively yellowing, browning, and blackening as the tool remains in contact with the virtual tissue. Figure 3 demonstrates a roller ablator instrument composed of 200 triangles cauterizing a virtual tissue composed of 2000 triangles.

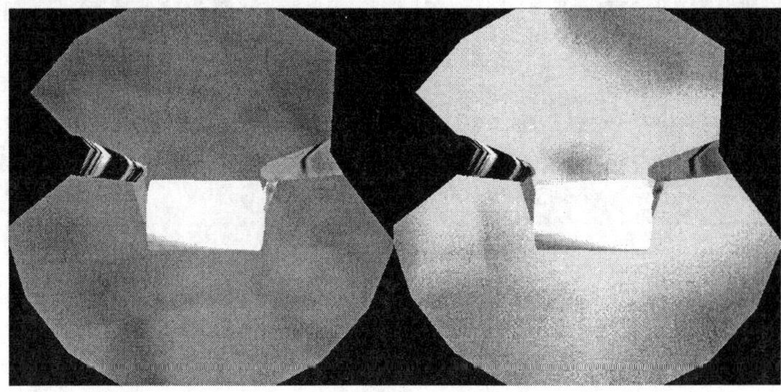

Figure 3. Cauterizing. [Left]: Before intersection. [Right]: Tissue is burned.

Cautery

When a virtual instrument (loop cautery) has been assigned the cauterizing interaction type, each object that it comes into contact with is eroded. Used in conjunction with an ablating interaction, this interaction is implemented by simply removing the triangles that are being intersected and ablating the boundary. Figure 4 demonstrates the use of an ablating tool composed of 200 triangles and a piece of virtual background tissue composed of 2000 triangles, with a polyp (foreground) of 881 faces.

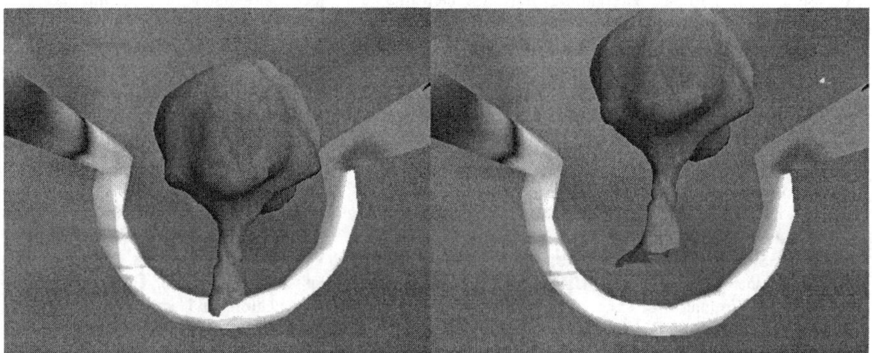

Figure 4. Cautery. [Left]: Searing through tissue. [Right]: Tissue disconnected after cautery.

A number of more abstract interactions are also implemented, such as selecting subparts of an object, coloring a subpart of an object, measuring distances and angles of an object, as well as texture manipulation.

3. Conclusions

We have demonstrated the implementation of several manipulations common to surgical simulation. These manipulations have been integrated into the *Spring* framework and are in use by several applications [9,10,11].

Acknowledgements

We wish to thank Richard Boyle and the Center for Bioinformatics at the NASA Ames Research Center for their support of this research. Special thanks to other staff members of the National Biocomputation Center, including Joel Brown, Steven Sorkin, Fredric Mazzella, Anil Menon, and Guillame Thonier. This work benefited greatly from discussions with a number of individuals, including LeRoy Heinrichs, Jean-Claude Latombe, and Michael Stephanides. This work was supported by grants from NASA (NCC2-1010), NIH (NLM-3506, HD38223), NSF (IIS-9907060), and a generous donation from Sun Microsystems.

References

[1]   H. Delingette. Towards realistic soft tissue modeling in medical simulation. In *Proceedings of the IEEE: Special Issue on Surgery Simulation*, pages 512–523, Apr. 1998.

[2]   C. Bosdogan, C. Ho, M.A. Srinivasan, S.D. Small, and S.L. Dawson. Force Interaction in Laparoscopic Simulation: Haptics Rendering of Soft Tissues. *Proc. Medicine Meets Virtual reality (MMVR'98)*, Jan. 1998, pp. 28-31.

[3]   S. Cotin, H. Delingette, and N. Ayache. A Hybrid Elastic Model Allowing Real-Time Cutting, Deformation and Force Feedback for Surgery Training and Simulation. *The Visual Computer*, 16(8):437-452, 2000.

[4]   Montgomery, K., Bruyns, C., Brown, J., Sorkin, S., Mazzella, F., Thonier, G., Tellier, A., Lerman, B., Menon, A.: Spring: A General Framework for Collaborative, Real-time Surgical Simulation, In: Westwood, J., et. al. (eds.): Medicine Meets Virtual Reality, IOS Press, Amsterdam, (2002).

[5]   Bruyns, C., Senger, S., Wildermuth, S., Montgomery, K., Boyle, R.: Real-time Interactions Using Virtual Tools. In: Niessen, W.J., et .al. (eds.) MICCAI 2001, LNCS 2208, Springer, Berlin Heidelberg, (2001) pp. 1349-1351.

[6]   Sorkin, S. Distance Computing Between Deformable Objects. Honors Thesis, Computer Science Department, Stanford University, June 2000.

[7]   Terzpoulos, D., Fleischer, K.: Modeling inelastic deformation: Viscoelasticity, plasticity, fracture. Computer Graphics, 22, (1998) 269-278.

[8]   Sundaraj, K., Laugier, C.: Fast Contact Localization of Moving Deformable Polyhedras. IEEE Conf. On Automation, Robotics, Control and Vision (ICARCV). Dec 5-8, 2000.

[9]   Bruyns, C., Montgomery, K., Wildermuth, S.,: A Virtual Environment for Simulated Rat Dissection. In: Westwood, J., et. al. (eds.) Medicine Meets Virtual Reality, IOS Press, Amsterdam (2001) pp. 75-81.

[10]   Wildermuth, S., Bruyns, C., Montgomery, K., Marincek, B., Virtual Colon Polyp Extraction (Simulation and Preoperative Planning), In: Niessen, W.J., et .al. (eds.) MICCAI 2001, LNCS 2208, Springer, Berlin Heidelberg, (2001) pp. 1347-1348.

[11]   Montgomery, K.; Heinrichs, L., Bruyns, C., Wildermuth, S., Hasser, C., Ozenne, S., Bailey, D.,: Surgical Simulator for Operative Hysteroscopy and Endometrial Ablation, In: Lemke, H., et. al. (eds.) Computer-Aided Radiology and Surgery, Elsevier, Amsterdam (2001) pp. 79-84.

Medicine Meets Virtual Reality 02/10
J.D. Westwood et al. (Eds.)
IOS Press, 2002

Generalized Interactions Using Virtual Tools within the *Spring* Framework: *Cutting*

Cynthia D. Bruyns[1,2] **Kevin Montgomery**[1]

[1]Center for Bioinformatics, NASA Ames Research Center, Moffett Field, CA 94035,
[2]National Biocomputation Center, Stanford University, Stanford, CA 94305

Abstract

We present schemes for real-time generalized mesh cutting. Starting with the a basic example, we describe the details of implementing cutting on single and multiple surface objects as well as hybrid and volumetric meshes using virtual tools with single and multiple cutting surfaces. These methods have been implemented in a robust surgical simulation environment allowing us to model procedures ranging from animal dissection to cleft lip correction.

1. Introduction

Cutting is a common manipulation encountered in simulations such as surgical training, clothing design and CAD/CAM manufacturing. A number of techniques have been developed to simulate cutting surface and volumetric meshes [1-17]. The number of intermediate steps required to recreate the cutting procedure often limits the level of realism offered by these methods, but intermediate steps have historically been necessitated by the inability to interactively update the underlying topological changes on large meshes.

The common element missing from these previous cutting tools is the ability to represent various forms of cutting using realistic tools on irregular meshes in real-time. The goal of this paper is to demonstrate how by using a very simple scheme, one can model widely differing behaviors of virtual tools within a real-time surgical simulation environment.

2. Methods

Starting with the most basic form of cutting, the following sections will describe the implementation of various cutting tools in a virtual environment. Since we start with a very general cutting scheme, each tool is an extension of the most basic cutting method requiring very little "special purpose" routines in order to model various forms of cutting. This method allows for any arbitrary cut to be made within an virtual object, and can simulate cutting surface, layered surface or tetrahedral objects using virtual scalpel, scissors, and loop cautery tools.

The basic engine for the cutting routine is collision detection, collision response, deformable object solution, and user interface information. This paper will describe the first two phases, the reader is directed to [18] for a detailed description of the last two phases.

Collision Detection

When modeling a cutting instrument one can either pre-compute the sharp regions of the mesh or choose which areas will be allowed to cut based on inspection of the model and included as information within the object's data file. This information can be a list of edges or faces [19].

Even if an object is visually composed of faces, for the sake of collision detection, we can create bounding volumes around other primitives to directly obtain the information important to cutting. If we choose to ignore intersections away from the sharp regions of a cutting instrument, we can enclose only the sharp primitives, reducing the number of intersection tests. If we choose more than one primitive to be sharp, the bounding hierarchy will enclose all of the sharp primitives. Since most tools will have fewer sharp primitives than the number of primitives in the overall geometry, this dramatically reduces the number of intersections tests that are necessary at each iteration.

When modeling cutting tools that are only composed of edges it is possible to pass over objects due to sampling latency. To solve this problem, we can choose to detect collisions not on the edge, but on the surface swept by the edge [20]. Furthermore, by enclosing the swept surfaces of the sharp edges by bounding volumes [21], we can still exploit the benefits of a binary search tree.

Currently we are storing intersection information as collision pairs with pointers to the objects that were in collision, the point at which collision occurred, and the primitives that were intersected. This list of collision pairs is then passed to the collision response scheme of the tool and provides us with the necessary information to perform a probing or a cutting manipulation.

Collision Response

The selection of sharp edges automatically defines a cutting direction, that is, the directions that the object can be moved that cause the tool to perform the specified action. For example, motion of a scalpel along the cut direction allows the cutting action to be implemented, while motion out of the allowed range causes the object to perform the probing action [22].

Cutting

The decision whether to cut a primitive is dependent on its state. These states are stored as information in the primitive class and used during re-meshing. For example, if the primitive has not been intersected before, then the intersection is recorded and the primitive is said to be in the *start* state. If at the next iteration the primitive is still in collision, then it is thought to be in the *update* state. In subsequent iterations, if the primitive is no longer in collision, then it is said to be in the *move* state and the primitive is cut based on the configuration of face and edge intersections that have been stored previously. The primitive state is determined by tracking which primitives the cutting edge was intersecting at the last iteration and checking that list against the list of primitives currently in collision. Figure 1 describes the cutting loop.

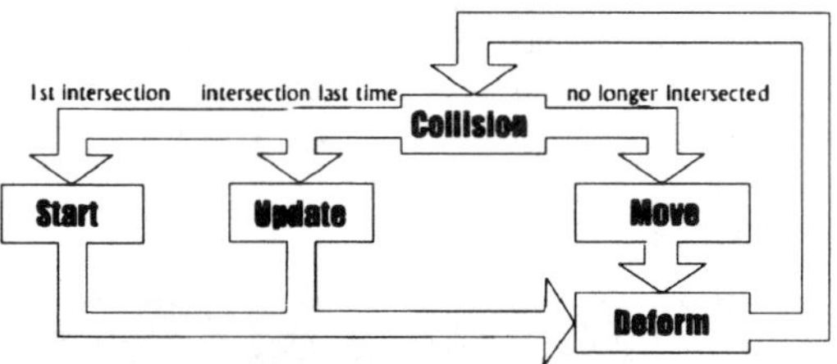

Figure 1. Flow diagram of the cutting loop.

As described in [18], each instrument has it's own dynamics and allowable behaviors. The following sections describe the results of implementing three kinds of instruments: a scalpel, a pair of scissors, and a cauterizing wire; on various mesh representations.

3. Results

On average, the simulation can detect collisions, compute the collision response, compute the deformation equations, update the bounding hierarchy and display the results on one processor of a Sun (Mountain View, CA) E3500 8x400 MHz UltraSparc workstation at 15 frames/second while the objects are intersecting. This frame rate increases to 70 frames/second if we display on one thread and run the simulation on another.

Scalpel Cutting

Single Surface

Figure 2 demonstrates the use of a single sharp edge to cut a single deformable object composed of 5,000 triangles.

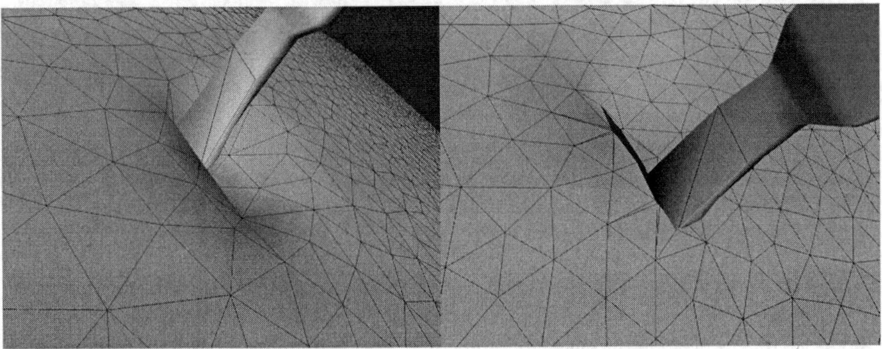

Figure 2. Edge states. [Left]: Surface deforms until the yield limit is reached. [Right]: The sharp edge cuts as the user moves the scalpel.

Multiple Surfaces

Because cutting is based on primitive states and not an object-wide state, it is possible to cut complex surfaces with folds, and objects that model a volume by extruding a surface thereby creating two surfaces connected by springs [23]. In these cases, the list of last primitives intersected might contain non-adjacent triangles and triangles with variable compliance and attributes. These triangles might also come from different objects. Figure 3 demonstrates the use of a single primitive to cut multiple surfaces. The deformable object is composed of 10,000 triangles.

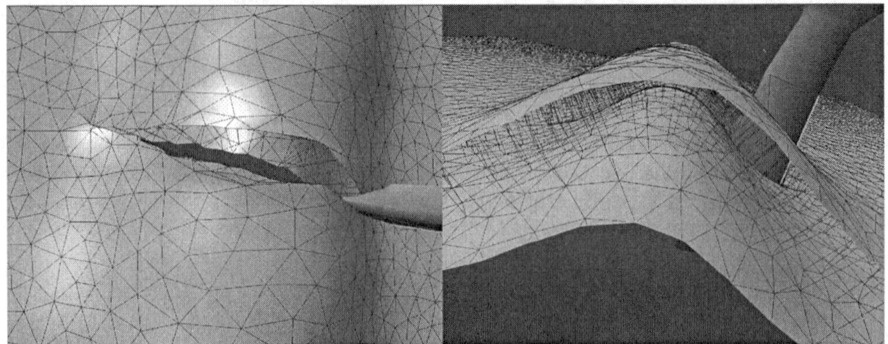

Figure 3. Cutting multiple surfaces. [Left]: Top View. [Right]: Side view.

Hybrid surface

In addition one might want to model separating a layer of a multiple surface object. In that case, one needs to use the hybrid method of collision detection enclosing the edges *and* faces of the surface with bounding spheres. In this case, the cutting scheme that is implemented is dependent on the type of primitive that is in collision. The triangular primitive is cut as before, however we choose to simply remove the intersected edges instead of subdividing it. This allows us to avoid creating edges with nodes that are not anchored and do not provide any structural or visual information to the model. Figure 4 shows a scalpel being used to cut a hybrid surface composed of 25,000 triangles.

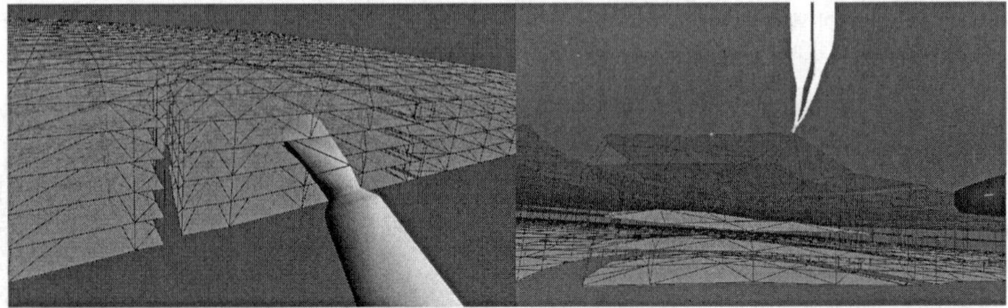

Figure 4. [Left]: Scalpel cutting away top layers of a multi-layered object. [Right]: Virtual forceps peeling back top layers.

Volume

When cutting an irregularly meshed volumetric object, tool motion is not as straightforward as moving across a surface. It is possible to be in several tetrahedra at once and when using a tool that is more complex than a single long edge [11], it is possible to partially intersect tetrahedra requiring additional re-tetrahedralizing cases. Another factor to consider when using tetrahedra is that since we only record face and edge intersections, internal motion and depth of cut information is lost *within the tetrahedral primitive*. If these motions inside a tetrahedral primitive are important to the given simulation scenario, one might want to use a progressive cutting option. Progressive cutting re-tetrahredralizes the original primitive as the user moves the tool within the original tetrahedra, instead of waiting to re-tetrahedralize once the tool has left the original tetrahedra. One must be aware however, that taking each of these internal motions literally will result in an increase in the number of tetrahedra unless additional mesh condensation schemes are employed. Figure 5 shows a scalpel cutting an irregular mesh of 300 tetrahedra.

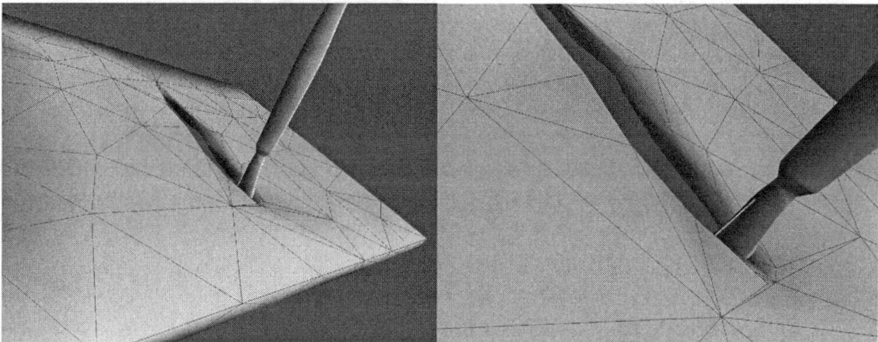

Figure 5. [Left]: A scalpel cutting a volumetric mesh. [Right]: Close-up on the cut path.

Scissors Cutting

When implementing scissors cutting, one must choose at least two edges as sharp. As mentioned previously, the allowable cutting direction is further restricted to permit cutting only when the cutting edges are moving towards each other. These two edges can either straddle the surface using the bottom edge to stabilize the surface while the top edge closes downward. Or if the edges are on the same side of the surface, the edges pinch the surface together until the two edges form a junction with the simulated tissue. Figure 6 shows a pair of virtual scissors cutting a deformable model consisting of 5,000 triangles. The figure also demonstrates how surface relaxes as the scissors are opened.

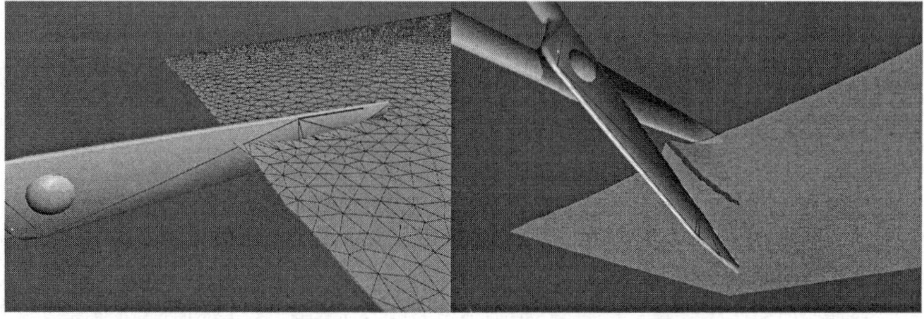

Figure 6. [Left]: Virtual scissors cutting. [Right]: Surface relaxing as scissors are opened.

Loop Cautery

When modeling a loop cautery tool, one needs to choose several edges as sharp. These edges have their own wire dynamics that must be modeled as well. Figure 7 shows a wire that has been assigned 20 cutting edges and is cutting a virtual polyp consisting of 5,000 triangles.

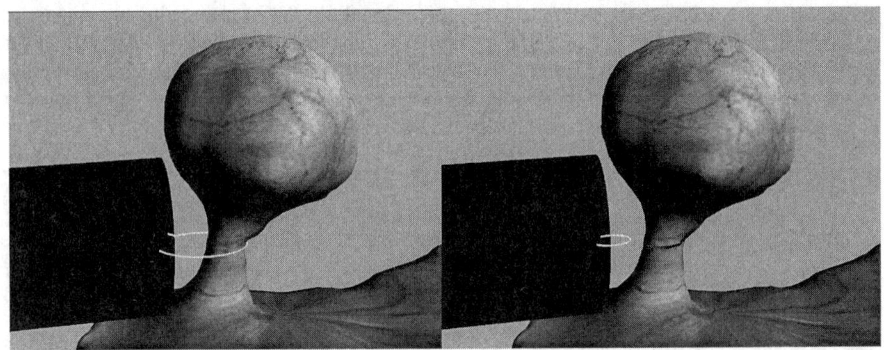

Figure 7. Loop cautery cutting. [Left]: Snaring a virtual polyp. [Right]: Resulting cut.

4. Conclusions

Creating cuts through very large meshes is extremely simple using the schemes presented in this paper. These schemes have been employed in a rat dissection simulation system [24], a virtual polypectomy simulator [25], and a virtual hysteroscopy simulation system [26].

Acknowledgements

We wish to thank Richard Boyle and the Center for Bioinformatics at the NASA Ames Research Center for their support of this research. Special thanks to the National Biocomputation Center and including Joel Brown, Steven Sorkin, Fredric Mazzella, Anil Menon, Jeremie Roux, Julien Durand, Bharat Beeedu, Guillame Thonier and Jean Claude Latombe. This work was supported by grants from NASA (NCC2-1010), NIH (NLM-3506, HD38223), NSF (IIS-9907060), and a generous donation from Sun Microsystems.

References

[1] Pieper, S., Rosen, J., Zeltzer, D.: Interactive Graphics for Plastic Surgery: A Task-level Analysis and Implementation. Symposium on Interactive 3D Graphics ACM Press, New York, (1992) pp.127–134.

[2] Song, G. and Reddy, N.: Tissue Cutting in Virtual Environments. In: Medicine Meets Virtual Reality. IOS Press, Amsterdam (1995) pp. 359-364.

[3] Keeve, E., Girod, S., and Girod, B.: Computer-Aided Craniofacial Surgery. Journal of the Int. Society for Computer Aided Surgery. 3 (1996) 6-10.

[4] Mazura, A., Seifert, S.: Virtual Cutting in Medical Data. In: Westwood, J., et. al. (eds.) Medicine Meets Virtual Reality. IOS Press, Amsterdam (1997) pp. 420-429.

[5] Wong, K. C., Siu, T. Y., and Heng, P.: Interactive Volume Cutting. Technical Report, Department of Computer Science and Engineering, Chinese University of Hong Kong (1998).

[6] Basdogan, C., Ho, C., and Srinivasan, M.A.: Simulation of Tissue Cutting and Bleeding for Laparoscopic Surgery Using Auxiliary Surfaces. In: Westwood, J., et. al. (eds.) Medicine Meets Virtual Reality. IOS Press, Amsterdam (1999) pp. 38-44.

[7] Bro-Nielsen, M., Helfrick, D., Glass, B., Zeng, X., Connacher, H:. VR Simulation of Abdominal Trauma Surgery. Westwood, J., et. al. (eds.) Medicine Meets Virtual Reality, IOS Press, Amsterdam (1999) pp.117-123.

[8] Voss, G., Hahn, J.K., Muller, W., Lineman, R.W.: Virtual Cutting of Anatomical Structures. In: Westwood, J., et. al. (eds.) Medicine Meets Virtual Reality, IOS Press, Amsterdam (1999) pp.381-383.

[9] Beisler, D., Gross, M.: Interactive Simulation of Surgical Cuts. Proceedings of Pacific Graphics, IEEE Computer Society Press, (2000) pp. 116-125.

[10] Neumann. P.: Near Real-Time Cutting. Siggraph 2000, Sketches and Applications. New Orleans, La. (2000).

[11] Ganovelli, F., Cignoni, P., Montani, C., Scopigno, R.: A Multiresolution Model for Soft Objects Supporting Interactive Cuts and Lacerations. Proceedings of the 21st European Conference on Computer Graphics. Blackwell, Cambridge (2000) pp. 271-282

[12] Mor, A., Kanade, T.: Modifying Soft Tissue Models: Progressive Cutting With Minimal New Element Creation. In: Niessen, W.J. et. al. (eds.) MICCAI 2000, LNCS 1935, Springer, Berlin Heidelberg, (2000) pp. 598-607.

[13] Schutyser, F., Van Cleyenbreugel, J., Nadjmi, N., Schoenaers, J., Suetens, P.: 3D Image-Based Planning for Unilateral Mandibular Distraction. In. Heinz. U., et. al. (eds.) Computer Assisted Radiology and Surgery, Elsevier, Amsterdam (2000) pp.899-904.

[14] Bruyns, C., Senger. S.: Interactive Cutting of 3D Surface Meshes. Computer and Graphics, 25 (2001) 635-642.

[15] Nienhuys, H-W., van der Stappen, A.F.: A Surgery Simulation Supporting Cuts and Finite Element Deformation, In: Niessen, W.J., et. al. (eds.) MICCAI 2001, LNCS 2208, Springer, Berlin Heidelberg, (2001) pp. 145-152.

[16] Meier, U., Monserrat, C., Parr, N-C., Garcia, F.J., Gil, J.A.: Real-Time Simulation of Minimally-Invasive Surgery with Cutting Based in Boundary Element Methods. In: Niessen, W.J., et. al. (eds.) MICCAI 2001, LNCS 2208, Springer, Berlin Heidelberg, (2001) pp. 1263-1264.

[17] Serby, D., Harders, M., Szekely, G.: A New Approach to Cutting into Finite Element Models. In: Niessen, W.J., et. al. (eds.) MICCAI 2001, LNCS 2208, Springer, Berlin Heidelberg, (2001) pp. 425-433.

[18] Montgomery, K., Bruyns, C., Brown, J., Sorkin, S., Mazzella, F., Thonier, G., Tellier, A., Lerman, B., Menon, A.: Spring: A General Framework for Collaborative, Real-time Surgical Simulation, In: Westwood, J., et. al. (eds.): Medicine Meets Virtual Reality, IOS Press, Amsterdam, (2002).

[19] Bruyns, C., Senger, S., Wildermuth, S., Montgomery, K., Boyle, R.: Real-time Interactions Using Virtual Tools. In: Niessen, W.J., et .al. (eds.) MICCAI 2001, LNCS 2208, Springer, Berlin Heidelberg, (2001) pp. 1349-1351.

[20] Boyse, J.W.: Interference Collision Detection Among Solids and Surfaces. Communications of the ACM 22 (1979) 3-9.

[21] Sorkin, S.: Distance Computing Between Deformable Objects. Honors Thesis, Computer Science Department, Stanford University, (2000).

[22] Bruyns, C., Montgomery, K.: Generalized Interactions Using Virtual Tools within the *Spring* Framework: *Probing, Piercing, Cauterizing and Ablating*, In: Westwood, J., et. al. (eds.): Medicine Meets Virtual Reality, IOS Press, Amsterdam, (2002).

[23] Mazzella, F.: Auto Acquisition of Elastic Properties for Surgical Simulation, http://biocomp.stanford.edu/papers/

[24] Bruyns, C., Montgomery, K., Wildermuth, S.,: A Virtual Environment for Simulated Rat Dissection. In: Westwood, J., et. al. (eds.) Medicine Meets Virtual Reality, IOS Press, Amsterdam (2001) pp. 75-81.

[25] Wildermuth, S., Bruyns, C., Montgomery, K., Marincek, B., Virtual Colon Polyp Extraction (Simulation and Preoperative Planning), In: Niessen, W.J., et .al. (eds.) MICCAI 2001, LNCS 2208, Springer, Berlin Heidelberg, (2001) pp. 1347-1348.

[26] Montgomery, K.; Heinrichs, L., Bruyns, C., Wildermuth, S., Hasser, C., Ozenne, S., Bailey, D.,: Surgical Simulator for Operative Hysteroscopy and Endometrial Ablation, In: Lemke, H., et. al. (eds.) Computer-Aided Radiology and Surgery, Elsevier, Amsterdam (2001) pp. 79-84.

Medicine Meets Virtual Reality 02/10
J.D. Westwood et al. (Eds.)
IOS Press, 2002

Volumetric Implant-Planning Based on Symmetry Considerations

Oliver Burgert[+], Tobias Salb[+], Tilo Gockel[+], Rüdiger Dillmann[+],
Stefan Hassfeld[*], Joachim Mühling[*]

[+] *Industrial Applications of Informatics and Microsystems (IAIM)*
Chair Prof. Dr.-Ing. R. Dillmann
Building 07.21, Department for Computer Science
Universität Karlsruhe (TH), 76128 Karlsruhe, Germany
Tel.: ++49 721 608 4261, Fax: ++49 721 608 8270
Email: burgert@ira.uka.de, WWW: http://wwwiaim.ira.uka.de/

[*] *Department of Oral and Maxillofacial Surgery*
University of Heidelberg, 69120 Heidelberg, Germany

Abstract. Symmetry Considerations can be used not only to plan the desired shape of reconstructured bone structures, but also to generate prototypes for soft tissue implants. The poster describes a system which allows to calculate a symmetry plane in the facial area automatically and computes proposals for implants or transplants. The system presented has been used to calculate soft tissue implants and a replacement for parts of the lower jaw.

1 Introduction

The goal of the system presented in this paper is to support facial surgeries which are aiming to transform an asymmetrical face to a symmetric one. There are two main techniques to achieve this goal: Producing an artificial implant or adding and removing of soft-tissue or bone at certain facial regions. In both cases planning steps are nowadays performed on 2D-datasets, real models and in many cases live at the surgical table by inserting an implant, visually inspecting the result and than milling it closer to the desired shape [1], [2].

These steps are time consuming and cost intensive so it would be desirable to virtually produce an implant, check it's functional behaviour and produce the real implant according to the simulation result [3].

2 Methods

The first task is to determine the area which should be reconstructed. In many cases, this can be done using symmetry considerations. The system described in this paper is based on volumetric CT or MRI. If the volumetric data is not yet segmented, it will be segmented for bone and soft tissue using a simple threshold-algorithm.

After this, the symmetry-plane must be determined. This can be done either by the surgeon or by an automatic calculation of the best mirroring plane [4]: The automatic approach uses a simulated annealing process for determining the best plane. This algorithm takes an initial plane, calculates the sum of certain tissue structures on each side and moves the plane corresponding to this result [5].

$$\Psi(b_1,b_2) = \sum_{i_1=0}^{z_{max}-1} \sum_{i_2=0}^{y_{max}-1} \sum_{i_3=0}^{x_{max}-1} \xi(i_1,i_2,i_3)$$

$$\xi(i_1,i_2,i_3) = \begin{cases} 1, \text{if } b_2(i_1,i_2,i_3) \in A(b_2) \wedge b_1(i_1,i_2,i_3) \notin A(b_1) \\ 0, \text{else} \end{cases}$$

Figure 1: Function used to evaluate the symmetry plane

After determining the symmetry plane, the deficit on one side of the face can be calculated. This can be done either on the whole volume dataset or just based on the segmented tissue structures, for example to produce soft tissue implants or bone implants. All of these steps are done on the volumetric data, not on reconstructed surfaces.

This calculated deficite is used to produce an initial implant. Therefore, thin and unneeded parts of the deficit have to be eleminated. This is done using the morphologic operators erosion and dilatation. Using this techniques, we get a proposal for an implant.

This initial implant can be inserted virtually to determine its functional correctness. For example, an implant should not cover the teeth of a patient. These errors in the automatically calculated implant have to be removed manually by the surgeon [6].

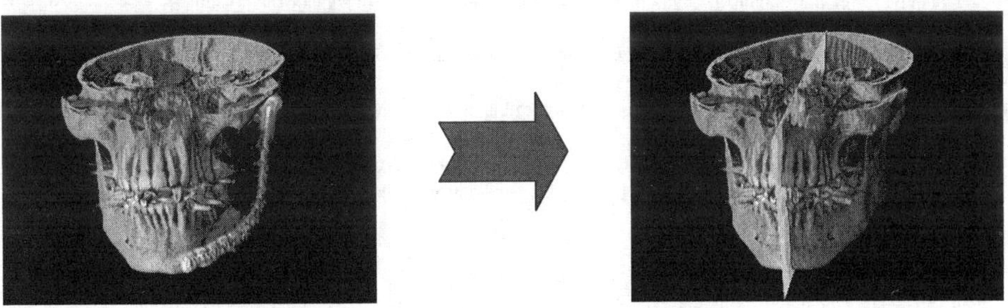

Figure 2: Symmetry plane applied to a patient with defect of the lower jaw

3 Results and Discussion

The automatic calculation of the symmetry plane gives aesthetically good results, if there are defects mainly on one side of the face and if there are enough correct facial structures recognizable. We are getting in trouble, if there are too much metal artifacts in the region of interest as they are destroying nearly every information contained in the CT data.

The initial implant is shaped well as a basis for the final implant. We have used the system to calculate soft tissue implants for a patient with various defects in the facial area (see figure 3) and to calculate a replacement for parts of the lower jaw (see figure 1).

The system presented in this paper helps producing patient specific implants if there are defects on one side of the face. It can be easily used to perform similar calculations in other parts of the body, like hip replacements or the shoulder joint.

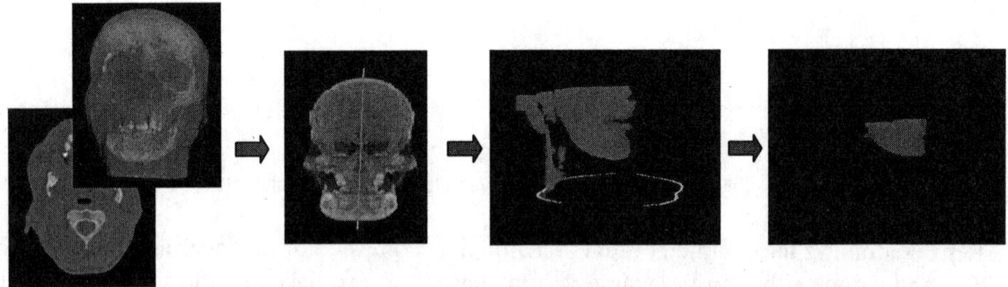

Figure 3: Original data set, calculated symmetry plane, deficite and resulting sot tissue implant

References

[1]   Richard A. Robb, Ph.D., Bruce Cameron: VRASP: Virtual Reality Assisted Surgery Program, http://www.mayo.edu/bir/repprints/VRASP2.html, Mai 2001.

[2]   Schramm, A. et al.: Non-invasive registration in computer assisted craniomaxillofacial surgery, Workshop "Rechner- und Sensorgestützte Chirurgie", Heidelberg, 19.-20. Juli 2001.

[3]   Burgert, O. et al.: A Haptic System for Simulation and Planning of Plastic Surgeries, ITEC 2000, The Hague, Netherlands.

[4]   Burgert, O. et. al: A System for Facial Reconstruction using Distraction and Symmetry Considerations, CARS 2001, Berlin, Juni 2001.

[5]   Sandberger, B.: Symmetriebetrachtungen am menschlichen Gesichtsschädel, Diplomarbeit, Universität Karlsruhe (TH), 2000.

[6]   Burgert, O., Salb, T., Dillmann, R.: Modellierung von Gewebestrukturen und Simulation risikominimierender chirurgischer Eingriffe, Workshop „Rechner- und Sensorgestützte Chirurgie", Heidelberg, Juli 2001.

Medicine Meets Virtual Reality 02/10
J.D. Westwood et al. (Eds.)
IOS Press, 2002

Clinical Test for Attention Enhancement System

Baek-Hwan Cho, Jeonghun Ku, Dongpyo Jang, Jaemin Lee, Myungjin Oh, Hun Kim, Janghan Lee[1],
Jaeseok Kim, Inyoung Kim, Sunill Kim

Department of Biomedical Engineering, College of Medicine, Hanyang University, Seoul, Korea
[1]Department of Psychology, Chung-Ang University, Seoul, Korea

Abstract. Attention Deficit Hyperactivity Disorder (ADHD) is a childhood syndrome characterized by short attention span, impulsiveness, and hyperactivity, which often leads to learning disabilities and various behavioral problems. The prevalence rates for ADHD varied from a low of 2.0% to a high of 6.3% in 1992 statistics, and it may be higher now. Using Virtual Environments and Neurofeedback, we have developed an Attention Enhancement System for treating ADHD. And we made a clinical test. Classroom-based virtual environments are constructed for intimacy and intensive attention enhancement. In this basic virtual environment, subjects performed some training sessions. There are two kinds of training sessions. One is Virtual Reality Cognitive Training (VRCT) and the other is Virtual Reality Neurofeedback Training (VRNT). In VRNT, we made a change in the virtual environment by Neurofeedback. Namely, if the Beta ratio is greater than the specified threshold level, the change as positive reinforce is created in the virtual environment. 50 subjects, aged 14 to 18, who had committed crimes and had been isolated in a reformatory took part in this study. They were randomly assigned to one of five 10-subject groups: a control Group, two placebo groups, and two experimental groups. The experimental groups and the placebo groups underwent 10 sessions over two weeks. The control group underwent no training session during the same period of time. While the experimental groups used HMD and Head Tracker in each session, the placebo groups used only a computer monitor. Consequently, only the experimental Groups could look around the virtual classroom. Besides that, Placebo Group 1 and Experimental Group 1 performed the same task(Neurofeedback Training), and Placebo Group 2 and Experimental Group 2 also performed the same task(Cognitive Training). All subjects Continuous Performance Task(CPT) before and after all training sessions. In the number of correct answers, omission errors and signal detection index (d'), the subjects' scores from CPT showed significant improvement (p<0.01) after all of the training sessions, while control group indicated no significant change. And experimental groups showed significant difference (p<0.01) with placebo groups. Lastly, the Virtual Reality Neurofeedback training group and the Virtual Reality Cognitive training group indicated not significant difference. Our System is supposed to enhance subjects' attention and lead their behavioral improvement. And also, we can conclude that virtual reality training (both Neurofeedback training and Cognitive training) has an advantage for attention enhancement compared with desk-top training.

1. Introduction

Increased computer usage in Medicine and Rehabilitation has changed the way health care is delivered. Virtual surgery, VR anatomy trainers, on-line patient databases, pre-surgery simulations, digital radiography, expert systems, and remote consultation are possible today using powerful computers [1]. And Virtual Reality Therapy (VRT) is an innovative paradigm of VR in Medicine [2]. VRT is based on exposure therapy, which provides phobic stimuli for the patient who cannot otherwise imagine well. VRT has an added advantage of greater control over graded exposure stimulus parameters as well as greater efficiency and economy in delivering the equivalent of in vivo exposure within the therapist's office [3,4,5].

Rizzo proposed the Virtual Classroom for the assessment and rehabilitation of attention deficits. This study shows that VR can be used in the assessment of attention as well as cognitive training and can offer better predictive information regarding performance in the real environment [6].

A lot of psychologists are still debating what attention is, and what it does for our mental processes. But they agree on the central premise that attention is an information management process in which intensiveness, sustainability, selectiveness and controllability combine and interact [7]. Although psychostimulant medication has been widely used for many years, current findings suggest that, as the sole treatment for attention deficit, it is an inadequate form of intervention. The main reasons are as follows. First, stimulants do not work for all children, and stimulant therapy is rarely sufficient to bring children into a normal range of academic and social function. Second, psychostimulant effects are limited to the period in which the drugs are physiologically active. Finally, without exception, studies that have followed children treated with psychostimulant medication for periods of up to 15 years have failed to provide any evidence that the drugs improve the long-term prognosis of children with Attention Deficit Hyperactivity Disorder (ADHD) [8].

Behavioral treatment is another approach that has been used to overcome the limits of psychostimulant medication in the treatment of ADHD. Since the mid-1970s, a number of studies have been conducted to evaluate the efficacy of behavior modification and therapy for children with ADHD. Behavioral interventions effect short-term amelioration of ADHD symptoms and these effects are comparable in some aspects to those obtained with low doses of stimulant medication. However, behavioral modification techniques are complicated and time consuming, and lack of consistency and follow-through can further reduce their effectiveness.

For the last few decades, Electroencephalography (EEG) has emerged as another potential diagnostic assessment and treatment technique for ADHD. Winkler, Dixon, and Parker revealed that there was more diffuse, rhythmically slow wave, specifically theta activity (4-8 Hz), and less faster wave beta sensorimotor rhythm (SMR) activity (12-20 Hz) in ADHD patients. They also found a greater incidence of abnormal transient discharges in the group exhibiting scholastic and behavioral problems [9]. EEG biofeedback treatment outcome studies for ADHD have reported promising results not only in significant reductions in hyperactive, inattentive, and disruptive behaviors, but also improvements in academic performance and IQ scores [10,11]. Recently, Othmer and Kaiser proposed the use of EEG Biofeedback, or Neurofeedback, with Virtual Reality [12]. According to this research, it is reasonable to project that implementation of more immersive and multi-modal feedback, leading ultimately to full virtual reality implementations, including realistic portrayals of physiological activity, should enhance patient commitment, comprehension, task engagement, and training efficiency.

In this study, we implemented an Attention Enhancement System using Virtual Reality and Neurofeedback and performed a clinical trial to demonstrate the efficacy of immersive VR in attention enhancement.

2. Attention Enhancement System

2.1. The Virtual Environment – A Classroom

Since children and adolescents spend a significant amount of time in their classroom, it is necessary that they are attentive to the lecturer and classroom tasks. Therefore, in this research, we developed a classroom-based virtual environment for intimacy and intensive attention enhancement.

The virtual environment consists of a small classroom with a whiteboard, a desk on which there are red, yellow and violet flags, a teacher avatar, a female friend avatar, a large window looking out onto a playground with a child exercising on a horizontal bar, a door, several pictures hanging on the walls, a sofa, a ceiling light, and a wooden floor. Subjects can see themselves, a self-avatar sitting at a desk. That is, subjects can feel as if they are in a real classroom. Subjects will perform some training sessions in this basic virtual environment.

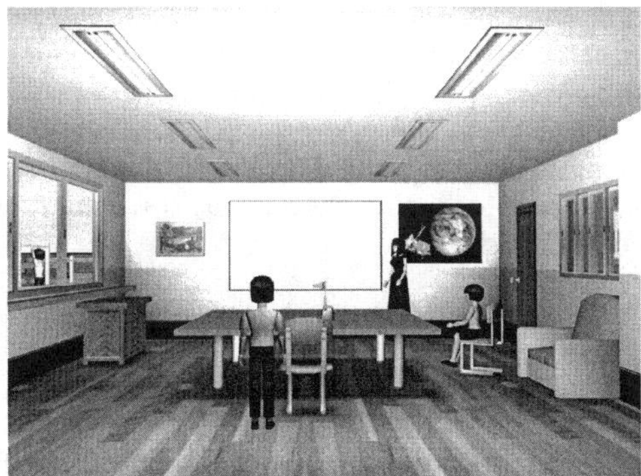

Fig. 1.　A Basic Classroom Virtual Environment

2.2. Virtual Reality Cognitive Training

We developed two cognitive training courses: Virtual Reality Comparison Training and Virtual Reality Sustained Attention Training.

These cognitive training sessions are similar to other ADHD assessment tools such as the Continuous Performance Task (CPT), Test of Variables of Attention (TOVA) or Wisconsin Card Sorting. Furthermore, there is not a repetition effect when using these assessment tools. The most important difference between these assessment tools and our cognitive training sessions is that the latter incorporate performance levels. In our cognitive training sessions, subjects know their performance level; therefore, they must endeavor to make progress to the next level. The higher the level of training session, the more difficult it is to complete.

A subject sits at the virtual desk and can see three flags (red, yellow and violet) that are lying on the desk. In both cognitive training courses, after stimuli are presented; the red, yellow and violet flags are erected in that order. Only once the violet flag is erected are the subjects permitted to respond. This technique is used to control hyperactive responses. If the subject violates this rule, they will hear a warning sound (beep) in the virtual environment.

Virtual Reality Comparison Training (VRCT) is used to enhance the focused attention and selective attention of a subject. When the training session starts, a subject can see two 3D objects on the desk. For example, a sphere and a square pillar. Those objects are sometimes identical and sometimes different. If identical objects are presented, one of those is occasionally yawed, pitched or rolled slightly. Therefore subjects should pay careful attention. If a subject decides that objects are identical, then he or she is instructed to press the left mouse button. Otherwise, the subject is to press the right button. For each session, a subject repeats this routine 60 times. The number of correct answers and the response times are recorded. If the number of correct answers is over 57, the subject will go to the next level in the following session. As the subject progresses through the levels, the length of time he or she can see the objects decreases gradually and the objects provided are less distinguishable: for example, a triangular pyramid and a quadrangular pyramid. There are 10 stages in total. Figure 2 shows an example of this training.

As indicated by its title, Virtual Reality Sustained Attention Training (VRST) is for enhancing sustained attention. In general, a routine VRST procedure is similar to that of VRCT. As the operator starts the training, a subject will see an Arabic numeral on the desk (Fig. 3). The subject is encouraged to press the left mouse button when the numeral '0' is presented after any digit other than '8'. Otherwise, the subject is instructed not to respond. In this procedure, advancement to higher levels is the same as in VRCT. But, unlike VRCT, as the subject progresses, the length of time that the stimuli (numerals) are presented increases gradually. Consequently the subject requires more endurance and must pay attention to the task continuously.

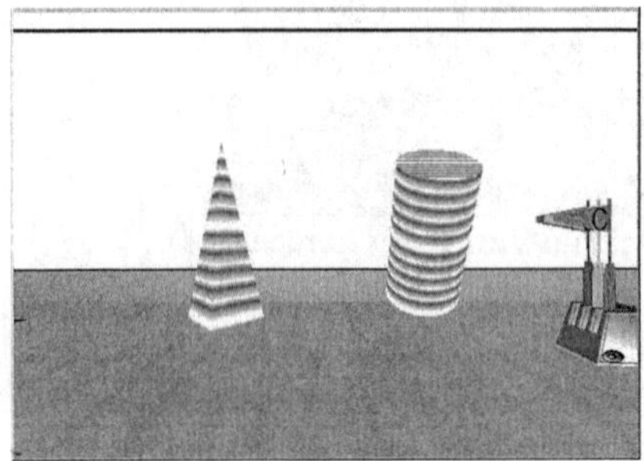 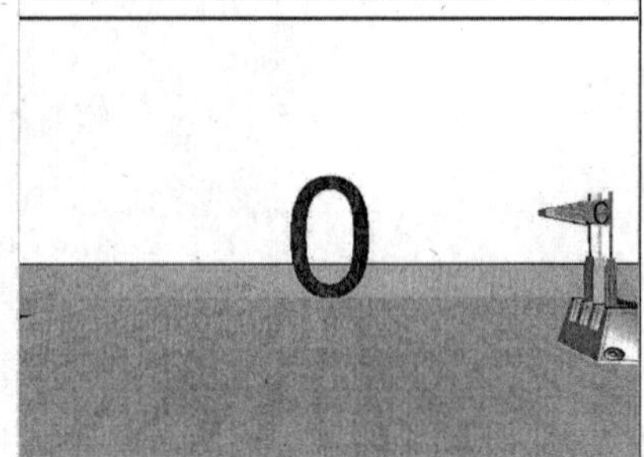

Fig. 2. An Example of VRCT   **Fig. 3.** An Example of VRST

2.3. Neurofeedback Training

Neurofeedback subjects are connected to the EEG signal acquisition device using three electrodes attached to the scalp at the placement of Cz and grounded at the right and left ears. Before analyzing the EEG signal, we preprocessed it by Notch and Lowpass Filtering. After that, Fast Fourier Transforms are used to analyze the latest 3-seconds of acquired EEG signal data in the frequency domain. Then frequency parameters are extracted such as Delta (0.5~3Hz), Theta (4~7Hz), Alpha (8~12Hz), SMR (12~15Hz), and Beta (15~18Hz).

Each frequency parameter is displayed as a bar graph by the EEG analysis program.   The operator can control the threshold levels of the parameters (Fig. 4).

By controlling the threshold levels, the virtual environment is changed. In this pilot study, if the Beta wave is greater than the specified threshold level, a positive reinforcement change is created in the virtual environment.

Before each training session, we measure the subject's EEG base line because it may vary according to emotional or physical conditions. If the subject wearing an HMD with attached EEG electrodes pays attention to the VE, the Beta wave goes over the specified threshold, the score increases and the VE is changed. When the subject is not able to be attentive and the score does not improve, the operator either encourages the subject to be more attentive or lowers the threshold level.

As the score progresses, a dinosaur egg rises from the desk. Then the egg is splits into two pieces. From the broken egg, one part of a dinosaur picture appears gradually from the whiteboard. If the score reaches '100' and all six parts of the picture are put together, the subject can hear the dinosaur roaring (Fig. 5).

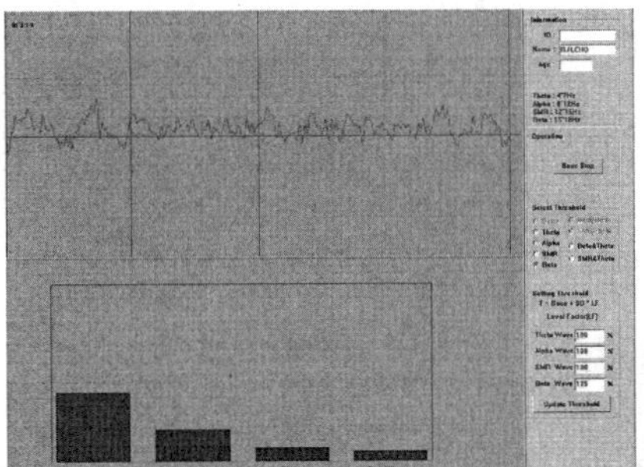

Fig. 4. EEG Biofeedback Analysis Module   **Fig. 5.**   An Example of Neurofeedback training

3. Experiments

Fifty subjects, aged 14 to 18, who had committed crimes and had been isolated in a reformatory, took part in this study. They had histories of learning difficulty and they were inattentive, impulsive, hyperactive and distracted. They were randomly assigned to one of five 10-subject groups: a control group, two placebo groups, and two experimental groups. Each group consisted of 10 subjects, respectively. The experimental groups and the placebo groups underwent 8 sessions over two weeks, which were each approximately 20 minutes in length.   The control group underwent no training during the same period.

Our hypothesis is that Virtual Reality is helpful for improving attention. We also posit that VR-EEG Biofeedback training and our cognitive training courses also support attention enhancement. Accordingly, we divided the subjects into five groups. The placebo groups were established to prove the efficacy of VR. While the experimental groups used a HMD and head tracker in each session, the placebo groups used only a computer monitor. Consequently, only the experimental groups could look around the virtual classroom. The placebo group 1 and experimental group 1 performed the same task (EEG Biofeedback Training), while the placebo group 2 and experimental group 2 also performed cognitive training task. For the cognitive training groups, Virtual Reality Concentration Training was employed in odd sessions and Virtual Reality Sustained Attention Training in even sessions.

All subjects were trained to become accustomed to the virtual environment by performing a Continuous Performance Task (CPT) before and after each session.

4. Results

The number of correct answers in CPT showed significant differences after training. The experimental and placebo groups has improved after the training ($F(1,32)=93.760$, $p<0.01$). And the experimental groups improved more than the placebo groups ($F(1,32)=4.193$, $p<0.05$). Finally, The EEG Biofeedback groups showed a relatively increased improvement than the cognitive training groups ($F(1,32)=3.121$, $p<0.10$). According to Figure 6, the Virtual Reality EEG Biofeedback group (Experimental Group 1) presented the greatest improvement and the desk-top cognitive training group (Placebo Group 2) presented the smallest change.

Figure 7 indicates that response sensitivity (d') of the experimental groups improved slightly more than that of the placebo groups ($F(1,32)=149.538$, $p<0.1$). Experimental Group 1 was also the most improved group in this case.

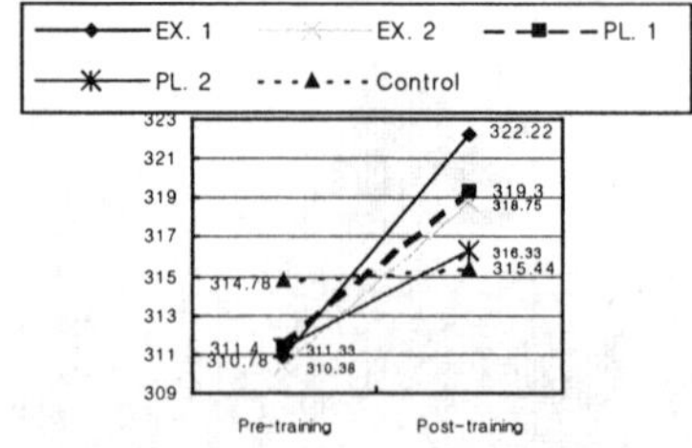

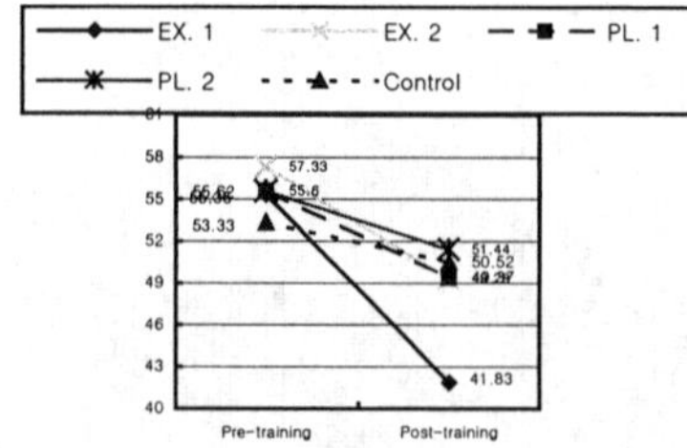

Fig. 6. The mean number of correct answers in CPT   **Fig. 7.** The mean response sensitivity in CPT

For the EEG Biofeedback groups, there was no significant change in completion time. However, completion time decreased slightly as the subjects progressed through the sessions with the completion time of the VR group decreasing more than that of the desktop group (Figure 8).

For the Cognitive groups, there was also no significant improvement in the number of correct answers in cognitive training. The number The number increased from the first to the third session, but it subsequently decreased after the fourth session. Still, the VR group demonstrated more improvement than the desktop group (Figure 9).

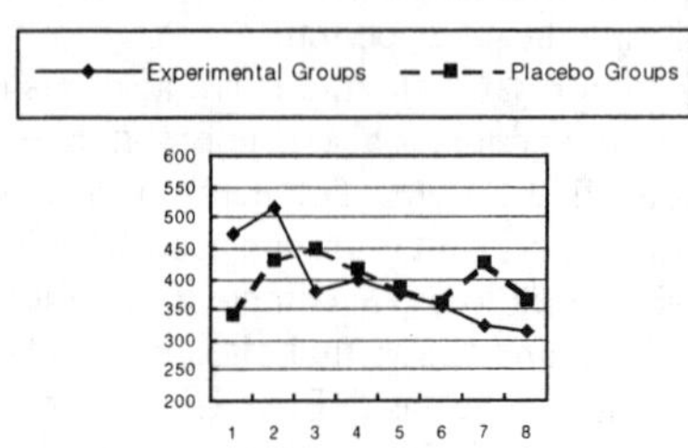

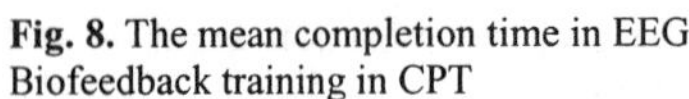

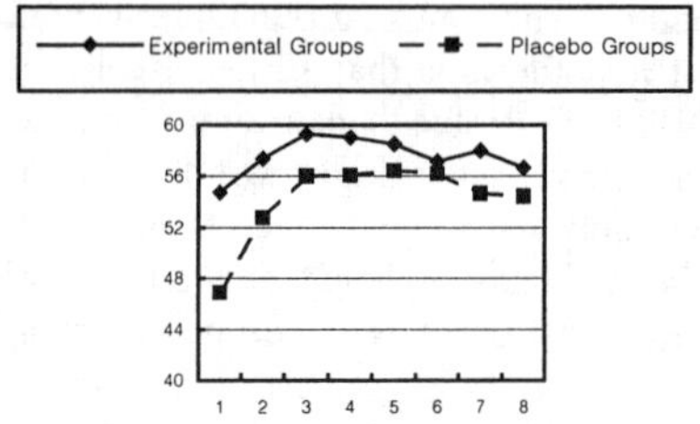

Fig. 8. The mean completion time in EEG Biofeedback training in CPT

Fig. 9. The mean number of correct answers in cognitive training

5. Conclusions and Discussions

We developed the prototype of an Attention Enhancement System using Virtual Reality technology and EEG biofeedback. From our clinical experiment, we can conclude that inattentiveness in the experimental groups declined and they were consistently attentive. We also demonstrated that our prototype was able to improve the attention span of subjects with attention deficits.

Immersive VR may be an effective tool for attention enhancement. Some subjects indicated that training only with a monitor, that is desktop VR, was tedious and uncomfortable. The subjects with a HMD, however, were more motivated and engaged. The combination of EEG Biofeedback training and cognitive training is also applicable to attention enhancement. In certain respects, EEG Biofeedback training is tiresome and difficult for children and adolescents. Immersive VR can supplement such training and keep it interesting for the subject.

In future research, we will enhance our training methods and environment improving the graphic quality of the VE. In addition, we are considering the incorporation of gaming in the development of attention enhancement therapies.

Acknowledgements

This study was funded by the National Research Laboratory(NRL) Program at Korea Institute of Science & Technology Evaluation and Planning

6. References

[1] R. Taylor, S. Lavellee, G. Burdea and R. Moesges, *Virtual Computer Integrated Surgery*, MIT Press., USA, 1994.

[2] M. North, S. North and J. Coble, *Virtual Reality Therapy: An Innovative Paradigm*, IPI Press, Colorado Springs, 1996.

[3] Strickland, D., Hodges, L. F., North, M. M., & Weghorst, S. "Overcoming Phobias by Virtual Exposure", Communications of the ACM, 40(8), 1997.

[4] Rothbaum, B. O., Hodges, L. F., Kooper, R., Opdyke, D., Williford, J. S., & North, M. "Virtual Reality Graded Exposure in the Treatment of Acrophobia: A Case Report. Behavior Therapy", 1995, 26, 547-554.

[5] Rothbaum, B. O., Hodges, L. F., Kooper, R., Opdyke, D., Williford, J. S., & North, M. "The efficacy of virtual reality graded exposure in the treatment of acrophobia" American Journal of Psychiatry, 1995, 152, pp. 626-628.

[6] Rizzo A. et al, "The virtual classroom : A virtual reality environment for the assessment and rehabilitation of attention deficits", CyberPsychology and Behavior. 3(3), 483-500

[7] G. Underwood, *The Psychology of Attention*, Edward Elgar Publishing Company, USA, 1993.

[8] W. Pelham, S. Sams, "Behavior Modification", *Child and Adolescent Psychiatric Clinics of North America*, Vol. 1, No. 2, 1992, pp. 505-918

[9] A. Winkler, J. Dixon and J. Parker, "Brain function in problem children and controls: Psychometric, neurological, electroencephalogic comparisons", *American Journal of Psychiatry*, 127, 1970, pp. 94-105

[10] M. Linden, T. Habib and V. Radojevic, "A controlled Study of the Effects of EEG Biofeedback on Cognition and Behavior of Children with Attention Deficit Disorder and Learning Disabilities", *Biofeedback and Self-Regulation*, Vol. 21, No. 1, 1996, pp. 35-49.

[11] V. Monastra et al, "Assessing Attention Deficit Heperactivity Disorder via Quantitative Electroencephalography: An Initial Validation Study", *Neuropsychology*, Vol. 13, No. 3, 1999, pp. 424-433

[12] S. Othmer, D. Kaiser, "Implementation of Virtual Reality in EEG Biofeedback", CyberPsychology and Behavior. Vol. 3, Num 3, 2000, 415-420.

Medicine Meets Virtual Reality 02/10
J.D. Westwood et al. (Eds.)
IOS Press, 2002

Training and Pretreatment Planning of Interventional Neuroradiology Procedures – Initial Clinical Validation

Chee-Kong Chui[1], Zirui Li[1], James H. Anderson[2], Kieran Murphy[2],
Anthony Venbrux[2], Xin Ma[1], Zhenlan Wang[1], Philippe Gailloud[2],
Yiyu Cai[3], Yaoping Wang[1], Wieslaw L. Nowinski[1]

1. Medical Imaging Lab, Kent Ridge Digital Labs, Singapore
2. Johns Hopkins University School of Medicine, Baltimore, USA
3. Mechanical and Production Engineering, Nanyang Technological University, Singapore

Abstract. A PC based system for simulating image-guided interventional neuroradiological procedures for physician training and patient specific pretreatment planning is described. The system allows physicians to manipulate and interface interventional devices such as catheters, guidewires, stents and coils within 2-D and hybrid surface and volume rendered 3-D patient vascular images in real time. A finite element method is employed to model the interaction of the catheters and guidewires with the vascular system. Fluoroscopic, roadmapping and volume rendered 3-D presentations of the vasculature are provided. System software libraries allow for the use of commonly employed catheters, guidewires, stents and occluding coils of various shapes and sizes. The results of an initial clinical validation suggest that the experience gained from our simulator is comparable with that of using a vascular phantom. We are conducting further validation with the aim of providing patient specific pretreatment planning.

1. Introduction

Interventional neuroradiology is a medical subspecialty in which the physician utilizes medical imaging, usually X-Ray fluoroscopy or computerized tomography (CT), to deliver therapy in the cerebral circulation in a minimally invasive manner. Such procedures usually involve manipulating plastic catheters and guidewires through blood vessels to the site of the lesion and then treating the lesions by means of devices or drugs delivered through the catheters. Planning image-guided vascular interventional procedures requires a full knowledge of the patient's vasculature and a thorough understanding of physician's techniques such as navigation of the catheter and the strategy of placing therapeutic devices. Knowledge of the vascular anatomy and pathology usually requires 2-D displays of real time images from X-Ray angiography (fluoroscopy or CT) or magnetic resonance angiography (MRA). It is difficult to preoperatively plan a treatment by mentally extracting blood vessels from 2-D images and reconstructing the 3-D vasculature. It is also difficult to predict the result of various treatment approaches when there is concern about the choice and delivery of devices. An effective pretreatment planning system should provide interventional neuroradiologists with tools to examine patient-specific anatomy through 3-D visualization and to interact with the vascular images in real time to realistically simulate the catheterization and treatment processes using specific devices. We have developed an interventional neuroradiology pretreatment planning system called *NeuroCath* [1][2] to provide the above capabilities. This PC based system provides integrated functionalities for both training and patient-specific pretreatment planning. Virtual reality based simulation technology is especially suited for interventional radiology because the image guided procedures involve viewing video monitors and places the interventional radiologist's hands manipulating instruments at a distance from the actual anatomical treatment site being treated [3].

In this paper, we discuss our initial clinical validation of *NeuroCath*, and its results. The results clearly show that the clinicians are ready to accept advanced simulator of this type for training and subsequently patient specific pretreatment planning.

2. Simulation for Training and Pretreatment Planning

NeuroCath is an advanced simulator for training and pretreatment planning. It provides a pretreatment planning environment closely resembling the angiography suite and allows clinicians to interact with patient specific vasculature in virtual space using actual interventional devices. Patient medical image datasets are acquired from rotational X-Ray angiography (XRA), computerized tomography angiography (CTA) or from vascular images obtained from MRA. The vascular images are extracted to construct 3-D geometrical models. The vascular network is segmented and traced in 3-D space and the central line of the vascular tree is identified. A reach-in device of 6 degrees of freedom is used to interact with the 3-D volume dataset in virtual space and to define essential points that are used to construct a topology model of the vasculature [4][5]. Physical properties of therapeutic devices, such as catheters and guidewires, stents and occluding coils are modeled using Finite Element Methods [6,7,8]. Figure 1 shows a physical setup of the system used in this initial clinical validation.

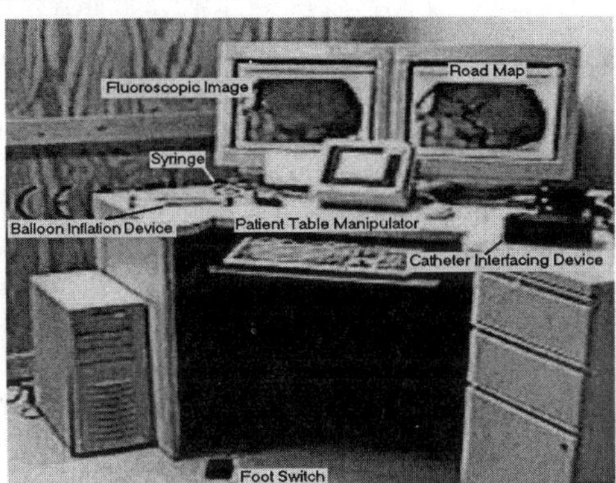

Figure 1. Setup of *NeuroCath* for initial clinical validation.

An interface device [9] provides the physician with the opportunity to advance, retract and rotate catheters and guidewires independently or together within the 2-D and 3-D modeled vasculature and view their movements in real time. This provides realistic hand-eye coordinated functions that can be of great value in training and evaluating individual skills. We are also developing haptic interface components to provide the user with tactile feedback during the catheterization procedure. The simulator predicts the behavior of these devices when navigated within blood vessels to treat the specific lesions identified in the patient image datasets. For example, a catheter tip shape deforms in a predictable manner when advancing through tortuous vessels and when encountering vascular constraints such as lumen narrowing, branch point bifurcation, etc. Figure 2 shows the graphical user interface of *NeuroCath*. The user can selectively display fluoroscopic, 3D, cross-sectional planar or roadmap images of the medical data and devices.

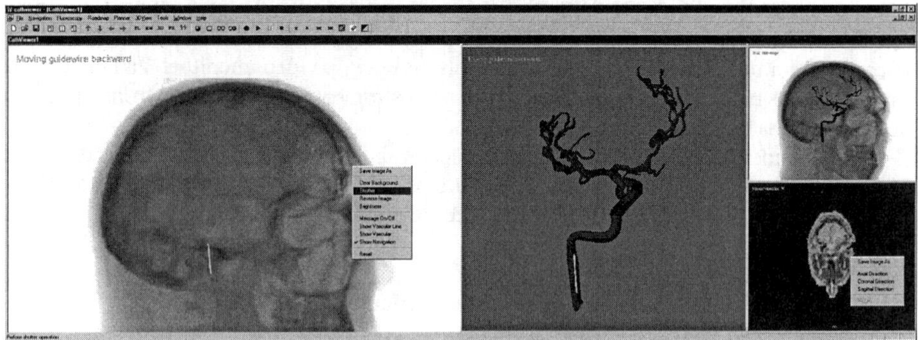

Figure 2. Graphical user interface of *NeuroCath* with multiple displays

3. Experiments and Results

The experiments were carried out on medical images of both patients and vascular phantoms. The availability of a virtual phantom in the simulator provided a mean for clinicians to compare the experience they had with the simulator with that of a phantom. This provides some form of ground truth although our emphasis is on patient specific treatment planning. In this section we describe the medical images of both patients and phantom used in this study, the method of evaluation, and the results.

3.1 Medical Images and Image Acquisition

The datasets used for this initial clinical study were acquired using various imaging modalities ranging from MRA, CTA and XRA. We decided to focus on two brain datasets because that most of the clinicians used our simulator for the first time, and hence, were not familiar with the simulator. The validation period was quite short - we had allocated only one month for this initial clinical study.

Figure 3(a) is a volume rendered image of the selected patient data which was used extensively in gathering feedback from the clinicians. This dataset was code named "GE-Carbic". GE-Carbic consists of cerebral vasculature of an unidentified patient who had a medium size and clearly visible aneurysm. The data was acquired using three-dimensional rotational angiography (3DRA) from GE Medical Systems. 3DRA is a relatively new technique for imaging blood vessels in the human body [10]. Using a standard C-arm imaging system, this technique yields high-resolution isotropic 3D datasets reconstructed from 2D X-ray angiography images acquired during a rotation of the X-ray source-detector combination following a single injection of contrast material. The data had a resolution of 512 x 512 pixels, 10 bits per pixel.

The availability of a segmented data allows us to focus more on the provision of computer modeling and simulation. 3DRA is a promising imaging technique and we expect more clinical examination to be performed using this imaging modality. On the other hand, there was now a need to register GE-Carbic with a human head, so that the rendered fluoroscopic images as shown in Figure 3(b) are realistic. We had chosen CT data from the VHD Male Project for this purpose. Note that the interventional neuroradiologists rely mainly on the fluoroscopic images in the navigation. The registration was done manually by clinicians and researchers using combination of our customized software and PhotoShop version 4 that is commercially available. Figure 4 shows the second dataset from another unidentified human for this study. We again registered the vasculature with the CT data from the VHD Male Project. The vascular structure in the second dataset was normal and with no obvious pathology.

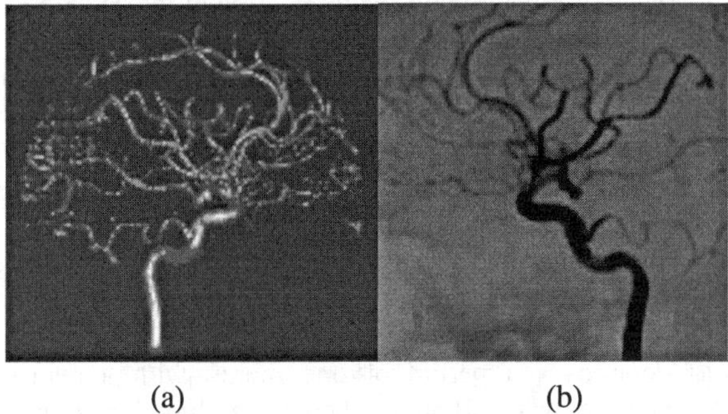

(a)　　　　　　　　　　　　　　　(b)

Figure 3. (a) Volume rendered image of GE-Carbic dataset. (b) Rendered fluoroscopic image of GE-Carbic and VHD Male datasets.

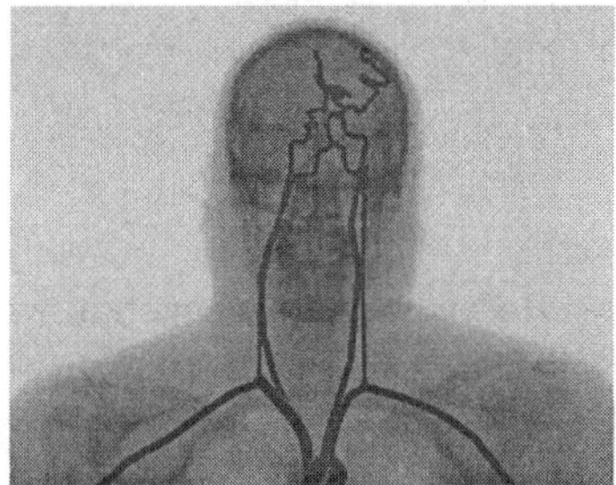

Figure 4. Normal human vasculature for simulation.

The phantom we used in the study was an intracranial anthropomorphic vascular phantom with a berry aneurysm at the tip of the basilar artery. It represents average dimensions of the corresponding vascular structures in the human body. The dome diameter of the aneurysm is 12.9 mm and the diameter of the aneurysmal neck is 2.6 mm. These diameters are important since their ratio has been suggested as guideline in selection of a surgical or an endovascular treatment. This is a typical phantom used in the residential training of interventional neuroradiology procedures. The phantom was filled with CT contrast (50%-50%) and scanned at a resolution of 256x256x130. The inter-slice interval was 3 mm. Figure 5 shows volume rendered images of the phantom.

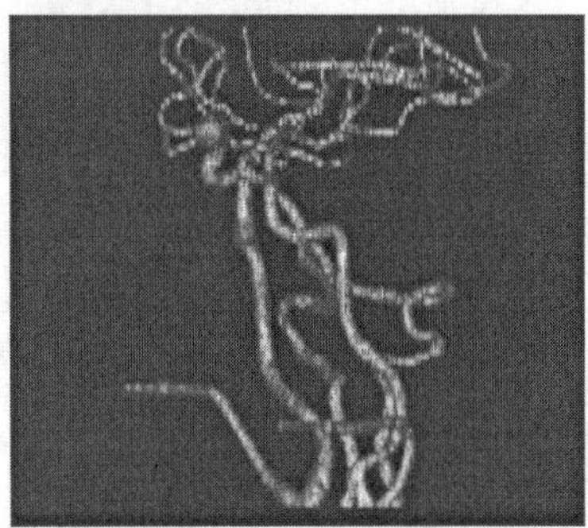

Figure 5. Volume rendered image of the scanned intracranial anthropomorphic vascular phantom

3.2 Method of Evaluation

Our initial validation involved assessing clinician acceptance of *NeuroCath* and the realism of the hand-eye coordinated real time interaction of the catheters and devices being navigated through the modeled vasculature. We are currently developing a program where physicians can compare the functionality, realism and value of the system with the actual procedures performed in the patients from which the image datasets were obtained.

We measured the turn around time, defined as the processing time between acquiring patient's imaging data and the availability of a respective biomechanical model for pretreatment planning. We determined the accuracy and interactivity of the simulator by focusing on realistic representations and real-time hand-eye coordinated catheterization of selected vessels. We also estimated the completeness of our system based upon the features available.

The study was done over a period of one month with a neuroradiologist and a peripheral vascular interventional radiologist being the clinical champions. The simulator .was installed in a hospital and was used routinely by several clinicians. *NeuroCath* was executing on an Intel Pentium III 1GHz processor, with 512 Mbytes of main memory, and an OpenGL graphic acceleration board supporting dual monitor display. The OS of the system was MS Windows NT 4.0 service pack 6. The software and data took up to 300 Mbytes of hard disk space.

3.3 Results

Depending upon the modality and quality of medical images, various methods were employed to extract vasculature from a patient-specific dataset. Such methods include automatic segmentation with Digital Subtraction Angiography (DSA) or 3DRA, and manual extraction using reach-in device with visualization of low resolution MRA. For the former, the targeted turn around time is 4 hours. We are convinced that this is possible with the advancement in noise reduction and reconstruction techniques especially with the availability of 3DRA.

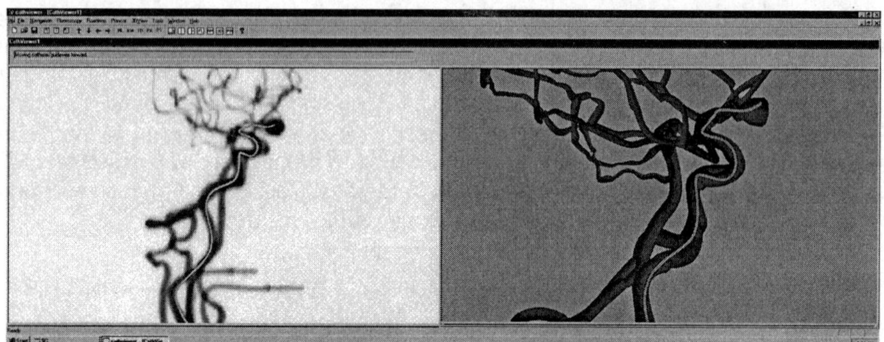

Figure 6. Catheter navigation with the virtual phantom

NeuroCath delivers a mean refresh rate of 15 frames per second. There is no or negligible delays for catheter manipulation. Clinician feedback evaluation of the current system indicates that it already has 70% - 75% of the desired features. This is sufficient for *NeuroCath* to be useful as a training system. By comparing vascular catheterization with a conventional plastic phantom and the corresponding visual model on our system, clinicians' feedback revealed that the interactive experience gained is comparable, while the virtual model is superior by providing patient-specific vasculature with various pathologies. Some clinicians were excited with the possibilities of introducing more arbitrary aneurysms into the virtual phantom for the purpose of training. Figure 6 shows interactive catheter navigation with the virtual phantom using *NeuroCath*. Table 1 summarizes the results according to the criteria that we have stated prior to the commencement of this study.

Table 1. Summary of results

Criteria	Clinical Feedback
Acceptance – Training	Good
Acceptance – Pretreatment planning	Potential acknowledged. Needs further clinical validation.
Interactivity – Visual	Acceptable
Interactivity – Catheter tracking	Acceptable
Reality – Visual	Needs improvement, particularly on the rendered fluoroscopic image featuring the vasculature.
Reality – Tactile	Force feedback may be required.
Features – Training	70% - 75%
Features – Pretreatment planning	Potential acknowledged. Need further clinical validation.
Turn around time	Depends on the availability of various image modalities. Needs further clinical validation.

Additional features and extensions that clinicians suggest as needed include modeling of physiological functions such as motion and cardiac pulsation that is applicable to intervention cardiology in contrast media injections. The clinicians also like to see improvement with our haptic force feedback components in the user interface and additional refinement in the modeling of the interactions of devices with the vasculature. Haptic interface technology is important because interventional radiological procedures rely heavily on hand-eye coordinated skills.

For the purpose of training and certification, we need to have a larger library of patient data, and to include a mechanism for users to introduce new datasets into the library on their own. We are currently acquiring new clinical cases of various vascular pathologies not restricted to brain vasculature. This human vasculature library will grow, as a function of time and provide trainees with the opportunity to practice catheterization and interventional procedures on a large variety of clinical cases. We anticipate that in time, a national (or even international) registrar could be formed where 3-D volume rendered patient specific datasets could be available for training or teaching purposes.

4. Conclusions

NeuroCath provides an efficient, comprehensive approach to understand the complexity of the interaction of vascular structures, therapeutic devices and required techniques to perform interventional procedures. *NeuroCath* could be customized for peripheral vascular and cardiac applications. Each of these applications has its own unique requirements, but each also draws on basic fundamental image processing and modeling principles that are generic and can be utilized for all applications. We are currently focusing on the development of cerebral circulation. We are also developing metrics that can be used to measure how the system benefits training and improves user skills by either reducing procedural time or decreasing complications based on simulation provided knowledge of favorable treatment approaches. Further validation is in place with the aim of integrating this treatment planning system into the angiography suit.

Acknowledgement: Support of this research development by National Science and Technology Board of Singapore is gratefully acknowledged. We are grateful to Dr. E. Maurincomme of GE Medical Systems for the provision of medical data, and A/Prof. L.-S. Wong of Kent Ridge Digital Labs for his assistance in securing the financial support of this study. The segmentation supports from Dr. Q. Hu and Mr. S. Huang of Kent Ridge Digital Labs are also acknowledged.

References

[1]   Z Li, CK Chui, JH Anderson, X Chen, X Ma, W Hua, Q Peng, Y Cai, Y Wang, WL Nowinski, Computer environment for interventional neuroradiology procedures, Simulation and Gaming – An Interdisciplinary Journal of Theory, Practice and Research 32(3) (2001), 405-420.

[2]   WL Nowinski and CK Chui, Simulation of interventional neuroradiology procedures, Proc. Medical Imaging and Augmented Reality MIAR2001, IEEE Computer Society Press (2001), 87-94

[3]   JH Anderson, R Raghavan, Y Wang and CK Chui, daVinci - A vascular catheterization simulator, Journal of Vascular and Interventional Radiology 8(1) Part 2 (1997), 261.

[4]   W Hua, CK Chui, Y Wang, X Chen, Z Wang, Q Peng and WL Nowinski, A semiautomatic framework for vasculature extraction from volume image, Proc. 10th International Conference on Biomedical Engineering (2000), 515-516.

[5]   X Chen, CK Chui, SH Teoh, SH Ong and WL Nowinski, Automatic modeling of anatomical structures for biomechanical analysis and visualization in a virtual spine workstation, Proc. Medical Image Computing and Computer-Assisted Intervention MICCAI2001, Springe-Verlag, (2001), 1170-1171.

[6]   Y Wang, CK Chui, HL Lim, Y Cai and KH Mak, Real-time interactive surgical simulators for catheterization procedures, Computer Aided Surgery 3(5) (1999), 211-227.

[7]   CK Chui, H Nguyen, Y Wang, R Mullick, R Raghavan and JH Anderson, Potential field and anatomy vasculature for real-time computation in daVinci, Proc. 1st Visible Human Conference (1996), 113-114.

[8]   Y Cai, CK Chui, Y Wang, Z Wang and JH Anderson, Parametric eyeball model for interactive simulation of ophthalmologic surgery, Proc. Medical Image Computing and Computer-Assisted Intervention MICCAI 2001, Springe-Verlag, (2001), 457-464.

[9]   CK Chui, P Chen, Y Wang, M Ang Jr and Y Cai, Tactile Controlling and Image Manipulation Apparatus for Computer Simulation of Image Guided Surgery, Recent Advances in Mechatronics, Springe-Verlag, (1999), 423-443.

[10] R. Anxionn et al., 3D angiography: clinical interests - first applications in interventional neuroradiology, Journal of Neuroradiology 25 (1998), 251-262.

Medicine Meets Virtual Reality 02/10
J.D. Westwood et al. (Eds.)
IOS Press, 2002

Navigation by Walking Around: Using the Pressure Mat to Move in Virtual Worlds

Warren Couvillion, Roger Lopez, Jian Ling
Southwest Research Institute, San Antonio, TX

Abstract. This paper describes a new virtual reality (VR) locomotion input device, the Pressure Mat, which allows a simulator user to navigate/traverse a virtual environment (VE) using similar motions as in the real world; i.e., walk, run, crawl. The device consists of an array of pressure sensitive resistors covered by a thin, flexible mat. The resistor array is connected to a personal computer (PC) that uses a real-time pattern recognition algorithm to determine if the user is standing still, or walking forward, backward, left or right. The information from the Pressure Mat was used to allow users to navigate in a VE. The Pressure Mat may also be useful in the diagnosis of a variety of conditions and/or in rehabilitative therapy.

1. Introduction

Methods of navigating in VEs have run the gamut from unnatural methods that are easy to implement and inexpensive, (e.g., using a joystick, or flying where the finger is pointing), to more natural methods using elaborate devices that move the surface under the user's feet or otherwise offer resistance to his movement. We wanted to develop a device that sits between these extremes. Our device was to use motions similar to those used in the real world, and make the user exert himself. Thus, increasing his sense of immersion while still being relatively inexpensive and have low maintenance.

This paper describes internal research performed at Southwest Research Institute (SwRI) that resulted in a prototype locomotion input device known as the Pressure Mat. The Pressure Mat returns the amount of pressure applied to several fixed points. To confirm that the pressure patterns generated as users walked were distinct and repeatable, we developed visualization techniques to isolate features of the pressure patterns, making them human readable.

After confirming pressure patterns could be used to detect user actions, we developed a pattern-recognition algorithm to detect which of a set of predefined gestures the user was making. Once we were able to detect which direction and at what rate the user was walking, we were able to integrate the Pressure Mat into an application that allows users to navigate in a VE.

Finally, we will also discuss why in addition to its use as a VR locomotion device, the Pressure Mat could possibly be used for rehabilitative therapy to assess patient progress and diagnosing conditions ranging from brain lesions to depression.

2. Background

Ideally, a simulator user should be able to move through a VE using the same motions as in the real world. There have been several approaches to make a locomotion interface that uses natural walking motions. One approach required the user to sit on a unicycle-like device, pedaling instead of walking, and shifting his weight to change his orientation [6].

Another system, the virtual perambulator, put the user on a low-friction surface and tracked the motions of his feet to determine where and how fast he was walking [10].

There have been attempts to create treadmills that change the direction of their resistance [11]. Most resulted in an unnatural form of locomotion where the user either steered with his hands or had to adjust his style of walking to the device. Still another approach, Gaiter, tracked the user's feet using pressure sensitive devices mounted to his shoes and devices to track the motions of his knees [18].

All of these approaches, as well as the "Virtual Motion Controller" [20], worked only for users walking upright and required the user to either be supported or adjust the way he walked to compensate for the behavior of the input device. In addition, most required the user to wear tracking devices or other types of equipment on his lower body. None allowed the user to "go prone," i.e., crawling as close to the ground as possible.

Attempts to allow going prone have sacrificed natural motion. The Naval Air Warfare Center-Training Systems Division (NAWC-TSD) developed a simple foot-pedal interface similar to the accelerator of a car, although pivoted in the middle, rather than at one end. On pressing the foot pedal, the user moved relative to the center of his field of view of the VE. Thus, direction of gaze controlled the direction of motion. This interface allowed the user to navigate from any posture, as long as he could control the foot pedal.

Under the direction of NAWC-TSD and the United States Marine Corps, SwRI developed two locomotion devices which are manipulated with the user's hands. The first device was the weapon-mounted joystick. This device consisted of an elastomer button on top of a pressure pad. The second device, the finger sleeve, consisted of a pressure sensitive pad in a wearable finger sleeve. Both of these devices were demonstrated and tried by USMC subject matter experts. In both cases, the subject matter experts expressed extreme dislike for the invasiveness of the devices and their interference with weapon handling.

SwRI developed an improved omnidirectional foot pedal consisting of a disc outputting the direction and pressure applied by the user. Both the user's waist and head were tracked with direction of motion determined by the waist. This allowed the user to look at his virtual surroundings without changing his direction of travel. The omnidirectional foot pedal allowed the user to move sideways. The user had to change his orientation in the real world to change his direction of travel, yielding a greater sense of immersion. However, the omnidirectional foot pedal did not require him to take steps or lift his feet as in the real world.

3. Technical Approach

The complete Pressure Mat system consists of the Pressure Mat, a computer to read the mat and determine the pressure patterns and an image generator (IG) for rendering the VE (see Figure 1).

Using techniques developed for pattern recognition, we determine if the user is walking forward, backward, right, or left, as well as the rate of travel. These data are sent to an image generator that renders a VE to a head-mounted display (HMD). The user's head and waist are tracked to provide an accurate view of the VE and proper direction of travel.

Resistor spacing was a compromise between sampling density and mat size. We placed sixty-four pressure sensitive resistors (PSRs) on a thick Lexan® sheet in an area about twelve inches by twenty-four inches, then covered them with a protective rubber mat. Small rubber knobs were placed on the border of the measurement area so that a user immersed in a VE could feel when he was leaving the measurement area (see Figure 2).

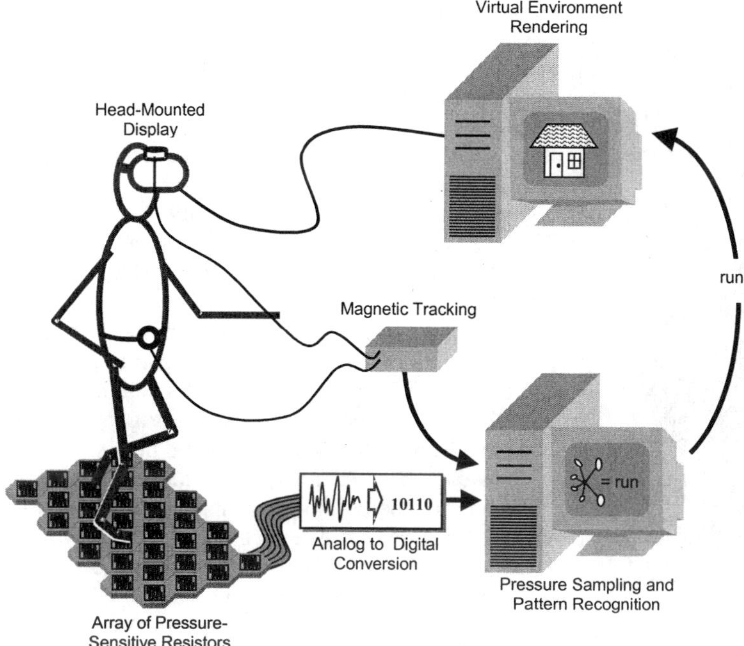

Figure 1. Pressure Mat System

The resistors were arranged in a hexagonal grid so that each sensor was equidistant from its nearest neighbors. This arrangement reduced directional bias that would occur with a rectangular grid [8]. For example, if a user's feet were along the diagonal of a square grid, his feet would touch about 30% fewer resistors than if he were standing aligned with one of the grid axes.

The pattern recognition algorithm classifies the gestures based on the features extracted from the pressure pattern generated by the feet [13] [17]. To simplify the pattern recognition task, we decided to use a set of defined motions (gestures) to indicate the direction of travel.

The pressure image is first rotated according to the direction the user's waist is pointing (as returned by the tracking device). The image is rotated around the image center to place the toe on the top and the heel on the bottom. This adjustment allowed the pressure pattern to be placed in a consistent orientation, greatly simplifying feature extraction.

The pressure image is then filtered to reduce noise, and "threshholded" to determine foot regions [4]. The threshold was determined using data of several users.

Several features are extracted from the pressure image. Those varying most across the set of gestures and least, and least within a gesture [19] are used to determine which step a user is taking.

Data from four subjects were used as training data to calculate the statistics. Seven features were finally selected to form the classifier: 1) the duration difference of the left and right (foot) supporting half-cycle; 2) the average toe area of a half-cycle; 3) the ratio between average toe area and heel average area of a half-cycle; 4) the peak (maximum) toe area in a half-cycle; 5) the ratio between average toe pressure and heel average pressure of a half-cycle; 6) the change of centroid vertical locations during a half-cycle; and 7) the average toe pressure of a half-cycle.

Once these features are extracted from the image, they are weighted by values determined from the training data described above. From these weighted values, the type of step made by a Pressure Mat user is determined. (A more detailed explanation of pressure image processing and gesture classification can be found in [5].)

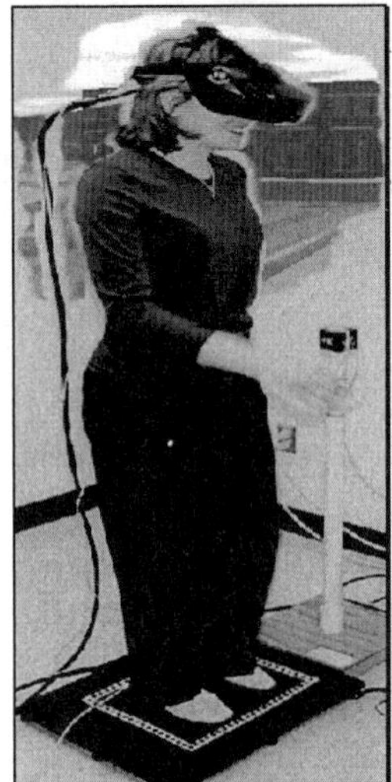

Figure 2. User on the Pressure Mat

For some users, the gestures for walking sideways and walking forward were very similar; so, many false readings would occur. We attempted to filter out the false readings by assuming a gesture different from a sequence of gestures was in error. To improve responsiveness when starting or stopping, filtering was not applied to transitions to or from standing. Rarely was standing reported as a false gesture; so, this did not harm the filter's effectiveness. The gesture filter weeded out many false steps.

Finally, we integrated the Pressure Mat into an existing VR application, allowing the user to navigate in a VE with walking motions. The VE application loaded a simple model of a town, and allowed the user to walk around. Figure 2 shows someone using the Pressure Mat while immersed in a VE.

Rendering the VE and performing pattern recognition was too taxing for the desktop personal computer we were using to read the Pressure Mat. We used our desktop PC to read the input devices (the Pressure Mat and the magnetic tracker), perform pattern recognition, and then send that information via Ethernet to another computer, the image generator, dedicated to rendering the VE. (A faster or dual processor PC could perform both the pattern recognition and rendering·the VE.)

4. Results

The Pressure Mat was successfully integrated into a VR application. The project did not include a formal evaluation of the Pressure Mat, but it was demonstrated to several people. Their subjective evaluations are described below.

Users were able to use the mat to traverse a virtual town. They were able to pick out objects in the VE and get to them by walking in the various directions and reorienting themselves. Physical exertion is known to affect a user's sense of immersion [2]. Many users commented on how long it took to get to their objective; but the times were reasonable, given the distances covered. The slow speed perceived by the users was probably caused by the limited field of view of their HMDs, rather than their locomotion device [3]. Users still get a better sense, not only of the time required to perform a task requiring traversal of a VE, but the amount of effort required. A particularly good use for this would be architectural walkthroughs of malls and stadiums. For example, designers could get a real idea of what it takes to get to a restroom.

We were successful in recognizing five gestures: standing, walking forward, walking backward, walking left, and walking right. Due to the size limitation of the prototype Pressure Mat, going prone was not feasible. Walking backward and forward worked particularly well. Walking sideways, while usable, was less successful, with many false forwards and backwards, even with the filtering described above. User response to gesture filtering was mixed. Some users accepted the slightly sluggish response when changing directions, preferring the fewer false steps. Others thought this was an unacceptable tradeoff.

The pressure sensitive resistors quickly hit their minimum resistances at relatively low pressures. We were hoping subtle changes of the pressure pattern could be detected as the user shifted his weight in preparation of taking a step. However, because the resistance so quickly bottomed out, changes in pressure were not detected until shortly before the user's foot was lifted from the mat.

Undersampling was a problem. For example, we were unable to determine the user's orientation solely from the pressure pattern. This would be possible with a more highly sampled pressure pattern, as feet are not symmetric.

5. Future Work

Future pattern recognition algorithms could be improved by designing a nonlinear classifier using neural networks or fuzzy logic. More training data would also make for a more robust classifier. The pattern algorithms need to be able to handle the image from a much larger Pressure Mat to include cases of walking, crawling, etc.

The pressure data captured by the pressure mat could be used to diagnose a variety of conditions. Digital motion-capture data have been used to diagnose depression [1]. The same effects measured by digital motion capture would affect the distribution of weight on the ground, and thus could be detected by the Pressure Mat. While the Pressure Mat would not provide as much data as digital motion capture, it requires fewer sensors be attached to the patient (if the patient is not using an HMD and remains in a single orientation, no sensors are required at all). This would make the patient less conscious of the testing apparatus so that his motions would be less affected. The Pressure Mat may serve useful for early screenings, with motion capture or video used for a more thorough examination of the patient's motions.

Motion capture data have also been used to assess arm motor deficits after brain lesions [12]. For conditions affecting the lower extremities, balance, or any condition affecting the user's distribution of weight on the ground, data from the pressure mat could be studied to determine a patient's progress. Similarly, the pressure mat could used to gather some of the same data as the "Rutgers Ankle" [7], a device that provides six degrees of freedom feedback and resistance. The Rutgers Ankle allows patients to perform exercises while playing VR games, while simultaneously providing data to the therapist. While the Pressure Mat cannot offer resistance, it can still provide diagnostic data for exercises requiring no resistance, while serving as an interface for VR games.

The visualizations developed to determine if pressure patterns are distinct and repeatable could have uses in rehabilitative therapy for patients with damaged proprioception. Extensive research has shown that people with hearing disorders can improve their pronunciation by viewing visualizations of their voices, and comparing them to those of normal speakers [9] [14] [15] [16]. Similarly, someone with impaired proprioception could view his pressure pattern visualization and confirm that he is distributing his weight correctly as he retrains himself to walk or stand, or other actions.

6. Conclusions

The pressure mat has numerous applications including training, architectural walk-throughs, and computer gaming. The pressure mat could be used as a diagnostic tool for condition affecting the way a user distributes his weight on the ground. The visualizations of pressure patterns could be used in rehabilitative therapy for patients who have lost sensation (particularly proprioception) in their lower bodies. While going through exercises, patients could reassure themselves that they are performing actions correctly by matching visual patterns.

The advantages of the pressure mat are that it is low cost and requires very few sensors be attached to the user. It could easily be expanded to accommodate crawling or "going prone" without requiring additional sensors to be attached to the user.

7. References

[1] Alessi, N.; Huang, M., "Digital Motion Phenomenology of Depression", *Medicine Meets Virtual Reality 2001*, J. D. Westwood *et al.* (Eds.), IOS Press, 2001.

[2] Allison, R., Harris, L., Jenkin, M., Pintilie, G., Redlick, F., Zikovitz, D. (2000) "First Steps with a Rideable Computer". *Proceedings. IEEE Virtual Reality 2000.* pp. 169-175.

[3] Banton, T.A.; Steve, J.; Durgin, F.H.; Proffitt, D.R. (2000). The Calibration of Optic Flow and Treadmill Speed during Treadmill Walking in a Virtual Environment. *Investigative Ophthalmology and Visual Science*, 41(4), S718.

[4] Castleman, K. (1996). "Digital Image Processing". Prentice Hall.

[5] Couvillion, W., Lopez, R.; Ling, J. (2001). "The Pressure Mat: A New Device for Traversing Virtual Environments Using Natural Motion" *Proceedings Interservice/Industry, Simulation and Education Conference 2001.*

[6] Darken, R. (1997). "Navigation in Virtual Environments". *Course Notes: Applied Virtual Reality.* SIGGRAPH 1997.

[7] Girome, M.; Burdea, G.; Bouzit, M.; Popescu, V. "Orthopedic Rehabilitation Using the 'Rutgers Ankle" Interface", *Medicine Meets Virtual Reality 2000*, J. D. Westwood *et al.* (Eds.), IOS Press, 2000.

[8] Glassner, I. (1995). "Chapter 10: Survey of Sampling and Reconstruction Techniques". *Principles of Digital Image Synthesis.* Morgan Kaufmann Publishers. Inc.

[9] Hatzis A., Green P.D., and Howard S. (1997), "OPTICAL LOGO-THERAPY (OLT) : A Computer-Based Real Time Visual Feedback Application for Speech Training.", Proc. EUROSPEECH 1997

[10] Iwata.H. and Fujii.T. (1996). "VIRTUAL PERAMBULATOR: A Novel Interface Device for Locomotion in Virtual Environment". *Proceedings of IEEE 1996 Virtual Reality Annual International Symposium.*

[11] Iwata. H. (1999). Walking About Virtual Environments on Infinite Floor. *Proceedings of IEEE 1999 Virtual Reality Annual International Symposium.*

[12] Piron, L.; Cenni F.; Dam, M. "Virtual Reality as an assessment tool for arm motor deficits after brain lesions", *Medicine Meets Virtual Reality 2001*, J. D. Westwood *et al.* (Eds.), IOS Press, 2001.

[13] Lord, M. (1981), "Foot Pressure Measurement: A Review of Methodology". J. Biomedical Engineering. Vol. 3, No. 2. pp91-99.

[14] Maki J. (1983), "Applications of the speech spectrographic display in developing articulatory skill in hearing impaired adults", in Speech of the hearing impaired: research, training and personnel preparation, ed. M.N. Osberger, University Park Press, Baltimore, MD.

[15] Pratt S., Heintzelman A.T., and Deming S. Ensrud (1993), "The efficacy of using the IBM Speech Viewer vowel accuracy module to treat young children with hearing impairment", Journal of Speech and Hearing Research, vol. 36, pp. 1063-1074.

[16] Reynolds J., and Tarassenko L. (1993), "Learning Pronunciation with the Visual Ear", Neural Computing & Applications (1993) 1: pp 169 - 175

[17] Soames, R. (1985) "Foot Pressure Patterns During Gait". J. Biomedical Engineering. Vol. 7, No. 2. pp120-126.

[18] Templeman, J., Denbrook, P., Sibert, L. (1999). "Virtual Locomotion: Walking in Place Through Virtual Environments". Presence. Volume 8, Issue 6. December 1999.

[19] Tou, J., Gonzalez, R., (1974) "Pattern Recognition Principles". Addison-Wesley.

[20] Wells, M., Peterson. B., Aten. J. (1997). "The Virtual Motion Controller: A Sufficient-Motion Walking Simulator". *Proceedings of VRAIS '97*. pp. 1-8.

Medicine Meets Virtual Reality 02/10
J.D. Westwood et al. (Eds.)
IOS Press, 2002

Intraoperative guidance of pre-planned bone deformations with a surface scanning system

*Sascha Däuber, *Harald Hoppe, **R. Krempien, ***S. Hassfeld, ***J. Brief
and *Heinz Wörn

*University of Karlsruhe (TH), Institute for Process Control and Robotics, Kaiserstraße 12,
76128 Karlsruhe, Germany*
**University of Heidelberg, Dept. of Clinical Radiology*
*** University of Heidelberg, Clinic of Cranio-Maxillo-Facial Surgery*

Abstract: Computer- and robot-based systems to support interventions become more and more important in modern surgery. In general these systems provide methods to plan an intervention pre-operatively [1,2,13] and to execute it with support from a autonomous robot-system [3,4]. Due to the principle restriction of a robot to comparatively simple work steps, there are some complex work steps which the surgeon may plan but which he/she has to execute manually. In craniofacial surgery osteotomised bone segments are deformed by hand to a shape given by the planning system. We support the execution of pre-planned deformation by comparison of the actual shape of an object with the target shape. The actual shape is obtained intra-operatively with a surface scanning device, the deviation from the target shape are visualised by projecting colour-coded error values directly on the object to be deformed. The surgeon uses these projections to adjust further deformation steps. The system is therefore able to validate the correct execution of planned deformations, especially of bony structures.

1. Introduction

Malformations of the skull's skeletal structures may occur for different reasons. Examples are accidents, tumor resection or craniosynosthoses, a disease of the cranial sutures. Figure 1 (left) shows an approx. one year old male patient with craniosynosthoses. The malformations, especially at the temples can be easily noticed. Furthermore, due to the restricted growth of the skull the intra-cranial pressure is increased which will cause severe damage to the patient if untreated. The disease is surgically treated at the University of Heidelberg, Clinic for Cranio and Maxillofacial Surgery. The surgery is called Frontal Orbital Advancement (FOA). Primary aims of the intervention are to increase the intra-cranial volume to decrease pressure and to restore a typical (sex, age) shape of the patient's skull[10]. This is achieved by an osteotomy and spatially advanced refixation of different bone segments. Position and orientation of the bones are changed. For optimal fixation which takes into account the functional as well as the esthetic aims of the surgery, it is necessary that the surgeon deforms the bone segments. An operation planning system provides methods and virtual tools to define dissection trajectories and new positions and shapes for the bone segments [1]. Figure 1 (right) shows a typical execution where the

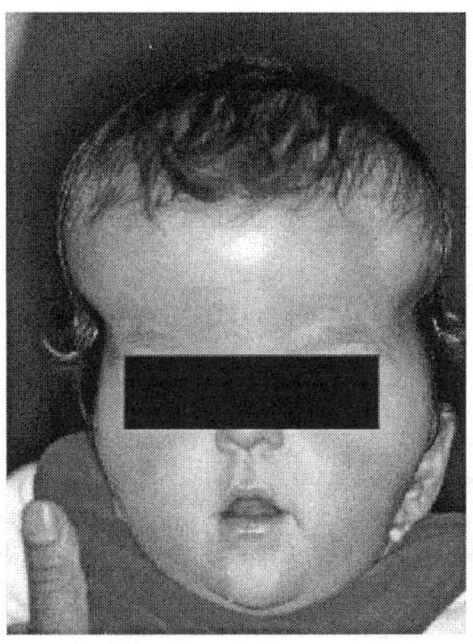 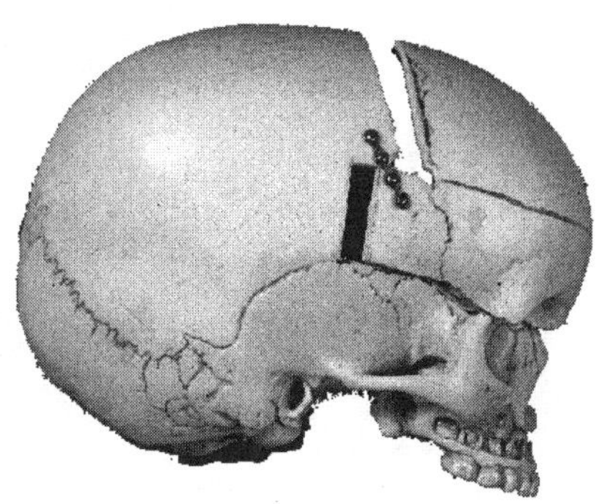

Figure 1: Patient with craniosynosthoses (left) and typical osteotomy (right)

bones are refixated with osteosynthesis plates. For a full description of the invention see
[9].

To transfer the generated plan optimally, it's necessary to support the exact execution of
the deformations. This work presents a system by means of the main bone segment, the
calotte, which guides the surgeon to the deformation process. The system compares the
target shape of the bone with the actual shape. The actual shape is obtained intra-
operatively with a surface scanning device. After evaluating the deviation from the target
shape with a standard computer system, the deviation values are visualised by projecting
them colour-coded directly on the bone. The surgeon uses this projection to adjust his next
deformation step as long as he consider the shapes to match.

2. Methods

The whole process is shown in figure 2. In the pre-operative phase a triangle mesh of the
skull is build with the initial CT-data. The model is used to plan the exact contours of the
calotte and how it's to be deformed. Along with the intra-operative osteotomy of the real
calotte this process is described in paragraph 2.1. In the intra-operative phase the real
calotte as well as the virtual target shape are available. After an initial deformation step,
manually performed by the surgeon (s. paragraph 2.4), the actual shape of the bone segment
is gathered with a surface scanning device (s. paragraph 0). Paragraph 2.3 describes the
comparison of the target with the actual shape and how we project differences. If the
degree of congruence isn't sufficient another deformation step will be necessary, if it is the
process will stop and the bone segment can be refixated. Now its shape matches the pre-
planned shape.

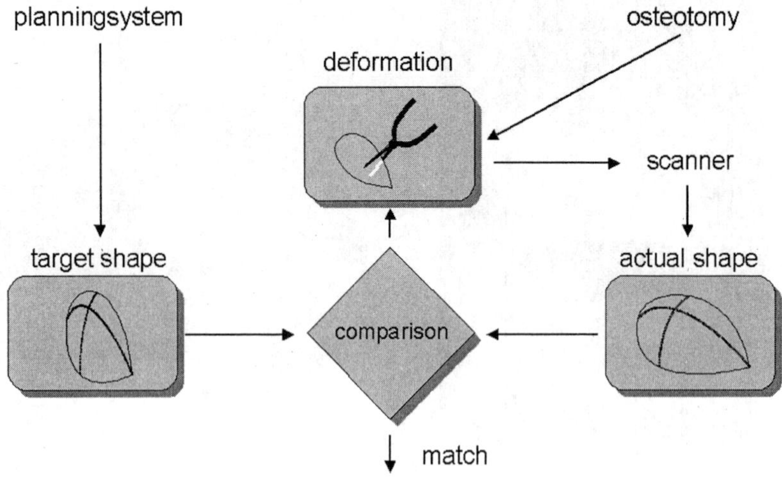

Figure 2: Process chain of the system

2.1 Preparations

Preparations are divided in a pre- and an intra-operative part. In pre-operative planning
stage a CT-scan of the head is segmented interactively, especially the bony structures. In
general we use simple threshold methods ore region growers. Afterwards a three-
dimensional mesh (triangles) of the skull is generated. We basically follow the way
described in [7]. The mesh is used to virtually cut, move and deform the bone segment
(figure 3).

During the intervention the surgeon is supported by an autonomous robot [14] or
augmented reality [12] to cut the bone segments in the pre-defined way.

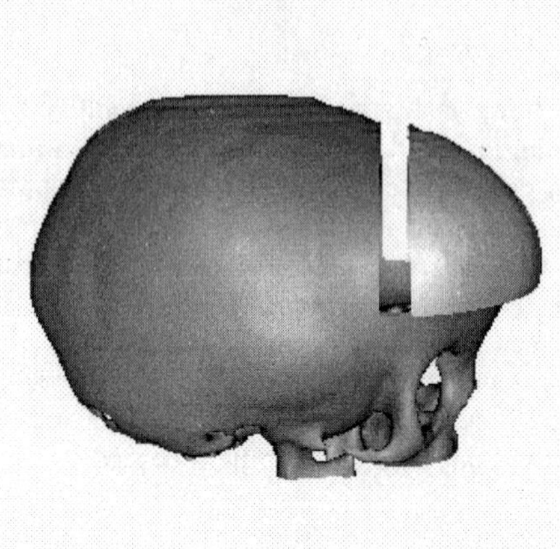

Figure 3: Mesh of the skull and planned (position and shape) calotte

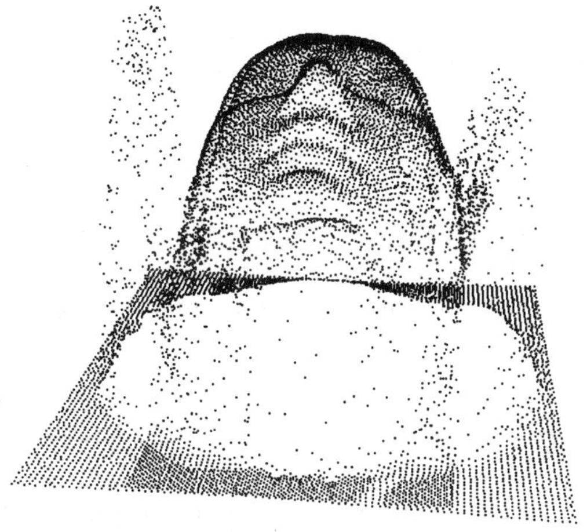

Figure 4: Intra-operatively gathered point cloud of a patient's head

2.2 Intra-operative Imaging

The hardware system consists of an off the shelf video projector, two CCD-cameras and a state-of-the-art PC (800 MHz CPU, 256 MByte RAM). The system is used to intra-operatively generate a 3D point cloud of an object's surface. This is done by projecting a sequence of stripe patterns (coded light) on top of the region of interest with the aid of the integrated video projector. The corresponding images are acquired by the cameras, analysed in consideration of emerging Moiré-patterns and yield a 3D point cloud of the scanned object [12] (s. figure 4).
Out of it we reconstruct the three-dimensional shape of the calotte. The real as well as the planned calotte are then available as triangle meshes.

2.3 Visualising deviations

To compare the triangle meshes it's necessary to match them as far as possible. As we work intra-operatively we use a simple register algorithm based on mass moments. It matches both models within one second but succeeds only in ca. 95%. If it fails the calculation will be redone, slightly changed. After five iterations the method succeeds in all cases (n ≈ 200). Next step is the calculation of the deviations. We cover the model of the actual calotte with a series of equally spaced points. For each point the orthogonal distance to the target is calculated. Alternatively a scalar criterion is available by accumulating all single distances.

To visualise the differences a variety of methods exists. Each point of the mesh can be assigned to a colour representing the distance to the target shape. Alternatively vectors can be visualised. The visualisation with the video projector normally uses the colour representation. For a description of the exact method to project virtual data on real objects see [12]. Ongoing research is engaged to develop methods to give the surgeon an idea not only where deviations of target and actual bone segment are, but how he/she should deform to reach a sufficient match easily and fast.

2.4 Deformation of the calotte

The surgeon manually deforms the bone segment. For a detailed description see [9]. When all bone segments match their associated planned model, the deformation process is stopped and the bones are positioned and fixed to the skull (figure 1, right) with osteosynthesis plates.

3. Results & discussion

A prototype of the above described system is in the last stage of technical tests. Bone segments are simulated using commercially available plasticine. The system allows an accurate shaping of planned bones with only a few iteration steps. To further decrease these steps we currently develop optimised visualisation techniques to indicate deviations fast and in a way that gives the surgeon an idea where and how to deform. Guidance should be as extensive as possible. To use the system in clinical practice there are some questions of accuracy and security to be answered.

The system extends the possibilities of current planning, simulation and execution procedures of surgical interventions. Whenever an object, medical or not, has to be brought in a specific target shape this system may be useful. It's easy to handle, comparatively small and easy to install in the operation room. In addition it's cheap. It enhances the accuracy and finally the quality of rearranging osteotomies as the post-operative appearance is an important goal of these interventions.

4. Acknowledgement

The work presented in this paper is part of the Sonderforschungsbereich 414, funded by the Deutsche Forschungsgemeinschaft (DFG).

5. References

[1]   J. Münchenberg, H. Wörn, J. Brief, C. Kübler, S. Hassfeld, J. Mühling: A Pattern Catalogue of Surgical Interventions for Computer-Supported Operation Planning, Medicine Meets Virtual Reality (MMVR), J.D. Westwood et al. (Eds.), pp. 227-229, 2000.

[2]   A. Lahmer, M. Börner, A. Bauer; Experiences with an image-guided planning system (ORTHODOC) for cementless hip replacement; Proceedings of First Joint Conference on Computer Vision, Virtual Reality and Robotics in Medicine and Medical Robotics and Computer Assisted Surgery (CVRMed-MRCAS '97), Grenoble, France, 1997.

[3]   Lueth et. al. ; A surgical Robot System for Maxillofacial Surgery. IEEE Int. Conf. On Industrial Electronics, Control and Instrumentation (IECON), Aachen, Germany, Sep.1998, pp. 2470-2475.

[4]   H. Wörn, J. Raczkowsky, D. Engel; Chirurgieroboter - eine Herausforderung an die Robotik; Robotik 2000, Berlin, 29.-30. Juni, 2000.

[5]   St. Haßfeld, J. Brief, R. Krempien, J. Raczkowsky, J. Münchenberg, H. Giess, H.P. Meinzer, U. Mende, H. Wörn, J. Mühling: Computerunterstützte Mund-, Kiefer und Gesichtschirurgie; Zeitschrift "Radiologe" 2000, Springer-Verlag, 2000, 40:218-226.

[6] H. Gärtner: Quantitative 3D-Vermessung mit codierter Beleuchtung. Institut für Technische Optik, Universität Stuttgart, 1998.

[7] Lorensen: „Creating Models From Segmented Images With VTK"; http://www.crd.ge.com/~lorensen/seg12/.

[8] Stephen Fedtke, Stefan Haßfeld, Joachim Mühling: Computerunterstützte Chirurgie; Vieweg, Wiesbaden, 1994.

[9] J. Mühling: *Kraniofaziale Chirurgie*. In: Kirschnersche allgemeine und spezielle Operationslehre; J.-E. Hausamen, E. Machtens, J. Reuther (Hrsg.); pp403-426; Springer Berlin-Heidelberg-New-York, ISBN 3-540-53865-8; 1995.

[10] S. Däuber et. al.: Creating a statistical atlas of the cranium; MMVR 2002

[11] H. Hoppe, J. Brief, S. Däuber, J. Raczkowsky, S. Haßfeld, and H. Wörn: *Projector Based Intraoperative Visualization of Surgical Planning Data*; ISRACAS 2001, Israeli Symposium on Computer-Aided Surgery, Medical Robotics, and Medical Imaging, Tel-Aviv, 2001

[12] H. Gärtner, "Quantitative 3D-Vermessung mit codierter Beleuchtung", Institut für Technische Optik, Universität Stuttgart, 1998.

[13] O. Schorr, J. Münchenberg, J. Raczkowsky, H. Wörn: *KasOp - A Generic System for Pre- and Intraoperative Surgical Assistance and Guidance*; In: H.U. Lemke, M.W. Vannier, K. Inamura, A.G. Farman, K. Doi; Proceedings of the 15th International Congress and Exhibition of Computer Assisted Radiology and Surgery (CARS).

[14] Dirk Engel, Jörg Raczkowsky, Heinz Wörn: *A Safe Robot System for Craniofacial Surgery*; ICRA 2001: IEEE International Conference On Robotics And Automation, Seoul, Korea, 2001

Medicine Meets Virtual Reality 02/10
J.D. Westwood et al. (Eds.)
IOS Press, 2002

Creating a statistical atlas of the cranium

*Sascha Däuber, **R. Krempien, *Michael Krätz, **Thomas Welzel and *Heinz Wörn

*University of Karlsruhe (TH), Institute for Process Control and Robotics, Kaiserstraße 12,
76128 Karlsruhe, Germany
**University of Heidelberg, Dept. of Clinical Radiology*

Abstract: Normative data is very important for simulation procedures in craniofacial surgery [1]. While treating e.g. a malformed skull the surgeon seeks to reconstruct its natural and harmonic shape. Atlas or normative data of the skull could support the surgeon in this effort [2], as it would provide a standard model of the skull which gives an idea of the natural shape. We create a standard skull by averaging regularly formed skulls in a shape space spanned by spherical harmonics. While state-of-the-art methods use landmarks to define the shape and mean shapes [4,5,6,14], this method is deterministic, i.e. it manages averaging without landmarks and it provides a complete description of the shape. In addition the shape space can be used to classify shapes to identify different types of an anatomy.

1. Motivation

Malformations of the skull's skeletal structures may occur for different reasons. Examples are accidents, tumor resection or craniosynosthoses, a disease of the cranial sutures. The latter one is surgically treated at the University of Heidelberg, Clinic for Cranio and Maxillofacial Surgery. Different bone segments are dissected, manually deformed and afterwards refixated in different positions. Figure 1 (left) shows an approx. one year old male patient with craniosynosthoses. The malformations, especially at the temples can be easily noticed. Figure 1 (right) shows typical dissection lines and refixation positions. For a full description of the invention see [7]. An important goal is to reconstruct the natural and harmonic shape of the patient's skull.

While deciding how to correct the bone malformation, the surgeon have to rely only upon his knowledge, experience and his sense of aesthetics. But to achieve non-subjective results of the postoperative skull it would be necessary to have an objective standard of the natural skull shape. An atlas or normative data of the skull shape could be such an objective standard. It would improve planning procedures in providing an image or model of the skull as it would appear, if the patient was healthy.

Generally speaking the lack of accurate normative data or atlases is the most significant obstacle for current simulation procedures in craniofacial surgery [1]. This work is engaged to create an atlas of skull shapes.

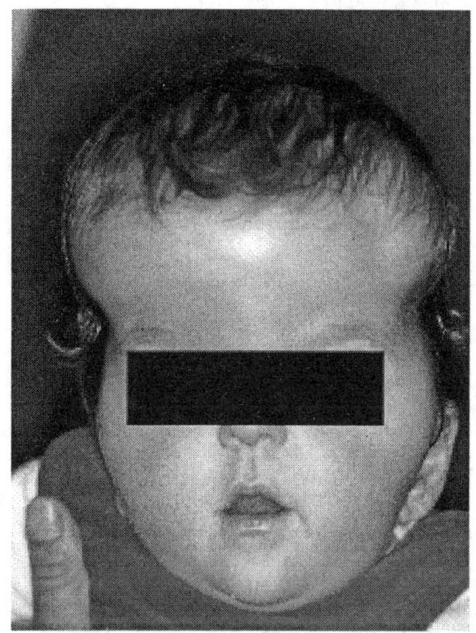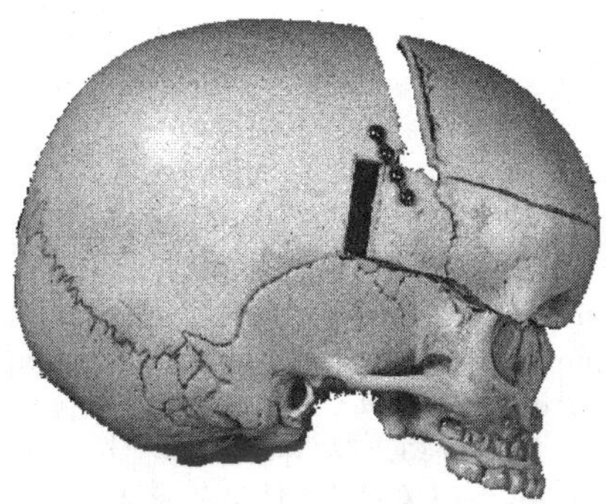

Figure 1: Patient with craniosynosthoses (left) and typical osteotomy (right)

2. Method

The basic idea is to collect a number of CT/MRT Scans of physiological patients, classify their skull shapes and calculate a mean of each class. The data is taken in daily routine, where the patient is scanned for diagnostic reasons and his/her skull shape turned out to be normal.

To calculate the mean, the shape has to be transformed to a representation which you can use to perform statistics. Most methods use landmarks [4,5,6,8] to do so. Unfortunately, it's impossible to find a sufficient amount of homologous landmarks [3] on the skull, especially on its back. It would be necessary to have landmarks equally distributed all over the head. A further drawback is that the set of the used landmarks determines the shape described with it. That makes the shape dependent on availability and choice of landmarks. Different sets of landmarks on the same object could describe a totally different shape. The method presented in this work describes the shape of an object completely, i.e. in a deterministic way.

2.1 Shape description

We use a complete set of orthogonal functions $Y_i(\vartheta,\varphi)$ and a linear transformation (1) to develop the function $r(\theta,\varphi)$ of the shape, defined on the unit sphere, into a series (2). The function $r(\theta,\varphi)$ specifies the distance of the origin to the margin of the shape along the direction defined by θ and φ.

$$c_i = \iint Y_i(\vartheta,\varphi)^* r(\vartheta,\varphi)\, d\vartheta\, d\varphi \tag{1}$$

$$r(\vartheta,\varphi) = \sum_i c_i Y_i(\vartheta,\varphi) \tag{2}$$

The coefficients c_i of the series describe the shape completely thus forming the so-called shape spectrum. We use the canonical spherical harmonics (3) as basis functions, a method first proposed by Brechbuehler [9]. The symbol j denotes the imaginary unit and P_l^m an associated Legendre polynomial. $Y_i(\vartheta,\varphi)^*$ denotes the complex conjugate of $Y_i(\vartheta,\varphi)$.

$$Y_i(\vartheta,\varphi) = \sqrt{\frac{(2n+1)(l-m)!}{4\pi(l+m)!}}\, P_l^m(\cos\vartheta)\, e^{jm\varphi}, \text{ where} \tag{3}$$

$$l = 0,1,2,\ldots$$

$$m = -l,-l+1,-l+2,\ldots,l-1,l$$

$$i = 2l+m$$

The accuracy of the provided description depends mainly on the amount of calculated coefficients. Theoretically the description is complete only if an infinite number are calculated. In practice you can terminate the series after a certain amount. The exact termination index is assessed by use of equation (2), the inversion of (1). Figure 2 shows the precision of the method. The left part shows the shape of a skull by means of a point cloud. That is the starting of the Shape analysis and is calculated with standard methods (e.g. dividing cubes [10]). The right part shows the reconstructed point cloud using 1300 coefficients. At the viscerocranium large variations occur, especially at sharp edges, but the back of the head shows good congruence (variation < 1mm). This is equivalent to the scale behavior of fourier (frequency) series.

2.2   Averaging shapes

The averaging of shapes is now realized using the coefficients of equation (1). At first the objects that ought to be averaged are analyzed, i.e. the shape spectra are calculated. For each index the mean coefficient is calculated using equation (4).

$$c_{i,mean} = \frac{1}{N}\sum_{n=1}^{N} c_{i,n} \tag{4}$$

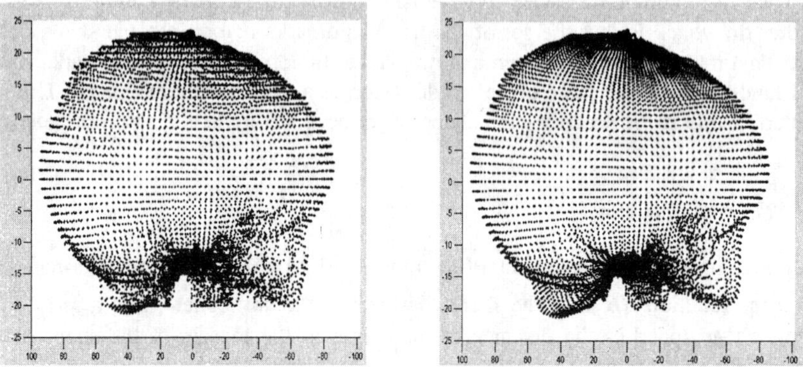

Figure 2: Original (left) and reconstructed shape (right)

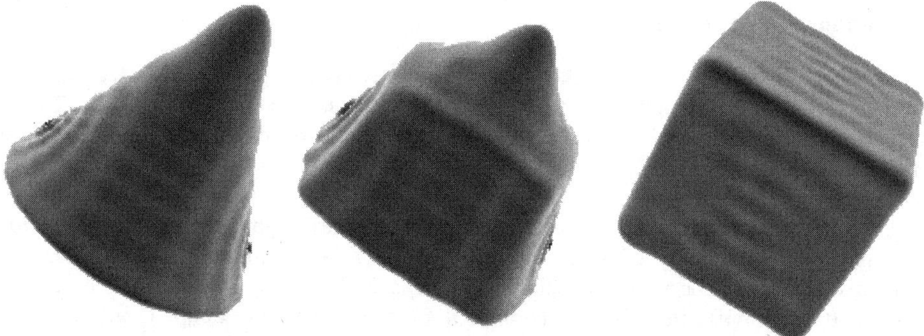

Figure 3: Two objects (cone and cube) and their calculated mean shape

By using the mean spectrum $c_{i,mean}$ and equation (2) to reconstruct the shape we receive a mean shape. For validation we use simple objects that we merge together, because on the basis of these simple shapes it's easier to find errors than on the basis of the far more complex skulls. Figure 3 shows two simple objects and the calculated shape in between. As common sense let you expect such a result, we consider the averaging process (4) to be valid.

2.3   Classifying shapes

As the coefficients give a full description of the shape, they can also be used to classify them. The spherical harmonics span a vector space where the coefficients form the coordinates. Each shape take up a single point in this high-dimensional shape space. Clusters of shapes could now be identified thus defining different shape classes. By creating the mean of all shapes in an individual class, we create the typical representation, the standard of this class.

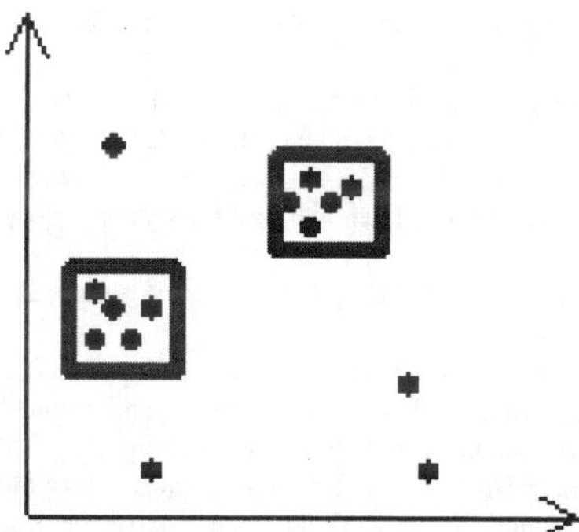

Figure 4: Classification in shape space: The frames contain accumulations of shapes thus defining classes

3. Summary and Conclusion

We present a method to describe the shape of an object in a volumetric data set (e.g. CT-scan). The description can be used to do statistics on the shapes. The method doesn't need any landmarks, hence the typical drawbacks of landmark methods (high degree of interaction, incomplete description, homology) can be avoided.
We use the shape description for averaging and to classify skull shapes. The mean shapes shall be calculated using physiological (healthy) skulls. They ought to be used in simulation and planning procedures of bone displacing surgical interventions as a standard or normative data of the desired postoperative appearance. We propose other applications, e.g. the classifying calcifications of the mamma[13], lung nodules[11] or tumors[12].

[1]   Altobelli DE, Kikines R, Mulliken JB, et al.: *Computer-assisted three dimensional planning in craniofacial surgery*, Plat Reconstr Surg 1993; 92:576-584

[2]   G. E. Christensen, S. C. Joshi, M. I. Miller: *Individualizing Anatomical Atlases of the Head*, in: K. Höhne, R. Kikinis (Hrsg.) Proceedings of 4th International Conference on Visualization in Biomedical Computing, Hamburg Germany, Lecture Notes in Computer Science 1131, Springer-Verlag Berlin, Heidelberg, September 1996, S. 343 - 348

[3]   F. L. Bookstein: *Landmark Methods for Forms Without Landmarks: Localizing Group Differences in Outline Shape*, IEEE Proceedings of MMBIA '96, 1996

[4]   Per Rønsholt Andresen*, Fred L. Bookstein, Knut Conradsen, Bjarne Kjær Ersbøll, Jeffrey L. Marsh, and Sven Kreiborg: *Surface-Bounded Growth Modeling Applied to Human Mandibles,* IEEE Transactions on Medical Imaging, vol. 19, no. 11, November 2000

[5]   Heinze, P.; Meister, D.; Kober, R.; Sungu, M.; Wörn, H.: *Statistischer Atlas zur Segmentierung des Kniegelenkes*; Rechner- und Sensorgestützte Chirurgie; Proceedings zum Workshop 19.-20. Juli, Heidelberg, 2001: 174-180

[6]   Lorenz, C.; Krahnstover, N.: *3D statistical shape models for medical image segmentation,* 3-D Digital Imaging and Modeling, 1999. Proceedings. Second International Conference on, 1999, Page(s): 414 – 423

[7]   J. Mühling: *Kraniofaziale Chirurgie.* In: Kirschnersche allgemeine und spezielle Operationslehre; J.-E. Hausamen, E. Machtens, J. Reuther (Hrsg.); pp403-426; Springer Berlin-Heidelberg-New-York, ISBN 3-540-53865-8; 1995.

[8]   Beil W, Rohr K und Stiehl S: *Investigation of Approaches for the Localization of Anatomical Landmarks in 3D Medical Images*, Comp Ass Rad Surg. Proc 11th Internat Symposium and Exhibition: 265-270. 1997

[9]   Ch. Brechbühler and G. Gerig and O. Kübler: *Parametrization of closed surfaces for 3-D shape description*; Computer Vision and Image Understanding: CVIU, 61(2), pp. 154-170, March 1995.

[10]   W. J. Schroeder, K. M. Martin und W. E. Lorensen: *The Visualization Toolkit: An object-oriented approach to 3D graphics*, 2nd Edition, Prentice Hall PTR New Jersey, USA (1998), ISBN 0/13/954694/4.

[11]   Reeves AP, Kostis WJ; Computer-aided diagnosis of small pulmonary nodules; *Semin Ultrasound CT MR* 2000 Apr;21(2):116-28

[12]   Handels, H. Roßmanith, C., Rinast, E., Weiss, H.-D. und Pöppl, S.J., „Objektbezogene Bildanalyse von Hirntumoren zur Unterstützung der neuroradiologischen Diagnostik", H.J. Trampisch und S. Lange (eds.), Medizinische Forschung – Ärztliches Handeln, MMV Medizin Verlag, München, 1995

[13]   Lori Mann Bruce: *Classifying Mammographic Mass Shapes Using the Wavelet Transform Modulus-Maxima Method*, IEEE Transactions on Medical Imaging, vol. 18, no. 12

[14]   Dean D, Bookstein FL, Koneru S, Lee J-H, Kamath J, Cutting CB, Hans M, Goldberg J: Average African American three-dimensional computed tomography skull images: the potential clinical importance of ethnicity and sex; J Craniofac Surg 1998 Jul; 9(4): (Page(s): 348-358)

Augmented Reality and Training for Airway Management Procedures

Larry Davis[†], Yonggang Ha[†], Seth Frolich[‡], Glenn Martin[‡], Catherine Meyer[†], Beth Pettitt[◊], Jack Norfleet[◊], Kuo-Chi Lin[‡], and Jannick P. Rolland[†]

[†]*School of Optics/CREOL University of Central Florida*
4000 Central Florida Blvd Orlando, FL 32816-2700

[‡]*Institute for Simulation and Training*
3280 Progress Drive Orlando, FL 32826

[◊]*U.S. Army Simulation, Training, and Instrumentation Command*
12350 Research Parkway, Orlando, FL 32826

Abstract: Augmented reality is often used for interactive, three-dimensional visualization within the medical community. To this end, we present the integration of an augmented reality system that will be used to train military medics in airway management. The system demonstrates how a head-mounted projective display can be integrated with a desktop PC to create an augmented reality visualization. Furthermore, the system, which uses a lightweight optical tracker, demonstrates the low cost and the portability of the application.

1. Introduction

Airway management is a common practice and critical skill for paramedics. To safely secure the airway during cardiopulmonary resuscitation (CPR) and ensure immediate ventilation and/or oxygenation, paramedics often perform a rapid sequence of endotracheal intubation (ETI), which consists of inserting a tracheal tube through the mouth into the trachea and then sealing the trachea so that all air passes through the tube.

However, there are inherent difficulties with ETI. In the case of severe trauma patients, emergency airway management is classified as a cause of pre-hospital (before emergency arrival at a hospital) death trauma by the American Heart Association [1]. A study by Orlando Regional Healthcare showed that out of 108 ETI patients who arrived at the Orlando Regional Medical Center emergency room from May 1 to Dec. 31, 1997, 27 had tubes that were placed mistakenly in either the esophagus or the voice box. Of the 27 patients with misplaced tubes, 13 died in the emergency room [2]. Moreover, in a 16 hospital study conducted by the National Emergency Airway Registry between August 1997 and October 1998, out of 2392 recorded ETIs, 309 complications were reported, with 132 of these difficulties resulting from intubation techniques [3].

The skills required to intubate a patient are not easily practiced, deteriorate over time, and can be costly with limited resources available. Due to the complex structure of the tube, extensive instruction and training are required in order to ensure its correct placement within an acceptable time frame. Intubation failure rates are caused more often by a lack of training than by the choice of airway devices themselves [4].

Thus, there is international concern for the need for extensive training of paramedics for pre-hospital emergency situations both in Europe and in the United States [5]. Current training methods for airway management procedures involve videos, printed media, classroom lectures and training on mannequins to develop the necessary skills. However, from the data presented, it appears that other efforts may be necessary to increase the rate of successful ETIs.

In an effort to improve airway management training, we present an augmented reality (AR) system that allows paramedics to practice their skills and provides them with visual feedback they could not otherwise obtain. Utilizing a human patient simulator from Medical Education Technologies, Inc. (METI) combined with three-dimensional (3D) visualization of the airway anatomy and the endotracheal tube, paramedics will be able to obtain a visual and tactile sense of proper ETI.

In the following sections, we review previous medical AR research, describe the methods used to realize the anatomical visualization for ETI, detail the airway visualization, and discuss observations made within the course of the research.

2. Previous Medical AR Research

There have been numerous AR applications developed for use in medicine. Peuchot et al. developed a system to aid surgeons in correcting scoliosis in patients [6]. State et al. applied video and ultrasound technology to develop an AR system for ultrasound-guided biopsies of breast lesions [7]. An enhanced version of the system developed in [7] was later used by Fuchs et al. in a laparoscopic surgical application that used structured light patterns for tracking within the application [8].

DiGioia et al. merged CT data with real world images using a flat-paneled monitor and a half silvered mirror that was not head-mounted, tracking the head of the user to display CT data from the correct point of view [9]. As an improvement to the system presented in [9], Stetten and Chib presented a method to overlay ultrasound data that was also not head-mounted but tracked user position using an ultrasound stylus [10]. Grimson et al. presented an AR system to aid brain surgeons [11] and Edwards et al. developed a system to project features from MR and CT data in a stereo microscope to assist with visualizing complex structures during surgery [12].

Outside of the realm of surgery, a fetal visualization AR system, using a video see-through HMD, was developed by Bajura et al. [13]. There have also been efforts to use AR to overcome ambulatory difficulties associated with Parkinson's Disease [14].

Within our research group, it was suggested by Wright et al. that virtual reality could be used to teach medical practitioners about the complex motion of anatomical joints [15]. In this context, Baillot et al. created a physical model of knee motion that resulted in realistic knee joint animations at interactive speed [16]. The research in [16] lead to an augmented reality implementation of the VRDA Tool, an AR system designed to allow medical practitioners to dynamically visualize internal joint anatomy [17] [18]. The methods presented in [17] and [18] constitute a basic theoretical framework that we are further developing to create a desktop AR visualization of anatomical airways, now detailed.

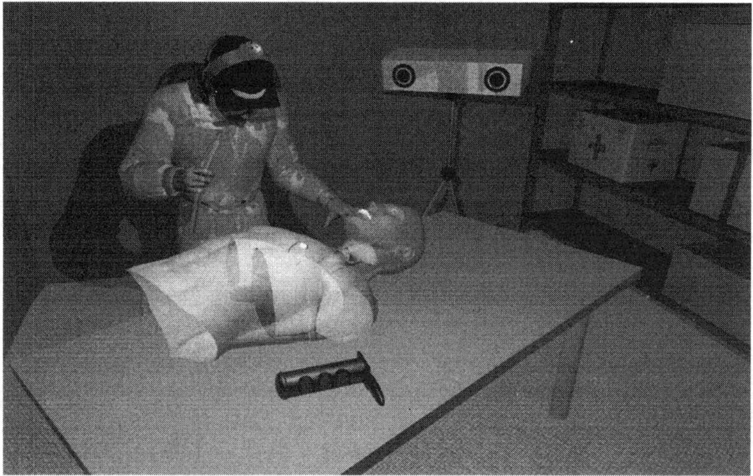

Fig. 1: Conceptual intubation of a HPS with superimposed anatomy

3. Method Overview

The AR system integrates a head-mounted projective display (HMPD) with a desktop PC to visualize internal airway anatomy on a human patient simulator (HPS). The concept of the HMPD will be reviewed in Section 4. The advantages of using a HMPD in this application are the lightweight optics (8g per eye) and the high quality images obtained from projection optics as opposed to eyepiece optics employed in conventional, optical see-through HMDs [19]. The location of the HPS, the trainee, and the endotracheal tube are obtained with a tracking system. A curvature measurement device is also used to assist in tracking the endotracheal tube. The HPS is a mannequin with several simulated human functions, including respiration, heart beat, and eye movements. Moreover, with respect to the airway, the HPS is anatomically correct. The trainee wears the HMPD and is able to see the internal airway anatomy due to retro-reflective material that has been placed on the throat and chest of the HPS. Thus, the trainee can see the airway anatomy, see the endotracheal tube, and feel normal bodily functions while practicing an intubation. A conceptual diagram of the application setting is shown in Fig. 1 and a picture of the intubed HPS is shown in Fig. 2.

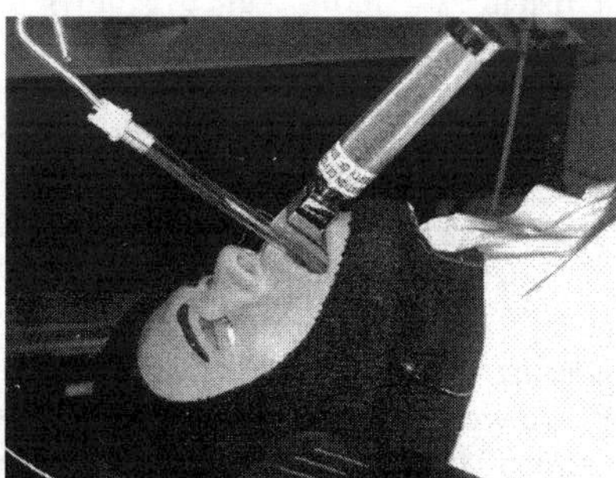

Fig. 2:The HPS with endotracheal tube and intubation tool

4. Visualization of the Airway

With the exception of the HMPD, the airway visualization is realized using commercially available hardware components. The computer used for computations and stereoscopic rendering has a 1GHz AMD Thunderbird CPU and uses Red Hat Linux 7.0 as its operating system. The graphics card used is a dual-head, Asus GeForce2MX. The tracking system used is a Polaris hybrid optical tracker, capable of tracking up to three objects simultaneously. The tracking data obtained is updated at 40 Hz. The current system configuration is shown in Fig.3.

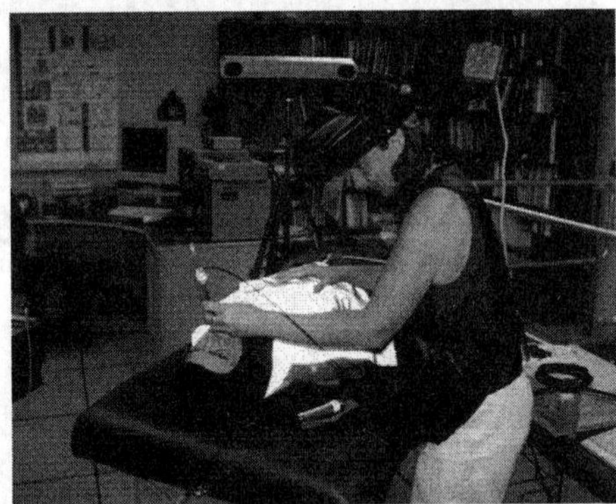

Fig. 3: The system setup, consisting of an optical tracker, desktop computer, HMPD, and curvature measurement device

Head-mounted projective displays are a novel type of HMD. They differ from conventional HMDs in that the images are formed using projection optics. Similar to a LCD projector, a HMPD projects computer-generated images into the environment. However, a HMPD uses a retro-reflective screen instead of a diffusing projection screen. In a HMPD, the image from the LCD is projected to a beam splitter, directed by the beam splitter toward the retro-reflective screen, reflected back in the same direction by the retro-reflective screen, and passes through the beam splitter to the eye of the user. The concept and design of a HMPD as well as a discussion of engineering and perceptual issues can be found in [20].

The HMPD used in this application has a diagonal, binocular field of view of 52 degrees. Retro-reflective material is placed on the neck and chest of the HPS to see the computer models. The HMPD displays images at a resolution of 640x480 and the models are rendered at a distance of 1m from the eyepoints. The airway model is 665 kB with 1.4 MB of texture and transparency enabled. The endotracheal tube model is 80 kB. The application is currently implemented in Open Inventor 2.0.

5. Observations and Future Work

In the course of this research, we made several observations. The first was that the quality and speed of rendering was excellent, considering the consumer-level pricing of the system. Moreover, we were able to use an operating system and software that, aside from the expenditure of time, was free and available to the general public. These two events lead us to believe that high-fidelity desktop stereoscopic rendering is possible. We also observed that a side benefit of using a HMPD is that some of the occlusion effects are preserved [20]. Specifically, objects passing between the user and the retro-reflective material occlude the computer-generated objects, as opposed to other see-through head-mounted displays.

In addition to the observations made, we gained valuable knowledge. We learned that there are substantial amounts of time and resourcefulness required for AR development on the Linux PC platform. We had to overcome hardware driver incompatibility issues. Specifically, to interface with the curvature measurement device and the tracking system, we had to write a Linux driver and API, respectively. Furthermore, the display parameters had to be adjusted to specify the resolution of the system, the color depth, the use of OpenGL, and the locations of the stereoscopic windows within the frame buffer. However, these issues will likely improve as more Linux development occurs.

As part of future research, we plan to make various enhancements to the airway management training system. We anticipate the availability of full, 3D curvature measurement devices and plan to integrate such a device in the system to allow modeling of throat dynamics. We also plan to improve the HMPD illumination via enhanced materials, with the end goal of full daylight visualization capability. In addition, the HMPD will become wireless, adding to the overall deployability of the system. An implementation in Open Performer 2.4 will be investigated and compared to the Open Inventor implementation to allow broad dissemination of the research. Finally, we shall begin perception and performance studies with combat medics to gauge the effectiveness of AR airway management training.

6. Acknowledgments

The authors thank Yann Argotti and Valerie Outters for their work in developing a first implementation of the Open Inventor visualization. The authors also thank Stephen Johnson and Ben Del Vento for their assistance. The application presented was funded by the U.S. Army Simulation, Training, and Instrumentation Command (STRICOM) and the Florida Education Fund. Furthermore, the overall virtual environment research that supports many components of the research presented is supported by the National Institute of Health under grant 1-R29-LM06322-01A1 and the National Science Foundation under grants EIA-99-86051 and NSF/ITR IIS-00-83037.

References

[1] American Heart Association. Guidelines for Cardiopulmonary Resuscitation and Emergency Cardiac Care – Part II : Adult Basic Life Support. *Journal of the American Medical Association*, 268:2184–2198, 1992.

[2] R. Suriano. "Intubation Major Issue for Paramedics". *The Orlando Sentinel*, February 16 2001.

[3] R. Walls, E. Barton, and A. McAfee. 2,392 Emergency Department Intubations: First Report of the Ongoing National Emergency Airway Registry Study (Near 97). *Annals of Emergency Medicine*, 26:364–403, 1999.

[4] P. Pepe, B. Zachariah, and N. Chandra. Invasive Airway Techniques in Resuscitation. *Annals of EmergencyMedicine*, 26:364–403, 1993.

[5] European Resuscitation Council and the American Heart Association (AHA) in collaboration with the International Liaison Committee on Resuscitation (ILCOR). International Guidelines for Cardiopulmonary Resuscitation andemergency cardiac care-An International Consensus on Science. Technical Report 102, European Resuscitation Council (ERC), 2000. Supplement 1:22-59.

[6] B. Peuchot, A. Tanguy, and M. Eude. Virtual Reality as an Operative Tool During Scoliosis Surgery. In *Proceedings of CVRMed '95*, pp. 549–554, 1995.

[7]   A. State, M. Livingston, W. Garrett, G. Hirota, M. Whitton, E. Pisano, and H. Fuchs. Technologies for Augmented Reality Systems: Realizing Ultrasound-Guided Needle Biopsies.

[8]   H. Fuchs, M. Livingston, R. Raskar, D. Colucci, K. Keller, A. State, J. Crawford, P. Rademacher, S. Drake, and A. Meyer. Augmented Reality Visualization for Laparoscopic Surgery. In *Proceedings of MICCAI '98*, pp. 934–943. Springer-Verlag, 1998.

[9]   A. DiGioia, B. Colgan, and N. Koerbel. Computer Aided Surgery. In: R. Satava (ed.), Cybersurgery. Wiley Press, 1998.

[10] G. Stetten and V. Chib. Real Time Tomographic Reflection with Ultrasound: Stationary and Hand-Held Implementations. Technical Report CMU-RI-TR-00-28, Carnegie Mellon University, 2000.

[11] W. Grimson, R. Kikinis, F. Jolesz, and P. Black. Image Guided Surgery. *Scientific American*, 282(1):63–69, 1999.

[12] Edwards, P.J. and A.P. King and C.R. Maurer and D.A. de Cunha and D.J. Hawkes and D.L.G. Hill and R.P. Gaston and M.R. Fenlon, A. Jusczyzck and A.J. Strong and C.L. Chandler and M.J. Gleeson. Design and Evaluation of a System for Microscope-Assisted Guided Interventions (MAGI). *IEEE Transactions on Medical Imaging*, 19(11):1082–1093, 2000.

[13] M. Bajura, H. Fuchs, and R. Ohbuchi. Merging Virtual Objects with the Real World: Seeing Ultrasound Imagery within the Patient. In *Proceedings of SIGGRAPH '92*, pp. 203–210. ACM SIGGRAPH, July 1992.

[14] S. Weghorst. Augmented Reality and Parkinson's Disease. *Communications of the ACM*, 40(8):47–48, 1997.

[15] D. Wright, J. Rolland, and A. Kancherla. Using Virtual Reality to Teach Radiographic Positioning. *Radiologic Technology*, 66(4):167–172, 1995.

[16] Y. Baillot, J. Rolland, K. Lin, and D. Wright. Automatic Modeling of Knee-Joint Motion for the Virtual Reality Dynamic Anatomy (VRDA) Tool. *Presence: Teleoperators and Virtual Environments*, 9(3): 223–235, 2000.

[17] Y. Argotti, V. Outters, L. Davis, A. Sun, and J. Rolland. Technologies for Augmented Reality: Calibration for Real-Time Superimposition on Rigid and Simple-Deformable Real Objects. In *The Fourth International Conference on Medical Image Computing and Computer-Assisted Intervention (MICCAI '01), Utrecht, The Netherlands*. Springer-Verlag, October 2001.

[18] Y. Argotti, L. Davis, V. Outters, and J. Rolland. Dynamic Superimposition of Synthetic Objects on Rigid and Simple-Deformable Real Objects. In *The Second IEEE and ACM International Symposium on Augmented Reality (ISAR '01), New York, NY*. IEEE Computer Society, IEEE Press, October 2001.

[19] J. Rolland, W. Gibson, and D. Ariely. Towards Quantifying Depth and Size Perception in Virtual Environments. *Presence:Teleoperators and Virtual Environments*, 4(1):24–49,1995.

[20] H. Hua, A. Girardot, C. Gao, and J. Rolland. Engineering of Head-Mounted Projective Displays. *Applied Optics*, 39(22):3814–3824, 2000.

Medicine Meets Virtual Reality 02/10
J.D. Westwood et al. (Eds.)
IOS Press, 2002

Multimodal Simulation of Laparoscopic Heller Myotomy Using a Meshless Technique

S. De[1], M. Manivannan[1], J. Kim[1], M. A. Srinivasan[1] and D. Rattner[2]
[1]Laboratory for Human and Machine Haptics,
Massachusetts Institute of Technology, Cambridge, MA 02139

[2]Division of General and Gastrointestinal Surgery,
Massachusetts General Hospital, Boston, MA 02114

Abstract. In this work we focus our attention on developing a surgical simulator for performing laparoscopic Heller myotomy using force feedback. A meshless numerical technique, the method of finite spheres, is used for the purpose of physically based, real time haptic and graphical rendering of soft tissues. Localized discretization allows display of deformations in the vicinity of the tool tip as well as interaction forces at high update rates (kHz). Novel cutting algorithms are implemented using point-based representation of anatomical models. Graphical rendering is accomplished by using a recently developed volumetric rendering technique known as splatting.

1. Introduction

Over the past few years, laparoscopic esophageal myotomy (Heller myotomy) has emerged as the surgical treatment of choice for the management of a rare esophageal motility disorder known as achalasia (see Figure 1). During the laparoscopoic procedure the outer longitudinal muscle layer and the inner circular muscle layer surrounding the lower esophageal sphincter (LES) are incised allowing it to open more easily. Benefits of this approach include five small incisions instead of one large abdominal incision, shorter hospital stay, reduced postoperative pain and a shorter recovery time of a few days.

The success of a laparoscopic surgeon depends heavily on his or her training. In this work we focus on the development of a multimodal virtual environment system that allows the user to perform laparoscopic Heller myotomy using his/her senses of vision as well as touch. Such a system will not only result in customized practice environments for surgical residents, but will also reduce the use of animals and cadavers that are currently used for such training.

One major requirement of such a surgical trainer is real time performance [1]. For real time visual display an update rate of 30 Hz is sufficient. We use a Phantom haptic interface device that records the position and orientation of the user's hands and conveys to him/her forces resulting from the interaction of the virtual laparoscopic tool with the computer model of the esophagus. For stable simulation, the haptic loop requires an update rate of about 1kHz. This imposes severe restrictions on the complexity of the models that can be rendered haptically.

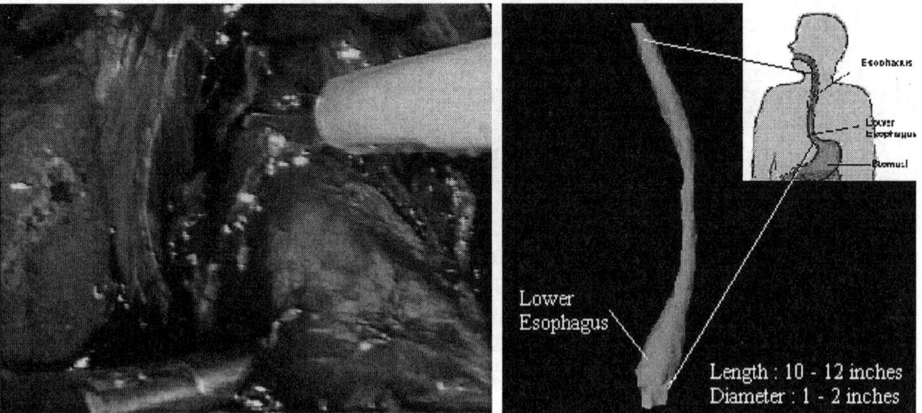

Figure 1. A snapshot of the Heller myotomy procedure is shown on the left. A model of the esophagus is shown on the right.

The material modeling of the soft tissue that comprises the esophagus is quite challenging. Soft tissues exhibit complex material properties [2]. They are nonlinear, anisotropic, viscoelastic, nonhomogeneous and layered. It is quite difficult to obtain *in vivo* material properties of the esophagus. We have performed *in vivo* experiments on the esophagus of pigs and developed linear elastic material models that have been used in our simulations. See [3] for details regarding the experiments and results.

Several researchers have applied finite element techniques for real time surgical simulations [1, 4, 5]. However, finite element techniques suffer from certain drawbacks in real time simulations. First, the contact between tool and tissues must occur only at nodal points. Therefore, to prevent loss of resolution, the density of nodal points should be sufficiently high. This requires extensive memory resources and high computational overhead. Second, cutting or tearing requires an expensive remeshing process during simulation. This means precomputed data of the object becomes, at least locally, invalid and all the data displayed to the user must be computed in real time. The computation time increases approximately as the cube of the number of nodal unknowns. This poses significant obstacles in real time applications, given the high rate of force updates required.

In [6] we presented a meshless numerical scheme, the method of finite spheres, for laparoscopic surgical simulation that does not suffer from these problems. In this technique nodal points are sprinkled locally around the surgical tool tip and the interpolation is performed by functions that are nonzero only on spheres surrounding the nodes. The governing partial differential equations of elasticity are applied at the nodal points only (a technique known as "collocation"). A force extrapolation technique was then used to obtain real time performance.

In this paper we use a point-based discretization of the geometric model and use the meshless technique to compute local deformations. We use splatting techniques to render our point-based geometrical model. Recently, a number of researchers have demonstrated the efficiency of splatting for rendering geometrically complex objects [7,8]. Splatting is a technique for representing continuous texture function of the surface of point-based models. With each point a reconstruction kernel (called a splat) is associated, which is usually a Gaussian distribution. Therefore, a single point is mapped to multiple pixels, and the resulting color of the pixel is the cumulative of all the contributing pixel colors. We have introduced splatting techniques to simulate cutting in this paper.

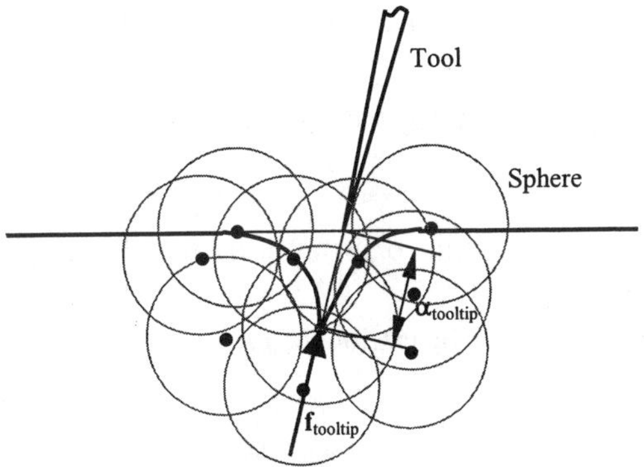

Figure 2. A laparoscopic surgical tool interacting with the surface of an organ. MFS nodes are distributed in the vicinity of the tool tip to obtain a localized discretization. $\alpha_{tooltip}$ and $f_{tooltip}$ are the prescribed displacement and reaction force at the tool tip, respectively.

In the next section we briefly introduce the MFS technique we have adopted in computing the deformation fields and reaction forces. In section 3 we discuss the technique we use to implement surgical cutting in the context of laparoscopic Heller myotomy.

2. The computation of deformation fields and reaction forces

In this section we briefly summarize the method of finite spheres. In this technique, we distribute nodal points around the surgical tool tip and define spherical "influence zones" around each node (see Figure 1). The approximation u_h of a variable u (e.g. displacement), using 'N' spheres, may be written as

$$u_h(\mathbf{x}) = \sum_{J=1}^{N} h_J(\mathbf{x})\alpha_J \tag{1}$$

where α_J is the nodal unknown at node J. The nodal shape function $h_J(\mathbf{x})$ at node J is generated using a moving least squares technique

$$h_J(\mathbf{x}) = W_J(\mathbf{x})\mathbf{P}(\mathbf{x})^T \mathbf{A}^{-1}(\mathbf{x})\mathbf{P}(\mathbf{x}_J) \qquad J=1,\ldots,N \tag{2}$$

where

$$\mathbf{A}(\mathbf{x}) = \sum_{I=1}^{N} W_I(\mathbf{x})\mathbf{P}(\mathbf{x}_I)\mathbf{P}(\mathbf{x}_I)^T . \tag{3}$$

The vector $\mathbf{P}(\mathbf{x})$ contains polynomials ensuring consistency up to a desired order (in our implementation we have chosen $\mathbf{P}(\mathbf{x}) = \{1,x,y,z\}^T$ to ensure a first order accurate scheme in 3D, similar to bilinear finite elements). W_J is a quartic spline radial weighting function at node J. We assume linear elastic tissue behavior and satisfy the elasticity equations only at the nodal points to obtain the discretized set of equations

$$\mathbf{KU} = \mathbf{f} \tag{4}$$

where $\mathbf{K}$ is the stiffness matrix and $\mathbf{f}$ is the vector containing nodal loads.

A node is placed at the tool tip ($\mathbf{x}_{tooltip}$) and we use a singular weighting function

$$\widetilde{W}_{tooltip} = W_{tooltip} \left\| \mathbf{x} - \mathbf{x}_{tooltip} \right\|_0^{-p} \;\; ; (p{>}0 \text{ is an integer and } \left\| \cdot \right\|_0 \text{ is the Euclidean norm}) \qquad (5)$$

at this node to enforce that the displacement computed at the tool tip using equation (1) is the one prescribed at the tool tip ($\mathbf{U}_{tooltip}$).

The stiffness matrix in Eq (3) may be partitioned as

$$\mathbf{K} = \begin{bmatrix} \mathbf{K}_{aa} & \mathbf{K}_{ab} \\ \mathbf{K}_{ba} & \mathbf{K}_{bb} \end{bmatrix} \qquad (6)$$

corresponding to a partitioning of the vector of nodal parameters as $\mathbf{U} = \begin{bmatrix} \mathbf{U}_{tooltip} & \mathbf{U}_b \end{bmatrix}^T$ where $\mathbf{U}_b$ is the vector of nodal unknowns which maybe obtained as $\mathbf{U}_b = -\mathbf{K}_{bb}^{-1}\mathbf{K}_{ba}\mathbf{U}_{toooltip}$. The reaction force to be delivered to the haptic interface device is obtained as $\mathbf{f}_{tooltip} = \mathbf{K}_{aa}\mathbf{U}_{tooltip} + \mathbf{K}_{ab}\mathbf{U}_b$.

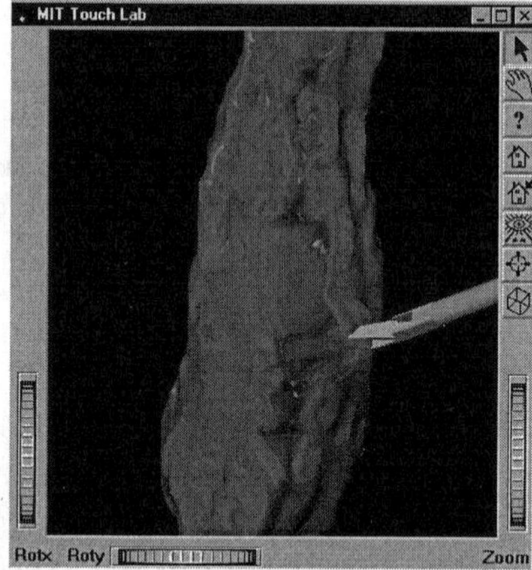

Figure 3. A snapshot of Heller myotomy simulation. Photorealistic textures are applied to the surface of an esophagus model.

3. Simulation of meshless cutting using splats

The concept of representing objects as a set of points and using these as rendering primitives has been introduced in a report by Levoy and Whitted [7]. Splatting, one of the recent image based volume rendering algorithms introduced by Lee Westover [8] in 1990, performs a front-to-back object-order traversal of the voxels in the volumetric dataset. Each voxel's contribution to the image is accumulated. Since this procedure is very similar to throwing a snowball (voxel's contribution to image) at a flat surface it is called splatting, where the amount of snow at the center of impact will be high and it drops off further away from the center. A reconstruction kernel determines the contribution of each voxel and the projection of this kernel into the image buffer is known as a footprint. The size of the footprint is proportional to the volume and the image to be generated and its shape is usually Gaussian.

This has the effect of increasing the contribution from voxels near the center of projection and reducing from those far from the center.

Use of points as geometric primitives is quite a deviation from the traditional use of triangular primitives that have connectivity information. Therefore, the primary challenge of point-based rendering is the reconstruction of this connectivity information from point clouds, i.e., reconstructing the continuous surface. The reconstruction algorithm should guarantee that there are no holes left on the surface [9]. While reconstruction algorithms guarantees that there are no holes left on the surface, cutting in point-based models involves deliberately creating discontinuities or holes by selecting regions of interest.

The first stage in the haptic rendering of cutting operation involves finding the point of contact or collision detection. Collision detection algorithms available in the literature are only for polygonal meshes. Haptic rendering or collision detection algorithms for point-based models are not known. We have developed a Z-buffer based [10] collision detection technique for point-based models.

To detect collision we shoot a ray from the camera to the tip of the force feedback device. The Z-buffer value at the intersection of this ray with the surface is used to decide whether there is indeed a collision. Collision occurs when: (a) the Z-buffer value of the tip is greater than that of the splats at the intersection while the back face is culled; and (b) the Z-buffer value is less than that of the splats at the intersection while the front face is culled.

Once collision is detected the tissue is deformed using the method of finite spheres. When the reaction force at the tool tip exceeds a critical value, the tissue is cut. Traditionally, cutting task is defined and simulated as splitting polygonal surfaces along a collection of marked edges and vertices [11]. Since point-based models do not have this connectivity information, we have developed special algorithms to find the neighboring points and move those points accordingly. After the tissue is cut, the layer beneath the surface is visible and the points are splat-rendered.

Figure 4 shows a schematic diagram of the point-based rendering paradigm and a snapshot of an esophagus model, generated using 4770 points and being cut using the scheme just described. Part of the code is used from Qsplat [9], a point rendering system that was designed to render large data sets produced by modern scanning devices.

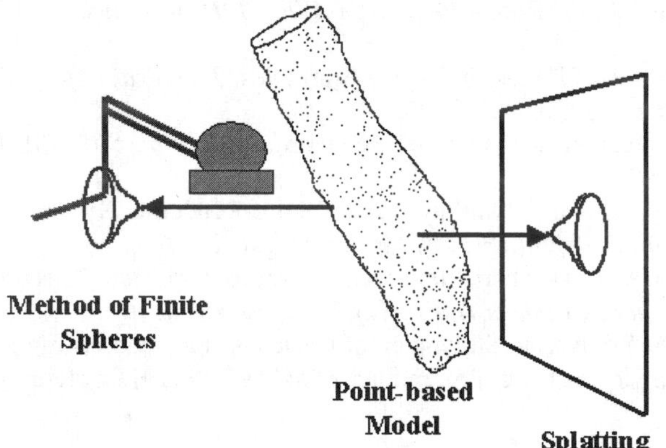

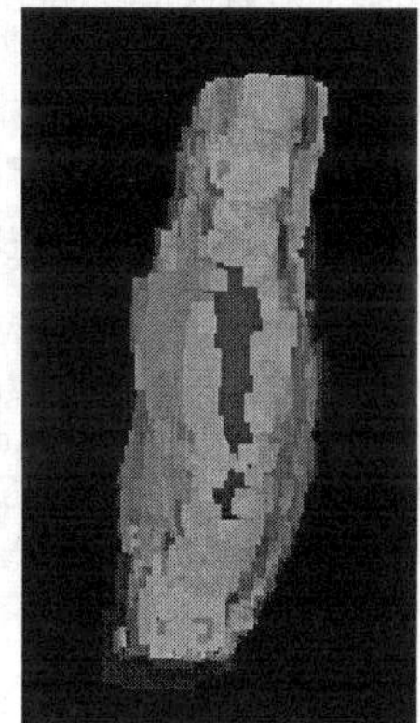

Figure 4. Schematic diagram of mashless cutting using splats (left). The actual cut esophagus is shown on the right.

4. Concluding remarks

In this paper we present a point-based paradigm for representing soft objects during multimodal medical simulations in general, and laparoscopic Heller myotomy, in particular. While a localized point based method of finite spheres is used to compute the deformation fields and reaction forces, a meshless cutting technique is implemented using splats. A new collision detection algorithm using the Z-buffer is also presented. The techniques are quite general and powerful. Further improvements in implementation may be achieved by coupling the localized method of finite spheres with a global discretization (which may be quite coarse) of the organ.

Acknowledgements: This work was supported by a grant from Harvard Center for Minimally Invasive Surgery.

References

[1] C. Basdogan, C. H. Ho and M. A. Srinivasan, Virtual Environments for Medical Training: Graphical and Haptic Simulation of Laparoscopic Common Bile Duct Exploration, *IEEE/ASME Trans. on Mechatronics*, (2001) Vol. 6, No. 3.

[2] S. De and M. A. Srinivasan, Thin Walled Models for Haptic and Graphical Rendering of Soft Tissues in Surgical Simulation, *Proceedings of MMVR 7 Conference* (1999) 94-99.

[3] B. K. Tay, S. De, N. Stylopoulos, D.W. Rattner and M. A. Srinivasan, *In vivo* Force Response of Intra-Abdominal Soft Tissue for the Simulation of Laparoscopic Procedures, *Proceedings of MMVR 2002 Conference* (2002)

[4] M. Bro-Nielsen and S. Cotin, Real Time Volumetric Deformable Models for Surgery Simulation Using Finite Elements and Condensation, *Proceedings of Computer Graphics Forum, Eurographics 96* (1996) 57-66.

[5] S. Cotin, H. Delingette, J. M. Clement, V. Tassetti, J. Marescaux and N. Ayache, Geometric and Physical Representations for a Simulator of Hepatic Surgery, *Proceedings of MMVR 4 Conference* (1996)139-151.

[6] S. De, J. Kim and M. A. Srinivasan, A Meshless Numerical Technique for Physically Based Real Time Medical Simulations, *Proceedings of MMVR 2001Conference* (2001), 113-118.

[7] M. Levoy and T. Whitted, The Use of Points as Display Primitives, *Technical Report TR 85-022, UNC at Chapel Hill, Dept. of Comp. Sc.* (1985).

[8] L.A. Westover, Footprint Evaluation for Volume Rendering, *Proc. of SIGGRAPH Conference'91*, pp. 275-284, 1991.

[9] S. Rusinkiewicz and M. Levoy, QSplat: A Multiresolution Point Rendering System for Large Meshes, *Computer Graphics (SIGGRAPH 2000 Proceedings)* (2000).

[10] E.A, Karabassi, G. Papaioannou & T. Theoharis, Intersection Test for Collision Detection in Particle Systems, *ACM Journal of Graphics Tools*, 4(1), 1999, pp. 25-37.

[11] C. Basdogan, C-H. Ho, and MA Srinivasan, Simulation of tissue cutting and bleeding for laparoscopic surgery using auxiliary surfaces, Proceedings of MMVR (1999) Conference, 1999.

Medicine Meets Virtual Reality 02/10
J.D. Westwood et al. (Eds.)
IOS Press, 2002

Imaging and Visualization of Pathology Beneath the Retinal Surface

Ann E. ELSNER, Ying Jie SI, Mariane Ballester Mellem-KAIRALA,
and Masahiro MIURA

*Schepens Eye Research Institute, Harvard Medical School,
20 Staniford St., Boston, MA, 02114*

Abstract. Pathology beneath the highly reflective surface, such as the human retina, is key in the detection and management of disease. Advanced imaging techniques can help reveal these. Visualization and guiding the imaging to the appropriate area still remain as problems, in part due to the small scale of the pathology with respect to the potential area to be covered.

1. Introduction

The imaging and visualization of pathology beneath a highly reflective surface such as the human retina presents a problem for the early detection and management of disease. The eye is transparent compared with many organs, but disease can produce changes that do not have sharp borders or high contrast. The problem is similar to visualization using endoscopy, in which there is a potentially reflective surface such as a mucous membrane and tissues of interest that can have pathology that is neither superficial nor in a plane. A chief example of a disease with pathology lying mostly beneath the retina is Age-related Macular Degeneration, the most common cause of irreversible blindness in industrialized countries [1]. The chief pathological changes are thought to begin in the photoreceptor/retinal pigment epithelial layer, which lies beneath the highly reflective boundary of the vitreous and retinal nerve fiber layer. An example is hyperpigmentation, the accumulation of dense retinal pigment epithelial cells and debris, usually elevated, which is an important sign of severe damage [2]. Similarly, uncontrolled new vessels that cause severe vision loss often arise from these deeper layers. Yet, most diagnostic tools in widespread use have been optimized for visualization of superficial tissues such as the nerve fiber layer or retinal vasculature. Clinical viewing with visible wavelength light is typically binocular and stereoscopic, while most advanced imaging techniques are monocular and depend upon computations and graphical representation for depth information.

Advanced imaging techniques, such as multiply scattered light imaging or confocal imaging, can reveal deeper structures as the contrast of the deeper structure is enhanced with respect to the superficial layers [3-4]. New visualization strategies are needed to enhance their clinical use. Recently, we found that for large networks of new vessel growth beneath the retina, retinal specialists preferred images that included overlying retinal structures [5-6]. Adding retinal structures to an image lowers the contrast of the underlying lesions. However, retinal structures provide contextual information useful for localizing lesions, and are potentially necessary for stereoscopic visualization. Retinal structures are large compared with some of the lesions in the early stages of disease, and a scale problem is introduced as well as the contrast one.

2. Methods

Imaging data were acquired from 100 patients in our longitudinal study of early Age-Related Macular Degeneration. The patients at study entry were 71 yr of age, on average, with 61 females and 39 males. Inclusion criteria were for the eye of test: early age-related macular degeneration with no exudation, only minimal atrophy, 20/60 or better visual acuity, and < 6 diopter ametropia so that uncontrolled new vessel growth would not be attributed to high myopia. The patients had no diabetes, glaucoma, or previous ocular trauma. History of heart disease or hypertension was permitted. All subjects signed a consent form and followed a protocol approved by the Institutional Review Board of the Schepens Eye Research Institute. The subjects were treated according to the Document of Helsinki.

We compared color photography with multiply scattered light imaging for a criterion feature of hyperpigmentation [2]. In these patients, clumped hyperpigmentation is predictive of significant vision loss at 5-year follow-up.

We acquired color fundus photographs, collected as slides. Color fundus photographs are considered the research standard, while for clinical use color digital images are available at increasingly more, but not all, centers. We scanned these in to provide digital data, using a 12-bit per color slide scanner at approximately 2500 x 2500 pixels (Polaroid Sprint Scan, Cambridge, MA), and without image compression. This produced data for digital image analysis. These were viewed on a 21 inch monitor for color grading. The images were also split into 3 channels, red, green, and blue for further analysis using 8 bit grayscale (Photoshop, Adobe, San Jose, CA).

We acquired multiply scattered light images as 8-bit grayscale, using a Scanning Laser Ophthalmoscope (Rodenstock, Ottobrun-Riemerling, Germany) at 633 nm to help visualize abnormalities in melanin. We used less than 75 microwatts at the cornea. A fixation cross was presented with graphics to the patient so that the area of best vision would be clearly marked. This instrument features point-by-point scanning and a detector that collects light from one illuminated position at a time. This reduces unwanted, long-range scattered light that greatly reduces contrast when longer wavelengths, not readily absorbed by the superficial layers of the ocular fundus, are used. An annular aperture with an 800 micron central stop in the plane of the retina blocks the light returned directly from the region of interest, but allows light that has scattered multiple times before arriving at, then passing through, to the detector. The operator sets the plane of focus at the retinal surface. Then the structures beneath the retina, i.e. pathological structures and normal choroidal blood vessels, are nearly all that should be seen in the multiply scattered light image. The result is that the scattered light collected to form an image is not from the retinal plane, nor is it scattered over long distances. In the ocular fundus, there are few structures in the relatively clear vitreous, so that the multiply scattered light image reveals structures below the plane of focus, such a hyperpigmentation. The overlying retinal vessels, that dominate the color pictures, are barely seen, if at all in multiply scattered light imaging. The rim of the optic nerve head is also visible, but not the smaller structures on or within it. These structures, however, normally provide landmarks for diagnosis and treatment.

The two types of data, those from the color slides and from multiply scattered light imaging, were analyzed interactively, using a 3-point grading scale (Table 1). The worst grade in each eye for the central 3000 x 3000 microns of retina, centered on the fixation cross. The worst region determined the overall grade. The region of interest that determined the grade, roughly 200 microns wide, is similar in scale to retinal landmarks. A typical retinal vein is about 180 microns.

Table 1. Hyperpigmentation grading scale

Hyperpigmenation Grade	Criterion
0	minimal hyperpigmentation
1	significant hyperpigmentation > 10 grayscale units change within 200 microns on the retina
2	grade 1 and pigment clumping

For quantification, the mean grayscale of the region of interest that determined the hyperpigmentation grade was sampled (200 x 200 microns). A control region was also sampled, which was not over an obvious landmark such as a blood vessel. The Michaelson contrast was computed for each hyperpigmentation sample: (Lmax − Lmin)/(Lmax + Lmin), where Lmax is the brighter sample and Lmin is the dimmer one. The mean contrast was computed for all the patients with grades 1 or 2.

This is an example of the comparison of two methods, one that is a standard but non-optimal method, and the other that is a newer method. One method may fail to detect hyperpigmentation that the other method succeeds in detecting. Thus, for the quantitative data, only grades 1 or 2 had enough gray scale change for a region of interest labeled hyperpigmentation to be sampled. When hyperpigmentation was seen with the multiply scattered light imaging, the newer method, but not in the color imaging or the grayscale imaging from the color slides, a value of 0 was not entered into the average value for contrast for the latter method.

3. Results

With multiply scattered light imaging, more patients had significant or clumped hyperpigmentation than found by either the original color data or grayscale data obtained from the color data (p < 0.0001). The multiply scattered light method indicated 48 eyes with the worst grade, but at most only 27 for the color data, graded from the slides. For the green channel, graded onscreen as grayscale, 21 eyes received grade 2, and 13 eyes received grade 1. This is not significantly different from viewing the slides. These data imply that the appearance of hyperpigmentation with clumping was not as great in the color images as it was with multiply scattered light imaging. Further, with multiply scattered light imaging, few superficial retinal features were visible, while with the color imaging, retinal features were apparent and masked the deeper structures.

Better detectability using the multiply scattered light might imply a higher contrast for these features. When we used the same size for the region of interest that we used previously [7], the average grayscale contrast was 0.116 for color data from the green channel. This was not significantly lower than in the patient's multiply scattered light images (p = 0.2773) when the feature was recognized in both types of images.

4. Conclusions

This work provides the comparison for very small features seen with a novel imaging technique, multiply scattered light imaging, to color photography. The color slides missed a large proportion of the features graded as hyperpigmentation using the multiply scattered light images. Thus, sampling for the location of hyperpigmentation could not be guided as readily using these images.

Small features can be detected by trained observers using advanced imaging techniques. The features may those indicating severe damage, such as the hyperpigmentation in the present case, or portions of a new vessel membrane [7]. Either of these is indicative of risk for severe vision loss. The new vessel membrane can be further analyzed for elevation over adjacent, more normal tissues, or overall thickness. However, localization of these features to date has been performed with trained observers.

With the goal of automating the detection of such features from the images, the factors necessary to automate the detection and localization of key features must be considered. Although using an advanced optical method improved detection significantly, the lack of a difference in contrast may seem paradoxical. Spatial scale must be considered. We used a fairly small scale, with samples about 40,000 sq. microns, compared with a sampling area of 9,000,000 sq. microns, but 25 sq. cm for the area that might need to be examined. A trained observer knows which portions of this immense region are crucial for vision and how to look carefully within them. A simple algorithm based on a decrement in contrast and coarse spatial filtering is unlikely to succeed. Further, the imaging method, multiply scattered light imaging, reduced the visibility of unwanted features in the retina, which may not necessarily lower contrast, but could be a source of the poorer detection of hyperpigmentation. The larger of these retinal features may be separated from the deeper structures, stereoscopically, but only if there are features large enough for fusion and transparent enough to still reveal the image components of the deeper layers.

In summary, advanced optical techniques are now available that greatly improve the detectability of pathological features, when compared with the standard clinical techniques that are still used in grading studies. Visualization schemes for small features, which are risk factors for vision loss, are needed to provide clinical utility.

5. Acknowledgements

The Retina Consultants of SW Florida recruited, screened, and imaged all the patients in this study as a part of an ongoing longitudinal study, supported by NIH NEI EYO7624 to A.E.E.

References

[1] H. Leibowitz et L., The Framingham Eye study Monograph: an ophthalmological and epidemiological study of cataract, glaucoma, diabetic retinopathy, macular degeneration and visual acuity in a general population of 2631 adults, *Survey of Ophthalmology* **24** (Suppl) (1980) 335-610.
[2] J. P. Sarks et al., Evolution of soft drusen in age-related macular degeneration, *Eye* **8** (1994) 269-83.
[3] A.E. Elsner, Infrared imaging of subretinal structures in human ocular fundus, *Vis Res* **36** (1996) 191-205.
[4] L.M. Kelley et al., Scanning laser ophthalmoscope imaging of age related macular degeneration and neoplasms, J. *Ophthal. Photography* **3** (1997) 89-94.
[5] A.E. Elsner et al., Scanning laser reflectometry of retinal and subretinal tissues, *Opt. Express* **6** (2000) 243-250.
[6] A.E. Elsner, Multiply scattered light tomography and confocal imaging: detecting neovascularization in age-related macular degeneration, *Opt. Express* **7** (2000) 95-106.
[7] M.Miura, Three dimensional imaging in age-related macular degeneration. *Opt. Express* **9** (2001) 436-443.

Medicine Meets Virtual Reality 02/10
J.D. Westwood et al. (Eds.)
IOS Press, 2002

'Putting It on the Table'

Direct-manipulative interaction and multi-user display technologies for semi-immersive environments and augmented reality applications

L. Miguel Encarnação and Oliver Bimber
Human Media Technologies
Fraunhofer Center for Research in Computer Graphics
321 South Main St., Providence, RI 02903, USA; me@crcg.edu

Abstract. Collaborative virtual environments for diagnosis and treatment planning are increasingly gaining importance in our global society. Virtual and Augmented Reality approaches promised to provide valuable means for the involved interactive data analysis, but the underlying technologies still create a cumbersome work environment that is inadequate for clinical employment. This paper addresses two of the shortcomings of such technology: Intuitive interaction with multi-dimensional data in immersive and semi-immersive environments as well as stereoscopic multi-user displays combining the advantages of Virtual and Augmented Reality technology.

1. Motivation

The fatalities of September 11, 2001 at the World Trade Center and Pentagon and subsequent bioterror attacks are moving the need for distributed virtual response environments into the spotlight, in anticipation of realizing the so-called Cybercare [11] paradigm on a global scale. Such environments seem to be a promising approach to improve and ensure the availability, assignment, flexibility and response time of available medical resources such as personnel, medication, and treatment facilities. One function of such a virtual environment will be the remote expert consultation, treatment planning and tele-medical interventions, which require the visualization, correlation, and analysis of a wealth of detailed patient information so that medical personnel can rapidly and confidently create a 'complete' mental image of patient anatomy, physiology and pathology. Virtual and Augmented Reality promised to provide valuable means for interactive data analysis, but the underlying technologies still create a cumbersome work environment that is inadequate for clinical employment. A major shortcoming of such environments is still a lack of perceptive, direct-manipulative, multi-modal interaction with the displayed data set. Moreover, Virtual and Augmented Reality technologies tend to grow its users 'lonely' by restricting them from sharing the same perspective onto a data set (due to the limitation of the display hardware to generate perspectively correct stereoscopic imagery for multiple users) or by prohibiting direct social interaction among users, e.g., in fully-immersive setups employing head-mounted display (HMDs), thus ruling out collaborative decision making.

In realization of these shortcomings of Virtual and Augmented Reality technologies, we are focusing our research and development efforts [1] onto two main areas: Intuitive interaction with multi-dimensional data in immersive and semi-immersive environments combines the advantages of the familiar 2D (WIMP) interfaces with the superiority of virtual environments with respect to direct manipulation and perception.

Stereoscopic multi-user displays combining the advantages of Virtual and Augmented Reality technology address the need for collaboration in decision-making processes such as diagnosis and treatment planning.

The following sections will summarize some of our current efforts.

2. Technological Background

Augmented Reality (AR) allows the superimposing of computer-generated graphics (i.e. the virtual scene) onto the user's view of the real (physical) world. In contrast to VR, AR techniques allow both virtual and real objects to coexist within the same space. Comparable to VR, the display technology that is employed for AR has its own inherent limitations. The display characteristics of Head Mounted Displays (HMDs) for example, such as resolution and field-of-view, greatly effect the ergonomics of its use. HMDs in general have reduced resolution and focal length capability when compared to large-surface VR –display characteristics that are essential elements of user perception. Optically translucent display systems additionally lack in image brilliance, since contrast and brightness of the displayed graphics is tightly coupled to the lighting conditions of the surrounding real environment. Finally, high performance see-through HMDs available today, which approach the resolution necessary for immersive perception, must sacrifice field of view and are cost prohibitive for widespread use.

Conversely, VR display devices fill a large portion of the user's field of view. While perceptively immersive, filling the user's field of view also isolates him from the surrounding physical environment. It is this isolation of the user from the real world which prevents the prevalent use of VEs in the workplace. Table-like display devices and wall-like projection systems—despite their limited viewing space—seem in this regard more promising since they allow the user to simultaneously perceive the surrounding real world while working with a virtual environment. UNC's "Office of the Future" vision is a consequent extension of this concept.

The current employment of VR display technology is not readily suitable for mixed-reality (MR) applications. In the case of rear-projection display systems, real-world objects are always located between the observer and the projection plane, thereby occluding the projected graphics and consequently obstructing the virtual environment. Front-projection has the advantage in that physical models can be augmented with projected graphics directly onto the surface of those objects, instead of displaying them in viewer's visual field. This technique, known most commonly as spatially-Augmented Reality (SAR), is still limited in so far as the user obstructs projected imagery when approaching the physical objects. This limits the use of the SAR concept to visualization, making it not suitable for complex interaction with virtual and augmented real objects.

3. The Virtual Table

The output device used for the following applications is a Barco BARON Virtual Table (cf. Fig. 1) [7]. It consists of an integrated RGB-projector that displays a 54" x 40" image on the backside of a ground glass screen. To gain the correct three-dimensional impression of the projected scene, we have applied head tracking using an electro-magnetic tracking device (e.g., an Ascension Flock of Birds [8]) and stereoscopic viewing in combination with shutter-glasses (e.g., Stereographics' CrystalEyes [9] or NuVision3D's 60GX [10]).

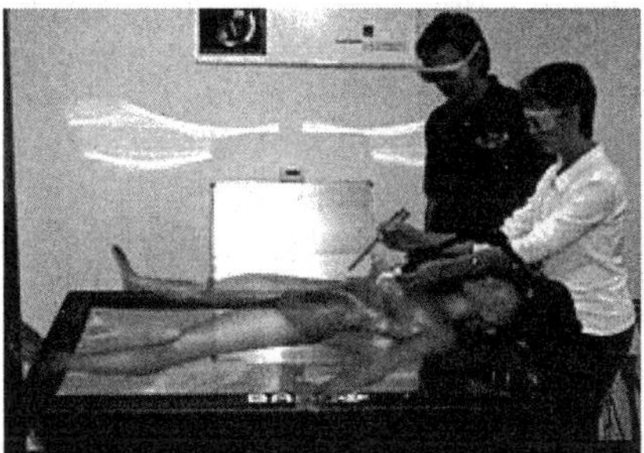

Figure 1: The Virtual Table.

The described technological developments are, however, not limited to the BARON but apply to any kind of backprojection technology with stereoscopic display capabilities.

4. MediDesk

The developed MediDesk system is a combination of an interaction–rich VR system and a volume-rendering system and is designed to enable users to view and analyze the data in stereoscopic projection. The interactive virtual reality techniques that have been developed enable users to process the parameters of data records directly. The developed interaction technologies use transparent props (pen and tablet) for two-handed interaction with a Virtual Table (VT) [2,3].

Our interaction framework unifies several previously isolated approaches to 3D user interface design, such as two-handed interaction and the use of multiple coordinate systemssupporting the following features:

– two-handed interaction
– multi-purpose physical props
– embedding 2D in 3D
– use of multiple coordinate systems (i.e., of the table and the pad)
– transparent tools, especially window-tools and through-the-plane tools (such as sketching).

Each of the listed properties allows the design of distinct forms of interaction, which in conjunction provide for a very rich user interface design space.

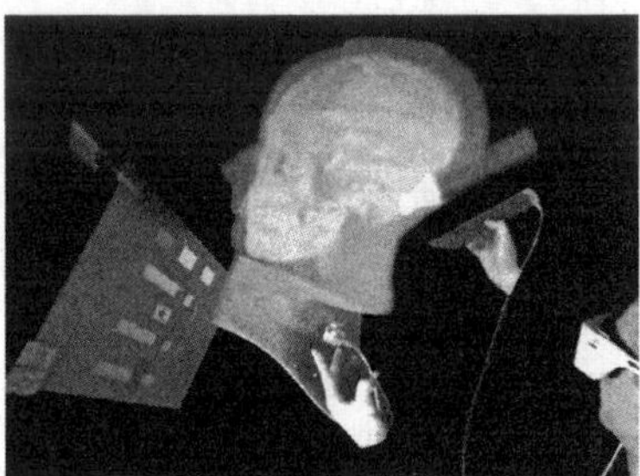
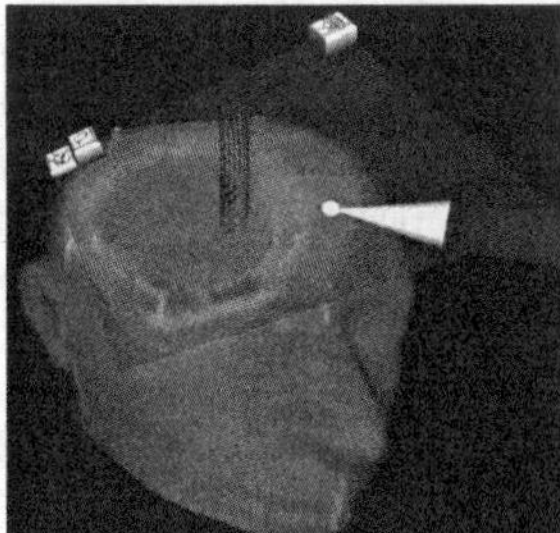

Figure 2: Intuitive, two-handed interaction with a medical data set in 3D space.

The system provides a natural three-dimensional interaction environment for dealing with three-dimensional volume data, which can be superior to two-dimensional volume rendering (cf. Fig. 2). The see-through pad is tracked and allows for user-defined display of virtual menus and context-sensitive information. The pen, which is also tracked, is used as a pointing device. These tools provide natural means of interaction for rotating, scaling or cutting a volume. Currently, MediDesk supports two-handed 3D interaction as well as gesture-based input. In the future speech input and haptic input devices will be integrated.

5. The Transflective Pad

Two fundamental problems of semi-immersive rear-projection devices are the limited viewing that is caused by relatively small projection planes, and their inability to combine real objects with displayed virtual ones. This is due to the fact that real objects always occlude the projection planes and consequently the displayed virtual environment, thus prohibiting traditional augmented reality tasks from being supported by such devices. To overcome both problems, we developed the transflective pad –a hand-held half-silvered mirror– that, on the one hand, allows to interactively increase the limited viewing volume (cf. Fig. 3) [5], and, on the other hand, enables rear-projection devices to support basic augmented reality tasks (cf. Fig. 4) [6].

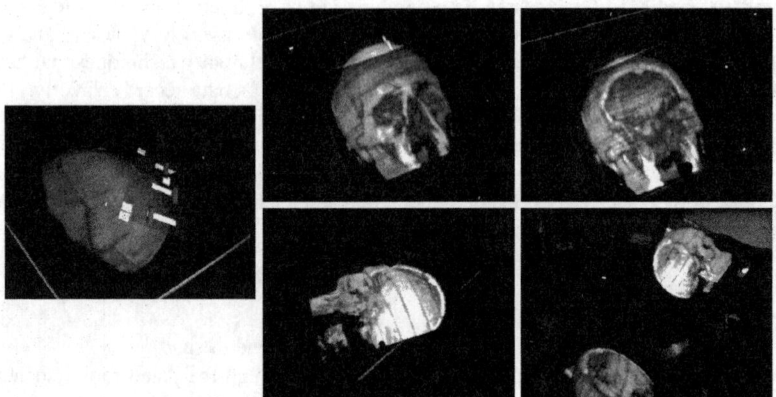

Figure 3: The Transflective Pad used in an opaque mode to interactively increase the limited viewing volume of the applied rear-projection system.

The presented approach allows an intuitive and effective application of immersive or semi-immersive virtual reality tasks and interaction techniques to an augmented surrounding space. We use a tracked mirror beam-splitter as optical combiner that merges the reflected graphics, which are displayed on the projection plane, with the transmitted image of the real environment.

Medicine Meets Virtual Reality 02/10
J.D. Westwood et al. (Eds.)
IOS Press, 2002

Quantitative Image Analysis of the Cartilage in Virtual Reality

K.-H. Englmeier[1], M. Siebert[1], T. Stammberger[1], R. v. Eisenhardt-Rothe, H. Graichen[2], F. Eckstein[3], M. Reiser[4]

1. GSF – National Research Center for Environment and Health, Institute for Medical Informatics and Health System Research, Ingolstaedter Landstr. 1, 85764 Neuherberg, Germany
2. Research Group for Kinematics and Biomechanics, Department of Orthopaedic Surgery, University of Frankfurt, Marienburgstr. 2, 60528, Frankfurt, Germany
3. Musculoskeletal Research Group, Institute of Anatomy, Ludwig-Maximilians-University, Pettenkoferstrasse 11, 80336 Munich, Germany
4. Department of Diagnostic Radiology, Klinikum Grosshadern, Ludwig-Maximilians-University, Marchioninistrasse 15, 81377 Munich, Germany

Abstract: The objective of this work is to develop image processing methods for analysing the morphology of the joint cartilage with magnetic resonance imaging. Quantitative data on the morphological distribution of the joint cartilage are of great interest for both research as well as for diagnosis. The cartilage thickness provides information on the local cartilage occurance and may therefore be helpful in early and objective diagnosing degenerative cartilage changes, monitoring the pathogenesis of osteoarthritis, and controlling the success of chondroprotective treatment. In biomechanics, the thickness distribution serves to analyse the functional adaptation or the compression of the cartilage under loading and may be used for numerical simulation of load transmission in the joint.

1. Keywords

Quantitative image analysis, cartilage thickness, image registration,

2. Introduction

Articular cartilage is subjected to forces of several times body weight during normal physical activity, dedicating it an important role for the proper function of diarthrodial joints [1]. The study of the deformational behavior of cartilage under mechanical loading is therefore of great interest for quantifying biomechanical properties of cartilage and for better understanding the pathogenesis of osteoarthritis. Whereas the deformation of articular cartilage has been investigated extensively in cartilage explants [1,2] and in indentation [1,3], relatively little is known about its compression in an intact joint and, in particular, on the microstructural changes of cartilage components during deformation.

A very promising, nondestructive technique to obtain data on microstructural cartilage components is magnetic resonance imaging (MRI). Together with adequate postprocessing, MRI has also been shown to be an accurate and reproducible method for determining the cartilage volume [4,5].

In the present paper we have extended the technique developed by [7] to measurements of MR signal intensity during a cartilage compression. The specific objectives of this paper are:

1) To quantify the average signal intensity changes of the whole 3D cartilage plate, determined from serial images, as a function of the mean cartilage deformation.

2) To develop image processing methods to delineate and register the cartilage boundaries in consecutive 2D MR images, in order to identify corresponding ROIs throughout the loading experiment.

3) To measure the MR signal intensity within these ROIs and its temporal evolution during the loading experiment as a function of the local cartilage deformation.

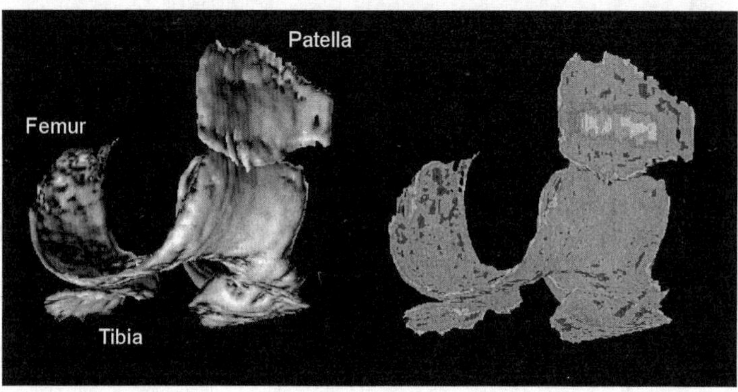

Figure 1: 3D reconstruction of the articular cartilage surfaces (left) for quantitative morphological measurement. The 3D cartilage thickness distribution is projected as a color map onto the cartilage surfaces (right).

3. Material and Methods

For image acquisition, a high resolution, fat-suppressed FLASH 3D sequence was applied that had been shown previously to permit an accurate delineation of the cartilage boundaries [5]. Complete 3D data sets were collected from three normal knee-joint specimens, before compression as well as when the load had been applied. at time intervals of 10 min for up to 4 hours. One 2D transverse image plane was selected in the centre of the joint for detailed analysis and for the tracking of ROIs. Exactly at the same slice position, two additional 2D spin echo images were acquired, each once before and after the compression experiment. In order to quantify the time dependent signal intensity changes as a function of cartilage deformation from consecutive 2D MR images, the following image processing steps have to be accomplished: Both the cartilage surface and the bone-cartilage interface were segmented separately using a B-spline snake algorithm demanding only minimal user interaction [8]. This method has been applied to the segmentation of the 3D images as well as for the consecutive 2D images. The cartilage-bone interface at the different compression stages (here referred to as "deformed" contours) are registered to the initial cartilage-bone interface before loading on the basis of the geometric distance between both interfaces. For this purpose, an Euclidean distance map is computed from the initial interface, using the Euclidean distance transformation [6,9,10,11] that assigns to every pixel in the image the minimal distance to the nearest interface pixel.

As a consequence of the compression, the cartilage-bone interface itself is distorted within the image plane relative to the scanner geometry. Since potential deformations of the bone tissue can be considered to be much smaller than the resolution of the MR images, these distortions can be modelled as rigid body transformation , permitting only rotation and translation of points on the segmented cartilage-bone interface.

To meet the demands and requirements of visualization, we introduced a new level of detail (LOD) algorithm to reduce the number of displayed polygons without visible loss of accuracy, and applied new volume rendering methods using volume texture mapping. An algorithm was developed which allows the simultaneous visualization of the 3D morphology of the cartilage as well as the colour coded cartilage thickness (fig. 1).

4. Results, Conclusion

The image analysis and visualization techniques described above are applied to the MR images in order to quantify and track signal intensity changes as a function of cartilage deformation. Whereas the 3D analysis of signal intensity changes within the complete cartilage plates is computationally straight forward, particular steps have to be taken when analysing changes within various tissue sectors.

The important distortions forced by the loading require further processing by the application of a registration procedure. The registration algorithm is based on the Euclidean distance transformation [9,10,11], which is a very efficient way to calculate distances in digital images since the computational complexity scales only linearly with the number of pixels. The similarity of two contours after their alignment, expressed as mean mutual distance, was below 0.5 pixel for all contour pairs, this being below the in-plane resolution. This high matching accuracy justifies retrospectively the modelling of the distortions as rigid transformation assuming the bone to be a rigid body.

References

[1]   A. Goldsmith, A. Hayes and S. Clift. Application of finite elements to the stress analysis of articular cartilage. Med. Eng. Phys., 18(2):89-98, 1996.
[2]   Y. Kim, J. Bonassar and A. Grodzinsky. The role of cartilage streaming potential, fluid flow and pressure in the stimulation of chondrocyte biosynthesis during dynamic compression. J. Biomech., 28:1055-1066, 1995.
[3]   R. Spilker, J. Suh and V. Mow. A finite element analysis of the indentation stress-relaxation response of linear biphasic articular cartilage. J. Biomech. Eng., 114:191-201, 1992.
[4]   C. G. Peterfy, C. F. van Dijke, D. L. Janzen, C. C. Gluer, R. Namba, S. Majumdar, P. Lang and H. K. Genant. Quantification of articular cartilage in the knee with pulsed saturation transfer subtraction and fat-suppressed MR imaging: optimization and validation. Radiology, 192:485-491, 1994.
[5]   F. Eckstein, A. Gavazzeni, H. Sittek, M. Haubner, A. Loesch, S. Milz, K.-H. Englmeier, R. Putz and M. Reiser. Determination of knee joint cartilage thickness using three dimensional magnetic resonance chondro-crassometry (3D MR-CCM). Magn. Reson. Med., 36:256-265, 1996.
[6]   T. Stammberger, F. Eckstein, K.-H. Englmeier and M. Reiser. Determination of 3D cartilage thickness from MR imaging – computational method and reproducibility in the living. Magn. Reson. Med., 41 (3) 529-536 (1999)
[7]   C. Herberhold, T. Stammberger, S. Faber, R. Putz, K.-H. Englmeier, M. Reiser and F. Eckstein. A MR-based technique for quantifying the deformation of articular cartilage during mechanical loading in an intact cadaver joint. Magn. Reson. Med., 39:843-850, 1998.
[8]   T. Stammberger, S. Rudert, M. Michaelis, M. Reiser and K. Englmeier. Segmentation of MR images with B-spline snakes: A multi-resolution approach using the distance transformation for model forces. In Proceedings of the 2nd workshop on Image Processing for Medicine, BVM'98, pages 164-168, Aachen, Germany, 1998.
[9]   P.-E. Danielsson. Euclidean distance mapping. Computer Graphics and Image Processing, 14:227-248, 1980.
[10]   G. Borgefors. Distance transformations in digital images. Computer Vision, Graphics and Image Processing, 34:344-371, 1986.
[11]   H. Embrechts and D. Roose. A parallel Euclidean distance transformation algorithm. Computer Vision and Image Understanding, 63(1):15-26, 1994.

Medicine Meets Virtual Reality 02/10
J.D. Westwood et al. (Eds.)
IOS Press, 2002

Using Mixed Reality, Force Feedback and Tactile Augmentation to Improve the Realism of Medical Simulation

J. Brian Fisher, Susan M. Porter
Southwest Research Institute, San Antonio, Texas

Abstract. This paper describes an application of a display approach which uses chromakey techniques to composite real and computer-generated images allowing a user to see his hands and medical instruments collocated with the display of virtual objects during a medical training simulation. Haptic feedback is provided through the use of a PHANTOM™ force feedback device in addition to tactile augmentation, which allows the user to touch virtual objects by introducing corresponding real objects in the workspace. A simplified catheter introducer insertion simulation was developed to demonstrate the capabilities of this approach.

1. Introduction

Effective medical simulation requires that visual/haptic feedback be correctly correlated to train the motor skills needed to perform medical procedures. Inconsistent visual/haptic registration can result in inter-sensory conflict leading to limited, and in the worst case, negative skill transfer. Yokokohji, et al. describe a system employing a WYSIWYF (What You See Is What You Feel) technique to ensure correct visual/haptic registration so that what the user sees is consistent with exactly what he/she feels via a haptic device [1][2][3]. In this approach, chromakeying techniques are used to capture real images of the user's hands, and to composite those images with the virtual environment. The work described in this paper builds upon this basic approach to simulate the insertion of a catheter introducer. In this application, force feedback is applied via a PHANTOM™ device, and tactile augmentation is used to allow the user to grasp a mannequin overlaid with virtual images allowing the user to train a procedure in a natural manner.

2. System Description

This application combines the effects of visual, haptic and simulation systems to produce a realistic environment for practicing medical procedures. The overall system configuration is illustrated in Figure 1. As can be seen in the illustration, the user places his/her hands below a liquid crystal display (LCD) monitor assuming the normal posture used in an actual procedure. The visual system captures images of the hands and medical instruments and blends them with images generated by the simulation system into a composite image displayed on the LCD. The haptic and simulation systems act together to generate the appropriate haptic feedback as the user performs the simulated procedure.

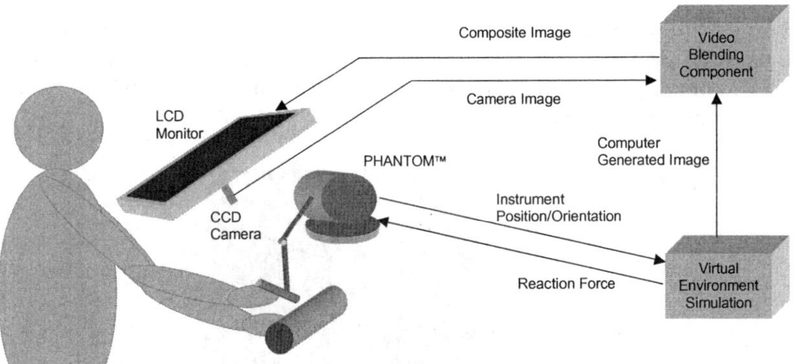

Figure 1: System Configuration

2.1 Visual System

The visual system consists of the components required to create, capture, and blend the real and computer generated images of the workspace. Computer generated images are rendered in real-time using the GHOST SDK and a combination of VRML models and OpenGL. For this system, images are rendered using a desktop PC configured with an NVidia GeForce2 Ultra 64MB graphics card. Graphics update rates of at least 30 frames per second were easily achieved with this system.

The video blending component performs operations to mix the computer-generated images with live video images which are captured with a charge coupled display (CCD) camera. The blending process is accomplished using a chromakey technique whereby one video source is overlaid onto another by choosing a key color. The video blending component substitutes the computer-generated video image everywhere the camera records the key color. The mixed video is then output to the LCD monitor which is positioned in such a way as to allow the user to assume a natural posture while interacting with the objects in the virtual environment.

The CCD camera captures real time video of the user's hands and any real object(s) with which he or she may be interacting with in the workspace. The camera is mounted to the back of the LCD monitor and is aligned with the line-of-sight of the user. The camera is carefully placed to provide a realistic view of the real objects behind the LCD monitor. Because the camera is not at the same location as the user's eye, a wide field of view is used to avoid having the image of the user's hands appear overly large. The field of view was selected so that the hands appear the appropriate size at the position where the procedure is conducted. A chromakey background is used to hide the area surrounding the display stand, and to produce the key color that is recorded by the camera. The video blending component processes this color in order to determine the mixture of real video with computer-generated video. Components that are not to be visible in the final blended image are covered with the key color, and, in this case, include the haptic device and a mannequin hand.

2.2 Haptic System

The haptic system provides feedback in two forms. Force feedback is applied using the PHANTOM™, while tactile feedback is provided via a mannequin hand mounted in the workspace. A PHANTOM™ Premium 1.5A is used to provide six degree of freedom (DOF) tracking of the instrument and the application of forces in three DOF. An actual catheter introducer, minus the needle, is mounted to the gimbal assembly of the PHANTOM™ device which was modified to limit the interference between the gimbals and the mannequin as the virtual introducer needle is inserted.

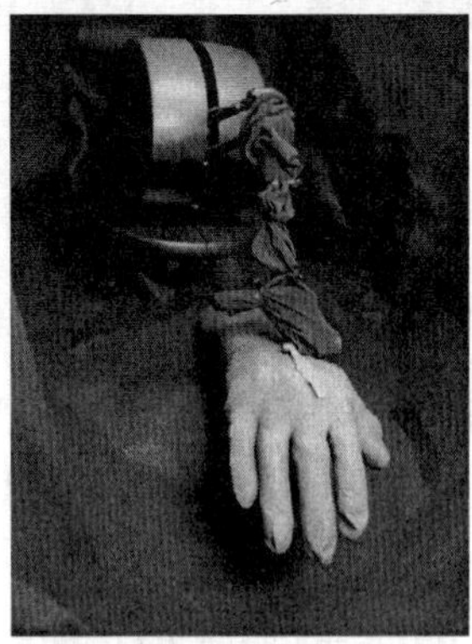

Figure 2: Haptic System Configuration

The PHANTOM™ applies the appropriate force feedback based on collisions between the virtual needle extending from the introducer and the virtual hand as detected by the simulation system described in the next section. The mannequin hand provides tactile feedback for the user's "off-hand" thus allowing the user to grasp the patient's hand as is done in the actual procedure. The mannequin is covered by the chromakey color so that a virtual image may be overlaid. Allowing the user to touch virtual objects is referred to as passive haptics or tactile augmentation. Previous research has shown that this can lead to more realistic and thus more effective simulation [4] [5] [6].

2.3 Simulation System

The simulation system is responsible for detecting collisions, computing the appropriate visual and haptic responses, and registering real and virtual objects. Collision detection is performed to determine contact and/or penetration of the various surfaces of the virtual hand by the virtual needle. The GHOST SDK was used and extended as needed to compute these collisions. Once a collision is detected, the simulation determines the type of surface contacted and computes the appropriate force based on the corresponding surface properties set by the user. For this application, three types of surfaces were modeled, the skin, bones, and veins. Properties of these surfaces can be set interactively using sliders controlling the surface friction, stiffness and puncture force threshold. When the simulation determines that the skin has been punctured, an additional viscous force is computed to further resist motion of the needle. The simulation also applies a simple visual deformation scheme to provide a visual cue signifying when the needle contacts and deforms the skin. When the needle is successfully inserted into a vein, feedback is provided to the user by changing the color of the virtual needle to simulate back flow.

The simulation software must also provide a mechanism to correctly register the real and virtual objects. Two assumptions were made which simplify the registration. First, it was assumed that the patient's hand would remain fixed in the environment. This eliminates the need to track the mannequin. It was also assumed that the user's head would remain in relatively the same position during the procedure, and can also be regarded as fixed. These assumptions greatly reduce the difficulty in the registration process. In this case, registration may simply be done at the start of the simulation, and is straightforward once the position of the camera and mannequin hand are known in the workspace. Software controls are provided which allow the user to interactively modify the virtual scene through positioning and scaling of the virtual objects, and the setting of the virtual camera properties to closely match the real and virtual scenes. The only moving objects that need to be registered are the virtual needle and the real introducer mounted to the PHANTOM™. This is straightforward as the position and orientation of the introducer are mechanically tracked by the PHANTOM™ and this information is readily available through the GHOST SDK. For this registration to be accurate, it is important that the PHANTOM™ be initialized correctly at its assumed origin as all measurements are relative to its starting position. Any errors in the initialization will result in registration errors between the real and virtual objects.

3. Results

A simplified catheter introducer insertion simulation was developed to demonstrate the capabilities of this approach for medical training. The demonstration has shown that chromakeying works well to combine real camera images and computer generated images to produce a realistic view of the hands in the virtual environment (see Figure 3).

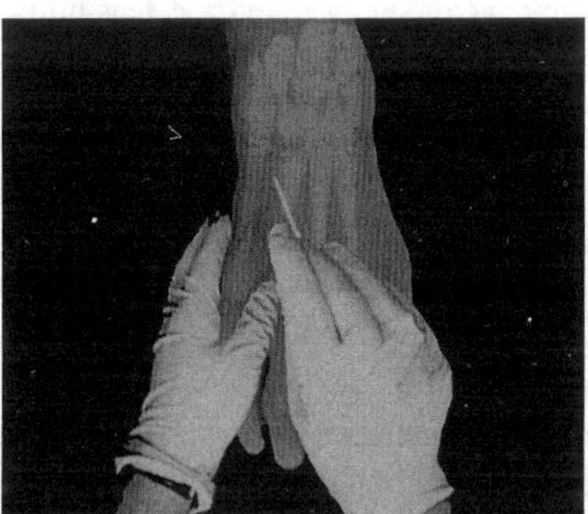

Figure 3: Sample Composite Image Blending Real and Computer Generated Imagery

The use of chromakeying allows the user's hands to be displayed without the need to track the position, orientation, and finger angles using an instrumented glove. This reduces the complexity of the system and is less restrictive to normal movements by the user. The use of the mannequin, in conjunction with the force feedback device, provides realistic feedback to both hands. This allows the user to grasp the virtual patient with one hand, while inserting the needle with the other, in much the same way as is done in the actual procedure. While the physical model used is fairly simple, the force feedback provided does simulate a realistic "pop" as the needle is inserted. In addition, a great deal of flexibility to simulate a wide range of physical characteristics is provided through the ability to interactively change the properties of the virtual patient. The corresponding visual representation may be changed simply by applying a different texture to the graphical model of the virtual hand.

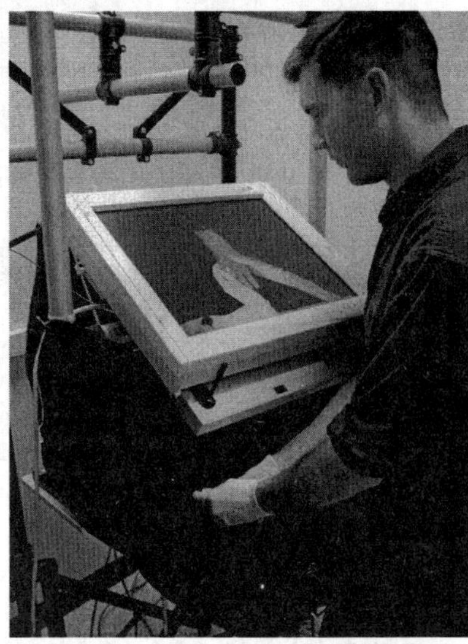

Figure 4: Demonstration System

4. Conclusions

The results of this work have demonstrated the feasibility of combining mixed reality techniques with haptic feedback in a small workspace environment to simulate a medical procedure in a natural and realistic manner. The ultimate goal of this work is to use this approach to improve the effectiveness of medical simulation for a broad range of training applications. Further work will concentrate on the following areas:

- Evaluation of the demonstration system by experts
- Development of instructor/training capabilities
- Resolving registration issues due to camera distortion
- Development of more sophisticated physical models
- Application of this method to simulate other types of procedures

The next step is an evaluation of the demonstration system by experts in the field. Plans are in work to have the system evaluated by medical personnel within the coming months. This evaluation will focus on the potential use of this approach not only for the application developed, but for its potential use in simulating other procedures as well.

Because the primary goal of this work was to demonstrate the application of this approach, little effort was made to facilitate the use of the system as a training device. Additional functionality should be added to provide instructor controls to make the simulation part of a complete training session, including the ability to record data during the procedure to provide immediate and meaningful feedback following a training session.

One of the issues identified during the construction of the demonstration system was that due to the wide field of view, a significant amount of distortion exists in the real image captured by the CCD camera. The distortion of the image increases as the distance from the center of the camera field of view increases. This can contribute to poor registration between the real and virtual world at the periphery. For this particular application, the actual working area is relatively small, and thus the distortion had little effect on the registration in the area of interest. However, to apply this technique to a wider range of applications, which may involve larger working areas, methods may need to be investigated to reduce and/or compensate for the distortion.

The physical model of the hand for this case is relatively simple but sufficient for this particular application. However, since the goal is to be able to apply this approach to other types of procedures, it may be necessary to employ more sophisticated physical models. The degree to which this is required will be dependent on input of expert medical personnel.

References

[1] Y. Yokokohji, R. L. Hollis and T. Kanade, What You can See Is What You can Feel - Development of a Visual/Haptic Interface to Virtual Environment, In *Proc., IEEE Virtual Reality Annual International Symposium (VRAIS '96)*, pp. 46-53 (1996).

[2] Y. Yokokohji, R. L. Hollis, T. Kanade, K. Henmi, and T. Yoshikawa, Toward Machine Mediated Training of Motor Skills - Skill Transfer from Human to Human via Virtual Environment, In *Proceedings of the RO-MAN '96: the 5th IEEE International Workshop on Robot and Human Communica*tion, (pp. 32-37).

[3] Y. Yokokohji, R. L. Hollis and T. Kanade, Vision-based Visual/Haptic Registration for WYSIWYF Display, In *Proc., IROS '96*, (1996)

[4] B. E. Insko, M. J. Meehan, M. C. Whitton, F. P. Brooks Jr, Passive Haptics Significantly Enhances Virtual Environments, Paper presented at the Fourth Annual International Workshop on Presence, Temple, PA, May 2001.

[5] H. Hoffman, J. Groen, S. Rousseau, A. Hollander, W. Winn, M. Wells, T. Furness, Tactile Augmentation: Enhancing Presence in Virtual Reality with Tactile Feedback from Real Objects, Paper presented at the meeting of the American Psychological Society, San Francisco, CA (1996).

[6] H.G. Hoffman, Physically Touching Virtual Objects Using Tactile Augmentation Enhances the Realism of Virtual Environments, *Proceedings of the IEEE Virtual Reality Annual International Symposium '98*, p. 59-63 (1998).

Medicine Meets Virtual Reality 02/10
J.D. Westwood et al. (Eds.)
IOS Press, 2002

Wireless Live Streaming Video of Laparoscopic Surgery: A Bandwidth Analysis for Handheld Computers

Alex Gandsas, MD[1], Katherine McIntire, MD[2], Ivan M. George[1], Wayne Witzke[1], James D. Hoskins, B.S.[1] and Adrian Park, MD[1]

[1] *Department of Surgery, University of Kentucky, 800 Rose Street Rd., Room #349, Lexington KY 40536*

[2] *Duke University Medical Center, School of Medicine, Durham, North Carolina*

Abstract: Over the last six years, streaming media has emerged as a powerful tool for delivering multimedia content over networks. Concurrently, wireless technology has evolved, freeing users from desktop boundaries and wired infrastructures. At the University of Kentucky Medical Center, we have integrated these technologies to develop a system that can wirelessly transmit live surgery from the operating room to a handheld computer. This study establishes the feasibility of using our system to view surgeries and describes the effect of bandwidth on image quality.

A live laparoscopic ventral hernia repair was transmitted to a single handheld computer using five encoding speeds at a constant frame rate, and the quality of the resulting streaming images was evaluated. No video images were rendered when video data were encoded at 28.8 kilobytes per second (Kbps), the slowest encoding bitrate studied. The highest quality images were rendered at encoding speeds greater than or equal to 150 Kbps. Of note, a 15 second transmission delay was experienced using all four encoding schemes that rendered video images.

We believe that the wireless transmission of streaming video to handheld computers has tremendous potential to enhance surgical education. For medical students and residents, the ability to view live surgeries, lectures, courses and seminars on handheld computers means a larger number of learning opportunities. In addition, we envision that wireless enabled devices may be used to telemonitor surgical procedures. However, bandwidth availability and streaming delay are major issues that must be addressed before wireless telementoring becomes a reality.

1- Introduction:

Handheld computer technology has been widely recognized for its potential to revolutionize healthcare. Sending medical data to portable devices using wireless protocols has been tested in a variety of medical contexts including patient triage[1], electronic medical record management[2], telecardiology[3] and data acquisition in critical care[4]. However, to date, wireless multimedia applications have not been fully explored for medical education.

At the University of Kentucky Medical Center (UKMC), we used streaming video technology and wireless protocols to create a broadcasting system that enables the transmission of live surgical procedures to handheld computers. This study was conducted to determine the smallest bandwidth required to render quality video images on the handheld display such that the transmitted surgery may be used for teaching purposes. Using five encoding bitrates, a live laparoscopic ventral hernia repair was transmitted to a single handheld computer, and the quality of the resulting streaming images was evaluated.

2- Materials And Methods:

After obtaining formal patient consent, a laparoscopic ventral hernia repair was transmitted live from a UKMC operating room to the handheld device using the following model, which integrated wired and wireless computer systems equipped with off-the-shelf software/hardware.

2.1 Model for live streaming video transmission (see Figure 1)

2.1.1 Wired Components and Configuration

The key hardware components of the wired system included a video monitor located in the operating room, a video HUB (provided by Stryker), a desktop computer (Optiplex by Dell) that functioned as a server, and a capture card (Belkin). ⹁ Important desktop computer software included Windows Media Encoder™. The operating room video monitor, the video signal source, was connected to the server (the desktop computer) via the in-house videoconference router. The server was equipped with a Pentium III 750 MHz processor, 128 MB of RAM, a Windows 2000 operating system, the capture card, and Windows Media Encoder™. The server's encoding bitrate was modified to the following five schemes: 28.8 Kbps, 56 Kbps, 150 Kbps, 250 Kbps and 300 Kbps. The desktop was connected to the private LAN, and the encoder was configured to stream video images at 15 frames per second (fps), the maximum streaming rate that the handheld computer's central processing unit (CPU) can process.

2.1.2 Wireless Components and Configuration

The key hardware components of the wireless system included a handheld computer (iPAQ 3670 by Compaq), a wireless PC card (RangeLAN 7410 CE by Proxim, Inc.), a wireless Ethernet Access point (RangeLAN2 by Proxim, Inc.), and a HUB/router device (Netgear) to establish a private LAN. Important handheld computer software included Windows Media Player™ version 7.1 for Windows CE.

The iPAQ 3670 was equipped with 64 MB of RAM, a 206 MHz Intel StrongARM 32-bit RISC Processor, a Pocket PC 2001 operating system operating on a Windows CE 3.01 platform and the Windows Media Player™ software. The iPAQ display technology included a 240 X 320 pixel touch screen and a color reflective thin film transistor (TFT) liquid color display (LCD) with 4,096 colors. The wireless PC card was connected to the iPAQ using an expansion pack compatible with type II PC cards. The wireless PC card was connected to the wireless Ethernet Access Point, which connected the iPAQ to the private LAN HUB/router. The wireless PC card and the Ethernet Access Point transmitted on a 2.4 GHz radio spectrum, the OpenAir standard, using the 802.11 b wireless protocol.

2.1 The working model (see Figure 1)

Analog video signals originating from the operating room monitor were transmitted to the server via the Stryker video HUB. The capture card received the analog signals and converted them into a digital format. Windows Media Encoder™ then encoded the digital video signals to streaming video format. In order to receive the streaming video images from the server, the researcher turned on the handheld device (the iPAQ connected automatically to the private LAN via the PC card/Access Point link described above) and launched Windows Media Player™. The researcher then entered the server's Intranet Address, and the real-time streaming video images were received and rendered on the handheld device.

Figure 1: Wireless Transmission of Live Streaming Video to a Handheld Computer

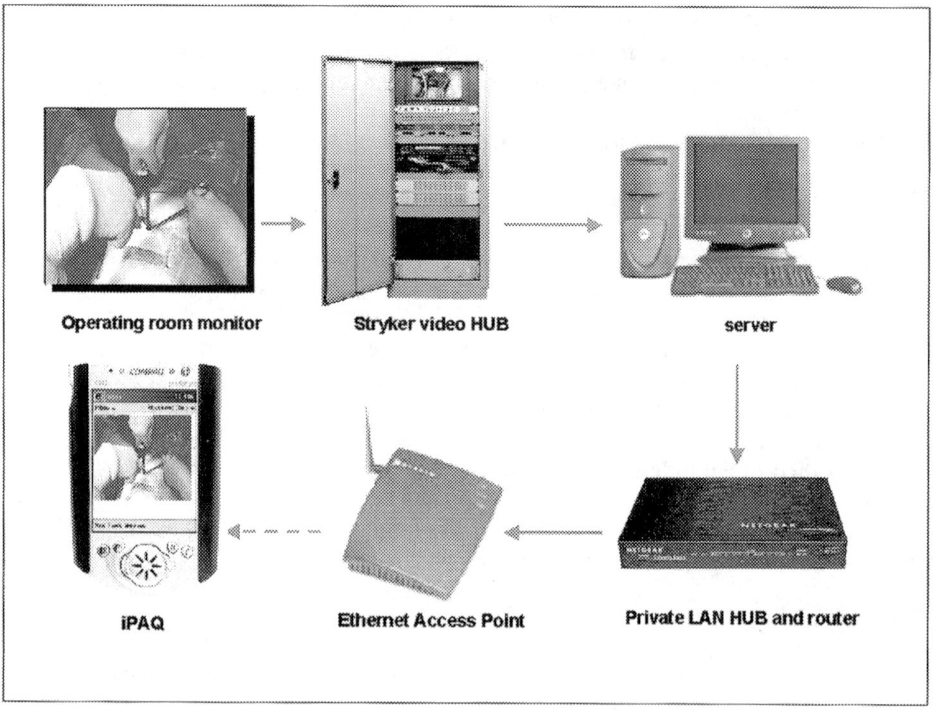

3- Results:

After entering the server's intranet address, 30 seconds were required for the iPAQ to connect to the server. Once connected, we attempted to transmit the surgery at five different encoding bitrates (28.8, 56.2, 150, 250 and 300 kbps) while the server's configured frame rate was held constant (15 fps). While transmitting at each encoding bitrate, overall video quality was subjectively assessed in terms of the image rendered and the continuity of motion. In addition, one objective parameter related to video quality was recorded, the resulting frame rate (see Table 1). Other parameters recorded during transmission included bandwidth availability and the transmission range.

In summary, sound and video images were successfully transmitted to the iPAQ using 4 out of the 5 encoding rates studied (56.2, 150, 250 and 300 kbps). At 28.8 kbps, only sound was transmitted. The highest quality video was achieved at bitrates greater than or equal 150 kbps. Significantly, video quality was not improved by increasing the bitrate from 150 to 250 to 300 kbps even though the resulting frame rate did increase slightly (13.1 to 14.0 to 14.3 fps). In addition, a 15 second video transmission delay was observed with all 4 encoding rates (56.2, 150, 250 and 350 kbps). The model accommodated a maximal radial transmission range of 500 feet around the Ethernet Access Point. The "bandwidth available" to carry the video data was always less than the configured encoding bitrate due to network traffic, which affected the frame rate.

Table 1: Video Quality, Bandwidth Availability and Frame Rate at Different Encoding Bitrates*

Encoding Bitrate (kbps)	Bandwidth Availability (kbps)	Frame rate (fps)	Video Quality
28.8	23.8	0	No video image rendered
56.2	36.7	11.3	Blurry Image, choppy motion
150	146.3	13.1	Crisp image, smooth motion
250	225	14.0	Crisp image, smooth motion
300	280	14.3	Crisp image, smooth motion

***Configured frame rate held constant at 15 fps**

4- Discussion:

Encoding bitrate and frame rate are two major determinants of what we perceive as video quality. Essentially, video is a sequence of still images known as frames that, when displayed in succession at high rates, are perceived as being in fluid motion. Encoding bitrate represents the amount of data transmitted in one second to create the still image. The higher the encoding rate, the clearer and more detailed the still image. As the frame rate (the rate at which still images are displayed) is increased, the motion of that image is perceived as increasingly fluid. High quality video such as that seen on television and in movie theaters is accomplished using frame rates of 30 and 24 fps, respectively. Therefore, to maximize video quality, one would ideally transmit data at the highest possible encoding bitrate and frame rate.

However, factors exist that limit the video quality rendered by our model. Currently, handheld computers are manufactured with central processing units that cannot render images at rates greater than 15 fps, the frame rate used in this study. In addition, the algorithm used by Windows Media Encoder™ to compress video and audio data into a specific bandwidth limits the encoding bitrate that can be used. Before analog video can be transmitted to a hand held computer, it must be digitized and then compressed so that the video data will fit within the bandwidth selected for smooth streaming. More importantly, using more sophisticated compression algorithms to increase the encoding bitrate also uses more hardware resources and increases the cost of transmission because more data must be delivered over the network.

Significantly, our study found that, given its limitations, our model was capable of transmitting a live surgical procedure to a handheld computer and that the video rendered was of sufficient quality to allow the researcher to easily follow the procedure from beginning to end. Therefore, the model may potential be used in surgical education. In addition, the study found that increasing the encoding bitrate from 150 to 300 kbps did not enhance the quality of the video, which was subjectively assessed. This information has economic implications for institutions with limited budgets that may plan use our model. Using an encoding bitrate of 150 kbps at 15 fps produces a video of similar quality to that rendered using a bitrate of 300 kbps at 15 fps without spending as twice as much.

Our model may be enhanced by incorporating software with more powerful compression algorithms. In 1998, the International Organization for Standardization (ISO) and the International Engineering Consortium (IEC) combined forces to create a new standard for the compression of audio and video signals known as Moving Picture Expert Group or MPEG. This group published several standards that allow video compression at rates ranging from 1.5 Mbps (MPEG-1) to 20 Mbps (MPEG-2). The MPEG-4 standard was first published in 1998 and enabled video encoding at rates as low as 5 kbps to a maximum of 5 Mbps. As a result, MPEG-4 compression algorithms provide high quality video that can be delivered over limited bandwidth to wireless-equipped handheld computers or cellular phones loaded   with video streaming software.

In addition to advances in data compression, developments have also been accomplished in data transfer using wireless protocols. In 1990, the Institute of Electrical and Electronics Engineers (IEEE) 802 Executive Group developed standard protocols for a wireless local area network (WLAN) that uses the 2.4 Ghz ISM (Industrial, Scientific and Medical) spectrum. The wireless link between the PC card on the iPAQ and the access point used the 802.11b standard with a total data throughput that ranged from 2.5 to 4Mbps.

During this experiment, although the data transmission was performed in real time, all video images were displayed on the handheld device with a 15 second delay. This is attributed mainly to the buffer effect of the software application that streamed the video images. This setback in data transmission will not limit the use of our model in education, which may include the transmission of lectures or courses, where real time transmission is not crucial. However, improved video interfaces with almost no delay are necessary if real time teleproctoring or even telementoring applications are sought.

In summary, we believe that the wireless transmission of streaming video to handheld computers has tremendous potential to enhance surgical education. Medical training keeps students and residents on the go and scattered throughout the hospital at any given moment, which can make it difficult for individuals to make group sessions and makes it impractical for individuals to rely on static computer terminals to access educational materials. Transmitting live surgery, lectures, courses and seminars to handheld computers overcomes the limitations of relying on static wired hardware to access content[1,5]. Receiving educational content on handheld computers means that medical students and residents may have more learning opportunities. Although telemonitoring of surgical procedures using wireless enabled devices is technically feasible, bandwidth availability and streaming delay are major issues that must be addressed before such applications are practical. Similarly, live broadcasts of surgical procedures can be performed successfully. However, further studies are needed to establish this technology as a tool that students can learn from.

Acknowledgments

This work was supported by STRYKER Communications (www.strykercom.com).
We would also like to thank Mr. Guillermo Palli for donating his time as a consultant in this project.

References:

[1] Gandsas A; Montgomery K; McIntire K. et al. Wireless vital sign telemetry to hand held computers. Stud Health Technol Inform . 2001; 81: 153-7

[2] Schneider S; Kostecke R; Tokazewski. Buying your first PDA. J. Fam Pract Manag. 2001;8(7): 50-1

[3] Sable C. Telecardiology: Potential impact on acute care. Crit Care Med. 2001; 29(8):159

[4] Lapinsky SE; Weshler J; Mehta.. Handheld computers in critical care. S. Crit Care. 2001;5(4):227-31

[5] Gandsas A, Altrudi R, Pleatman M and Silva Y. Live Interactive Broadcast of Laparoscopic Surgery Via the Internet. Surg Endosc. 1998;12, 252-255.

Medicine Meets Virtual Reality 02/10
J.D. Westwood et al. (Eds.)
IOS Press, 2002

Using Semi-automated Image Processing and Desktop Systems to Incorporate Actual Patient Volumetric Data In Immersive Surgical Planning and Viewing Systems for Multiple Patients

I. George, M. Mastrangelo, Jr. M.D., J. Hoskins, W. Witzke, J. Stich, J. Garrison,
D.B. Witzke, PhD., M. Nichols, M.D., A. Park, M.D.
The University of Kentucky Center for Minimally Invasive Surgery (UKCMIS)

Abstract: This paper describes how patient specific volumetric data are managed from image acquisition through final processing for the purposes of creating a 3D VR rendering of user selected and manipulated 3D models. The system described here allows for the development of quick, inexpensive, and clinician manipulated patient-specific models. The utility of this process is demonstrated by being able to move VRML models to desktop or immersive environments for both pre-operative planning and patient-specific surgical and anatomical training.

Introduction

Methods for the creation of 3D models used for surgical planning and education have been detailed in the past. (1,2) However, they typically lacked realism and clinical renderings lacked full manipulability. In some cases these limitations resulted in loss of required volumetric data. Typically, creation of these renderings was resource intensive requiring great expenditures of labor, software, and hardware. More importantly, the models were not easily or intuitively accessible by the end user or surgeon. In some instances the anatomy being studied was literally removed from the volumetric data by a technician in an effort to "clean up" the image. This limited the clinician's ability to traverse the anatomic landscape, because much of the data no longer existed for such review. These obstacles have limited the clinician in effectively using volumetric 3D imaging for procedural planning. A key feature of our image modeling system is that it accommodates patient-to-patient variability for any patient that has undergone appropriate radiographic studies. The focus of our process is to increase the realism of our surgical simulators by bringing accurate, rapidly implemented patient-specific data to the virtual reality (VR) or desktop environment.

Methods and Tools

Stage I: Image Acquisition and Processing

Specific patient data sets are taken from computerized tomography (CT) sources (e.g. Siemens Somatom Plus 4 CT scanner) and this information is outputted into a DICOM file. Images are then ported to recordable media and reviewed in axial view, analyzed for image quality, and processed with Amira 2.3 ®(Template Graphics Software, Inc., San Diego, CA). Images are cropped and segmented using semiautomatic or automatic techniques. Volumetric data are thresholded to reveal an image of a particular radiodensity range. Once the structures of interest are defined, a regular surface is created from the points that define the anatomical entity being studied. These images are then turned into the anatomical models that are to be studied in the VR session. The models created in Amira must be in a surface conformity that allows for export as a VRML object. Figure 1 depicts our modeling process.

Stage II: Second Stage Processing

The VRML file is then imported into Cosmo Worlds 1.0.3 ®(Computer Associates International, Inc., Islandia, NY) where the geometry is simplified and mated to other anatomical structures that may have been ported in for the same patient. Currently, Amira exports the VRML as four integrated geometries. This collateral information, unnecessary for our purposes, is easily removed and the geometry is converted to a single simplified model using CosmoWorld. Simplification takes place in the form of triangle mesh decimation. Finally, the viewable model is exported in a format easily accessible by a standard desktop PC with a VRML viewer. These models can also be viewed on a VR simulator like the University of Kentucky's Trainer for Surgical Preparation (TSP) in the immersive environment of the ImmersaDesk (Idesk) ® (Fakespace Systems, Ontario, Canada).

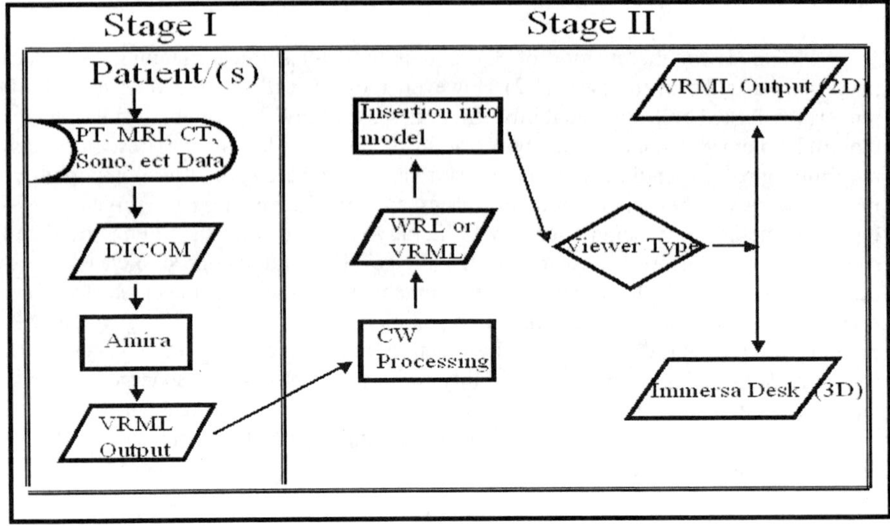

Figure 1. 3D Model Development Process

Results

We demonstrated a simple application for this process in surgical planning. Figure 2 shows an example of how we used this process to assist in the planning of trocar placement for laparoscopic nephrectomy. This example illustrates a simple patient model with the volumetric data of a patient's aorta, renal arteries, renal veins, and kidneys. We are able to travel through the ports and visualize how the view would look from the laparoscope and from an instrument perspective. Through this image we clearly gain insight into how we might approach the vessels and which port would provide for optimal approach to the renal vessels. We intuitively recognized basic and relative anatomic locations. We could use this model to predict where (approximate) optimal port placement might be, and to assist in anticipating procedural difficulties due to anatomy and positioning.

As a teaching aid, we provided anatomical simulations that were virtually dissected. Using this process in conjunction with standard techniques facilitated training.

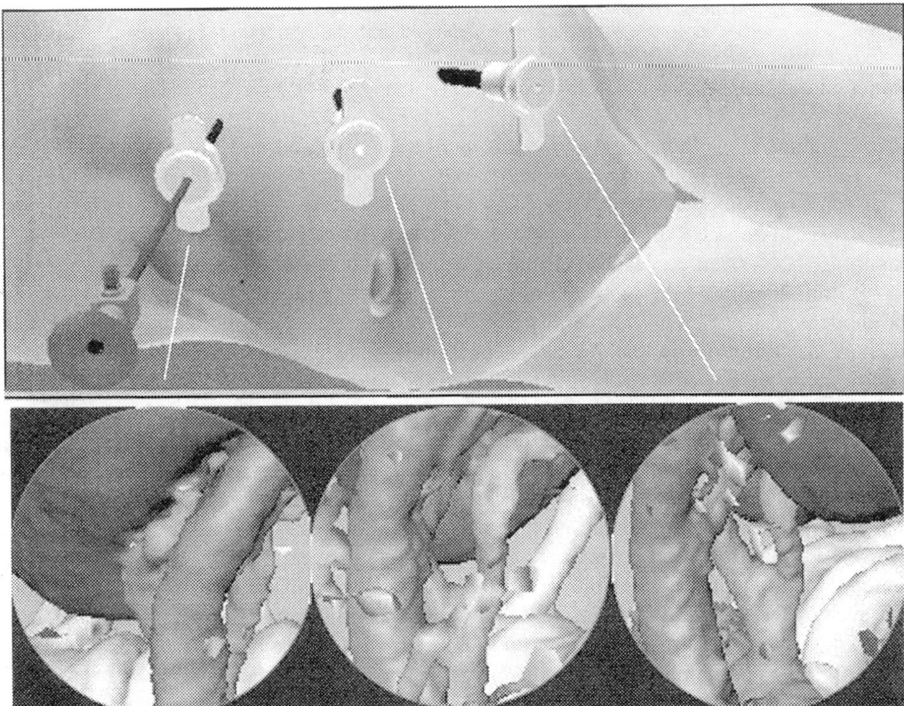

Figure 2. Laparoscopic views of renal vasculature

Processing an image using 0.5 mm CT slice data was done extremely quickly (i.e., in less than 15 minutes for most solid organs). The process timing included all the steps from acquiring the CT file in DICOM format to porting the VRML model into a target viewer (see Figure 1). The comparative cost and time requirements for model generation are detailed in Table 1.

	UKMIS System without Immersive VR (VRML Viewer and Desktop VR only)	UKMIS System with Immersive VR and VRML Viewer/desktop VR	CT scanner 3D imaging (integrated into scanner)	"Convention al Imaging Centers" VRML Viewer and Desktop only
Hardware	$2,100	$250,000	Itemized costs were not available.	
Software	$1,500	$1,500		
Staff excluding MD	$10	$10		
Total	$3,610	$251,510		
Image Cost	$10 15 min	$10 15 min	$450 45 min**	$850 and 3-30 days

Table 1. Cost Analysis*(excluding diagnostic scanner and output station)
*Approximations based on imaging of renal vasculature and also based on phone surveys conducted 10/17/01.
** Scanners are not available for patient imaging during this time with many scanners.

Conclusions

Actual 3D volumetric data/models can be incorporated into VR patients by means that facilitate teaching, technique or technology development, and surgical planning. These goals can be accomplished cost effectively and quickly using readily available software and hardware. This process also allows for ease of anatomic segmentation, and exportation of this information to either desktop or immersive VR environments.

Initially, in the development of our systems, we used only CT data sets. However, the model can incorporate both a physical 3-D geometry and a volumetric rendering with internal structures from either unimodal or multimodal imaging and registration systems. Additionally, we placed actual patient volumetric data (both 1st and 2nd generation [3]) in to a VR body (TSP). Using our method we reduced the processing time from days to minutes, reduced the need for super computing systems to desktop systems, and reduced our dependence on skilled anatomists and information specialists to render and interpret the final image. This was made possible as we moved from a manual segmentation process to semiautomatic and in some cases automatic segmentation.

Another important aspect of our process is that we used software that utilized standard Windows interfaces that are relatively easy to assimilate. The image manipulation process was facilitated by, but did not require a programmer/software specialist per se. As a result, the cost of our process is markedly less expensive than other means used to achieve similar, but less comprehensive, results.

The process we have detailed in this document is an important step towards the creation of comprehensive VR surgical preparation simulators and remote operative patient avatars. (4) The models created, image acquisition, and placement process are accomplished rapidly with off-the-shelf software and equipment. This allows for rapid placement into the immersive environment and subsequent 3D visualization. This process provides for immediate review of patient anatomy by the clinician via means less cumbersome than others described to date.

References

1.　　Robb, RA, *Biomedical Imaging, Visualization and Analysis.* New York, NY USA: VCH Press 2000: 326-328

2.　　Adachi, H. *Three-Dimensional CT Angiography.* Boston, USA: Little, Brown and Company Press 1995 1st Ed.

3.　　DB Witzke, JD Hoskins, MJ Mastrangelo, WO Witzke, UB Chu, S Pande, AE Park. Immersive virtual reality used as a platform for perioperative training for surgical residents. In JD Westwood, et.al. (Eds.) *Medicine Meets Virtual Reality, 2001.* Amsterdam: IOS Press. 570-576.

Medicine Meets Virtual Reality 02/10
J.D. Westwood et al. (Eds.)
IOS Press, 2002

Interactive Simulation
of the Teeth Cleaning Process
using Volumetric Prototypes

Tilo Gockel, Ulrich Laupp, Tobias Salb,
Oliver Burgert, Rüdiger Dillmann

Industrial Applications of Informatics and Microsystems (IAIM)
Chair Prof. Dr.-Ing. R. Dillmann
Building 07.21, Department for Computer Science
Universität Karlsruhe (TH), 76128 Karlsruhe, Germany
Tel.: ++49 721 608 7132, Fax: ++49 721 608 8270
Email: gockel@ira.uka.de, WWW: http://wwwiaim.ira.uka.de

Abstract. In this paper, an interactive simulation system for teeth cleaning is presented. This simulation system offers assistance for optimizing design and manufacturing of new toothbrushes. Data acquisition and pre-processing techniques for the model generation are shown and the mathematical method for modelling of the elastic behaviour of the toothbrushes parts is explained. Afterwards, a new approach to collision detection based on simple volumetric prototypes is described, user interaction is discussed and results of the project are shown.

1 Background

In this paper we present an interactive simulation system for teeth cleaning. This simulation system offers valuable assistance for optimizing the design and manufacturing of new toothbrushes. Benefit is also granted to researchers in Oral Health Care. The simulation system enables early tests of the functionality of future brush generations and enables the engineers to estimate the effects of design changes in an early state of the manufacturing process. Furthermore, the simulation system offers a cost-efficient way to experiment with different designs and functional properties in the development process of toothbrushes. It also allows to validate the efficiency of certain brush types and bristle configurations.

As far as we know, at present there's only one project dealing with the described task: the Virtual Toothbrush Simulator from Syseca [14]. Anyway, Syseca uses a much more simplified model, which is not capable of supporting more than one collision point or simulating bending of single bristles, therefore novelty of the presented system is granted.

First in this paper, data acquisition for jaw and brush models and preprocessing techniques for the model generation are shown. Then, modelling of the elastic behaviour of the handle of the toothbrush and the toothbrush's bristles is explained. Afterwards we describe a new approach to collision detection between bristles and teeth and we discuss the user interface of the system. The paper finishes with the presentation of the results.

2 Methods and Tools

2.1 Data Acquisition and Conversion

For a realistic simulation of the teethbrushing process three-dimensional models of the toothbrush and the jaw are needed. CAD models of different toothbrush handles were provided by our industrial partner. As the simulation is based on the Open Inventor Object Library [7,8], we had to convert the models into the Open Inventor data file format. This task was performed using the functionality of the ProEngineer CAD system. The bristle bundles on the toothbrushes head are modelled manually as rounded cylinders.

At the beginning of the project, CT scans of plaster casts from individual probands were used as jaw data sets with relatively poor results (1.4 mm slices), later on we used an optical pattern scanner that was developed exactly for this application and that delivered much more precise scans [3].

2.2 Modelling of Flexible Areas and Bristles

For modelling the flexible behaviour of the toothbrushes handle and bristles a basic Finite Element model is used [2,5,6,11]. First, the flexible area is divided into individual segments. Then, each of these elements is modeled as a bending beam. The analytical solution of the differential equation for one single bending beam is given by a polynomial function. Taking this polynom as an approach for the solution of the problem within the Finite Element Method, it provides precise functional values for the contact points between the different equidistant elements.

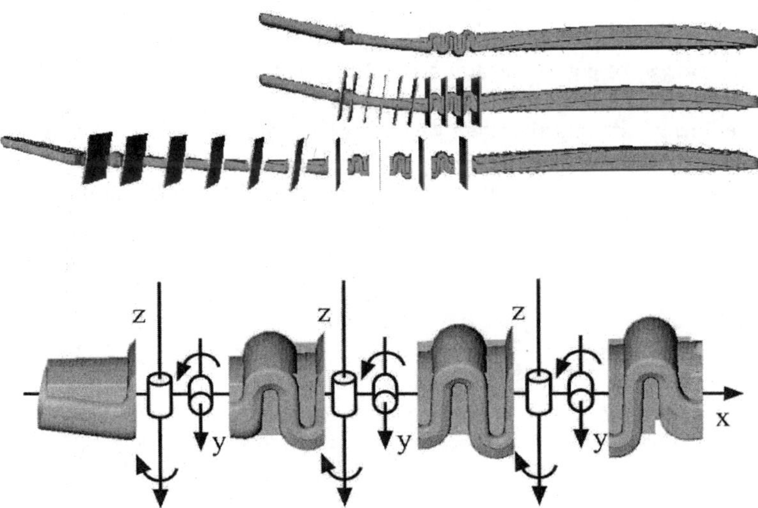

Figure 1: Sliced toothbrush dataset with inserted joints

A single bristle is currently modelled by five equidistant bending beams. Taking forces and momentums as input values and positions and angles as output values, a 10-dimensional equation system describes the relationship between these mathematical entities. Due to the dependencies between adjacent segments, a 10 x 10 matrix A, containing the single polynomial equations, represents the Finite Element model for a bristle. Considering additional conditions to be fulfilled by the equations, the resulting matrix A is a sparse matrix. The equation *Ax* = *b* represents the solution of the Finite Element calculation for a bristle whereby *b* is a *10*-dimensional vector that specifies the forces and momentums on each segment and *x* determines the new position and angle values of the segment after application of the forces and momentums. The emerging system of equations is solved using the *L/U*-decomposition. [5,6]

2.3 *Collision Detection between Toothbrush and Teeth*

The detection and visualization of collisions between the toothbrush and the teeth in the simulation system is of high importance for the whole project. With the delivered software library of the PHANToM haptoid (cp. *2.4, User Interface*), the GHOST library, it is impossible to handle more than one collision point (one bristle), so we had to implement a new volume-based algorithm for collision detection which is quite complex but nevertheless quite elegant: Given a (binary) voxel representation of the teeth, one can, using the Euclidian Distance Transformation, substitute the 1 or 0 in the representation of the object (inside or outside the object) with the length of the vector pointing directly to the surface of the object. This is the force vector, describing the reverse force effecting the colliding object, in our case the toothbrush.

Furthermore given a surface-model-based representation of the toothbrush and letting it literally "dive" inside the teeth, one can sum up all the force vectors that point backwards and one can calculate the resulting force vector $\mathbf{r}(V)$ for the system's user [15].

$$\mathrm{r}(V) = \int_V r_p(x)dx = \int_V r(\nabla Q(x))dx$$

This "diving" process of course has to be simulated via the FEM analysis as a bending of the bristles at the surface of the teeth.

After experiments with this algorithm we realized that the calculation was way to slow to permit interactivity and we decided not to use voxels but volumetric prototypes like spheres and cylinders as a representation of the surface model. The underlying algorithic idea is still the same but the calculation can be done much faster.

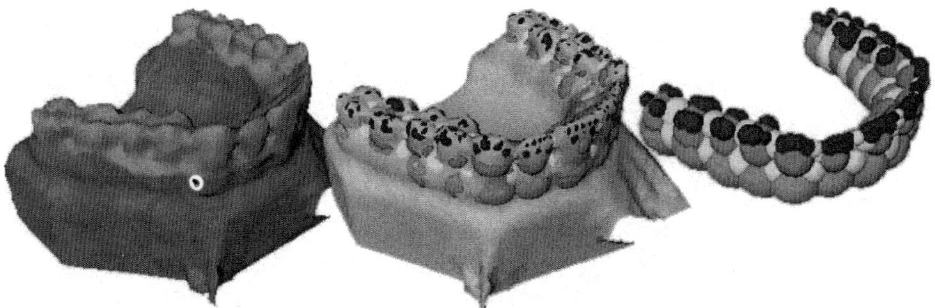

Figure 2: Teeth's surface data and overlay of the volumetrical representation

With this approach, a rapid collision detection is now possible. The frame rate of the visualization is directly proportional to the number of elements used (bristles and volumetric prototypes) and therefore the system is easily scalable with regard to the given computer power and the desired accuracy. [5]

2.4 User Interface

A fairly realistic behaviour of a simulation system can be achieved using an adequate user machine interface. At the beginning of the project, we integrated the PHANToM haptic feedback device in our simulation system [12,13]. Force-feedback can be simulated by programming a force field using the GHOST library delivered with the device. The force-feedback device plays the role of a virtual toothbrush. User interaction with the PHANToM worked well with one collision point [4,10] but was nearly impossible to realize with a reasonable response time with e. g. 30 bristles (one bristle representing one bristle bundle).

So we decided to return to user interaction via PC keyboard, using 12 keys to move the toothbrush in six degrees-of-freedom. At the moment we are working on a re-integration of the PHANToM with a second PC dedicated to this device and communicating via a socket interface with the PC managing the visualization.

3 Results and Discussion

A first prototype of our system has been established, using an SGI Octane SSI with a single R10000 processor. The software modules described above have been implemented and form a powerful simulation application. The bending lines of the toothbrush's handle and the bristles have been validated through overlay of the virtual toothbrush with a flatbed scan of a bended real toothbrush.

By now, it is possible to simulate the movements of the toothbrushes handle and of bristle bundles on the toothbrushes head considering the material properties specified by the user.

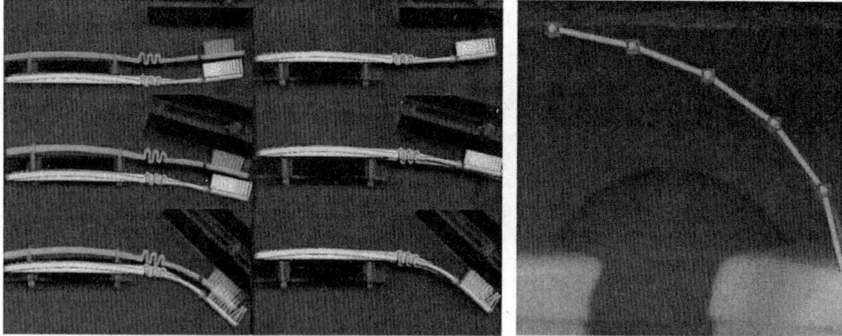

Figure 3: Validation of the bending line of the handle and the bristle
through overlay of simulated and real toothbrush (flatbed scan)

An interactive use of the simulation is still limited through the given computational power to approx. 20 to 30 bristles, but the system offers the possibility to record a trajectory and to do a second simulation run with more bristles without user interaction. In this offline-simulation a movie is recorded and can be viewed afterwards with an adjustable frame rate.

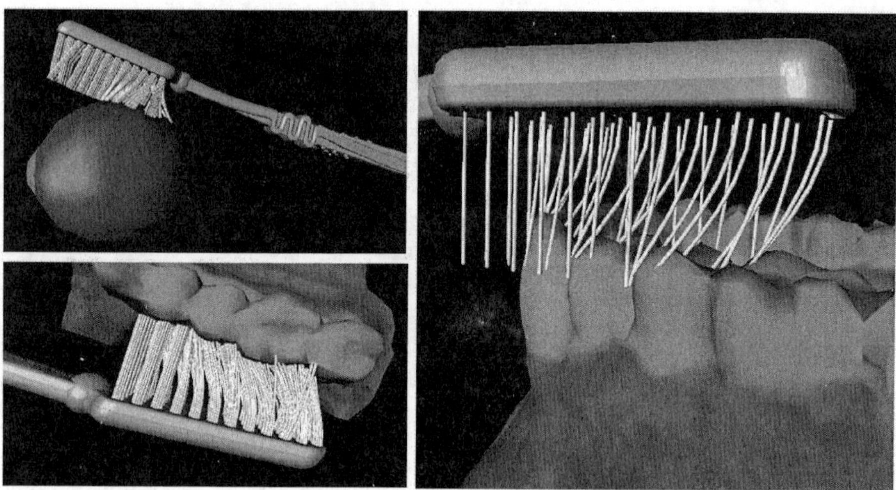

Figure 4: Screenshots of simulation sequences

4 Conclusion

In this paper a 3D simulation system for visualization and analysis of teeth brushing has been presented. The system is based on the Open Inventor Object Library. With the given import filters, standard jaw data sets may be used as well as patient individual data. Toothbrush datasets are modelled using original CAD data and specific bristle models. Behaviour of flexible elements of the brush like the bristles and parts of the handle is modelled using the Finite-Element Method.

First results are promising and the system will be refined. Future work will concentrate on re-integration of the PHANToM haptoid and the implementation of a reachability analysis for the brush and especially the bristles in order to control which points in the oral space are touched by the brush. Furthermore we are working on our own LASER-scanner for plaster casts to automatize and to speed-up the scanning process.

Acknowledgement

This research was performed at the IAIM Institute (Industrial Applications of Informatics and Microsystems) in the group of Prof. Dr.-Ing. R. Dillmann, Universität Karlsruhe (TH), Germany. This work was initiated and funded by an industrial partner of our institute.

References and Bibliography

[1]   Alcañiz, M., Grau, V., Monserrat, C., Juan, C. and Albalat, S. *A system for simulation and planning of orthodontic treatment using a low cost 3D laser scanner for dental anatomy capturing*. In: Medicine Meets Virtual Reality (MMVR), pages 8-14, San Diego, CA, IOS Press and Ohmsha, Jan 1999.

[2]   De Arantes e Oliveira, E. *Theoretical Foundations of the Finite Element Method*. In: International Journal of Solids and Structures, Vol. 4, 1968.

[3]   Girrbach-Dental Inc. *Product Description DIGIDENT - Teeth-Scanning and Milling of Replacements*. http://www.girrbach.de/D/ds/index.html. (German)

[4]   Gockel, T., Salb, T., Weyrich, T., Dillmann, R. *Interactive Simulation of Teeth Cleaning*. In: Computer Aided Radiology and Surgery (CARS), Berlin, Juni 2001

[5]   Laupp, U. *Modellierung und Simulation der Borstenbewegungen beim Zahnreinigungsvorgang*. IPR Institut for Process Control and Robotics. Diploma Thesis. Universität Karlsruhe, 2001 (German)

[6]   Nold, M. *Bewegungsanalyse und mathematische Modellierung des mechanischen Verhaltens einer Zahnbürste*. Universität Karlsruhe, IPR Institut for Process Control and Robotics. Diploma Thesis. Universität Karlsruhe, 1999 (German)

[7]   Open Inventor Architecture Group: *Open Inventor C++ Reference Manual*. Addison-Wesley, 1992.

[8]   Open Inventor Architecture Group: *The Open Inventor Mentor*. Addison-Wesley, 1994.

[9]   Salb, T., Brief, J., Burgert, O., Hassfeld, S., Mühling, J. and Dillmann, R. *An augmented reality system for intraoperative presentation of planning and simulation results*. In: 2nd EUREL Worskhop on Medical Robotics, Pisa, Italy, Sept 1999.

[10]   Salb, T., Ghanai, S., Burgert, O., Dillmann, R. *Interactive Simulation of Tooth Cleaning with an Interdental Brush*. In: MMVR (Medicine Meets Virtual Reality), San Diego, CA. IOS Press and Ohmsha, Jan 1998.

[11]   Schwarz, R. *Methode der finiten Elemente*. Teubner, 1994. (German)

[12]   SensAble Technologies Inc. *GHOST® SDK Programmer's Guide – Version 2.1*. Technical report, Cambridge, MA, 1999.

[13]   SensAble Technologies Inc. *PHANToM™ Haptic Interface – Hardware Installation and Technical Manual*. Technical report, Cambridge, MA, 1997.

[14]   Syseca   Inc.   *A   Virtual   Toothbrush   Simulator*.   http://www.syseca.thomson-csf.com/templates/section.asp?IDSECT=93&PAGE=4

[15]   Weyrich, T. *Kollision volumetrischer Körper mit einer als binäres Voxelbild gegebenen Umgebung*. Universität Karlsruhe, IPR (Institute für Process Control and Robotics), Internal Technical Report, IPR, 13. April 2000. (German)

Medicine Meets Virtual Reality 02/10
J.D. Westwood et al. (Eds.)
IOS Press, 2002

A Haptic Virtual Environment for Tele-Echography

Agnès Guerraz[1], Adriana Vilchis Gonzalez[2], Jocelyne Troccaz[2], Philippe Cinquin[2],
Bernard Hennion[1], Franck Pellissier[1], Pierre Thorel[1]
[1] France Telecom R&D, 28 chem du vieux chêne BP 98, F-38243 Meylan cedex
[2] TIMC/IMAG, Fac de Médecine, domaine de la Merci, F-38706 La Tronche cedex

Abstract. Having a haptic virtual environment for tele-echography will enable the medical expert with faster adaptation and especially facilitated immersion in what we could call a "virtual echographic examination cabinet". The innovation of this haptic control is to preserve medical expert proprioception and gesture feelings, which provide the users with indications that are synchronized with the echographic images. In this paper, we will focus on the telegesture module: we will detail several issues and solutions related to this particular problem of tele-robotic scan examination.

1. Introduction

Echographic examination which is mainly diagnosis-oriented turns out to be difficult and highly specialized. Several telemedicine projects have been launched to allow the remote assistance of an expert for such an examination when a patient cannot benefit from the best health care in the place where the examination should take place. These projects have faced communication problems since existing technology was not fast and robust enough at the time the projects started. Moreover, guiding an operator remotely is difficult. On one hand, the expert loses the haptic feedback of the probe moving onto the patient's body which is an important information; on the other hand, the non expert operator must interpret the 6D movement orders transmitted by the expert on a purely verbal way. In order to assist such an examination a French consortium has launched, the TER project [12], for robotic tele-echography.

The specific requirements for the tele-echography service are:
- Reliability of the systems
- Quality of the displayed images
- Proprioceptive control for fine and slow gestures of the remote probe
- High accuracy of gesture flows through the network
- Synchronization of echographic images and expert gestures
- Ease of use

We present a remote echographic system using haptic environment and providing a reliable solution for the practice of expert echographic examinations in distant geographical areas, or for emergency scenarios. The high value and performance of the medical gesture are the main reasons for haptic interface use.

During classical examination, the medical expert mentally rebuilds the 3D starting from the 2D echographic image and the gesture information. We must take into account physiological constraints of human gesture [13] so that telegesture is possible.

2. Method and Tools Used

The system can be briefly described as follows:
A virtual probe is mounted on the master interface device. The real probe is placed on the slave robot end-effector. Position and force information are transmitted bi-directionally (together with live visual and audio). Then, mainly based on the echographic images and force information he receives back, the expert operator can move the virtual probe to control the real one, see Figure 1. The slave robot executes the orders sent from the master site. A non-expert operator is located close to the patient and supervises the procedure that he can interrupt. The patient can at any time communicate with him or with the expert.
From clinician side, the haptic control station is developed to give more realistic environment and finer command of what remotely occurs. From patient side, the slave robot is remotely controlled by the medical expert, who handles his virtual probe via the force feedback robot.
The slave robot is an uncoupled parallel robot, composed of two independent parallel structures using artificial muscles McKibben [11] as actuators. This robot is equipped with a force sensor that makes it possible to control the force exerted in probe axis, [10], [12].

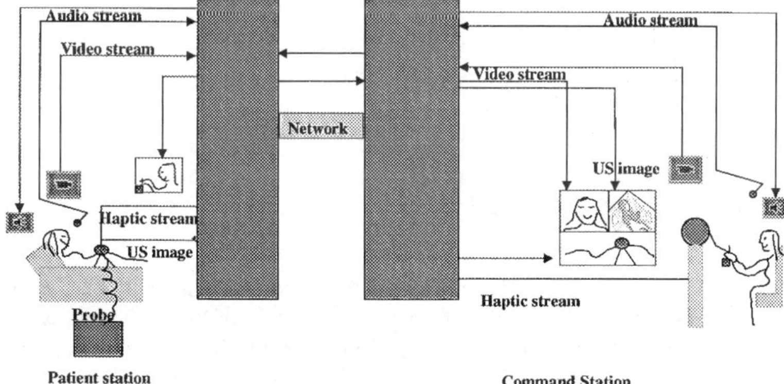

Figure 1 General and final architecture

We also use a virtual patient in order to make earlier experiments, see Figure 5 on the right. In that case, a software program simulates the patient. The 3D geometric model of the virtual distant patient is coded with a polygonal mesh. The force feedback is calculated starting from a physical model of the virtual 3D form that is touched. The material point is heavy, elastic and viscous. The state of the material point is governed by mechanical equations. The virtual patient is flexible, deformable and its mechanical characteristics: viscosity, rigidity, and mass can be adjusted.

3. The obstetrical scan examination

The obstetrical scan examination knew its first applications for the pregnancy woman at the end of the fifties, and its true development during the beginning of the seventies.
According to the stage of the pregnancy, this technique of medical imagery allows to visualize all or a part of the fetus, to measure it and to observe it. For the mother, the examination is simple, painless and without danger. A probe to pass on the maternal abdomen emits ultrasounds. According to the difference in acoustic density of the met bodies and members, the reflexion of the ultrasounds facts of appearing on the screen in a more or less clear or sunk way, in black and white or even color.

Each echography of the pregnancy, one per quarter in the French health care, has its reasons to be and brings the invaluable information, become irreplaceable within the framework of a monitoring of quality of the pregnancy.

The expert echographists advise to preferably pass this examination between 12th and 13th week of amenorrhoea, for the first examination, then during the 22nd week and the last at the 32nd week.

The general objective of the examination of echography is to provide the date of the beginning and the end of the pregnancy, to obtain measurements on the fetus in order to establish curves of growths and to compare them with curves of pre-established growths. It enables also the detection of anomalies on certain bodies.

In the case of problem, it happens that the attending practician prescribes additional echography, because they are now part of this new specialty, which is the antenatal diagnosis. The practician can thus act as soon as possible to establish a diagnosis. One will often distinguish the various types of echographic examinations: traditional examinations, of monitoring, for expertise, or urgently. These examination types are different by their context from application and the level of expertise necessary.

4. Gesture Analyze

The following observations are based on 11 different examinations, on various stages of the pregnancy: 11th week, 22nd week, and 32nd week of amenorrhoea. These echographic examinations proceeded in the cabinet of MD. Marc Althuser, with the agreement of the patients. These meetings were filmed so analyzed completely and precisely the movements necessary to the catch of the echographic sights.

4.1   The practician

The practician initially prepares the abdomen of the patient who will be the surface of work. Then it spreads out gel to allow an easy displacement of the probe but especially for facility the penetration of the ultrasounds. Initially, it practices the localization of the fetus by making translations length on broad the surface of work. From this moment, the study of the bodies of the fetus, but also of the mother can start. The activities of the traditional practician during the examination steps are the following ones:
-    Verbal interaction with patient
-    Application of gel on the abdomen of the patient
-    Gesture Interaction: position - orientation - pressure of the probe on the abdomen of the patient
-    Indications to the patient, for example: stop and resumption of breathing
-    Process of analysis of the echographic images
-    Rebuilding of information 3D by the means of images 2D and of gesture, proprioception information.

4.2   Gesture observation of traditional obstetrical echographic examinations

The movements most usually used in rising order: orientation and motionless pressure, pressure, motionless and pressure, side / longitudinal translation, orientation pitching, orientation rolling, orientation yawing, entering movement, zigzag movement.

The circular rotation is not necessary but it is used nevertheless.

4.3   The measurement of the variations of the efforts

We found that the main force exerted on the abdomen of the patient was the pressure. Due to the gel spread out over the abdomen, there are very few tangential forces.

The measurement of the effort variation during the examination:

Measuring apparatus used: a dynamometer
Method of measurement: the dynamometer is attached to the probe

Results:

- Gesture Work using of the minimal pressures: measurements from 0.6 to 0.7 dN
- Gesture Work using of the pressures standards: measurements from 0.8 to 1.1 dN
- Maximum Pressure: 1.3 dN
- Variation of Pressure exerted: 0.7 dN

These measurements do not reflect the reality of the exerted pressures in a precise way. However the results show the variations of the efforts authorized.

4.4　　The surface of work

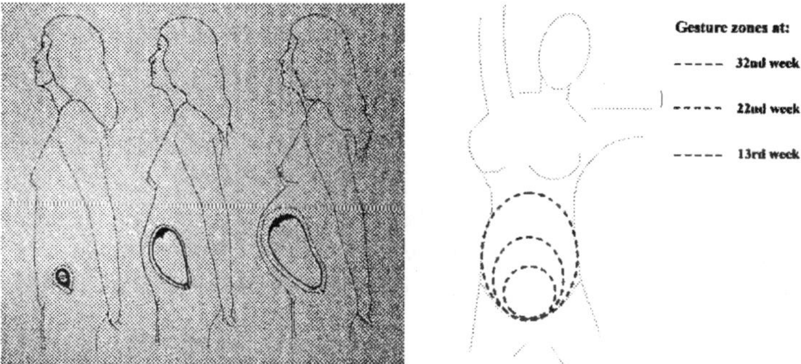

Figure 2 Gesture zones

The translations and gestures zones observed are used to define the surface of work used during the examination by the doctor this surface of work depends on the stage on the pregnancy. As the pregnancy evolves/moves, the surface of work becomes larger.
On the Figure 2, three stages of the pregnancy are shown; one notices the evolution of the place taken by the uterus. The surface of work is taken into account at the examination beginning according to the corpulence and the pregnancy stage of the patient.

5.　Our Virtual Reality Approach for the coding of these gestures

The 3D geometrical model of the patient is coded with polygonal objects. The grid is deformed under the gesture. The fine touch is the notion of touching free forms.

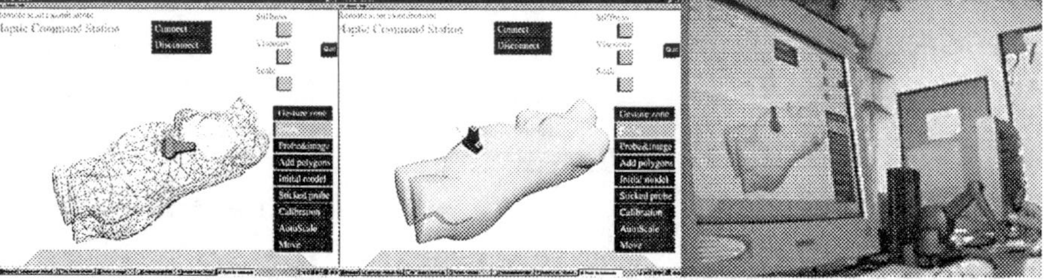

Figure 3 Haptic command station screen shot in local loop – without network connection

Touch of the facets: it is the calculation of the position of a point that is named the haptic point[1] , compared to a selection of facets to touch - when the scalar product between the normal to the touched face and the vector going from the haptic point to its projection

---

[1] The haptic point is the extremity of the phantom arm that is the point of application of the force, in the virtual world.

on the same face changes sign, the haptic point crosses the facet. The force will then be calculated as F = - K X. (K is the stiffness of the virtual object at the considered face and may be fixed or dynamically adjusted and X outdistance the haptic point to the facet). For this approach the continuity of the force is not induced and the processing of smoothing is necessary. Indeed, the force must be continuous when the user makes the handle slide along the surface of the object so that the haptic point projection changes facet.

We tried out two ways of feeling this modelling dependent on the contact with a polygonal object. The first one allows a force feedback according to the nearest polygon to the haptic point position. The second comes from the first one, and allows an effort feedback according to the polygon closer to the haptic point, but also according to its vicinity. In the Figure 3 on the center, the green segment materializes the intensity of the force perceived by the manipulator via the force feedback robot.

Gesture sequences can also be recorded to make a simulation, or to replay these sequences. We can build gesture cards.

6. Transport of these gestures

The tele-gesture is the achievement of a remote gesture, i.e. to touch a distant object, that is real or virtual, for example, a human body, and to feel its mechanical characteristics, sensitivity specific to the bones, muscles, tendons and joints which give information about its static, balance and the displacement of the body in space. To reach a good sensory perception of the distant scene, it is necessary to create a specific flow for the haptic data: position, orientations, and feedback forces. This flow presents intrinsically a bi-directional characteristic. Its quality is extremely dependent on the latency of the intermediary telecom network. To ensure an encoding of the gesture, it is advisable to use a virtual 3D object, of which it is necessary to build a coherent visual and haptic representation [4]. Each scene is duplicated on the two connected sites: on the local machine and on the distant machine.

The haptic device frequency is too high, typically 1KHz, so it would not be possible to go forwards and backwards through the network at such a rate! On each machine, one must thus establish a local loop operating at the rate of 1KHz, from which the data is extracted and sent to the network at a desired lower rate.

A SensAble PHANToM haptic robot is used. This device has 6 degrees of freedom and renders three-dimensional force information. It can track the position and orientation of the tool within a workspace of 16 cm wide, 13 cm high and 13 cm deep. The maximum exerted force is 6.4 Newton.

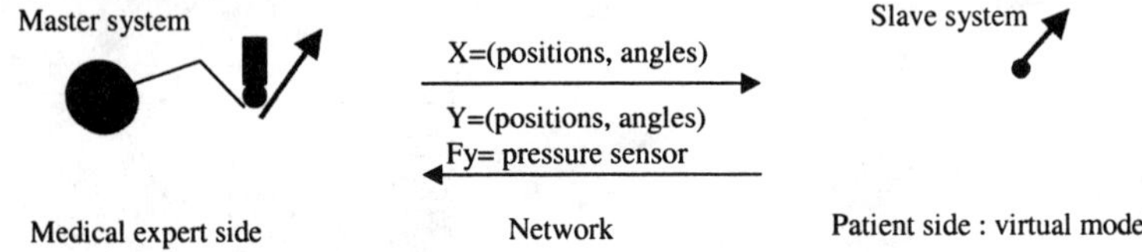

Figure 4 Diagram describing the networked gesture prototype

The gestures used in the traditional scan examination are possible with such haptic device. The effort variation is of the same order than the one observed during examinations. The maximum exerted force is smaller than the one measured during the examination. Thus the practician have to adapt a little, but the most important point is to feel variation of pressures.

The tele-echography is a case of static touch, with a pressure sensor on the patient abdomen. The command station, side of the medical expert, sends his position command and receives the position of the distant virtual probe as well as the pressure force calculated on the distant virtual patient, see Figure 3.

Figure 5 (on the left) shows the current interface of the haptic command station for tele-echography. The green segment materializes the intensity of the force perceived by the medical expert.

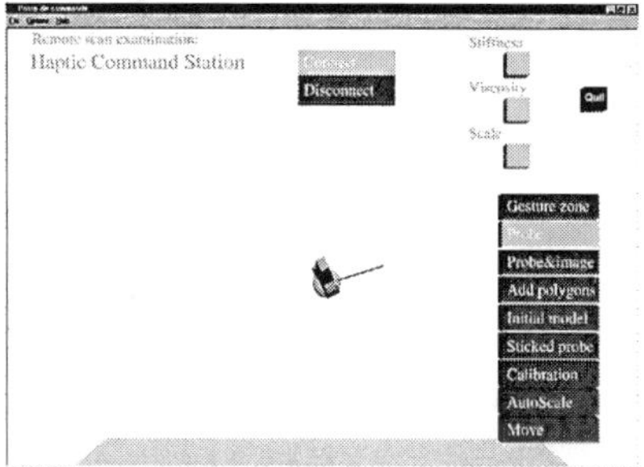
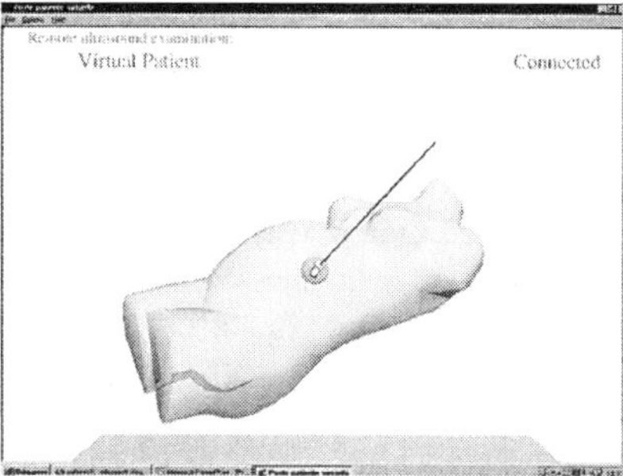

Figure 5 Screen shots of the haptic command station - expert side (on the left) and of the distant virtual patient (on the right) in network

Via the network the doctor feels mechanic characteristics of the abdomen: hardness, viscosity. That contributes to the recognition of fetus the positioning. This tactil feedback also makes it possible to get the 3D gesture in space by correlating it with the 2D echographic images, as during the traditional examination.

To improve gesture ergonomics of the expert within the tele-echography, we will create the virtual tangential forces, which increase quickly if the medical expert moves his hand too quickly, because the distant robot will have its own speed limits. The medical expert will feel the force exerted on the patient and measured with a sensor, perpendicularly. For the moment, the force exerted on the virtual patient is calculated according to a mechanical model and his mechanical characteristics, viscosity, rigidity, and mass can be adjusted.

7. Results

The different modules of our system have been tested separately. In particular, slave robot control and telegesture testing demonstrated encouraging results [10], [4]. Integration and testing of the whole system will be finished at the end of this year.

The first prototype of tele-echography on ISDN, Integrated Services Digital Network, using a virtual patient has been tested in Bristol - UK (Master system – Medical expert) through Grenoble – France (Slave system – virtual patient). During this experiment the latency of the network was 78 ms. The quality of the gesture was correct for slow gestures. Some oscillations appeared, but the haptic rendering was good.

Prototype of tele-echography on ISDN using a virtual patient results:

- Slow gestures with no limit in rotations and translations
- Ease of use and immersive feeling
- Traditional gestures are possible
- Presences of oscillations due to the latency of the network
- Interest of the network terminal for learning gestures: possibilities to record gestures - positions and pressure synchronized with the echographic images.

8. Conclusion

Compared to the tele-medicine systems [2], [5] [9], this system uses robotics for robot tele-operation and haptic for "rendering" the force exerted by the robot. The transport of the gesture data via the network allows an immersion even more complete and realistic for distant manipulators. This haptic command station preserves medical expert proprioception and gesture feelings. In the final architecture, it will give to the users, haptic indications that are synchronized with the echographic images.

9. Acknowledgements

We thank MD. Marc Althuser who allowed us: to film gestures, to evaluate the gesture efforts, and also who participates in testing the first prototype of tele-gestures. We also thank all his patients who accepted our presence and our experiments during their scan examinations.

References

[1] De Cunha D., Gravez P., Leroy C., Maillard E., Jouan J., Varley P., Jones M., Halliwell M., Hawkes D., Wells P.N.T., Angelini L., The midstep system for ultrasound guided remote telesurgery, in 20th Annual International Conference of the IEEE Engineering in Medicine and Biology Society, volume 20, pages 1266-1269,1998.

[2] Ferrer-Roca O., Sosa-Iudicissa M., Handbook of telemedicine, IOS Press, 1999.

[3] Gourdon A., Poignet Ph., Poisson G., Vieyres P., and Marché P., A new robotic mechanism for medical application, in IEEE/ASME International conference on Advanced Intelligent Mechatronics, pages 33-38, September 1999.

[4] Guerraz A., Hennion B., Vienne A., Belghit I., The tele-gesture: problems of networked gestures, in proceedings of the EuroHaptics 2001, pages 65-70, 2001.

[5] www.irisi-nordpasdecalais.org/acercles/loginat.htm.

[6] Masuda K., Kimura E ., Tateishi N. and Ishihara K. Development of remote echographic diagnosis system by using probe movable mechanism and transferring echograp via high speed digital network, in Procceding of IX Mediterranean Conference on Medical and Bilogical Engineering an Computing (MEDICON'01), Pula, pages 96- 98, juin 2001.

[7] Pierrot F., Dombre E., Dégoulange E., Urbain L., Caron P., Boudet S., Gariépy J., and Mégnien JL. Hippocrate : a safe robot arm for medical applications with force feedback, Medical Image Analysis, vol 3:285-300, 1999.

[8] Salcudean S.E., Bell G., Bachmann S., Zhu W.H., Abolmaesumi P, and Lawrence P.D. Robot-assisted diagnostic ultrasound-design and feasibility experiments, In Lecture Notes in Computer Science, Medical Image Computing and Computer-Assisted Intervention (MICCAI'99), pages 1062-1071, 1999.

[9] www.crcg.edu/projects/teleinvivo.html.

[10] Vilchis G. A., Cinquin Ph., Troccaz J ., Guerraz A., Hennion B., Pellissier F., Thorel P., Courreges F., Gourdon A., Poisson G., Vieyres P., Caron P., Mérigeaux O., Urbain L., Daimo C., Lavalle S., Arbeille Ph., Althuser M., Ayoubi M., Tondu B., and Ippolito S. TER : a system robotic tele-Echography, lecture Notes in computer Science, Medical Image Computing and Computer-Assisted Intervention (MICCAI'01), 2001.

[11] B. Tondu and P. Lopez, Modeling and Control of McKibben Artificial Muscle Robot Actuators, IEEE Control Systems Magazine, vol. 20, no.2, pp. 15-38, 2000.

[12] Vilchis G. A., Troccaz J., Cinquin Ph., Courreges F., Poisson G., and Tondu B. Robotic Tele-ultrasound System (TER): Slave Robot Control, in proceedings of TA'2001, IFAC Conference on Telematics Application in Automation and Robotics, July 2001.

[13] Wing A-M., Haggard P., Flanagan J-R., Hand and Brain - The neurophysiology and Psychology of Hand Movements, Academic Press, 1996.

Medicine Meets Virtual Reality 02/10
J.D. Westwood et al. (Eds.)
IOS Press, 2002

Cryotherapy Simulator for Localized Prostate Cancer

James K. Hahn, Ph.D.[1], Michael J. Manyak, M.D.[2], Ge Jin[1], Dongho Kim[1],
John Rewcastle, Ph.D.[3], Sunil Kim, Ph.D.[4], and Raymond J. Walsh, Ph.D.[2]

[1]Institute for Computer Graphics
[2] Department of Urology , School of Medicine and Health Sciences
The George Washington University
[3]Department of Radiology, University of Calgary and Endocare Inc.
[4]Department of Biomedical Engineering, Hanyang University

Abstract. Cryotherapy is a treatment modality that uses a technique to selectively freeze tissue and thereby cause controlled tissue destruction. The procedure involves placement of multiple small diameter probes through the perineum into the prostate tissue at selected spatial intervals. Transrectal ultrasound is used to properly position the cylindrical probes before activation of the liquid Argon cooling element, which lowers the tissue temperature below -40 degrees Centigrade. Tissue effect is monitored by transrectal ultrasound changes as well as thermocouples placed in the tissue. The computer-based cryotherapy simulation system mimics the major surgical steps involved in the procedure. The simulated real-time ultrasound display is generated from 3-D ultrasound datasets where the interaction of the ultrasound with the instruments as well as the frozen tissue is simulated by image processing. The thermal and mechanical simulations of the tissue are done using a modified finite-difference/finite-element method optimized for real-time performance. The simulator developed is a part of a comprehensive training program, including a computer-based learning system and hands-on training program with a proctor, designed to familiarize the physician with the technique and equipment involved.

1. Introduction

Prostate cryotherapy is a relatively new procedure for prostate cancer in which the prostate gland is treated in situ by freezing. The freezing and thawing process destroys the prostate glands, which are replaced by scar tissue following the procedure. This is accomplished by inserting several cylindrical cryoprobes into the gland under ultrasound guidance. Thermocouples are placed at strategic locations within and around the gland to monitor the formation of ice crystals around the cryoprobes which occurs when the cryoprobes are activated. The ability of a physician to deliver an efficacious freezing injury is largely dependent on clinical experience and the ability to create an area of treatment known as an 'iceball' that kills the target cancerous tissue without damaging surrounding tissues.

A prostate cryotherapy simulator has been developed to expedite the learning process associated with this technically demanding procedure. Three dimensional ultrasound images of the prostates from real patients are used. The physician can practice prostate cryotherapy in a clinically realistic manner by placing and operating the cryoprobes before actually treating a patient. During a clinical procedure the physician monitors the iceball growth on ultrasound and also uses the temperature measurements from the thermocouples

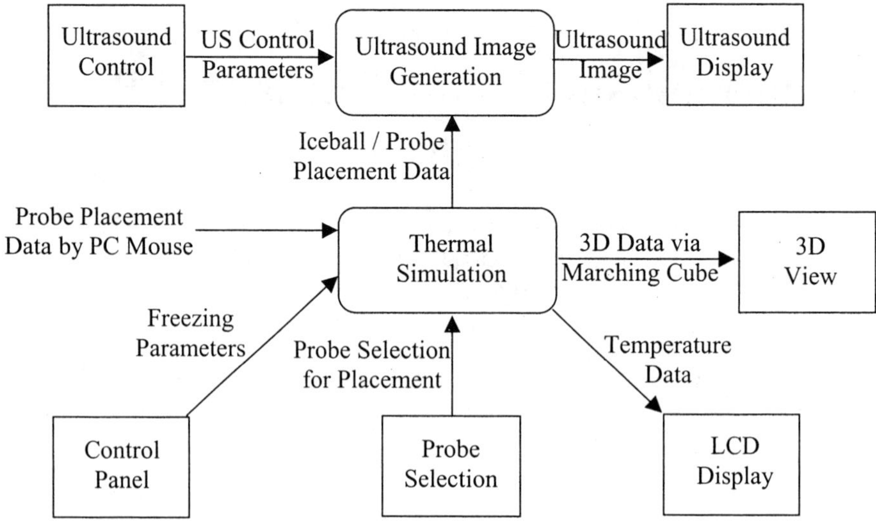

Figure 1: Diagram of Functional Modules

to assess the extent of the freezing injury. A mathematical cryotherapy simulation with verified accuracy is used to determine the temperatures surrounding the cryoprobes during the procedure simulation. Changes that occur in the ultrasound image when ice forms in tissue have been accurately reproduced. Combining this visual feedback with the thermocouple readings, the physician can judge the extent of freeze injury in both tissues targeted for destruction and tissues that must remain unfrozen.

This simulator allows a physician to gain a skill set previously attainable only with clinical experience. The simulation is being incorporated into the training process by Endocare Inc., a leader in the development of cryotherapy technologies. The current training process consists of a day of classroom instruction and the physician being proctored, on average, for their first six clinical cases. This is very inefficient from a cost perspective because of the need to provide an expert in cryotherapy as the proctor for each case. The simulator provides a physician an intuitive feel for the procedure and a solid understanding of how the freezing process will be visualized within the target tissue based upon placement and activation of the cryoprobes. Incorporation of the simulator into the training process is expected to reduce the number of cases that require oversight as the physician becomes comfortable with the procedure. Consequently, it is believed that this will result in a significant reduction of the cost associated with training [8].

2. System Design

The simulation system is composed of three main sub-systems:
1) the ultrasound image generator
2) the thermal simulator
3) the user interface components to control the simulation and the virtual instrumentation

Figure 1 shows the overall functional diagram of the simulator. In this figure, the rounded blocks denote internal function blocks, and rectangular blocks represent the

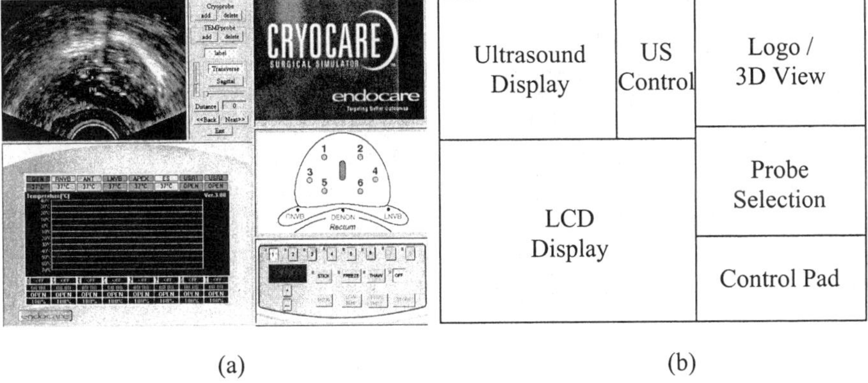

<table>
<tr><td rowspan="2">Ultrasound Display</td><td rowspan="2">US Control</td><td>Logo / 3D View</td></tr>
<tr><td rowspan="2">Probe Selection</td></tr>
<tr><td rowspan="2">LCD Display</td><td></td></tr>
<tr><td>Control Pad</td></tr>
</table>

(a)   (b)

Figure 2: (a) Overall interface (b) Functional diagram of the interface

functions of user interface components. The descriptions along the arrows denote the type of data flow.

3. User Interface (UI) Components

The interface to the system mimics the devices that the physician interacts with in a real procedure including ultrasound display and control, LCD screen for the cryoprobe instrumentation as well as thermocouples, and the control panel for controlling the temperatures of the cryoprobes. In addition, there is a 3D view pane that shows a bird's-eye-view of the prostate, position of the cryoprobes and the thermocouples, and the growing ice balls. This view is not available during a real procedure. This situational awareness is what an experienced surgeon deduces from inputs of the available instruments. However, giving the user this explicit view allows the user to gain an understanding of how to interpret the information he/she is given during the procedure. Figure 2 shows a screen shot of the simulator interface along with the functions performed by the user interface components. At the beginning of the simulation, the user selects from a number of case studies to give a rich variety of simulated experiences. A surgery planning software is incorporated into the simulator to give the ideal placement for a particular patient. A number of metrics can be recorded during the procedure to give the user a feedback on his/her performance.

3.1 Ultrasound Display

Ultrasound display and control are shown in the upper-left part of the screen. This display is generated from a cross-section of a 3D ultrasound volume data for the surgery area. The 3D volume data is obtained by a 3D ultrasound device. The cross sectional view is generated according to the control parameters given by ultrasound control user interface. The control for the simulated ultrasound mimics a real transrectal ultrasound device. A physician can switch between axial and lateral views. The position and orientation of the transducer are controlled by using the slide bars. In addition to the tissue, the inserted cryoprobes are rendered on the ultrasound. Optionally, labels can be shown on the ultrasound to identify the locations of particular cryoprobes. When tissue freezes, the area

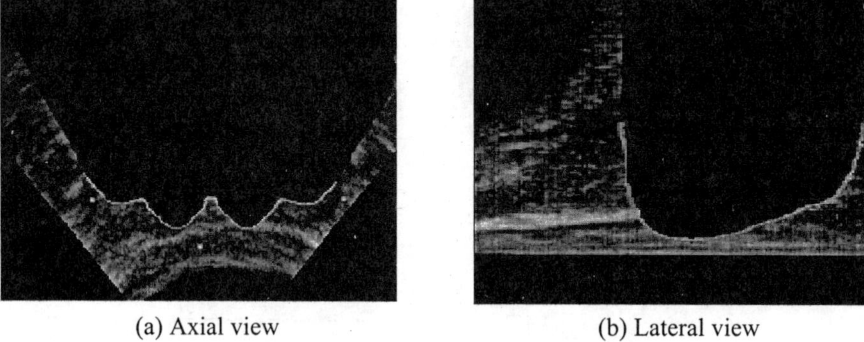

(a) Axial view   (b) Lateral view

Figure 3: Ultrasound images during the simulation

becomes opaque to ultrasound. The resultant shadows and diffraction is simulated (Figure 3). The virtual ultrasound view is generated in real time [1,2,6].

3.2 LCD Display and Control Pad

The freezing process in real cryotherapy is controlled by a remote control pad. The same interface is located in the lower right corner of the simulator's screen. With the control pad, the physician can set the operational mode for each of the cryoprobes. With the remote control, he/she can select a cryoprobe which is currently being operated. The operating mode can also be changed between stick, freeze, thaw, and off modes. The number denotes the duty factor which controls the amount of freezing for each cryoprobe.

The LCD display shows the information for the cryoprobes and current temperatures at the cryoprobes and thermocouples. The history of the temperatures for each thermocouple is shown on a graph. Figure 4 shows the LCD display with temperature graphs obtained during the simulation.

3.3 Cryoprobe Management

The interface shown in the middle-right area of Figure 2(a) enables the user to select a cryoprobe or thermocouple being currently controlled. Once the inserting position is determined, the operator can insert the probe by dragging the mouse. The probes are displayed in real time on the ultrasound display. The physician can practice the placement by dragging the probes while controlling the ultrasound device.

4. Thermal Simulation

The purpose of the simulator is to mimic the freezing process of real cryotherapy. In order to achieve this, thermal simulation is performed based on finite difference model. We use three dimensional grid structure to represent the thermal simulation elements. Each element contains current temperature, and interacts with nearby elements by giving and receiving thermal energy. The freezing process begins at the tips of the probes and neighboring elements are frozen as the simulation proceeds. The temperature information of the elements is always available so that it can be given to the user.

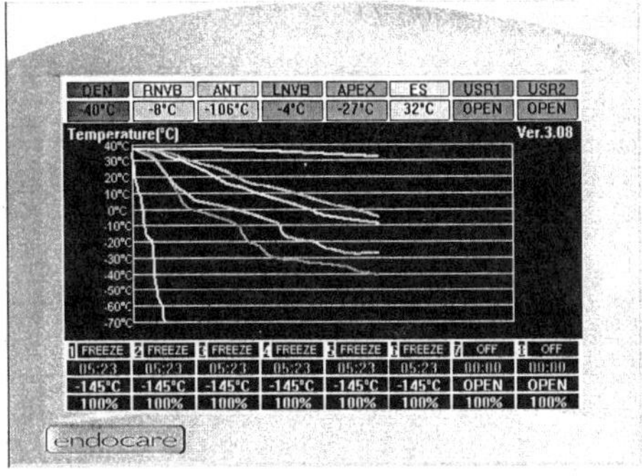

Figure 4: LCD Display

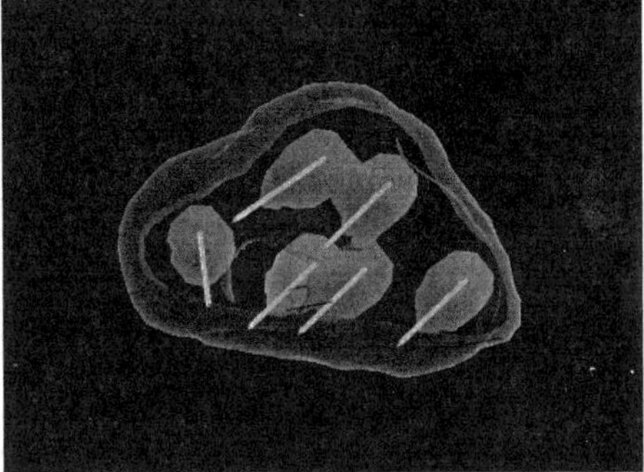

Figure 5: 3D View

The information about the current situation is given to the operator through the ultrasound image. During the simulation of cryotherapy, the ultrasound image is altered in order to reflect the changes made by the freezing process. Iceball regions are identified by the thermal simulation module as being opaque to ultrasound. Ultrasound shadows and reflection effects are added. Figure 3 shows the ultrasound display during the simulation of cryotherapy in axial and lateral views.

LCD display shows the current temperatures for all cryoprobes and thermocouples. The current operating modes of the cryoprobes are also provided. Figure 4 shows a screen shot of LCD display during the simulation. The graphs in the figure represent the temperature history for the cryoprobes.

The simulation status can also be seen in 3-D birds-eye-view. A typical result is shown in Figure 5. In this figure, the red object is a model of the prostate while yellow rods are cryoprobes. Iceballs are shown in two colors. The white iceballs are iso-surfaces for the temperature of -40 °C, and blue iceballs are for 0 °C. This view can be rotated or zoomed by simple mouse operations. The prostate model is obtained by segmentation before the simulation. The iceball objects are obtained by standard marching cube algorithm [5]. Once the user pauses the simulation, the marching cube algorithm extracts the iso-surface from thermal simulation grids and generates the iceball objects.

5. Conclusion

Despite the prevalence of surgical simulation systems, very few are actually being used routinely for training. The difficulty is not only technical but in engineering a system that fits the task. In this simulation system, we have taken the approach that many low-end flight simulators have taken in that we have concentrated on the intellectual learning component and left out the manual dexterity to be learned in actual procedures.

The simulation system has been developed and has gone through several iterations. Preliminary indications are that it is effective in training the user in the techniques and the instrumentation and is an important component in a coherent and comprehensive training program for the procedure.

References

[1] D. Aiger, D. Cohen-Or, "Real-Time Ultrasound Imaging Simulation," Real-Time Imaging, Volume 4(3), pp. 263--274, August 1998.

[2] Michael Bajura, Henry Fuchs, and Ryutarou Ohbuchi, "Merging Virtual Objects with the Real World: Seeing Ultrasound Imagery within the Patient," Computer Graphics (Proceedings of SIGGRAPH 92), 26 (2), pp. 203-210, Chicago, July 26-31, 1992.

[3] James G. Colsher, "Interative 3 Dimensional Image Reconstruction from Tomographic Projections," Computer Graphics and Image Processing, 6(6), pp. 513-537, December 1977.

[4] James Hahn, Roger Kaufman, Adam Winick, Thurston Carleton, Youngser Park, Rob Lindeman, Kwang-Man Oh, Nadia Al-Ghreimil, Raymond Walsh, Murray Loew, Joanne Gerber, and Siddarth Sankar, "Training Environment for Inferior Vena Caval Filter Placement," Medicine Meets Virtual Reality (MMVR '98), San Diego, CA, January 28-31, 1998, IOS Press.

[5] William E. Lorensen and Harvey E. Cline, "Marching Cubes: A High Resolution 3D Surface Construction Algorithm," Computer Graphics (Proceedings of SIGGRAPH 87), *21 (4)*, pp. 163-169, Anaheim, California, July 1987.

[6] Thomas R. Nelson and Todd Todd Elvins, "Visualization of 3D Ultrasound Data," IEEE Computer Graphics and Applications, 13(6), pp. 50-57, November 1993.

[7] http://www.endocare.com

Reliability and Validity of EndoTower, a Virtual Reality Trainer for Angled Endoscope Navigation

Randy S. HALUCK MD FACS[1], Anthony G. GALLAGHER PhD[2,3],
Richard M. SATAVA MD FACS[2], Roger WEBSTER PhD[4],
Thomas L. BASS MD[1], Cynthia A. MILLER BS[1]

[1]*Department of Surgery, Penn State College of Medicine, Hershey, PA   17033*
[2]*Department of Surgery, Yale University School of Medicine, New Haven, CT 06510*
[3]*School of Psychology, The Queen's University of Belfast, Belfast BT7 1NN, NI*
[4]*Department of Computer Science, Millersville University of Pennsylvania School of Science and Mathematics, Millersville, PA   17551*

Abstract. We hypothesized that a simulator designed to train surgical novices angled laparoscopic navigation would show an improvement in subjects' performance, a high test re-test reliability and high internal validity as measured by standardized coefficient alpha.   It was also predicted that simulator performance would be strongly related to objectively assess perceptual and visuospatial ability. EndoTower has good face validity in that it mimics precisely the performance of an angled laparoscope and previous studies suggest construct validity.   In this study, EndoTower is shown to be a trainer intended for laparoscopic skill than can test for inherent perceptual and visuospatial ability.

1. Background/Problem:

The Penn State EndoTower (EndoTower) is a PC based simulator/trainer that utilizes the Virtual Laparoscopic Interface (VLI, Immersion Corp., San Jose, CA).   An additional hardware component attached to the VLI device represents an angled laparoscope structure and function. It is designed to provide instruction and practice in the skills necessary for camera/laparoscope navigation for minimally invasive surgery [1].

All surgical procedures require some degree of visual navigation within an operative field. Laparoscopy presents additional challenges as visual and spatial cues are altered. Most commercially available angled laparoscopic camera and lens systems must be independently rotated, or not rotated by the user in order to achieve the desired angle of view while maintaining correct right-side-up orientation. This camera and angled rigid lens system is used in many different operations covering a number of surgical specialties.

The function, orientation, and correct manipulation of an angled laparoscopic lens in combination with an independently rotating camera system is not necessarily intuitive. As the surgeon performs the actual operation, the duty of camera navigation falls to the assistant, often a less-experienced team member. Robotic assisted camera navigation also requires that the surgeon have a fluid understanding of the workings of the optical system.

Several studies suggest that an inherent trait, visuospatial ability, correlate with a higher level of surgical skill [2-4]. Visuospatial abilities relate to the ability to mentally represent three-dimensional situation using key landmarks, and to have a clear mental picture of their relationship in space [5]. While other studies do not support this conclusion [6], it is apparent that some degree of visuospatial ability is required for surgical performance,

Surgeons using video assistance need to form visual impressions of three-dimensional structures, organs and instruments, from a two-dimensional television monitor. While this is often described as loss of binocularity [7], it is simpler and more accurate to call it pictorial perception. So-called primary cues – binocular disparity and convergence, accommodation, and motion parallax – are present in abundance. The difficulty is that the primary cues and other cues related to lighting and texture yield a conclusion that is inimical to surgery. The conclusion specified is that the structures in view form a single surface, virtually flat and usually vertical. The surgeon has to set aside that conclusion in order to register the information carried by subtler 'pictorial' cues and to reconstruct the structure that they specify despite the incompleteness of the information provided. Individuals differ in this ability and such differences could clearly contribute to performance differences for pictorially guided laparoscopic surgery.

Although EndoTower was designed to provide instruction in angled laparoscope navigation, we hypothesized that it would also serve as a testing platform to reliably assess visuospatial and perceptual ability. A simulation tool that is able to reliably assess these abilities, identifying levels of inherent ability in surgeons, while increasing skill acquisition may have additional value for surgical education.

2. Methods:

The task for the EndoTower testing session entailed identifying randomly placed arrows in the virtual "EndoTower". The EndoTower is a three-dimensional (3D) block tower with cylindrical holes within its various arms (Figure 1). The EndoTower provides a relatively complex three-dimensional structure for exploration with the virtual angled lens. In the simulator, 3D arrows of varying colors and directional orientation are randomly placed around the tower and inside the cylindrical cut-outs. Arrows were chosen as the targets so that participants would be required to maintain right-side-up orientation in order to be able to properly identify them. Arrows could have one of four colors and six directional orientations giving 24 possible combinations. Six arrows were randomly placed on and within the virtual EndoTower as part of the software program (Figure 2).

To operate the simulator, the subject held one of the VLI laparoscopic tools, modified to simulate the angled lens laparoscope. Rotation of this mock camera and lens rotated the horizon and angle of view from the longitudinal axis of the virtual laparoscope, respectively. The virtual world mimics the real world as the user's viewpoint is placed at the tip of the laparoscopic tool. Due to the 3D nature of the EndoTower and the cylindrical cutouts, identifying all the arrows entailed manipulating the laparoscope to many different and challenging orientations and positions.

Once a target arrow was found and identified, the student selected the matching arrow from a list using the foot-pedal function of the VLI. Any collision with the EndoTower caused the view to become fuzzy and blurry with 'red out', simulating touching the laparoscope to an organ and smudging the lens with blood. The learner was required to withdraw the virtual laparoscope and await a cleaning mode, thus penalizing the user's score in terms of time efficiency and also scoring an error. EndoTower mechanism recorded the amount of time to correctly identify the color and orientation of each arrow and the number of arrows.

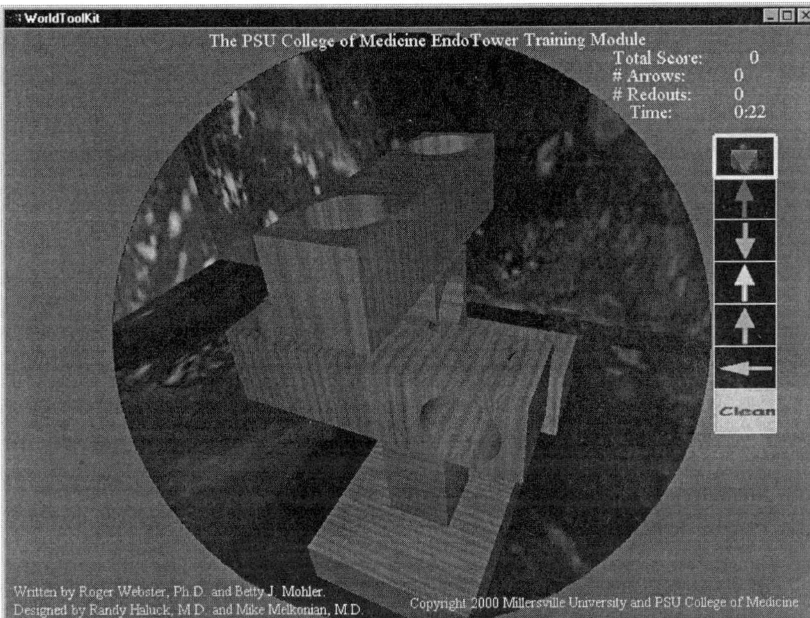

Figure 1: The three dimensional EndoTower

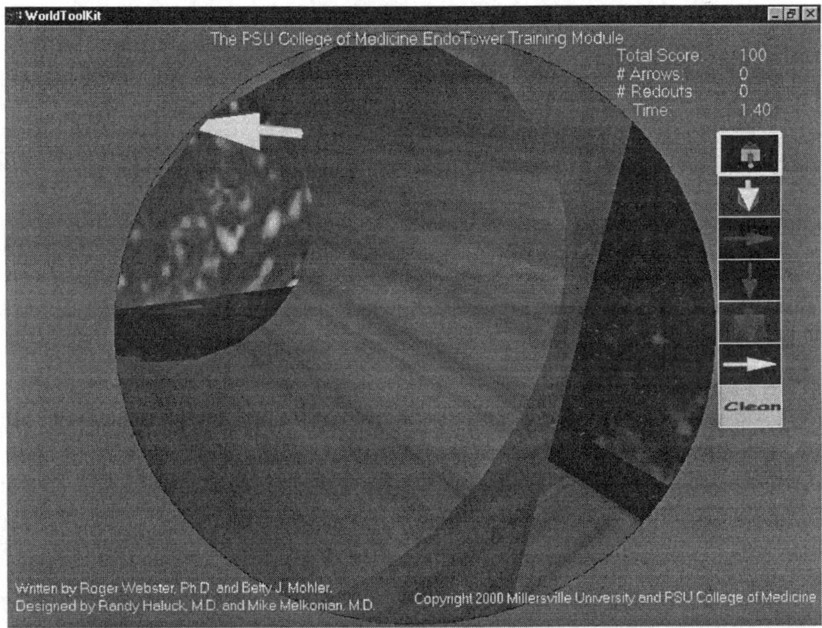

Figure 2: A randomly placed arrow within the virtual EndoTower

A time limit of four minutes was selected to complete the task of correctly identifying all six arrows. Computerized scoring was determined by the time to find all six of the target arrows plus the number of "red-out" errors multiplied by a factor of 10. If at the end of the four minute time limit, all of the arrows were not identified, the number of arrows not found was multiplied by 30 and added to the score. Therefore, a lower score indicated a better performance.

Twenty-five laparoscopic novices completed three trials on EndoTower. None of the subjects had ever used EndoTower or manipulated a rigid laparoscopic lens. All subjects received a brief and standardized instruction session on the goals and function of EndoTower. One testing was accomplished and the computer-generated score was recorded.

All subjects also completed the Pictorial Surface Orientation (PicSOr) test battery, a perceptual task that assesses the ability to reconstruct 3-D from 2-D perceptual cues [8]. They also completed three tests that assess fundamental visuospatial abilities, Card Rotation (CR), Cube Comparison (CC), and Map Plan (MP) [9]. Gallagher et al have reported that these tests are reliably associated with laparoscopic performance [10, 11]. The study was approved by the institutional review board with informed consent obtained from all participants.

3. Results:

The mean EndoTower scores were, trial 1 = 337 ± 50, trial 2 = 324 ± 73 and trial 3 285 ± 71. Subjects' performance improved consistently across the three trials. Analysis of variance for repeated measures showed that there was a statistically significant difference between the trials ($F(2, 24) = 13.05$, $p < 0.00001$). Differences between the different trials were compared for significance with Scheffe Post Hoc F-Tests. Although there was an improvement in scores between trial 1 and trial 2 this improvement was not statistically significant. The improvement in scores between trial 1 and 3 was statistically significant (Scheffe $F = 12.62$, $p < 0.0001$) as were the differences between trials 2 and 3 (Scheffe $F = 6.87$, $p < 0.01$). A statistically significant within subject effect was also observed. The within subject effect means that some subjects' EndoTower scores were statistically different from the mean EndoTower score ($F(2, 24) = 5.05$, $p < 0.0001$).

The test re-test reliability of EndoTower was calculated using Pearson's Product Moment Correlation Coefficient. The observed correlation coefficient was $r = 0.8$ ($F(1, 23) = 33.82$, $p < 0.0001$) and $r^2 = 0.6$.

To determine the internal validity or consistency of EndoTower as a measurement device Standardize Coefficient Alpha was calculated and was observed to be $\propto = 0.88$ ($F(2, 24) = 13.574$, $p < 0.00001$).

The correlations between EndoTower performance and PicSOr, CR, CC and MP were $r=0.591$, $r=0.296$, $r=0.354$ and $r=0.392$ respectively. However, when any single visuospatial test was combined with the PicSOr perceptual test in a multiple regression model the correlations increased dramatically. The results for the different regression models showed that for, PicSOr and CR, $r=0.658$, $r^2=0.43$ ($F(2,37)=14.2$; $p<0.00001$); PicSOr and CC, $r=0.701$, $r^2=0.49$ ($F(2,37)=17.89$; $p<0.00001$); and PicSOr and MP, $r=0.708$, $r^2=0.50$ ($F(2,37)=118.6$; $p<0.00001$).

4. Discussion / Conclusions:

A number of factors cumulate in the successful performance of an operation. Spencer suggested that "probably about 75% of the important events in an operation are related to making decisions, and about 25% to dexterity" [12]. Although this may be true, an operation is the result of manipulation of tissues ultimately requiring technical performance and skill. At this point in time, the acquisition of operative technical skill is poorly understood, both from the standpoint of the ingredients or abilities that serve as the basis for skill and which individuals might posses those ingredients. A test that replicates tasks for which surgical skill is required, yet can assess inherent abilities, may help to further the understanding of skill acquisition. One factor that will affect operative performance is practice.

The human brain has a limited capacity to attend to different sources and amounts of information. This means that the surgeon can only attend to a given amount of information at any given time. The more familiar the surgeon is with information, or the more frequently they have come in contact with it, the less attentional processing resources that information will require. The opposite is also true. This is important in surgery because attentional resources that are used on behaviors such as instrument navigation are not available for the most important aspect of surgery, i.e., surgical performance. We believe that simple but fundamental aspects of video assisted surgery such as camera navigation should be largely learned in the laboratory so that residents can hone their skills in the operating room rather than acquire them from basics.

One of the primary functions of a simulator, virtual reality or otherwise, is to improve performance. Another function of a virtual reality simulator is to provide objective assessment of performance, however, assessment cannot be accepted at face value. Satava [13] has suggested that if a virtual reality system purports to assess performance, validation metrics associated with that claim must be reported. In this paper we have reported that EndoTower has good face validity in that it mimics precisely the performance of an angled laparoscope. Interestingly, EndoTower also appears to be able to discriminate those individuals who have difficulty performing the task as indicated by the significant probability value for between subjects ANOVA results. It also has been demonstrated to have high test re-test reliability and a high alpha coefficient. In this study, we have also taken the validation a stage further.

Visuospatial ability and perceptual ability have been hypothesized and reported to be correlated with laparoscopic performance [10, 11]. These hypotheses appear sensible but need further experimental validation. In this study these abilities were found to be strongly related to EndoTower performance, particularly when included in a multiple regression model. In fact, simple regression models accounted for 43–50% of the variance. This is an important point because multimodal behaviors (e.g., perceptual, cognitive and psychomotor) required for complex real-world performance, such as surgery are unlikely to be explained by a simple correlation model, more likely a multiple regression model or ideally a Structural Equation Model.

Intuitively, it would seem that an ability to mentally reconstruct 3D from 2D cues and manipulate complex 3D structures and environments would be fundamental to performing operative manipulations. However, there is disagreement in the surgical literature regarding their ability to predict surgical skill. The study reported here shows that objectively assessed perceptual and visuospatial abilities predict angled scope navigation performance. This lends support to the hypothesis that these abilities are related to laparoscopic surgical performance. Furthermore, EndoTower assessment of these abilities has greater face validity for the assessment of a surgical skill, i.e., the test is simulated angled scope navigation. However, further validation work on this issue is required.

Virtual reality simulation has moved from 'is it pretty' to 'does it work and where is the evidence' to sophisticated metrics about performance parameters. Satava [13] has suggested that all virtual reality simulators must meet these fundamental criterion markers to be considered as a scientifically validated simulator. EndoTower has gone some way to meet these criteria however one of the major challenges for virtual reality remains, "Does training in the virtual environment transfer to the OR?" This work is currently underway in our laboratories and we are optimistic about the outcome.

5. Acknowledgements:

This project was funded in part by the Penn State Eberly Virtual Hospital Project and one of the authors (AGG) was supported by the Fulbright Distinguished Scholar program.

6. References:

1. Haluck RS, Webster R, Melkonian M, Mohler B, Dise M, LeFever A: A virtual reality surgical training module for instruction in angled laparoscopic lens navigation. Stud Health Technol Inform 2001;81:171-176.
2. Schueneman AL, Pickleman J, Hesslein MA et al: Neuropsychological predictors of operative skill among general surgery residents. Surgery 1984;96:288-295.
3. Gibbons RD, Baker RJ, Skinner DB: Field articulation testing: A predictor of technical skills in surgical residents. J Surg Res 1986;41:53-57.
4. Risucci D, Tortolani A, Horowitz M: Neuropsychological assessment of general surgery interns. Focus Surg Edu 1991;10:14-15.
5. DesCoteaux JG, Leclere H: Learning surgical technical skills. CJS 1995;38:33-38.
6. Francis NK, Hanna GB, Cresswell AB, Carer FJ, Cuschieri A. The performance of master surgeons on standard aptitude testing. Am J Surg 2001;182:30-33.
7. Reinhardt-Rutland AH and Gallagher AG. Visual depth perception in Minimally Invasive Surgery. In SA Robertson (Ed) Contemporary Ergonomics;1996:531-536.
8. Cowie R. Measurement and modeling of perceived slant in surfaces represented by freely viewed line drawings. Perception 1998;27:505–540.
9. Ekstrom RB, French JW, Harman HH, Dermen D. Manual Kit for Factor – Referenced Cognitive Tests. 1976 Princeton New Jersey: Educational Testing Service.
10. Gallagher AG, Crothers I, Satava RM. Comprehensive objective assessment of fundamental skills for laparoscopic surgery. Surg Endosc 2001; In Press.
11. Gallagher AG, Cowie R, Crothers I, Jordan JA, McGlade K, McGuigan J, McClure N. PicSOr: An objective test of perceptual skill that predicts laparoscopic performance in three separate studies. Surg Endosc 2001; In Press.
12. Spencer FC. Observations on the teaching of operative technique. Bull Am Coll Surg 1983;3:3-6.
13. Satava, RM. The need for metrics in surgical education. (1999) Surg Endosc; 13: 1082-1082

Medicine Meets Virtual Reality 02/10
J.D. Westwood et al. (Eds.)
IOS Press, 2002

Volumetric Virtual Body Structures

Paul Hatfield, BS, Bharti Temkin, PhD
Dept. of Computer Science, Texas Tech University
Lubbock, TX 79409,
(806) 742-3527, Bharti.Temkin@coe.ttu.edu

John A. Griswold, MD, Sammy A. Deeb MD,
Dept. of Surgery, Texas Tech University Health Science Center

Parvati Dev, Ph.D., W. LeRoy Heinrichs, M.D., Sakti Srivastava, M.D., Kenneth Waldron,
Ph.D.
*SUMMIT (Stanford University Medical Media and Information Technologies), Stanford
University School of Medicine*

Abstract

Understanding the visuospatial aspects of anatomic structures is one of the most important goals of gross anatomy. Creation of realistic three-dimensional structures of human anatomy has thus been a goal of medical doctors and computer scientists. In this paper, we describe a PC/NT based system in which a user can easily select anatomical structures to be created, along with the chosen connected structures. The system then constructs a three-dimensional volumetric model, a virtual body structure, slice-by-slide. Once the virtual structure is assembled it is possible to "walk" through the volume with coronal, sagittal, and transverse views, or at any angle. The dynamic nature of the system is unique in that it allows for real time choice of volumetric body structures to be created, their rapid generation, and the ability to manipulate the resulting visualization.

1. Introduction

In the past, computational complexity of volumetric visualization and interactive manipulation made it necessary to use high-end workstations to obtain detailed structural information (including internal structures) and visuospatial relations between body structures.

This paper describes a unique PC/NT based system, which creates interactive volumetric virtual body structures (V-VBS) in real-time using the Visible Human segmented data set. The system allows a user to easily 1) navigate through human body via sagittal and coronal slices. Labeling identifies organs within the slices. Navigational tools incorporated into the system allow users to quickly select the volume of interest. The system can also create a volume around specific chosen structures, if desired by the user. 2) Adding or deleting anatomical structures, from a list of structures within the volume, permits inclusion of connected (or proximal) structures to be created for interactive visualization. 3) Once the V-VBS is created, dynamic manipulations, such as zoom in and out, changes in resolution, translation and rotation, changes in transparency, etc. are easily performed allowing the user to see high level of anatomical details. Some of these details and the "waking through the volume" capability enhance the 3D experience that may be difficult to achieve with other modes of learning anatomy.

2. Volume and Organs Selection

Our system is dramatically different than most volume visualization systems. Current systems rely on static data files to load a restricting bounding volume such as the system described in a paper published by the university of erlangen-nuremberg [2]. Our system allows the user to define the volume. There are two ways of selecting the V-VBS to be generated. The first method uses an alphabetical list of organs within the database. Once structures are selected a pre-existing tightly fitting bounding box is used to initiate visualization. If a smaller, or a larger, volume is of interest, the pre-existing bounding box can be easily modified to create a new volume. The second method allows a direct traversing through coronal and sagittal views for choosing the x, y, and z values, Figure 1. System navigational tools are simple and interactive between the views. The organs can be labeled for navigational aid.

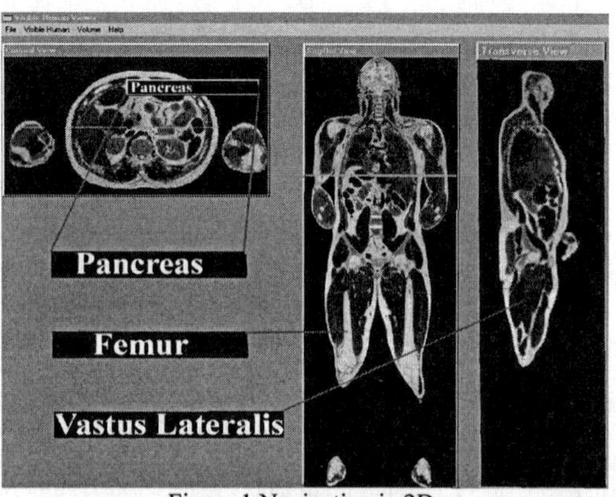

Figure 1 Navigating in 2D.

Once a volume is chosen the user selects the list of anatomical structures (and their connected structures) within the volume, Figure 2. The chosen structures will be opaque during visualization, with the level of opacity under user's control.

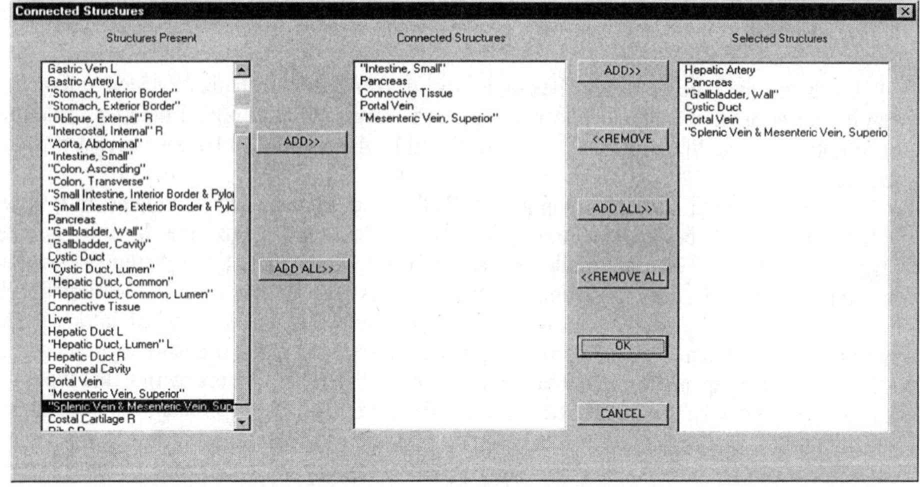

Figure 2 Choosing structures for visualization. The left, middle, and right columns respectively represent the organs within the specified volume, the organs connected or adjacent to the selected organ in the left column, and the organs selected for visualization.

3. Building and Manipulation of V-VBS

Once the structures are chosen, the system builds the volume slice by slice. The slice-by-slice construction process of a V-VBS can be animated to facilitate the learning experience that leads one to "build 3D models in the mind" [1]. Realistic color rendering of the volume is achieved via a database of RGB values for each pixel. Surface or slice rendering options are provided for faster manipulations. Switching to volume rendering provides greater level of detail. An example of a V-VBS is shown in Fig. 3. The gall bladder and pancreas were chosen as a single V-VBS. The realistic coloring and the ability to fly through the organs present more information in sharp contrast to surface based models. In addition, an option to make specified organs opaque and others transparent is available. The system allows for dynamic manipulations, such as zoom in and out, resolution change, translation and rotation, change of transparency, etc. 3D labeling system helps identify structures, which aids in accomplishing the key goal of the National Library of Medicine to link visual information to text-data [3].

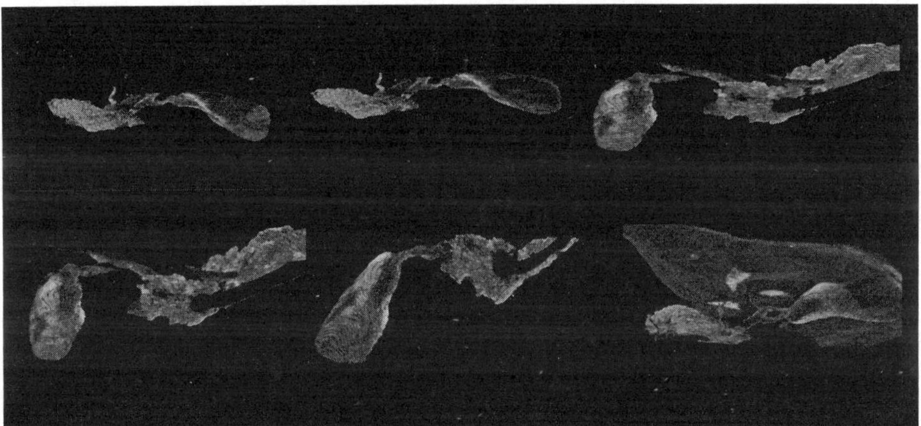

Figure 3 Gallbladder and pancreas manipulations.

4. Conclusion

Compared with other methods for volume visualization, our system offers rapid construction of user-defined volumetric virtual body structures from segmented Visible Human data set. The 3D models are not pre-existing in our system. The system is based on the concept of "what you want is what you get" for real-time assembly and efficient viewing, navigating, and manipulating of many organs, and their connected (or proximal) structures. The system allows for dynamic selection, creation, and detailed volumetric visualization of human body in real-time on PC/NT platform. The user does not have to have medical background to use this system and does not have to be a student to learn from it.

Our future efforts will include 3D labeling navigational tool to aid in understanding of what is being seen; employing larger regions of human body in real-time; networking V-VBS for collaborative environment; developing volumetric haptics for touching and eventually performing deformations and cutting that are the basics for surgical simulation.

5. References

[1] Bharti Temkin, Ph.D., Bryan Stephens, Eric Acosta, Bin Wei, Paul Hatfield. "Virtual Body Structures" http://www.nlm.nih.gov/research/visible/vhpconf2000/AUTHORS/STEPHENS/TEXTINDX.HTM, 2000.

[2] C. Rezk-Salama, K. Engel, M. Bauer, G. Greiner, T. Ertl. "Interactive Volume Rendering on Standard PC Graphics Hardware Using Multi-Textures and Multi-Stage Rasterization" In Proc. Eurographics/SIGGRAPH Workshop on Graphics Hardware, 2000.

[3] National Library of Medicine *The Visible Human Project.* http://www.nlm.nih.gov/pubs/factsheets/visible_human.html, 2001.

Medicine Meets Virtual Reality 02/10
J.D. Westwood et al. (Eds.)
IOS Press, 2002

Intraoperative 3D Shape Recovery of Abdominal Organs for Laparoscopic Data Fusion

Mitsuhiro HAYASHIBE[1], Naoki SUZUKI[1], Yoshihiko NAKAMURA[2]

Asaki HATTORI[1], Shigeyuki SUZUKI[1]

[1]Institute for High Dimensional Medical Imaging, Jikei Univ. School of Med

4-11-1, Izumihoncho, Komae-shi, Tokyo 201-8601 Japan

[2]Department of Mechano-Informatics, University of Tokyo

7-3-1, Hongo, Bunkyoku, Tokyo 113-8656 Japan

Abstract

Precise measurements of geometry should accompany robotic equipments in operating rooms if their advantages are further pursued. For deforming organs including the liver, intraoperative geometric measurements play an essential role in computer surgery in addition to pre-operative geometric information from CT/MRI. The laser-scan endoscope system acquires and visualizes the shape of the area of interest in a flash of time. Results of in-vivo experiments on the liver of a pig verify the effectiveness of the proposed system. In the next stage, we aim to make a data-fusion in laparoscopy.

1. Introduction

Endoscopic surgery forces surgeons to operate under mental tension with mechanical and visual constraints. The visual difficulties are due to the narrow area of view of endoscopes and the lack of depth perception. This means surgeons are required to extract a sense of orientation in the abdominal cavity from the anatomical structure and the direction of the laparocope, which leads to awkward operating technique for surgeons. As a result this may cause you misperception due to the difference in environment from open surgery.

Laparoscopic surgery would be technologically improved if surgeons were provided with a 3D representation of the internal geometry in an intuitive manner. Being integrated with real time interface, such technology would make a significant difference in the operational environments. We believe this would be effective under surgery directly operated by surgeons and robotic surgery. The technical advance of minimally invasive surgery has introduced more and more such equipped environments [1]. As there are many mechanical devices such as the laparoscope, with its holding arm and forceps, it would be important to make a position management for these devices from the viewpoint of safety. The 3D shape of the internal geometry can play an important role in enabling a surgeon to approach his target from the correct direction.

In the field of robotic surgery, master-slave robotic systems have recently been introduced in operating rooms. Da Vinci (Intuitive Surgical Inc[2]) and Zeus (Computer Motion Inc.[3]) have been applied to endoscopic cardiac surgery and laparoscopic surgery. Surgeons are now able to control two arms in the patient's body with two master devices outside from a distance. Even in these systems, the interface between the robotic systems and surgeons is only a straightforward one where the human interface is still limited to direct manipulation between master and slave robotics devices. We presented "Laser-Pointing Endoscope System for Natural 3D Interface between Robotic Equipments and Surgeons" [4] in MMVR2001. This paper showed the realization of *in-situ* 3D point registration from 2D image. An invivo measurement of a pig's liver was carried out and scanned data was automatically redescribed into VRML.

In this paper, we show a further developed system that has been extended from the previous paper. Using 3D geometric information, it would have the function of a safety management for laparoscopic surgery including the robot system. Now, we are introducing a second prototype. It is the intraoperative 3D shape recovery system for laparoscopic data fusion. Previous work dealt only with the surface geometry of the organ. However, the internal structure measured by CT/MRI is also essential geometric information for medical use. Therefore, we are developing a second prototype system that allows the data-fusion of 3D reconstructed internal structure for laparoscopy. Also, we propose a floating window that enables us to provide intuitive comprehension about the abdominal space. This device displays the virtually computed information onto the actual abdomen.

2. Intraoperative 3D Geometric Registration

Here, we depict the measured models by this system (first prototype). Please refer to the previous paper as to system configuration. In the sense of 3D measurement, the second prototype is similar to the first one. The second prototype configuration is shown in chapter 6.

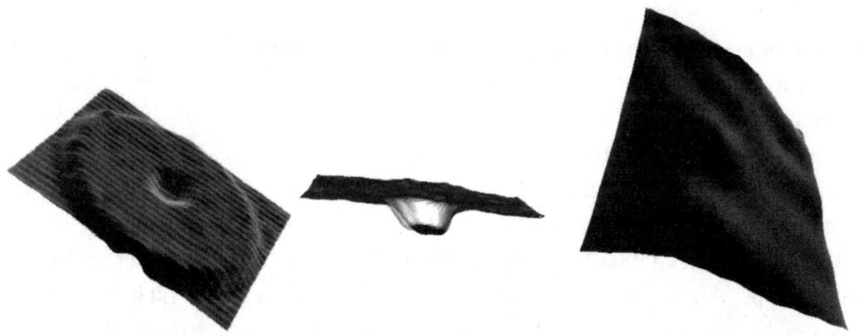

Fig. 1 Scanned surface of 50yen coin   **Fig. 2 Scanned VRML liver model in laparoscopy**

Figure 1 shows the scanned surface of a 50yen coin done by Laser-Pointing Endoscope. The hole on the 50yen coin could be measured and the error is within 1%. The scanned 3D data is automatically redescribed in VRML 2.0 by our developed program. The surface is composed of numerous triangle patches.

The scanned data of the previous paper was obtained after the abdomen was opened. The prime purpose of this research is to obtain 3D geometry under the laparoscopic surgery. We made an in-vivo experiment under the laparoscopy to obtain the intraoperative 3D geometry as shown in Fig.3. We scanned the area of 8cm square and obtained 400 points of data. Sampling time took 1.2ms for each point including the calculation time for the 3D position, and the total measuring time was 0.5 seconds. The intraoperative 3D geometry of the liver surface could be as quickly obtained as Fig.2.

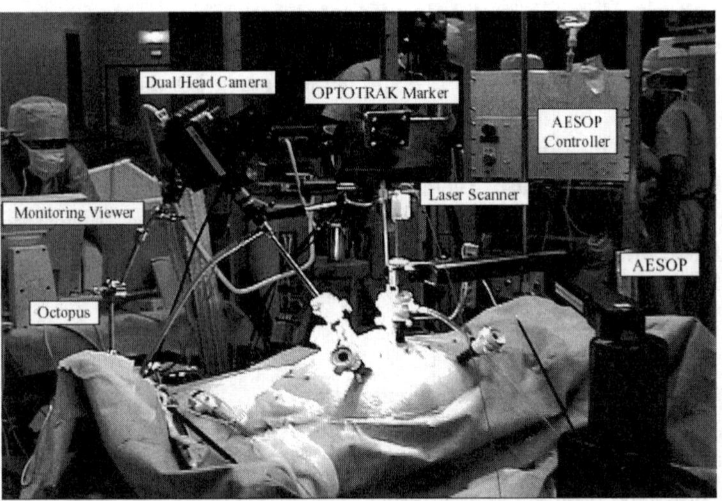

Fig.3 The in-vivo experiment using pig's liver in laparoscopy

3. Intraoperative Monitoring of Surgical Robot Motion

As I mentioned in the introduction, we propose the function of safety management for laparoscopic surgery including robot system. We think this is the best way to show the effectiveness of measuring the 3D shape of an organ's surface. From the computation of the 3D geometry inside the abdomen, it will enhance the safety management even in robotic surgery.

In this research, AESOP (Computer Motion Inc.) was adopted as surgical robot to hold forceps. AESOP is originally designed for laparoscope positioning. It has 6 joints including 2 passive joints. The link parameters of these 2 joints are passively decided by the constraint of the hole on the abdominal wall. To guide the forceps, we reprogramed the robot controller to control the 3D tip position of the forceps attached to AESOP. The modeling of AESOP is done based on the shape of link and link parameters. The geometric link shape is described in local link coordinates in VRML2.0.

As a command to AESOP, absolute 3D position extracted by the Laser-Pointing Endoscope is used to guide the tip of the forceps to the destination on the organ. The controller generates the linearly interpolated objective position from the initial position and destination every sampling time. Using synchronous flag, joint angles are transmitted to that of the virtual model in every 10ms. The controller always observes the emergency stop flag, which is raised if interference between the robot and the organ is detected. Fig.4 shows the activated virtual model synchronized with the motion of the real surgical robot.

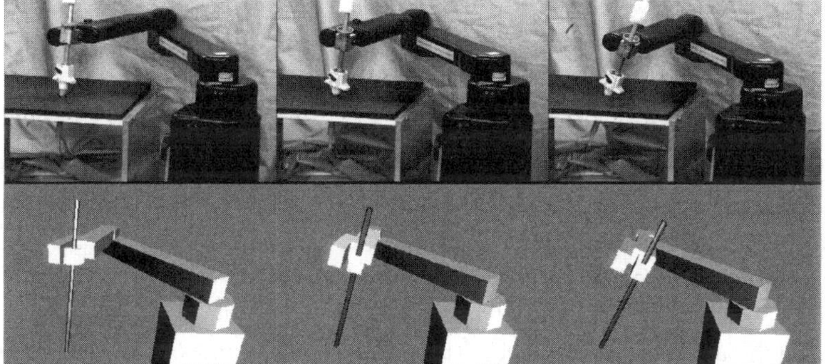

Fig.4 Synchronization with the virtual model

4. Safety Management

To prevent the forceps from colliding with the organ or endoscopes this system constantly checks the distances between objects. For the computation of the distances, we adopted the PQP, the Proximity Query Package [5]. PQP is a geometric computation library for proximity queries performed on polyhedrons composed of numerous triangles. The function of distance computation returns the distance between two models and the points establish the minimum distance for the models. The function of tolerance check can detect whether two models are closer or farther than a tolerance value, and it computes more quickly than distance computation.

Figure 5 shows the warning window for the surgeons to avoid collision. All surgical instruments and scanned 3D shapes are modeled on VRML 2.0 and the scene is drawn using OpenGL. If the distance between two objects is closer than the critical distance, it warns surgeons by changing background color and popping up a warning message. This enables the slave robot to be stopped in case of emergency, even in a situation where the surgeons fail to notice the closeness. For the navigation to avoid collision, it can also identify the shortest path between the closest points.

Surgeons will be able to figure out what happens even out of view of the endoscope by this intraoperative monitoring. In the lab experiment, surgical robot could be stopped in an emergency when the forceps approached the phantom organ within to 10mm as shown in Fig.6.

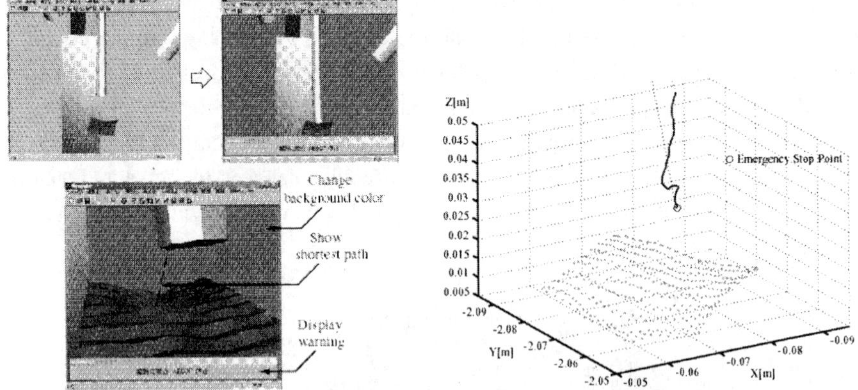

Fig.5 Warning window to avoid collision   **Fig.6 Emergency stop using geometric computation**

5. Non-Master-Slave Operation

The present interface of the surgical robot is limited to master-slave configuration. In the robotic tele-surgery using master-slave, the large amount of image data must be transmitted through a general network. This causes the difficulties of time delay. For the application of 3D pointing interface, the 3D point of destination for the surgical robot can be obtained from the 2D input on the touch screen. The surgeons have been able to guide the surgical robot to the place where it should approach at the end by the intuitive touch input on the endoscopic image. As shown in Fig.7, The forceps attached to surgical robot could be guided to the object by non-master-slave operation.

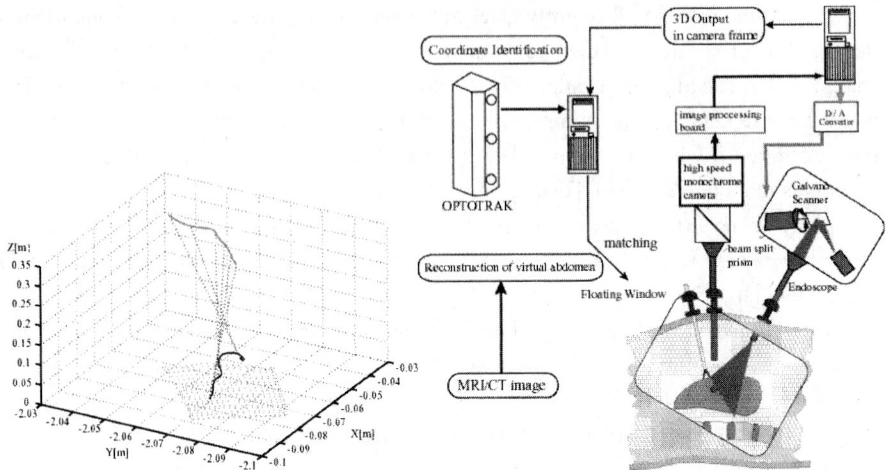

Fig.7 Guided forceps by non-master-slave   **Fig.8 System configuration(second prototype)**

6. Extension for the Laparoscopic Data-Fusion

The first system mainly focused on the surface geometric management. As a useful application, the effectiveness is shown in the field of robotic safety support. Now, we are trying to deal with the internal structure of the organ in order to realize data-fusion during laparoscopy. In laparoscopy, it is very difficult to get spatial perception. To supply a convenient interpretation in laparoscopy, we think it is useful to superimpose the deformed preoperative 3D model, which is reconstructed from CT/MRI, on the actual organ in the laparoscopic image. And we propose a floating window that enables us to provide intuitive comprehension about the abdominal space. This device displays the virtually computed information onto the actual abdomen like Fig.9.

The precise anatomical data of a patient is accessible using CT/MRI.The data is usually evaluated in the pre-operative conferences to discuss and plan the surgical procedures. One current issue is how to utilize such data in the operation room. The CT or MRI data shows geometrical inconsistency with the deformation due tothe change of patient's body postures. For deformation, a surgeon has to rely on his imagination to map the pre-surgical data onto the deformed one. If we scan the organ*in-situ* using the laser-scan endoscope, we can compute and estimate its internal defomation using the scanned data.

Three components are necessary to make intraoperative data-fusion for soft tissue. One is a laser-scan endoscope for the laparoscopic measurement. The development of a deformation/matching algorithm and floating window is required to enhance the virtualized reality. Fig.8 shows the system configuration of second prototype.

Being controlled by the mirror of a galvano scanner, a laser line is projected inside the patient's body through an endoscopic optic device. We used a closed-loop galvano scanner which responds up to 1kHz. The laser line pattern is captured by a 262fps high-speed camera (532*516 pixels, 256 gray scale) and a high-speed image processing board. The laser and camera coordinate systems are identified by OPTOTRAK attached to the devices. And 3D coordinates of the reference lines are reconstructed based on the triangulation between the high-speed camera image and the mirror angles of galvano scanner. The reconstruction computation is also processed in the sampling time of 4ms.

The image captured through the endoscope is distorted by the relayed lens inside. It is corrected and used to calculate the 3D position. The computed graphics are automatically produced from reconstruction of the scanned intraoperative 3D geometry. This image is projected onto a floating window to superpose onto the actual organ.

The concept of this system (second prototype) is to totally support the surgeon with an intuitive interface. Therefore, besides floating window, the surgical navigation program is also being developed as Fig.10. This program has the function of multi view interface. The surgeon is provided with laparoscopic view and his own point of view to see the intraoperative liver posture in transparence. The 3D model in the picture is the reconstructed liver model from pre-operative MRI images.

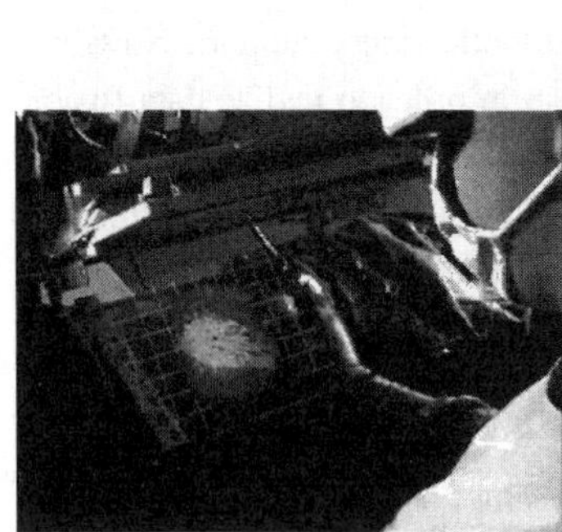

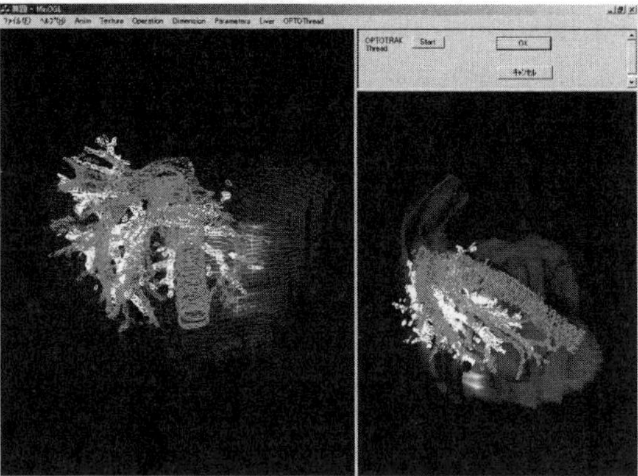

Fig.9 Floating window   **Fig.10 3D internal structure of liver**

Conclusion

The conclusion of this paper is summarized in the following four points:

(1) The intraoperative geometric information of the internal surface in laparoscopy was obtained successfully in the pig experiment. Preliminary results of in-vivo experiments verified the functionality and showed the performance.

(2) We proposed and realized the monitoring of the motion of the surgical robot and non-master-slave operation for the surgical robot.

(3) Safety management was carried out using intraoperative monitoringof the internal geometry in the virtual space. The recovered 3D surface of the liver was effectively used for geometric computation.

(4) The concept of laparoscopic data-fusion was proposed. We described the necessities of technology for the data-fusion. We try to develop the algorithm for the deformation and matching of the organ.

References

[1] Marc O. Schurr: "Robotic Devices for Advanced Endoscopic Surgical Procedures,"
Journal of the Robotics Society of Japan, Vol.18 No.1, pp.16-19, (2000).

[2] G S.Guthart: "The Intuitive Telesurgery System," Proceedings of the IEEE International Conference on Robotics and Automation, pp.618-621, (2000).

[3] Computer Motion Inc., "Internet Home Page," http://www.computermotion.com.

[4] Y.Nakamura, M.Hayashibe: "Laser-Pointing Endoscope System for Natural 3D Interface between Robotic Equipments and Surgeons," Medicine Meets Virtual Reality 2001, IOS Press, pp.348-354, (2001).

[5] Department of Computer Science, UNC Chapel Hill: "Fast proximity queries with swept sphere volumes, " technical report TR99-018, (1999).

[6] M.Hayashibe, Y.Nakamura: "Laser-Pointing Endoscope System for Intraoperative 3D Geometric Registration," 2001 IEEE International Conference on Robotics and Automation, pp. 1543-1548, (2001).

Medicine Meets Virtual Reality 02/10
J.D. Westwood et al. (Eds.)
IOS Press, 2002

Improved Haptic Rendering of Anatomical Data

Florian Heike, Andre Ley, and Robert Riener
Institute of Automatic Control Engineering, Technische Universität München, Germany

Abstract. We perform haptic rendering of a polygonal mesh at a high speed, independent of its face count, using a topologically structured data representation that avoids edge gap effects from small numerical errors. Constraints on the virtual proxy's position on the mesh give good results in rendering concave edges. The algorithm allows force shading and smoothing at convex corners and edges by an approach originally developed for graphic rendering.

1. Introduction

Simulation with force feedback is attractive for medical training, based on detailed anatomical data from medical. An anatomical object usually has an irregular shape, so that a polygonal representation is more easily constructed than one with larger, more complex patches such as NURBS. This work extends on the God-object-method introduced by Zilles and Salisbury [1], with solutions to some problems they describe, such as transition of the proxy past concave edges, real-time issues with a large polygon count, and numerical-error gaps at edges. Several workers have improved haptic rendering at convex edges. A popular approach is force shading [2]. Another is to smooth the surface before rendering. We implement a method originally used for graphics.

2. Methods

The anatomical model is a surface mesh of triangles. Colliding with it, for a cursor point **r**, is equivalent to penetrating its surface via some triangle **T**. Penetration depth and direction (which determine rendered force) are relative to the proxy **g**, the point nearest **r** on **T** (Fig. 1).

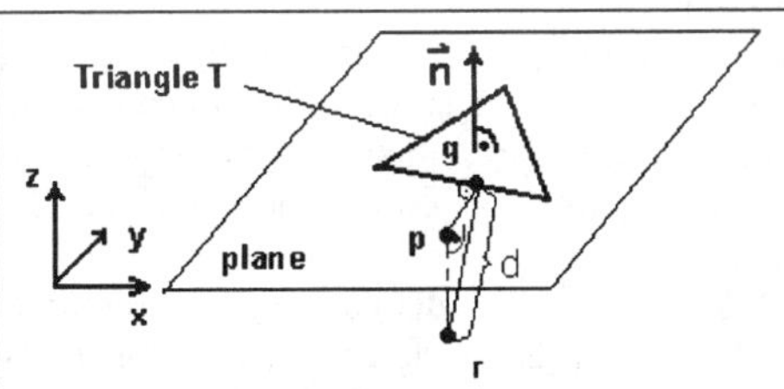

Figure 1: Virtual Proxy on a Triangle. The cursor point **r** projects to **p** in the plane of triangle **T**.

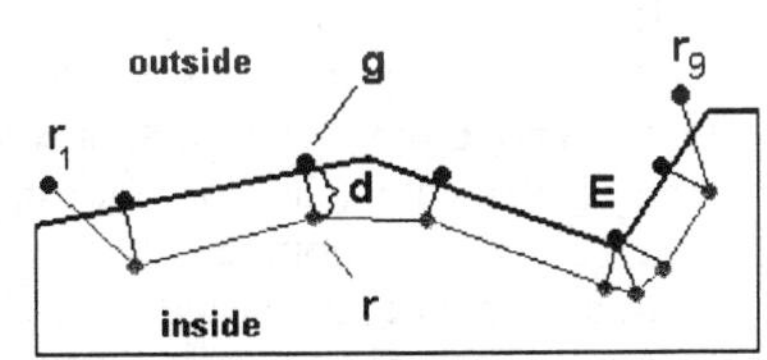

Figure 2: Path of physical and proxy position

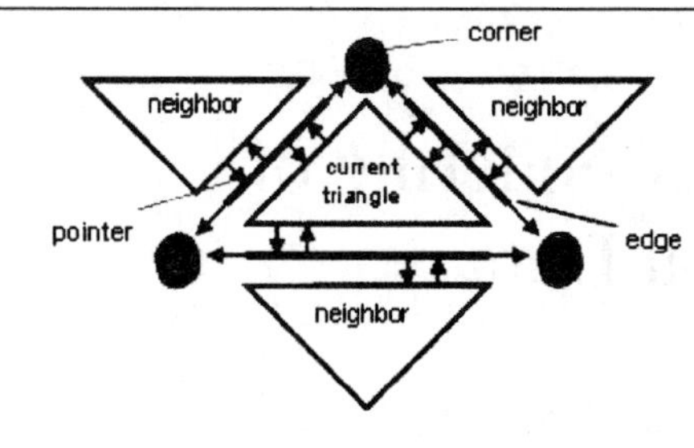

Figure 3: Data representation of triangles, edges and corners

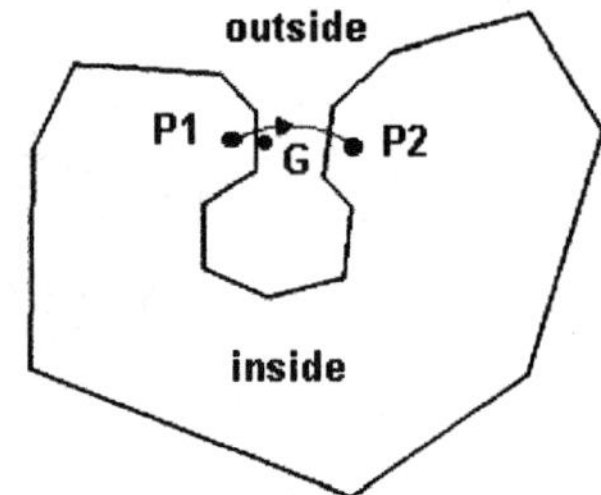

Figure 4: In this case the standard algorithm does not allow to track **P1**

If **g** is inside the triangle, it is identical to the god-object introduced by Zilles and Salisbury [1]. If not, it is on an edge or corner. The length d of the differential vector between **g** and **r** is the distance between **T** and the cursor. The haptic force feedback vector uses the triangle $\mathbf{T}_{near}$ with the least d. Once $\mathbf{T}_{near}$ is found, compute the force vector in the direction from **r** to $\mathbf{g}_{near}$, with magnitude using any contact model, using d_{near} as penetration depth. Fig. 2 shows a possible sequence of positions while stroking a surface. Note the behaviour around a concave edge **E**, where the force vector always points to **E**.

The major challenge for all haptic rendering algorithms is the real-time constraint of a repetition frequency of about 1000Hz, required for a smooth impression of a rendered object. This makes it essential to limit the number of triangles examined.

First, the *current triangle* $\mathbf{T}_{near}$ must be found. Since **r** cannot move infinitely fast, it is natural to search near $\mathbf{T}_{oldnear}$, the previous $\mathbf{T}_{near}$. We use the topology of the mesh rather than 3D proximity. Each triangle knows the indexes of its three edges (Fig. 3). Each edge knows the indexes of the two corners it connects, and each corner knows its three Cartesian coordinates. Doubly chained pointers between an edge and its two neighbouring triangles allow quick finding of the three triangles touching $\mathbf{T}_{oldnear}$ along an edge. These candidates for $\mathbf{T}_{near}$ are examined during one iteration. If a neighbour is located closer to the physical position, it becomes $\mathbf{T}_{near}$ for the next iteration. If penetration occurrs, the force vector is calculated as described before. In the less frequent case that two edges have been crossed in one iteration, as by crossing near a vertex, the proper proxy position is found after a few iterations. In order to track the proxy on the surface this method has to be applied whether or not penetration occurred. However, the algorithm can fail, as shown in Fig. 4. When the cursor moves from $\mathbf{p}_1$ to $\mathbf{p}_2$ the proxy **g** sticks near $\mathbf{p}_1$. Examining a randomly chosen fifth triangle *T* resolves this problem. If *T* is nearer the cursor than the topological neighbours, **g** jumps to it and then quickly steps to the nearest point.

The algorithm is fast and fully independent of the number of triangles of the object, since only the adjacent triangles and one distant triangle are considered. This enables the increase of triangle number to obtain a smoother surface representation. Two approaches have been implemented, one by Ruspini et al. [2], as well as corner cutting algorithm developed by Doo and Sabin [3].

The user interface consisted of a PHANToM™ haptic display and a monitor. Computation was shared by three Pentium 200 MHz PCs (connected via a 100Mbit LAN using a standard TCP-protocol) which separately controlled the PHANToM™, force vector calculation and visual feedback. The Maverik graphics C-library enabled effective graphic rendering. Human bone surfaces were extracted from CT images and saved in VRML format.

3. Results and Discussion

The system can display any closed mesh surface independently of its numbers of triangles. Dynamic performance did depend on triangle size, since the algorithm only crosses one edge per millisecond (1000Hz). This leads to a kind of "stickiness" when the structure is small compared to the speed of the moving end-effector of the haptic display. The force shading and the Doo-Sabin algorithms work independently of each other, since force shading is working on line and Doo-Sabin off line.

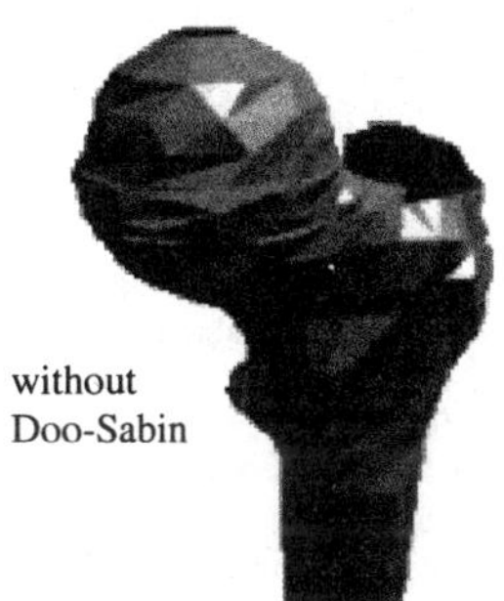

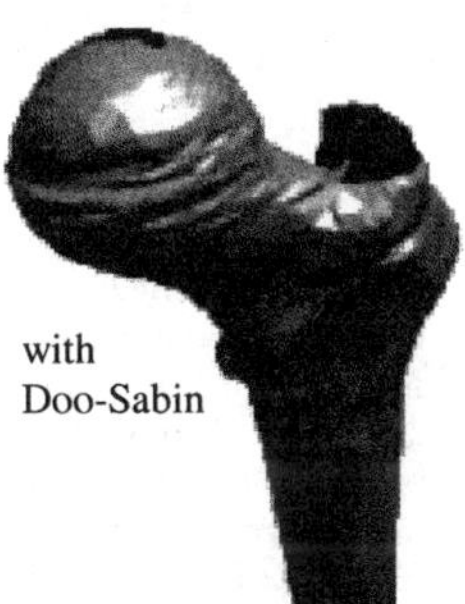

Figure 5: Graphical representation of the femur

Computational delays, due to temporary loss of tracking when moving the tool fast, can cause temporarily unrealistic force vectors. The use of a fifth, randomly chosen, triangle does not fully solve the problem of pushing through a flat object when the cursor approaches the rear, as reconvergence to the nearest triangle exaggerates the force discontinuity of this transition. Currently, the algorithm is limited to rigid objects. Further work is required to display soft tissues and deformable objects.

4. Conclusion

Parametric description of scanned 3D-data can be difficult. A fast algorithm independent of triangle count allows use of the data directly from a scan. It can enhance the details near the cursor position, by reducing real-time problems with real-time capable data representation.

References

[1] C. B. Zilles and J. K. Salisbury: A constraint-based god-object method for haptic display, Artificial Intelligence Laboratory, MIT, Cambridge, MA, 1995
[2] D. C. Ruspini, K. Kolarov and O. Khatib: The haptic display of complex environments, Stanford University, CA, Computer Graphics Proc., Annual Conference Series, 1997
[3] D. Doo and M. Sabin: Behaviour of recursive division surfaces near extraordinary points, Computer-Aided Design 10, pp. 356-360, 1978

Acknowledgements
The authors thank Prof. Schmidt and Jens Hoogen for their contributions, and the German Ministry of Education and Research (BMBF) for support in the frame of project VOR.

Medicine Meets Virtual Reality 02/10
J.D. Westwood et al. (Eds.)
IOS Press, 2002

Atlas-based segmentation of pathological knee joints

*Peter Heinze, **Dietmar Meister, **Rudolf Kober, *Jörg Raczkowsky, *Heinz Wörn
*University of Karlsruhe (TH), Institute for Process Control and Robotics,
Kaiserstraße 12, D-76128 Karlsruhe, Germany
**URS Ortho GmbH & Co. KG, Kehler Str. 31, D-76437 Rastatt, Germany*

Abstract. Efficiency, comparability and simplicity are key aspects for user acceptance of surgical planning systems in the long term. Automatic segmentation and identification of geometric reference systems of the anatomical structures are essential to fulfill these requirements. A statistical motivated shape atlas of the knee joint, based on 235 normal and abnormal MR and CT volume sets, is constructed for automatic segmentation of CT image data. In the first step of the atlas construction, the bony structures of the knee were segmented semi-automatically and processed into a dense and a sparse triangulated surface mesh to obtain training data sets. To establish an inter-individual correspondence, a skeleton-based registration method is used. The registered sparse surface meshes are retriangulated to estimate a pointwise inter-individual correspondence. The shape atlas is build upon these correspondences and integrated into a segmentation algorithm. An iterative segmentation scheme is proposed, which consists of a combination of the iterative-closest-point algorithm for spatial registration and of a downhill-simplex optimization procedure for deformation of the statistical motivated shape atlas to the image data. We expect the statistical shape model to be a robust and image modality independent method for the segmentation of pathological knee joints in CT image data.

1 Introduction

Efficiency, comparability and simplicity are key aspects for user acceptance of surgical planning systems in the long term. Automatic segmentation and identification of geometrical reference systems of the anatomical structures are essential to fulfil these requirements. In practice, the segmentation algorithms are confronted with a wide variety of imaging modalities, acquisition protocols, restricted acquisition areas, and image quality. As a matter of fact, image data of pathological cases, e.g. of arthrotic patients, makes the development of a robust segmentation algorithm more difficult, refer to figure 1.

Total knee replacement (*TKR*) is an orthopaedic surgical intervention with approximately 70.000 performed surgeries each year in Germany. The positive outcome of the surgery is strongly related to an correct placement of the knee prosthesis regarding several anatomical and biomechanical reference systems. Therefore, a steadily increase of computer assistance for the TKR intervention can be noticed over the last years. Up to now, more than 500 robot-assisted interventions have been performed in Germany. The computer-assisted TKR intervention is expected to be a major application for robot assisted surgery in the long run.

To improve the robustness and reproducibility of the computer-assisted planning of a TKR intervention, a statistical motivated anatomical shape atlas is developed to guide the segmentation process of pathological knee joints in CT-image data.

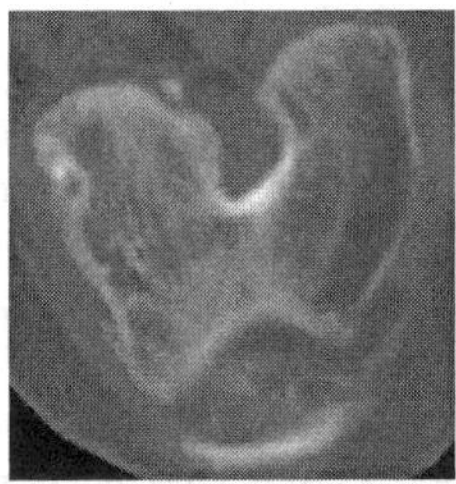 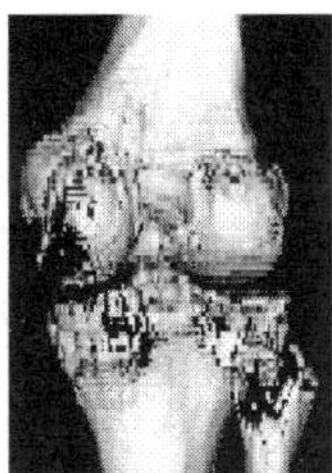

Figure 1: Transversal slice through a CT data set, showing the silhouette of a degenerated femur (*left*). Dorsal view of a threshold segmented knee joint (*right*). Large gray value differences lead to serious artifacts in the bone's surfaces.

Over the last years, several volume-based as well as surface-based anatomical models have been developed. However, many applications have been solely directed either towards a surface reconstruction task [1][2] or towards the segmentation of brain volume sets via an atlas matching [3][4].

2   Generation of the statistical shape atlas

The foundation of our statistical motivated shape model of the knee is a large database, consisting of 155 normal and 70 abnormal three-dimensional CT-volume sets. Additionally, 10 MR volume sets were acquired to include information of the ligaments and meniscii into the atlas. The legs of the patients were positioned in a physiologic hyperextension pose, i.e. the relative positions of the bones are individual reproducible.

The surface shape atlas itself is modelled within a point distribution model (*PDM*) framework [5]. Given a collection of N training shapes, where each instance is described by the same set of landmarks in cartesian coordinates $L_i = \{\vec{v_1}^{[i]}, \vec{v_2}^{[i]}, \ldots, \vec{v_k}^{[i]}\} \subset \mathrm{R}^3, 1 \leq i \leq N$, the mean shape $\overline{T}$ and its corresponding covariance matrix are calculated. A principal component analysis (*PCA*) results in a set of eigenvectors and eigenvalues which describe the most significant modes of variation of the examined shape. Most of the shape variation can be explained by a small number of modes. New instances of the anatomical object's class can be generated by adding a weighted sum of the estimated eigenvectors to the mean shape.

2.1   Data preprocessing

Every volume is segmented semi-automatically with the *ANALYZE* image processing software into the bony structures of the knee, namely femur, tibia, patella, and fibula. Additionally, the ligaments and the meniscii were segmented in the MR volume data sets. For each object in the segmented volumes, a triangular mesh $T = (V, F)$ with vertices $V = \{\vec{v_1}, \vec{v_2}, \ldots, \vec{v_k}\} \subset \mathrm{R}^3$ and facets $F \subset V^3$ is created with the marching cubes algorithm [6]. These high-resolution triangular meshes were further carefully processed with the surface processing software *POLYWORKS*. The processing included a hierarchical mesh reduction and the removal of topological errors, like self-intersections and degenerated edges. Finally, the shapes were classified by age, sex, patients side, normal and abnormal shape appearance.

2.2   Data alignment

For employing the PDM framework, it is necessary to obtain a description of each training shape with the same set of landmarks in cartesian coordinates. This property is not guaranteed by the surface creation and processing.

To simplify the determination of the common landmarks, all object shapes are first rigidly aligned (*registration*) in a common coordinate system (*reference coordinate system*). In fact, the estimation of this inter-subject registration transformation is an ill-posed problem. Common registration methods were not straight applicable for this kind of shape registration problem. The manual identification of landmarks for registration was impractical due to the high manual effort, whereas surface registration techniques did not produce acceptable results.

However, to obtain a natural and intuitive registration, the three-dimensional object skeleton was used in this study instead of the object's surface. The object skeleton describes hierarchical either the global as well as the local shape properties in a natural manner [7], see figure 2.2.

The object skeletons to be registered are determined in the volume data sets. All volume elements (*voxels*) in the volume data set belonging to the object are set to zero. All remaining "non-object" voxels are initialized with their maximal value. The application of a distance transformation [8] on this binary volume sets all "non-object" voxels to a value which is equal to the continuous distance to the nearest voxel on the object's surface. This is followed by the calculation of a nearest-neighbor-map, in which each voxel contains a 3D vector directing to the nearest surface voxel [9]. Finally, each voxel is examined, if it belongs to the skeleton or not. The membership criterion is defined over the enclosed angles between the nearest-neighbor vectors. A large angle between the nearest-neighbor vectors indicates that this voxel is member of the skeleton. The application of a threshold upon this criterion influences the detail of the desired skeleton.

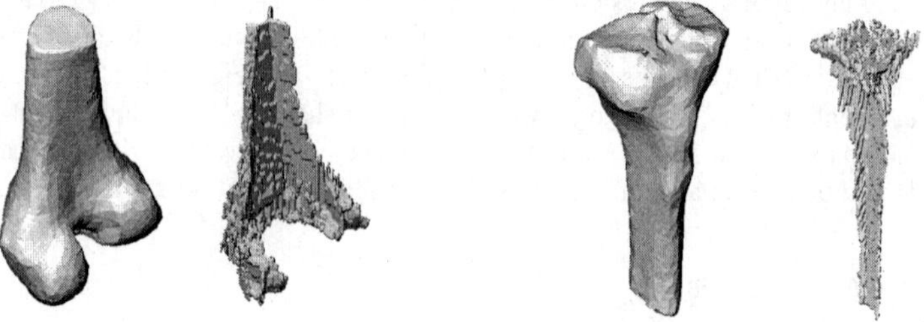

Figure 2: Triangulated surface of a femur and its corresponding skeleton (*left*). Triangulated surface of a tibia and its corresponding skeleton (*right*)

The skeleton of a complete shape of a knee joint, i.e. including the femoral head and the ankle joint, serves as a reference shape T_{Ref}. Each object skeleton is registered to this reference skeleton with the iterative closest point (*IPC*) algorithm [10].

2.3　Estimating the point distribution model

After aligning every individual object shape in the reference object coordinate system, the PDM can be determined. A sparse representation $T_{Ref}^{Reduced}$ of the reference surface T_{Ref} is used as a base for a retriangulation of the dense training surface meshes T_i. For each vertex $\vec{r_k}$ of the reduced reference surface $T_{Ref}^{Reduced}$ a corresponding vertex $\vec{v_k}$ on each training surface T_i is selected. The selection criteria is a cost function combining the euclidian distance between $\vec{v_k}$ and $\vec{r_k}$ with the enclosed angle of their associated vertex normals.

The identified and now sparse triangulated vertices $\vec{v_k}$ are used to obtain a more dense triangulation. The triangular subdivision of the sparse triangles of the reference surface $T_{Ref}^{Reduced}$ is transfered to the training data sets T_i. New vertices are created on the training data surface analogous to the subdivision scheme of the reference triangles and assigned to the corresponding reference vertices.

Consequently, the training data for the shape model consists of $N = 235$ knee shape instances, represented in a matrix by "polygonal models"

$$T_i = [v_{1_x}^{[i]}, v_{1_y}^{[i]}, v_{1_z}^{[i]}, \ldots, v_{K_x}^{[i]}, v_{K_y}^{[i]}, v_{K_z}^{[i]}], 1 \le i \le N \tag{1}$$

where K denotes the number of shape vertices. The mean shape and its corresponding covariance matrix are calculated as follows:

$$\overline{T} = \sum_{i=1}^{N} T_i; \qquad S = \frac{1}{N} * \sum_{i=1}^{N} (T_i - \overline{T})(T_i - \overline{T})^T \tag{2}$$

The principal component analysis on the covariance matrix S yields to the eigenvalues $\lambda_1 \ge \lambda_2 \ge \ldots \ge \lambda_{3K} \ge 0$ and eigenvectors $\phi_1, \phi_2, \ldots, \phi_{3K}$. As shown in [5], the eigenvalue problem of the dimension $3K \times 3K$ can be reduced to a problem of the dimension $N \times N$, the dimension of the reduced covariance matrix. With this in mind, a new shape can be generated by adding a weighted sum of the estimated eigenvectors to the mean shape:

$$T_{new} \approx \overline{T} + \omega_i * \phi_i, \qquad 1 \le i \le N \tag{3}$$

Thus, the weights ω_i span a parameter space in which many different instances of the trained anatomical object can be generated, e.g. in the deformation step of the following segmentation algorithm.

3　Application of the statistical shape atlas

The shape model is used to segment pathological knee joints in CT image data of varying imaging hardware. The segmentation process is performed for each single object in the following order: femur, tibia, patella, and fibula. Granted that the femur is segmented, it is possible to find a good initial position for the tibia and the other anatomical objects.

First, a rough initial position is estimated for the anatomical object. This is currently done via a simple user interaction, but will be automated in a later stage of the project. The optimization scheme consists mainly of two components. An ICP algorithm [10] is used for refining the spatial position of the shape model and a standard downhill-simplex optimization algorithm [11] for the determination of the best shape deformation with respect to the most important eigenvalues $\lambda_1, \ldots, \lambda_h, h \ll 3N$, resp. eigenvectors, refer to equation 3.

The determination of the best deformation and the estimation of the corresponding points for the ICP algorithm are based on an interpretation of gray-value profiles along the vertex normals of the shape model, directing inwards as well as outwards. The gray-value profiles are calculated for each new position of the deformed shape model, based on a tri-linear interpolation of the CT data. In the gray-value profile, the point of a possible edge is detected by considering either the gray-value information as well as its first and second derivative. This edge point depicts the corresponding spatial point to the examined shape model vertex for the ICP algorithm. The sum of all distances between edge points and shape model vertices is used as a cost function for the deformation optimization algorithm and as a termination criterion for the iteration process itself, refer to figure 3.

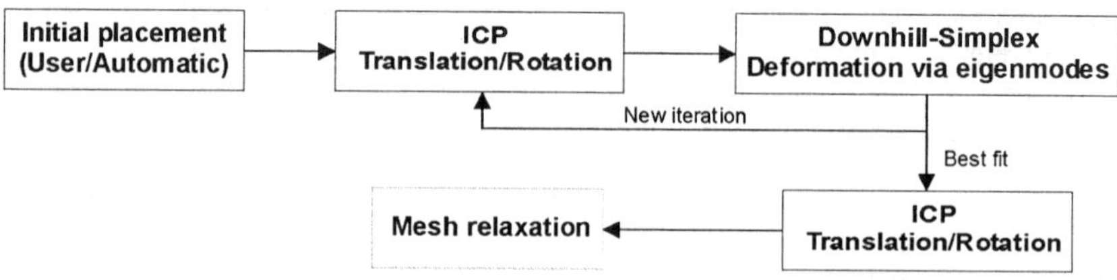

Figure 3: Scheme of the segmentation algorithm. Dotted line depicts not implemented process steps.

4   Discussion

In fact, it is not guaranteed that every anatomical shape of this anatomical object class can be exactly generated by the shape model. This is because the deformation is lead by the eigenmodes and therefore dependent on the underlying training data set. Nonetheless, the shape model will be a good approximation of the anatomical object to be segmented. Therefore, a following mesh relaxation with hard constraints can avoid this problem and lead to an exact segmentation, see figure 3. However, this functionality is not yet implemented.

The automatic landmark generation induces that no semantic information of the landmarks is incorporated in the statistical shape model. As a consequence, a postprocessing algorithm must determine the important geometrical reference systems on the segmented surface of the knee. For this reason and for reducing the amount of data describing the knee shape, the application of NURBS-surfaces will be examined in the near future.

Furthermore, the statistical shape model can be extended to incorporate gray value information. A statistical analysis upon this information gives better understanding in the bone density distribution in the knee joint, for improving the design of new knee implants.

To conclude, we expect the statistical shape model to be a robust and image modality independent method for medical image segmentation. Furthermore, it is a wide applicable common framework which is also transferable to other kinds of surgical applications. The high expenses to build such statistical model will be covered in addition by the benefits employing this method in several working fields, e.g. improved implant design. In summary, an overall quality improvement of the surgical planning procedure resp. the surgical intervention can be achieved by employing an anatomical atlas in computer assisted surgery applications.

References

[1] S.Däuber, J.Raczkowsky, J.Brief, S.Hassfeld, H.Wörn: Statistical analysis of the morphology of threedimensional objects and pathological structures using spherical harmonics; Medicine Meets Virtual Reality, 2001, pp. 103–105.

[2] M.E.Leventon: Statistical Models in in Medical Image Analysis. Dissertation, Massachusetts Institute of Technology, 2000.

[3] M.Chen: 3-D Deformable Registration Using a Statistical Atlas with Applications in Medicine. Dissertation, The Robotics Institute Carnegie Mellon University Pittsburgh, 1999.

[4] G.E.Christensen, R.D.Rabbitt, M.I.Miller: 3D brain mapping using a deformable neuroanatomy. Physics in Medicine and Biology **39** (1994), pp. 209–618.

[5] T.F.Cootes, C.J.Taylor: Statistical models of appearance for computer vision. Technical report, University of Manchester, Wolfson Image Analysis Unit, 2001.

[6] W.E.Lorensen, H.E.Cline: Marching cubes: A high resolution 3D surface construction algorithm. Computer Graphics (SIGGRAPH '87 Proceedings), **21** (1987), pp. 163–169.

[7] B.S.Morse: Computation of object cores from grey-level images. Dissertation, University of North Carolina, Chapel Hill, 1994.

[8] G.Borgefors: Distance Transformations in Arbitrary Dimensions. Computer Vision and Image Processing **27** (1984), pp. 321–345.

[9] E.Cuchet, J.Knoplioch, D.Dormont, C.Marsault: Registration in Neurosurgery and Neuroradiotherapy Applications. Proc. of the 2nd International Symposium on MRCAS, Baltimore (USA), 1995, pp. 31–38.

[10] P.J.Besl, N.D.McKay: A Method for Registration of 3-D Shapes. IEEE Transactions on PAMI **14(2)** (2000), pp. 239–256.

[11] W.H.Press, S.A.Teukolsky, W.T.Vetterling, B.P.Flannery: Numerical Recipes in C. Cambridge University Press, 1992.

[12] P.Golland, W.E.L.Grimson, R.Kikinis: Statistical shape analysis using fixed topology skeletons: Corpus Callosum study. Information Processing in Medical Imaging LNCS 1613, 1999, pp. 382–388.

[13] M.Näf, O.Kübler, R.Kikinis, M.E.Shenton, G.Székely: Characterization and recognition of 3D organ shape in medical image analysis using skeletonization. IEEE Workshop on Mathematical Methods in Biomedical Image Analysis, 1996.

[14] K.Siddiqi, S.Bouix, A.Tannenbaum, S.W.Zucker: The Hamilton-Jacobi Skeleton. International Conference on Computer Vision (Corfu, Greece), 1999.

[15] M.Styner, G.Gerig: Medial models incorporation shape variability for 3D shape analysis. Technical report, University of North Carolina Chapel Hill, Department of Computer Science, 2000.

[16] G.Subsol, J.P.Thirion, N.Ayache: A scheme for automatically building three-dimensional morphometric atlases: application to a skull atlas. Medical Image Analysis, **2** (1998), pp. 37–60.

Medicine Meets Virtual Reality 02/10
J.D. Westwood et al. (Eds.)
IOS Press, 2002

A New, Accurate and Easy To Implement Camera and Video Projector Model

Harald Hoppe, Sascha Däuber, Carsten Kübler, Jörg Raczkowsky, Heinz Wörn
Universität Karlsruhe (TH), Institute for Process Control and Robotics,
Kaiserstraße 12, D-76128 Karlsruhe, Germany, e-mail: hoppe@ira.uka.de

Abstract. In 2000, the Institute for Process Control and Robotics/Universität Karlsruhe (TH) has developed a prototype system for projector based augmented reality consisting of a state-of-the-art PC, two CCD cameras and a video projector which is used for registration and projection of surgical planning data. Tracking, registration as well as projection require an accurate calibration process for cameras and video projectors. We have developed a new, flexible, plain and easy to implement model, which can both be used for calibration of cameras and video projectors.

1 Camera and video projector model

Assume Z to be the optical center of the pinhole-like camera resp. video projector. The model now bacically uses the projection of the CCD- resp. LCD-Chip onto a parallel plane through the coordinate system's origin described by

$$\mathcal{C}: \quad \vec{x_d} = \vec{a}(n_d - n_0) + \vec{b}(m_d - m_0), \tag{1}$$

where n_d, m_d are the lense distorted pixel coordinates (as used by the computer). While $\vec{a}$ and $\vec{b}$ align with the boundaries of one pixel, n_0 and m_0 define the location of pixel $(0,0)$ in relation to the origin (see figure 1). Assuming the optical axis to be perpendicular to the CCD/LCD-plane, the center of lense distorsion F (focal point $\vec{f} = \vec{a}(n_f - n_0) + \vec{b}(m_f - m_0)$) is found by perpendicularly projecting Z onto $\mathcal{C}$. We concentrate on modelling radial lense distorsion, where the undistorted coordinate $\vec{x_u} \in \mathcal{C}$ results from

$$\vec{x_u} = \vec{f} + (1 + \kappa_0 r_d + \kappa_1 r_d^2)\vec{r_d} \quad \text{with} \quad \vec{r_d} = \vec{x_d} - \vec{f},\ r_d = |\vec{r_d}|. \tag{2}$$

Therefore, the undistorted radius $r_u = |\vec{x_u} - \vec{f}|$ depends on r_d by $r_u/r_d = 1 + \kappa_0 r_d + \kappa_1 r_d^2$. Tsai [1] supposes $r_u/r_d = 1 + \kappa_1 r_d^2 + \kappa_2 r_d^4 + \ldots$, thus neglecting the term proportional to r_d. We will show in section 2 that taking into account this terms yields better results. Inserting (1) into (2) yields $\vec{x_u} = \vec{a}(n_u - n_0) + \vec{b}(m_u - m_0)$ with the following undistorted pixel coordinates:

$$\begin{pmatrix} n_u \\ m_u \end{pmatrix} = \begin{pmatrix} n_d \\ m_d \end{pmatrix} + (\kappa_0 r_d + \kappa_1 r_d^2) \begin{pmatrix} n_d - n_f \\ m_d - m_f \end{pmatrix}. \tag{3}$$

Given an arbitrary world coordinate $\vec{x}$, the undistorted pixel coordinates can also be calculated by perspectively projecting $\vec{x}$ onto $\mathcal{C}$, thus solving

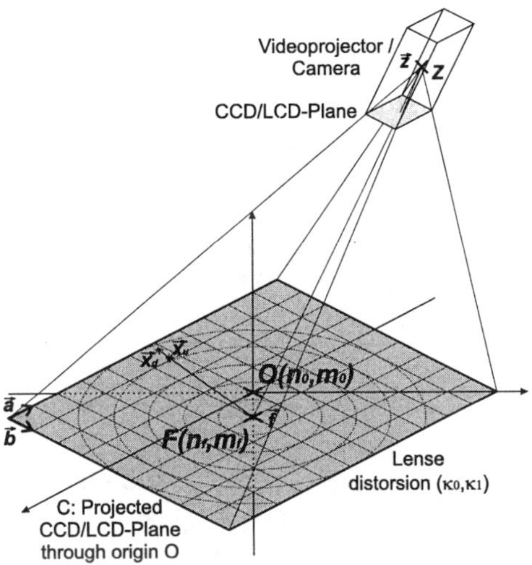

Figure 1: Schematic model configuration

$$\vec{a}(n_u - n_0) + \vec{b}(m_u - m_0) = \vec{x} + s(\vec{z} - \vec{x}). \tag{4}$$

Multiplying (4) with $\vec{a} \times (\vec{z} - \vec{x})$ resp. $\vec{b} \times (\vec{z} - \vec{x})$ and using the identity $\vec{a}(\vec{b} \times \vec{z}) = \vec{b}(\vec{z} \times \vec{a}) = \vec{z}(\vec{a} \times \vec{b})$ yields the following set of coupled equations

$$n_u \vec{x}\vec{k} - \vec{x}\vec{u} + n_0 = n_u \tag{5}$$

$$m_u \vec{x}\vec{k} - \vec{x}\vec{v} + m_0 = m_u, \tag{6}$$

where we introduced the abbreviations $\gamma := \vec{z}(\vec{a} \times \vec{b})$, $\vec{k} := \vec{a} \times \vec{b}/\gamma$, $\vec{c} := \vec{z} \times \vec{a}/\gamma$, $\vec{d} := \vec{z} \times \vec{b}/\gamma$, $\vec{v} := m_0\vec{k} - \vec{c}$ and $\vec{u} = n_0\vec{k} + \vec{d}$. Given a set of at least six non planar world coordinates $\vec{x}_i$ corresponding to appropriate pixel coordinates n_i, m_i, the model parameters can be found by solving the overdetermined linear equation system

$$\begin{pmatrix} n_1\vec{x_1}^T & -\vec{x_1}^T & \vec{0} & 1 & 0 \\ m_1\vec{x_1}^T & \vec{0} & -\vec{x_1}^T & 0 & 1 \\ n_2\vec{x_2}^T & -\vec{x_2}^T & \vec{0} & 1 & 0 \\ m_2\vec{x_2}^T & \vec{0} & -\vec{x_2}^T & 0 & 1 \\ \vdots & \vdots & \vdots & \vdots & \vdots \end{pmatrix} \begin{pmatrix} \vec{k} \\ \vec{u} \\ \vec{v} \\ n_0 \\ m_0 \end{pmatrix} = \begin{pmatrix} n_1 \\ m_1 \\ n_2 \\ m_2 \\ \vdots \end{pmatrix}. \tag{7}$$

Having solved the above equation, n_0 and m_0 are already known and the remaining model parameters $\vec{a}, \vec{b}, \vec{z}$ can be found by using $\vec{c} = m_0\vec{k} - \vec{v}$, $\vec{d} = -n_0\vec{k} + \vec{u}$ and

$$\vec{z} = \frac{1}{\gamma}\vec{z}\left[\vec{z}(\vec{a} \times \vec{b})\right] = \frac{1}{\gamma}(\vec{z} \times \vec{a})(\vec{z} \times \vec{b}) = \gamma\vec{c} \times \vec{d}. \tag{8}$$

Analogously you can find that $\vec{a} = \gamma\vec{c} \times \vec{k}$ and $\vec{b} = \gamma\vec{d} \times \vec{k}$ where γ can be determined by realizing that

$$\gamma = \vec{z}(\vec{a} \times \vec{b}) \quad \Leftrightarrow \quad \frac{1}{\gamma^2} = \frac{\vec{z}}{\gamma}\left(\frac{\vec{a}}{\gamma} \times \frac{\vec{b}}{\gamma}\right) \quad \Leftrightarrow \quad \gamma = \pm 1/\sqrt{(\vec{c} \times \vec{d})\left[(\vec{c} \times \vec{k}) \times (\vec{d} \times \vec{k})\right]} \tag{9}$$

To get a first approximation for the model parameters, the radial lense distorsion can be neglected. This is equivalent to considering the distorted pixel coordinates as undistorted and calculating the parameters as described above. Afterwards, the approximated undistorted coordinates $\vec{x_{ui}}'$ can be found by perspectively projecting $\vec{x_i}$ onto $\mathcal{C}$. Now the lense distorsion parameters can be determined by minimizing $f(\kappa_0, \kappa_1) = \sum_i (\vec{x_{ui}} - \vec{x_{ui}}')^2$ which is equivalent to solving the linear equation

$$\sum_i \begin{pmatrix} r_{di}^4 & r_{di}^5 \\ r_{di}^5 & r_{di}^6 \end{pmatrix} \begin{pmatrix} \kappa_0 \\ \kappa_1 \end{pmatrix} = \sum_i \begin{pmatrix} (\vec{r_{di}}\vec{r_{ui}}')r_{ui}' - r_{ui}'^3 \\ (\vec{r_{di}}\vec{r_{ui}}')r_{ui}'^2 - r_{ui}'^4 \end{pmatrix} \tag{10}$$

where we defined $\vec{r_{ui}}' = \vec{x_{ui}}' - \vec{f}$ and $r_{ui}' = |\vec{r_{ui}}'|$. Following iterations will not use the distorted pixel coordinates n_d, m_d but the undistorted ones calculated by using equation (3).

Please note that $\vec{a}$ and $\vec{b}$ are not assumed to be perpendicular. Therefore, after calculating the model parameters, $\vec{a} \cdot \vec{b} \approx 0$ can be taken as indication for a successful parameter calculation.

2 Results and Conclusions

Given three sets of 438, 429 and 1000 world coordinates that correspond to sets of camera (set 1 and 2) and video projector (set 3) pixel coordinates, we have compared Tsai's standard camera model to the one described above. The following table shows the average pixel deviation of original and computed distorted pixel coordinates:

Camera model	average pixel deviation (in pixel)		
	set 1	set 2	set 3
Tsai standard	0.351	0.361	0.096
Our approach	0.188	0.171	0.094

While we found out that our model can be implemented much easier and faster than Tsai's, it also shows better results. Furthermore, the algorithm neither requires initial parameter guesses nor system parameter specifications. Our model limits the calibration effort to a minimum, nevertheless providing best results.

References

[1] R. Y. Tsai: A Versatile Camera Calibration Technique for High-Accuracy 3D Machine Vision Metrology Using Off-the-Shelf TV and Lenses, IEEE Journal of Robotics and Automation, vol. RA-3, no. 4, 1987.

Medicine Meets Virtual Reality 02/10
J.D. Westwood et al. (Eds.)
IOS Press, 2002

An Investigation of Immersiveness in Virtual Reality Exposure Using Physiological Data

Dong P. Jang, In Y. Kim, Sang W. Nam[1], Brenda K. Wiederhold[2], Mark D. Wiederhold[3], Sun I. Kim

Department of Biomedical Engineering, Hanyang University, Seoul, Korea
[1]Department of Electrical & Computer Engineering, Hanyang University, Seoul, Korea
[2]center for Advanced Multimedial Psychotherapy, CA, USA
[3]Scripps Clinic Medical Group, Inc. La Jolla, CA, USA

Abstract. As virtual reality technology is increasingly attracting significant attention in clinical psychology, especially in the treatment of phobias, physiological monitoring is increasingly considered as an objective measuring tool for studying participants. However, there are few studies of the normal individual's physiological response to virtual environments, or their reactions to different virtual environments.

The goal of this study is to analyze non-phobic participants' physiological reaction to two virtual environments: driving and flying and to investigate the usefulness of heart rate variability. Eleven non-phobic participants were exposed to each virtual environment for 15 minutes. Heart rate, skin resistance, and skin temperature measurements were taken for physiological monitoring and Presence and Simulator Sickness Questionnaires were obtained after each exposure.

This study found that skin resistance and heart rate variability can be used to show arousal of participant exposed to virtual environments experience and that such measures generally returned to normal as time went by. The Study showed that skin resistance and heart rate can be used as objective measures in monitoring the reaction of non-phobic participants to virtual environments. Significantly, heart rate variability analysis in virtual environments showed that it could be useful for assessing the emotional states of participants.

1. Introduction

Virtual reality (VR) has been attracting increasing attention in clinical psychology, especially in the treatment of phobias [1-5]. At the same time, physiological monitoring has become important as an objective measuring tool for checking the state of participants [6-9]. Also, real-time physiological monitoring has been used as an indicator of excessive patient arousal and the need to be placed back at a lower level of the fear hierarchy or taken out of the phobic scenario altogether. Conversely, knowledge about the physiological consequences for users of virtual environments (VEs) is limited. Meehan stated that heart rate had a high and significant correlation with presence in VEs and could be used as an objective measurement of presence [9]. Also Wiederhold has demonstrated the differences between the non-phobic's physiological responses and the phobic's response when placed in VEs [10]. Although the number of participants was too small and the result could not clearly show the relationship among measures and physiology, this study has been considered as important work in that it revealed that physiological measures were related to presence, degree of realism, and immersiveness. Regenbrecht has described a 37-subject study in which the relationship between presence and fear of heights was analyzed [11]. The analysis showed that reported fear had a significant relationship with height anxiety (positive), height avoidance (negative), and presence (positive). That is, reported fear was significantly higher for subjects who reported higher presence and (pre-experiment) height anxiety. In this study, non-phobic participants' physiological reactions to VEs were analyzed and their physiological characteristics and trends were investigated in two virtual environments: driving and flying.

2. Methods

2.1. Subjects

Eleven volunteers (24.9±5.82) over 18 years of age were chosen as non-phobic participants for this study. A participant was excluded from the study if he or she had a history of heart disease, migraines, seizures, or a concurrent diagnosis of severe mental disorders such as psychosis or major depressive disorder as determined by interview.

2.2. Virtual Environment

Two virtual environments were used in this study. The first environment, a flying simulator for fear of flying had one interaction interface: a head motion tracking device. The second virtual environment for fear of driving had two interaction interface with the participant: a head motion tracking device and a driving control device. Therefore, the driving simulator was considered to be more interactive than the flying simulator.

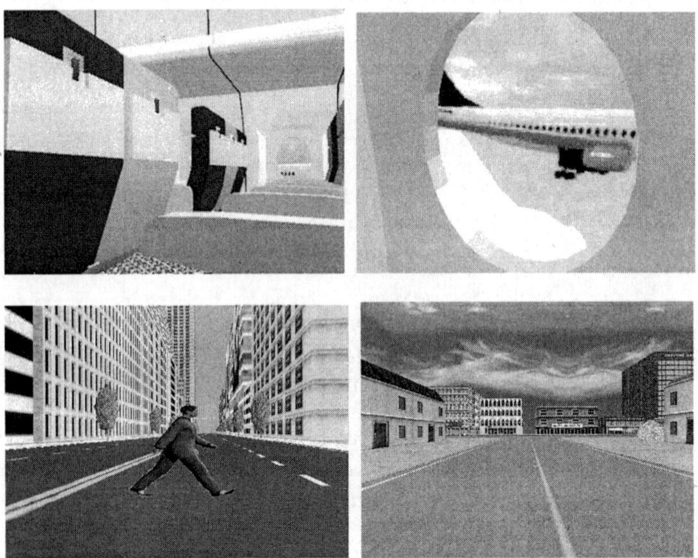

Fig. 1. Scene for the VE Flying Simulator and Scenes from the Driving Simulator

2.2.1. Virtual Environment for fear of flying

The VE for this study consisted of a head mounted display(VFX3D), a head tracker and a flight seat with a subwoofer that produced vibrations. It was designed by Drs. Hodges and Rothbaum of Virtually Better, Inc. (Atlanta, Georgia) who have previously performed VR treatment for acrophobia and fear of flying [1,12].

2.2.2. Virtual Environment for fear of driving

We also developed a Virtual Environment for fear of driving. It consisted of a head mounted display (VFX3D), a three degree of freedom head motion tracker, a steering wheel (Wingman Formula GT) and a vibration chair using sound produced by from computer. The driving software was developed on a Pentium 600 personal computer with a 3D accelerator graphics card. It largely consisted of three parts: an urban street, a secluded road, and a tunnel. The participant began to drive on a two-lane urban street and drove to the secluded road without buildings or people. There also was a long tunnel with traffic jam. The participant was stuck inside the tunnel, and the operator was able to control the traffic. The traffic lights and sounds mimicked those found in real world.

2.3. Measure

2.3.1. Physiology

Skin Resistance (SR) was measured to observe the changes in sweat gland activity. SR generally decreases as sweat gland activity increases. SR was monitored with two silver/silver chloride electrodes placed on the ring and index fingers of the left hand. For heart rate (HR), a small amount of electrode gel was placed on each of two disposable electrodes attached to the participants' right and left wrists.

2.3.2. Questionnaires

The Simulator Sickness Questionnaire (SSQ) provided measurements of simulator sickness [13]. The SSQ is a 16-item symptom checklist. The Presence & Realism Questionnaire (PRQ) rated the sense of presence and degree of realism felt in the virtual environment [14]. The PRQ consists of a 10-item presence and realism checklist as well as, overall rate of realism, and an overall rate of presence.

2.4. Virtual Reality Exposure Procedure

To begin with, a flying simulation of two virtual environments was experienced. A 5-minute eyes-open baseline then was taken in order to objectively analyze physiological response in the virtual environment. The participant was placed in a VFX3D head-mounted display (HMD). The participant was allowed to look around the virtual plane to become oriented for a short while before the flight began. The participant was instructed to look out of the left window during the entire 15-minute VR flight. The participant took a rest for 30 minutes after finishing the VR flying experience. After a 5-minute eyes-open baseline was taken, the participant was ordered to follow the direction signs, which showed where to go and to control the wheel with their right hand to minimize the movement noise in obtaining physiological data. During the 15-minute driving experience wearing a HMD, the participant felt the vibration of the chair through the subwoofer.

Measures	VEs	Statistics	Student-t Test	P
∇Skin Temperature	Flying	0.016±0.059	1.138	.282
	Driving	0.0013±0.033		
∇Skin Resistance	Flying	0.198±0.292	1.938	.081
	Driving	-0.103±0.486		
Simulator Sickness Questionnaire	Flying	2.9±1.66	1.892	.091
	Driving	11.2±13.6		
Presence	Flying	11.6±5.10	0.577	.578
	Driving	10.7±7.04		

Table1. The Student-t test of two virtual environments (flying and driving simulators) in Skin Temperature, Skin Resistance, Simulator Sickness Questionnaire, Presence Questionnaire.

3. Results

Table 1 shows the result of a conventional Student T-test of physiological responses and questionnaires between flying virtual environments and the driving virtual environments. Although the skin resistances in the two VEs did not show significant differences (P=.081) because of the small number sample size, the change of skin resistance over time presented very different reactions according to the particular VEs (Fig. 2). The study showed that the participants were initially aroused in the VE exposure, but returned to normal after approximately 7 minutes in each of the two VEs. The driving VE, however, required the participant's attention and alertness more than the flying VE, since the participants had to pay more attention to control the steering wheel. After habituation for 7 minutes, therefore, overall skin resistance reaction in the driving VE was more active than for the flying VE. This was matched with Slator's study which showed that individuals feel presence in active virtual environments which react to their movements or actions more than passive virtual environments [17]. Contrary to the results of the physiological response, however, there was no significant differences in the scores of the Presence Questionnaire.

The analysis of age and Simulator Sickness Questionnaires by Pearson Correlation showed that there was a significant correlation (r=.902, P=.0001) between age and SSQ after the driving VE, while there was no correlation (r=.390, P=.914) between age and SSQ after the flying VE. It meant that the older participants felt sickness in the complex virtual environments more than the younger participants. The driving VE had two control devices: a head motion tracker and a steering wheel and the view changes by those devices evoked sickness in the older participants.

In the analysis of heart rate variability, there were no significant differences between baseline and VE exposure except heart rates (P=0.004) in the driving VE. However, the trend of the LF/HF ratio demonstrated a similar pattern to the skin resistance response in Fig. 2. This ratio is well known for quantifying the overall balance between the sympathetic and parasympathetic systems. A higher number indicates increased sympathetic activity or reduced parasympathetic activity. Therefore, Fig. 3. shows that participants aroused at the beginning of exposure are habituated after around 8 minutes in that the LF/HF ratio returns to the baseline.

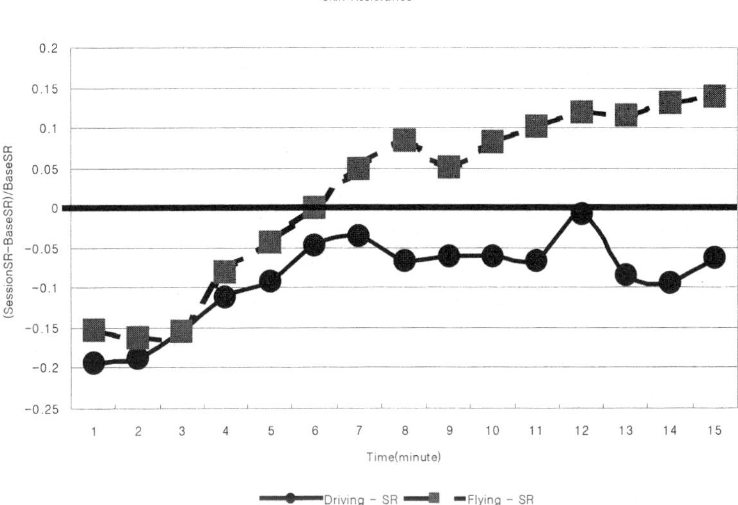

Fig. 2. The change of skin resistance over time. Values were the average of all of the participant's skin resistance change rates: (SessionSR – BaseSR)/BaseSR. The figure showed that the participants were aroused initially in VE exposure, and returned to the normal after approximately 7 minutes.

4. Discussion

Early in the last century, Carl Jung reported: "Every stimulus accompanied by an emotion produced a deviation of the galvanometer to a degree in direct proportion to the liveliness and actuality of the emotion aroused"[18]. We also found that skin resistance increase over time after around 7~8 minutes supporting the idea that subjects could become habituated VEs. The result showed again that skin resistance could be used as an objective measurement for checking the state of participants in the field of virtual reality psychotherapy.

Heart rate variability (HRV) has been generally used for the recognition of autonomic activity in various fields [20]. Although the HRV analysis about normal individuals in this experiment did not show significant differences in the two virtual environments owing to the small number of cases, there are a few things to consider and to be investigated in future work. One was that the LF/HF Ratio in exposure to VEs was higher than that in baseline. LF/HF Ratio refers to the ratio of the low frequency component and the high frequency component in the power spectrum density of heart rates. As previously mentioned, this is generally accepted for sympathetic balance. The higher value of the LF/HF Ratio reflects the change of that balance, that is, the response to a new and novel stimulus like a VE. Further, the trend of the LF/HF Ratio showed almost the same pattern with skin resistance.

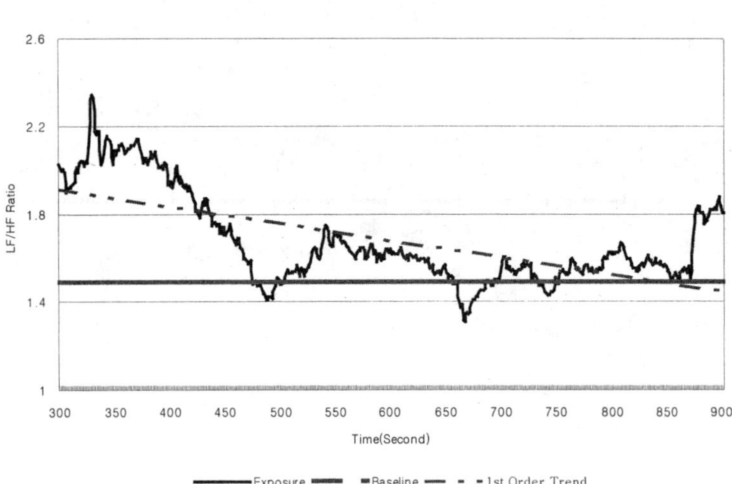

Fig. 3. The time-plot of the LF/HF Ratio was obtained by the average of the flying VE participants' LF/HF Ratios. The ratio value was calculated with the previous 5–minute by that time.

5. Conclusion

In this paper, the physiological responses to two VEs were analyzed. It showed that skin resistance and heart rate could be used as objective measures in monitoring reactions to virtual environments. Especially, the heart rate variability analysis in VEs showed that it could be useful for assessing the emotional states of participants, even patients in VEs.

Acknowledgements
This study was funded by the National Research Laboratory (NRL) Program at Korea Institute of Science & Technology Evaluation and Planning (2000-N-NL-01-C-159).

6. References

[1]	B. O. Rothbaum, L. F. Hodges, and R. Kooper, Virtual reality exposure therapy, Journal of Psychotherapy Practice and Research, **6** (1997) 291-296.

[2]	M. P. Huang, J. Himle, D.-I. K.-P. Beier, and N. E. Alessi, "Comparing Virtual and Real Worlds for Acrophobia Treatment," in Medicine Meets Virtual Reality, vol.,, J. D. Westwood, H. M. Hoffman, D. Stredney, and S. J. Weghorst, Ed: ed.: IOS Press and Ohmsha, 1998, pp. 175-179.

[3]	R. A. Klein, Virtual Reality Exposure Therapy (Fear of Flying): From a Private Practice Perspective, CyberPsychology & Behavior, **1** (1998) 311-316.

[4]	B. K. Wiederhold, R. Gevirtz, and M. D. Wiederhold, Fear of Flying: A Case Report Using Virtual Reality Therapy with Physiological Monitoring, CyberPsychology & Behavior, **1** (1998) 97-103.

[5]　L. F. Hodges, B. O. Rothbaum, R. Alarcon, D. Ready, F. Shahar, K. Graap, J. Pair, P. Hebert, D. Gotz, B. Wills, and D. Baltzell, A Virtual Environment for the Treatment of Chronic Combat-Related Post-Traumatic Stress Disorder, CyberPsychology & Behavior, **2** (1999) 7-14.

[6]　M. Lombard and T. Ditton, At the Heart of It All: The Concept of Presence, Journal of Computer-Mediated Communication, **3** (1997).

[7]　B. K. Wiederhold and M. D. Wiederhold, Clinical Observations During Virtual Reality Therapy for Specific Phobias, CyberPsychology & Behavior, **2** (1999) 161-168.

[8]　C. Dillon, E. Keogh, J. Freeman, and J. Davidoff, *Aroused and immersed: the psychophysiology of presence*, vol. 2001, ed.Prensece 2000-3rd International Workshop on Presence, 2000. http://www.presence-research.org

[9]　M. Meehan, *An Objective Surrogate for Presence: Physiological Response*, vol. 2001, ed.Prensece 2000-3rd International Workshop on Presence, 2000. http://www.presence-research.org

[10]　B. K. Wiederhold, R. Davis, and M. D. Wiederhold, "The Effects of Immersiveness on Physiology," in Virtual Environments in Clinical Psychology and Neuroscience, vol.,, G. Riva, Ed: ed.: IOS Press, 1998, pp. 52-60.

[11]　H. T. Regenbrecht, T. W. Schubert, and F. Friedmann, Measuring the Sense of Presence and its Relations to Fear of Heights in Virtual Environments, International Journal of Human-Computer Interaction, **10** (1998) 233-249.

[12]　L. F. Hodges, R. Kooper, B. O. Rothbaum, D. Opdyke, J. J. De Graaff, J. S. Williford, and M. M. North, Virtual Environments for Treating the fear of heights, Computer Innovative Technology for Computer Professionals, **28** (1995) 27-34.

[13]　R. S. Kennedy and N. E. Lane, Simulator Sickness Questionnaire: An Enhanced Method for Quantifying Simulator Sickness, The International Journal of Aviation Psychology, **3** (1993) 203-220.

[14]　C. Hendrix and W. Barfield, Presence within Virtual Environments as a function of visual display parameters, Presence:Teleoperators and Virtual Environments, **5** (1996) 290-301.

[15]　A. Tellegen and G. Atkinson, Openness to absorbing and self-altering experiences (absorption), a trait related to hypnotic susceptibility, Journal of Abnormal Psychology, **83** (1974) 268-277.

[16]　E. M. Bernstein and F. W. Putnam, Development, reliability and validity of a dissociation scale, Journal of Nervous & Mental Disease, **174** (1986).

[17]　M. Slater, A. Steed, J. McCarthy, and P. Maringelli, The Influence of Body Movement on Subjective Presence in Virtual Environments, Human Factors, **40** (1998) 469-447.

[18]　E. Neumann and R. Balanton, Tie early history of electrodermal research, Psychophysiology, **6** (1970) 453-475.

[19]　M. Meehan, "Physiological Reaction as an Objective Measure of Presence in Virtual Environments," in *The Department of Computer Science*, vol.,, Ed.^Eds., ed. Chapel Hill: the University of North Carolina, 2001, pp. 133.

[20]　M. Malik, Heart Rate Variability, Circulation, **93** (1996) 1043-1065.

Medicine Meets Virtual Reality 02/10
J.D. Westwood et al. (Eds.)
IOS Press, 2002

Using Stereoscopy for Medical Virtual Reality

Nigel W. John
Manchester Visualization Centre
University of Manchester, UK

Abstract. The use of stereoscopy to enhance the immersive experience obtained from a virtual environment is well known, and many medical applications can benefit from this technology. The stereoscopic projection sessions at the last two MMVR conferences contain many excellent examples. Stereoscopy need not be expensive to implement, and can easily be provided on a desktop PC. This paper looks at the different options available today, from active stereo, to passive stereo, to autostereoscopic displays, and their deployment on both high-end and low-end systems. The potential benefits of these different approaches are illustrated with examples from medical visualisation projects currently being carried out at the Manchester Visualization Centre (MVC).

1. Background

Just as in the real world, a stereoscopic image presents your left and right eye with a different perspective viewpoint. The human mind can fuse these two slightly different views into an image of the world with stereoscopic depth. Some people are able to do this with the unaided eye but many find this a difficult skill to master and need to use physical aids such as a stereoscopic display. The main techniques used by these display environments are summarized below. Note that as well as using perspective, the stereoscopic effect can be enhanced through the use of depth cues such as motion parallax (e.g. by rotating an object), light and shade, relative size, and texture.

Charles Wheatstone's stereoscope [1] is regarded as the first stereoscopic viewer. The stereoscope dates back to 1838 and used an ingenuous combination of mirrors to separate the left and right eye images. Modern equivalents of this device are still in use today (see Figure 1B), and are often used by chemists for visualizing drawings of molecules, for example.

The next generation for stereoscopy was the use of stereo photography, and stereo cameras have been obtainable from the 1920's onwards. Cinemas also joined the craze and is the 1930's and 1940's it was not unusual to be able to see the latest big film releases in 3D. Projectors were expensive and the quality was not great, however, and the demand for 3D films declined. With the advent of the IMAX and improved technology, the interest in this area is again growing.

Another popular and inexpensive way of presenting stereoscopy is to use an anaglyph. Here, contrasting colours (one red and the other blue-green) are used to render or print the left and right eye images. The images are superimposed on top of each other, producing a three-dimensional effect when viewed through two correspondingly coloured filters – usually red/blue cardboard glasses (Figure 1A). Comic books, films, and photographs have all used this technique and anaglyph images can easily be found on the internet.

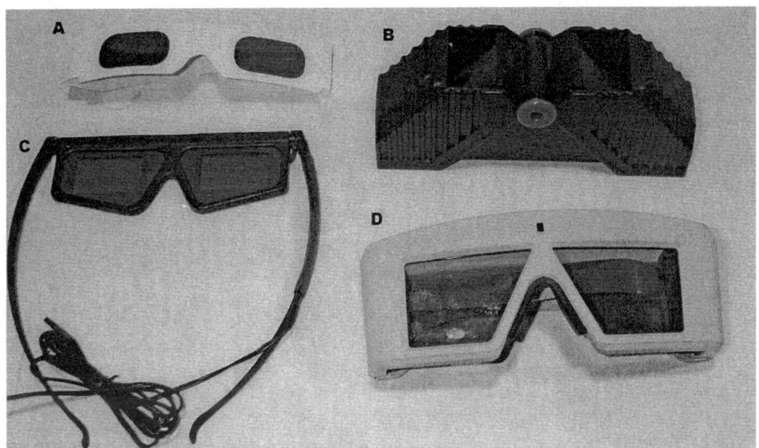

Figure 1: Stereo Glasses used at MVC - A: red/blue cardboard glasses; B: VCH Reflecting Stereoscope; C: VREX Visualizer shutter glasses; D: StereoGraphics CrystalEyes LCD shutter glasses

Modern electro-stereoscopic displays such as those available from StereoGraphics Corp. [2] (Figure 1D) have evolved from the Wheatstone stereoscope. Left and right images are alternated rapidly on the monitor screen. When the viewer looks at the screen using Liquid Crystal Display (LCD) shutter glasses, each shutter is synchronised to occlude the unwanted image and transmit just the wanted image. The result is that the left eye sees only the left perspective view, and the right eye sees only the right perspective view. If the images (often called fields) are refreshed fast enough (often at twice the rate of the planar display), the result is a flickerless stereoscopic image. This kind of a display is called a field-sequential stereoscopic display. Starting in the 1990s, high-end graphics computers such as those from SGI have been able to deliver stereoscopic projection. They use a double buffering technique operating at a refresh rate of 120Hz. Each field has a vertical blanking area associated with it to provide a synchronisation pulse. With electro-stereoscopic displays, you will also come across the terms "active" stereo and "passive" stereo. In an active stereoscopic system, the shutter glasses contain electronic components to interpret the synchronisation pulse – received through infrared or a direct connection. With passive stereoscopic systems, the glasses use polarized filters and have no electronic components (and so are much cheaper). A dual projector system is typically used in this case, with polaroid filters placed in front of the projector lenses. Passive stereo has been used at the stereoscopic sessions at MMVR.

Today, inexpensive PC graphics cards such as those from NVIDIA are capable of high refresh rates (greater than 100Hz) and also support stereoscopic projection using double buffering [3]. The graphics card driver using a hardware override can create the stereoscopic 3D views automatically, so no modifications need to be made to the application software. At the same time cheap LCD shutter glasses developed for the games market are becoming available (e.g. ELSA 3D Revelator, and VREX VR Visualizer System [4]). This type of stereoscopic system is now very affordable.

The newest generation of stereoscopic display technology is starting to become available commercially. These are the autosteroscopic displays, and they do not require the user to wear special glasses. The left and right eye images are interlaced vertically across the image. A special prism mask is placed over the display and directs every odd column in the image to the left eye, and every even column to the right eye. A stereoscopic image results – Figure 2 gives the impression of the effect that is achieved.

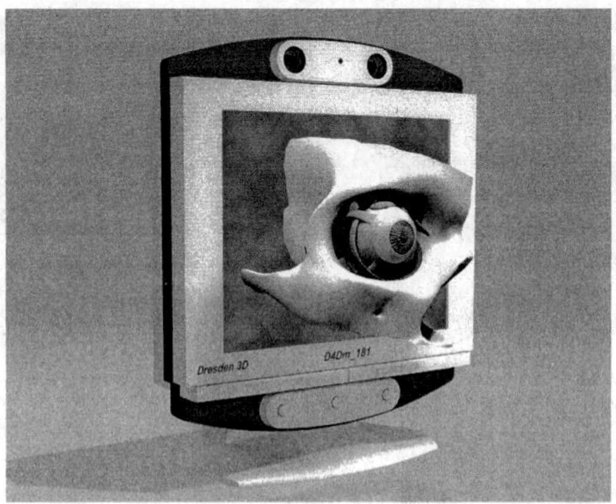

Figure 2: Autosterescopic Display - the user sees stereo images without having to wear special glasses. The image of the D4D digital display is courtesy of Dresden 3D GmbH.

The best quality 3D images are from optical holography, which uses the physical phenomena of interference and diffraction to record and construct a 3D image [5]. Research is already underway to compute holographic patterns for the generation of 3D holographic images at interactive speeds [6]. This will be the future generation of stereoscopic display technology, but is outside of the scope of this paper.

2. Methods & Tools

The Manchester Visualization Centre (MVC) has an extensive research programme that is applying visualisation and virtual reality techniques to medical applications. This section contains examples of how and why stereoscopy is being applied within these projects.

2.1 High End Stereoscopy

The premier visualization facility at MVC is an immersive projection theatre powered by an SGI Onyx supercomputer. It can seat 30 people comfortably, and all can experience high quality stereoscopy using an active stereo configuration. The images are projected onto a large cylindrical screen using three CRT projectors.

Two software applications are being used regularly in the VR theatre for medical visualisation. We have developed our own general-purpose volume visualisation tool – called *volumize*. We have also adapted a commercial visualisation package (AVS/Express) to be stereo aware and suitable for use in virtual environments. Both of these software environments require a powerful SGI workstation, and make use of the OpenGL Multipipe SDK programming interface [7] to implement the stereoscopy and multiple channel rendering support required.

Visualisation and Teaching Tool

The Volumize software utilises the OpenGL Volumizer API [8], which enables rendering of and interaction with large data sets in real time. A primary use of volumize is for the visualisation of medical data sets and its functionality has been designed with invaluable input from clinical colleagues. Examples include providing high quality visualisation of medical data that exhibit unusual features such as from a patient with a bidelphic uterine anatomy; and time variant data such as a 3D Ultrasound data set of a beating heart. Feedback received from clinicians indicates that seeing the data in stereo makes interpretation far easier for them.

A further use of volumize as a teaching tool is also promising. The Department of Anatomy at the University have already started using the VR Theatre for teaching their students. We can use stereoscopy to show them life-size renderings of data acquired locally, or from other sources such as the Visible Human Project. Recently, some of the anatomy students have selected a second year project that will create further VR anatomical models using the facilities at MVC. In due course this will provide further material that can be used in undergraduate teaching.

Endovascular Surgical Planning Tool

MVC is developing an Endovascular Surgical Planning (ESP) tool that can be used to help treat a patient suffering from a brain haemorrhage [9]. The commonest form of treatment involves packing the aneurysm with a small platinum coil. This is introduced into the body by a catheter inserted into the femoral artery in the groin and fed up into the brain and eventually into the aneurysm itself. This project has developed a visualisation application using the AVS/Express toolkit, that aims to provide renderings that simplify and accelerate the process of assessing the shape, size and position of the aneurysm and for selecting the optimal aneurysm views for the coiling procedure – see Figure 3.

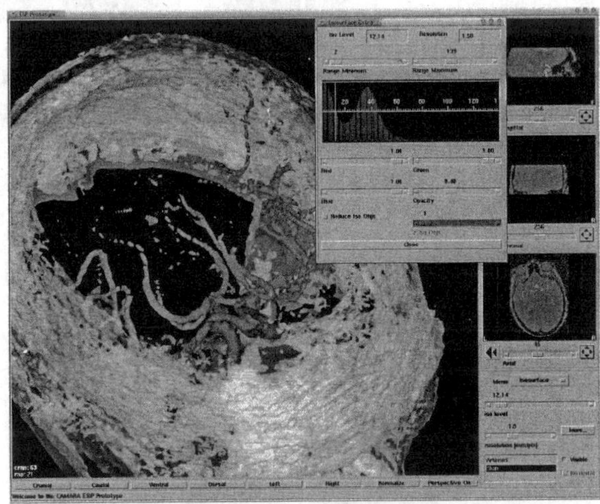

Figure 3: Monocsopic View of a 3D Rendering in the ESP software. The blood vessels are reconstructed from MRA data.

The ESP software conforms to a clinician's standard working practices but also integrates new and faster methods for examining and analysing MRA data. The ability to correlate different 3D views of the aneurysm structure with the angiography equipment used during the coiling procedure greatly helps the clinician's planning of the procedure. This is enhanced further when stereoscopy is used - the clinician has a clearer idea of how the coils should be placed to reduce the chance of aneurysm re-growth. Other benefits we hope to achieve are a reduction in time needed to both assess each case and for carrying out the procedure. In turn this means a reduction in the exposure to radiation for the patient.

2.2 Low End Steroscopy

Stereoscopy is not confined to the domain of expensive VR facilities. A combination of the latest PC graphics cards (such as the NVIDIA GeForce range) and cheap shutter glasses (primarily aimed at the games market) can deliver a low cost, but still effective, stereoscopy environment. We use this low end stereoscopy environment in the WebSET project, which is developing surgical procedure training tools delivered over the Web using the Virtual Reality Modeling Language (VRML) [10]. Figure 4 shows a snapshot from the Ventricular Catheterisation training tool that we have produced, presented as a stereo pair of images. It is straightforward to operate training tools such as these in stereo without making any modifications to the VRML source. The graphics card driver can automatically generate the stereo output required – both field sequential and anaglyph formats are possible (the stereo pair in Figure 4 is used for illustration only). We use the Cortona VRML plug-in from Parallel Graphics. It has to be set to full screen mode for the stereo output to be enabled.

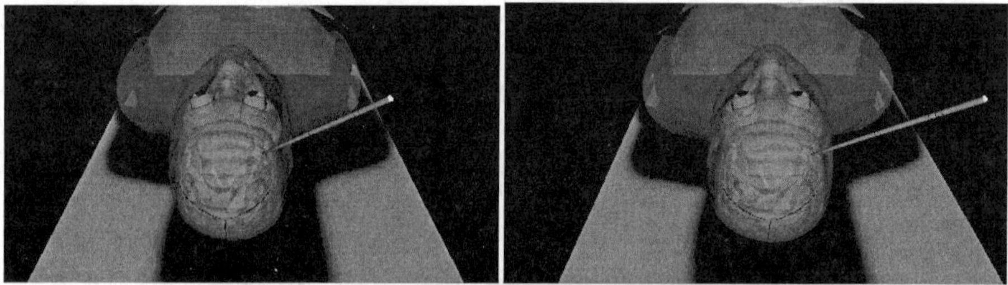

Figure 4: Stereo Pair View of the WebSET Ventricular Catheterisation Simulator. Can be viewed in stereo using a device such as the Reflecting Stereoscope (Figure 1B).

A key part of a procedure such as ventricular catheterisation is to position and orientate the cannula accurately before it is inserted through the brain. The ability to do this successfully is greatly enhanced when using stereoscopy. Further, once stereo output is enabled on the graphics card, any VRML content can benefit without any modifications being required.

2.3 Autostereoscopy

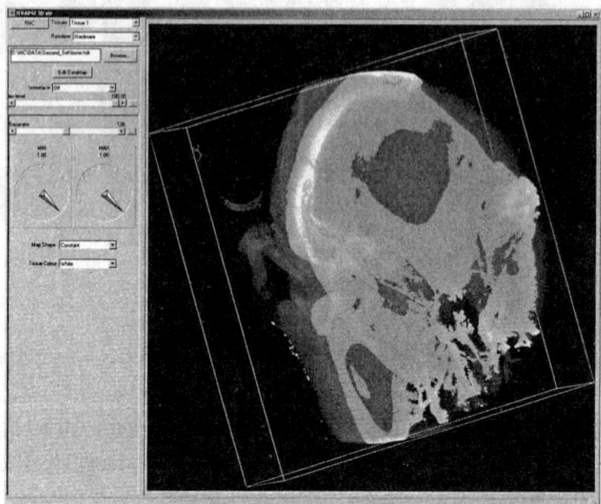

Figure 5 Monoscopic view of the IERAPSI Pre-operative Planning Environment

In the IERAPSI project [11] we are using the Dresden D4D autostereoscopic display [12] – see Figure 2. We are interested here in providing an easy to use stereoscopic environment that does not require the clinician to use special eyewear. The application being developed to use the D4D is a pre-operative planning environment for petrous bone surgery. It employs an advanced multi-dimensional classification technique to calculate tissue probability maps for bone, blood vessels and soft tissue [13]. The probability maps can then be visualised using direct volume and/or surface rendering techniques (Figure 5.). Note that only the 3D rendering can be viewed on the D4D. It is not suitable for the 2D widgets and menus of the user interface.

The pre-operative planning software is using the AVS/Express toolkit. Support for the vertical interlacing of the left and right eye images required for the D4D is built into the graphics card (an ATI FireGL3) and so no modification to the application code is required to obtain the stereo effect. The quality of the stereoscopy is not yet as good as that obtained from the field sequential technique, however.

2.4 Other Technologies

Another partner in the IERAPSI project is using a binocular environment to simulate the surgical microscope used for procedures such as a mastoidechtomy [14]. The virtual surgical microscope has been built using a high-resolution hand held display (the VB-30 from N.Vision, Inc.), which contains two small (0.7 inch) LCD displays – one for each eye. This does not provide stereoscopy as described in this paper, but is a related approach.

Also in use at MVC is a Reachin Display system [15]. The unique advantage of this system is that it co-locates active stereoscopy with a high quality force feedback joystick. We are porting the simulators from the WebSET project to this environment.

3. Results

The projects described above are all producing compelling stereoscopic images and gaining the general approval of our clinical end users. Several problems do exist with stereoscopic viewing, however, and these are highlighted in this section.

When using the field sequential stereoscopic techniques, users initially reported eyestrain and other negative symptoms if viewing in stereo for longer than 15 minutes. This is a well known problem and is due to the difference between viewing a stereoscopic image in reality versus viewing it on a monitor or screen. In the real world, your eyes will automatically focus and converge on an object at a particular depth. In the virtual world, the focal point is fixed at the depth of the monitor or screen surface, whereas the convergence depth is based on the object being viewed. The disparity between these two processes is initially uncomfortable. However, most users do get used to this over time and the eyestrain will disappear. Reducing the stereo separation between the two views can also help reduce eyestrain. Note that a big advantage of the new autostereoscopic displays is that they do not require eyewear and so do not cause eyestrain in this way.

Another common problem is with "crosstalk", where each eye sees some of the image from the unwanted perspective view. In a perfect stereoscopic system each eye sees only its assigned image. This is the case with the reflecting stereoscope as each image is optically separated from the other. However, with electronic displays there are two causes of crosstalk: departures from the ideal shutter in the eyewear, and CRT phosphor afterglow. Both are likely to be present to some extent. The autostereoscopic display is also prone to crosstalk and requires careful calibration to reduce this effect.

Although high end stereoscopy generally gives higher quality results (particularly compared with the current quality of an autostereoscopic display), there are also problems specific only to this medium. Active stereo systems rely on CRT projectors, as other technologies cannot deliver the high frame rates required. A CRT projector is typically bulky and difficult to calibrate. It also needs to use fast phosphor tubes to support a 120Hz refresh rate, a downside of which is that high brightness levels are difficult to achieve. There is also a common problem with ghosting at the bottom of the imaging area resulting from the finite time required for the electron beam to scan from the top to the bottom of the image.

4. Conclusions

This paper has outlined the main stereoscopy techniques in use today and is intended to provide pointers for others to use when considering making use of stereo for the first time. The applications described in this paper show that the use of stereoscopy with medical visualisation can be a useful aid for diagnosis, planning, training and teaching. There are many ways in which stereoscopy can be achieved, and it need not be expensive. Problems do exist with stereoscopic technology, but these can be minimised and new solutions are appearing on the market all of the time. The author is confident that in a few years time the use of stereoscopy for medical visualisation will be the *de facto* choice for most applications.

References

[1]   C. Wheatstone, On some remarkable, and hitherto unobserved, phenomena of binocular vision (Part the first). Philosophical Transactions of the Royal Society of London, 1838, pp371-94.
[2]   StereoGraphics Corporation Web Site http://www.stereographics.com/
[3]   NVIDIA 3D Stereo Technical Brief. Web site:
      http://www.nvidia.com/docs/lo/539/SUPP/3D_Stereo_Tech_Brief.pdf
[4]   VREX Web Site http://www.vrex.com/
[5]   P. Hariharen, Optical Holography. Cambridge University Press, 1984.
[6]   M. Lucente and T. A. Galyean, Rendering Interactive Holographic Images. Proc. of SIGGRAPH 95 (Los Angeles, CA, Aug. 6-11, 1995). In Computer Graphics Proceedings, Annual Conference Series, 1995, ACM SIGGRAPH, pp. 387-394.
[7]   P.G. Lever et al., Design Issues in the AVS/Express Multi-Pipe Edition, *IEEE Visualization 2000*, Salt Lake City, Utah, October 2000
[8]   OpenGL Volumizer Web site: http://www.sgi.com/software/volumizer/
[9]   J.S. Perrin et al., A Visualization System for the Clinical Evaluation of Cerebral Aneurysms from MRA Data, In: *Short Presentations Proceedings, Eurographics 2001*, Manchester, September 2001, ISSN 1017-4656
[10] N.W. John, et al., Web-based Surgical Educational Tools, In J. D. Westwood, editor, Medicine Meets Virtual Reality 2001, IOS Press Amsterdam, January 2001.
[11] N. W. John, et al., An integrated simulator for surgery of the petrous bone. In J. D. Westwood, editor, Medicine Meets Virtual Reality 2001, IOS Press Amsterdam, January 2001.
[12] A. Schwerdtner and H. Heidrich, Dresden 3D Display: A Flat Autostereoscopic Display, Electronic Imaging / Photonics West 1998, San Jose, California, 1998.
[13] M. Pokric, et al., Multi-dimensional Medical Image Segmentation with Partial Voluming. Proceedings of Medical Imaging Understanding and Analysis, July 2001
[14] M. Agus, et al., Mastoidectomy Simulation with Combined Visual and Haptic Feedback, Submitted to Medicine Meets Virtual Reality 2002, IOS Press Amsterdam, January 2002.
[15] Reachin Web site: http://www.reachin.se

Acknowledgements

The following MVC staff and students are contributing to the projects described above: Nicolas Antoine, Matt Cooper, Andrew Dodd, James Perrin, Maja Pokric, and Mark Riding. The IERAPSI Project is part funded by the European Community under the IST Project IST-1999-12175. The WebSET Project is part funded by the European Community under the IST Project IST-1999-10632. The ESP software is being developed as part of the CAMRAS project, which is funded by the Sir Jules Thorn Charitable Trust.

Medicine Meets Virtual Reality 02/10
J.D. Westwood et al. (Eds.)
IOS Press, 2002

A Virtual Environment for Esophageal Intubation Training

T Kesavadas PhD[1], Dhananjay Joshi[1], James Mayrose PhD[2], Kevin Chugh PhD[3]

[1]Virtual Reality Lab, Department of Mechanical and Aerospace Engineering
[2]Department of Emergency Medicine
[3]New York State Center for Engineering Design and Industrial Innovation

State University of New York at Buffalo
Buffalo, NY 14260

Abstract: Esophageal intubations are performed for urgent airway control in injured patients. Current methods of training include working on cadavers and mannequins, which lack the realism of a living human being. Work in this field has been limited due to the complex nature of simulating in real-time the interactive forces and deformations which occur during an actual patient intubation. This study addressed the issue of intubation training in an attempt to bridge the gap between actual and virtual patient scenarios. The two haptic devices along with the real-time performance of the simulator give it both visual and physical realism. The three dimensional viewing and interaction available through virtual reality make it possible for physicians, pre-hospital personnel and students to practice many esophageal intubations without ever touching a patient. The ability for a medical professional to practice a procedure multiple times prior to performing it on a patient will both enhance the skill of the individual while reducing the risk to the patient.

1. Introduction

Development of Virtual Environments for Medical research is a multi-disciplinary effort, aimed at advancing the state of art in health and emergency care. Virtual Reality (VR) (also called Virtual Environments, VE) has many definitions but is best described by Cruz-Neira [1] as follows: "Virtual Reality refers to immersive, interactive, multi-sensory, view-centered 3-D computer generated environments and the combination of technologies required to build these technologies". VR applications now offer unprecedented avenues by using several areas of engineering such as computer technology, sensory data acquisition and controls, force feedback and real-time visualization to provide engineering solutions to medical problems. Such systems are good example of what Dr. Fred Brooks, one of the pioneers of VR, calls "intelligence amplification".

Esophageal intubations in the emergency department or in the pre-hospital setting are performed for urgent airway control in injured patients. Typically medical personnel have just minutes to perform an endotracheal intubation on a patient in the field. If the procedure is not successful on the first attempt the medical personnel have to try again with ever diminishing chances of success. The best way to prepare for this procedure, according to doctors, is to do as many intubations as possible. Given the delicate condition of the patients it is not the best time to train a paramedic or a resident. Another feature of this process is that it requires accurate manipulation of the laryngascope blade and intubation tube. If this two-handed procedure is not practiced often, it may result in an incorrect intubation or worse yet, additional injury to the patient. The circumstances surrounding these intubations are often less than controlled, with the pre-hospital setting posing perhaps the most adverse conditions both in terms of environmental factors and patient's clinical presentations [1]. In addition, definitive airway control in the pre-hospital setting is most often done by physician extenders who have demonstrated a misplaced endotracheal tube rate of up to 9% [2]. It was the misplaced endotracheal tube rate that gave us the idea for the development of a real-time esophageal intubation simulator. Most recent attempts to create a model for intubation training purposes have been based on physiologically responsive patient simulator models which lack the realism necessary for appropriate training [3]. Although great care is taken to make the physical properties of the simulator as close to that of a human subject, the training is far from realistic. A definite improvement can be made in the quality of training by using a Virtual Reality based simulation for intubation.

In most of the surgical simulators we see in the market place as well as research labs today, the one thing that is common to them all is the type of interaction the user has with the virtual environment. In these simulators, the tool's the user uses to interact with the virtual environment are assumed to be rigid. The tools interact through a point during suturing for example or through a line during a cutting application. The intubation simulator developed here differs from the others in a fundamental way. Having a rigid virtual endotrachial tube with just a point or a line contact will not allow us to realistically simulate the intubation procedure. Consequently we must have the following basic properties for a physically based intubation simulator. First, we use a surface contact or have an approximation for the surface contact. Second, we have a Physical model of the endotrachial tube which allows for dynamic and real-time deformation within the virtual environment. The deformation of this tube is not localized in certain parts but spread over its entire length. The final version of this intubation simulator will have other characteristics such as audio and video overlays similar to other surgical simulators on the market today.

2. Methods

The goal of our effort is to eventually develop a simulator based on the comparatively in-expensive personal desktop computer platform. The Reachin Display by Reachin AB (Stockholm, Sweden) offers a generic platform for development of surgical simulators in the PC environment. This platform significantly improves the immersion characteristics of the simulation. The Reachin Application Programming Interface (API) offers a generic software tool for rapid development of medical simulators. Included in the reaching display architecture is the Phantom Haptic feedback device developed by

SensAble Technologies, Inc. (Woburn, Massachusetts). Figure 1 represents the system architecture of the intubation simulator developed in this study.

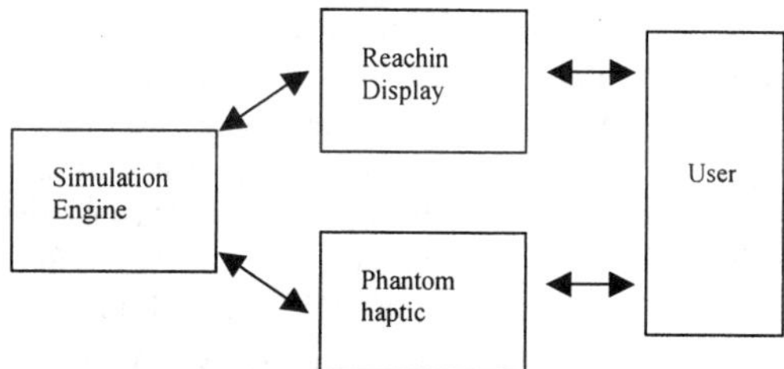

Figure 1: The system architecture for virtual intubation simulator

The simulation engine runs on a Pentium III Dual processor PC with a GVX 210 graphics accelerator card from 3Dlabs.

2.1 Physical Model

Many methods have been employed over the years to simulate dynamic deformation and direct manipulation of non-physical geometry. Mass spring models and continuum models using Finite Element Methods (FEM) are two of the most widely used methods. Non-physical methods for modeling deformation are limited by the expertise and patience of the user. Deformations must be explicitly specified and the system has no knowledge about the object being manipulated. FEM has limited application in real-time simulation due to the computationally intensive nature of the calculations. A Mass spring model is one physically based technique that has been used widely and effectively for modeling deformable objects [4]. An object is modeled as a collection of point masses connected by springs in a lattice structure. The springs are linear though non-linear springs can also be used. Newton's Second law governs the motion of a single mass point in the lattice. Depending on the current position of the particle various forces are found.

$$\begin{pmatrix} force \\ on \\ particle \end{pmatrix} = \begin{pmatrix} force \\ due \\ to \\ spring \end{pmatrix} + \begin{pmatrix} force \\ due \\ to \\ gravity \end{pmatrix} + \begin{pmatrix} force \\ due \\ to \\ damping \end{pmatrix} \tag{1}$$

The new velocity for the particle is found using the combined forces shown in Equation 1 along with the elapsed time of the event. Using this velocity the new position of the particle is found. This method can also be applied to a system of particles in order to determine the overall deformation. A variety of numerical integration techniques are available to calculate the new positions and velocities as a function of time, the simplest being Euler Integration. Mass-spring systems are a simple physical system with well understood dynamics. They are easy to construct and can be animated at rates not possible with other methods. Mass spring models have been implemented for a variety of applications from animation of the human face to simulating the movement of woven cloth. The implementation of the mass spring model for our case was fairly trivial because the endotracheal tube was already tessellated as triangles in a Virtual Reality Markup Language (VRML) file. The masses were added at the vertices of the triangles and the topology of the springs were easily available from the VRML data. The stiffness of springs was taken from the physical data of the material used for the endotracheal tube. The 3-dimensional model of the upper torso and head of the human body were also tessellated as triangles, so determination of the positions of the particles in the mass spring model is possible using simple point-plane intersection tests. Take for instance the equation of a plane $Ax+By+Cz+D=0$ and a point $P(x',y',z')$. Point P collides with the plane if $Ax'+By'+Cz'+D < \varepsilon$, where ε is a very small number. This test was carried out for the plane of each triangle as well as with the plane normal to the triangle and passing through each side of the triangle to determine the collision of the particle with the triangle. Thus, it is possible to determine completely the behavior of the virtual endotracheal tube using a mass spring model and simple collision tests.

2.2 Binary Space Partitioning

To achieve real-time graphic update rates, we used Binary Space Partitioning (BSP). BSP is a well-known technique in the field of computer graphics. It is used in the preprocessing stage to divide the object space into a binary tree. Using partitioning hyper-planes that are defined by the user the BSP algorithm is used to segment the total hyperspace into mutually exclusive subspaces. A hyper-plane for a 2-D geometry is a line. For a 3D geometry that we all live in, the hyper-plane is a plane. The applications include determination of visibility and collision detection to name a few. We have implemented the BSP tree for the triangles that constitute the soft tissue of the virtual human patient (Figure 2). That is the triangles of the virtual tissue have been partitioned into a binary tree. The immediate benefit of this endeavor is to reduce the complexity of the algorithm for collision detection [$O(n^2)$ to $O(n\log n)$]. The preprocessing stage is itself $O(n)$ in most cases and $O(n^3)$ in the worst case, n being the number of triangles [5]. Consequently the amount of time required to solve the system is reduced and real-time graphics update rates are achieved.

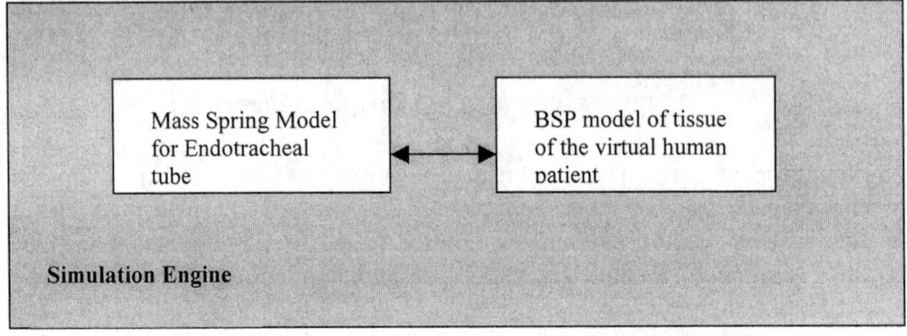

Figure 2: The simulation engine for the virtual intubation simulator

We have implemented and tested the algorithm for a vastly simplified virtual environment (Figure 3). The straight white tube shown at the left of Figure 3 is used to interact with the curved gray tube in the center. Both the tubes are made up of 400 triangles each. The frame rate for this system without using BSP is approximately 1 frame per sec (fps). After applying the BSP technique, we obtained a frame rate upwards of 60 fps.

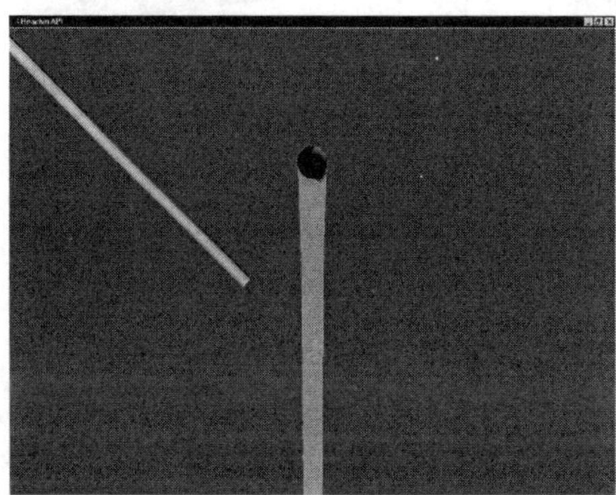

Figure 3: A simplified version developed to test the algorithm

2.3 Atomic Unit Method

A 3-dimensional, volumetric, model of the human head and neck was developed using the Visible Human Data-set provided by the National Institutes of Health. The individual tissue and cartilage that make up these regions were broken down into cubes called atomic units. The Atomic Unit Method is designed to compute force-displacement relationships for soft tissue deformations in real-time [6,7]. Traditional approaches perform these calculations by computing the effect that every discrete unit of tissue has on every other discrete unit of tissue. These approaches use one master computational engine which iterates through each piece of data. Using an object oriented methodology, the atomic unit method distributes the computation into many individual computational engines, which has both tangible and intangible benefits. The tangible benefit is that this simplified model allows for very fast and robust computation. It is fast, again, because each unit performs some constant time calculation. It is also robust because the individual atomic unit classes can be customized to achieve tissue-specific behaviors. The intangible benefit of this method is that all coding and design are done at the atomic unit level. This means that a divide-and-conquer approach is taken wherein a large computational task is accomplished by breaking it into very small parts and assembling a large set of small computational units (atomic units). Programming at this low level is much easier and cleaner than programming one master computational engine. With the Atomic Unit Methodology, each discrete tissue volume is modeled as an atomic unit, and each atomic unit has its own behavior (Figure 4). Forces are handed off from atomic unit

     T. Kesavadas et al. / Virtual Environment for Esophageal Intubation Training

to atomic unit, and the global behavior of the tissue model is computed by aggregating the atomic unit behaviors.

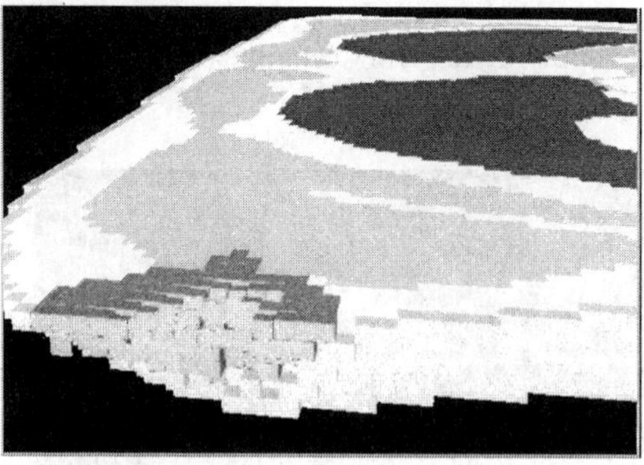

Figure 4: Atomic Unit Tissue Model

3. Conclusions and Future Work

This study has shown that it is possible to get a real-time dynamic deformation for the endotracheal tube even in a fairly large virtual model. The immediate future work is to apply the algorithm to a virtual human patient based on the visible human dataset shown in Figure 5. Future work will include the implementation of haptic feedback to the user. The use of sounds and video overlays will be added to the simulator in order to give it a more realistic look and feel. Once the simulator is complete, human subject testing will be conducted in order to ascertain the validity of our hypothesis that a Virtual Reality based intubation simulator is a viable alternative to mannequin models for training medical professionals.

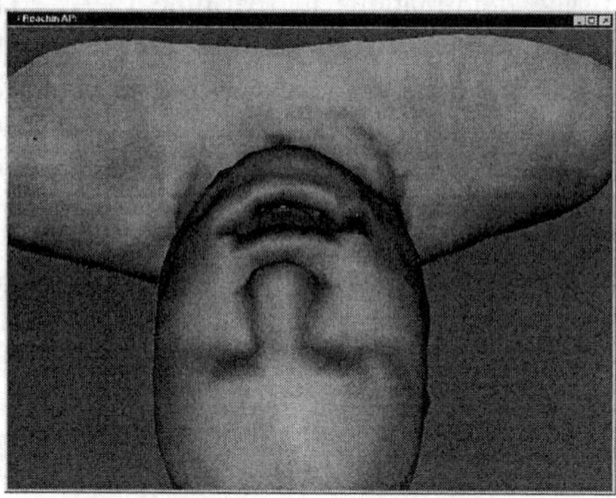

Figure 5: 3-dimensional Virtual Human Patient

4. Acknowledgements

This study was funded in part by a grant from the Federal Highway Administration No. DTFH61-98-X-00103 as awarded by the Center for Transportation Injury Research (CenTIR).

5. References

[1] Jenkins WA, Verdile VP, Paris PM: The Syringe Aspiration Technique to Verify Endotracheal Tube Position, American Journal of Emergency Medicine 1994; 12(4)

[2] Stewart RD, Paris PM, Pelton GH, et al: Effect of varied training techniques on field endotracheal intubation success rates. Ann Emerg Med 1984; 13:1032-1036

[3] Thalmann, N.M., D. Thalmann: Towards virtual humans in medicine: A prospective view. Computerized Medical Imaging & Graphics, 18:97-106, 1994

[4] Sarah.F.F.Gibson, Brian Mirtich, A survey of deformable modeling in computer graphics, MERL TR-97-19

[5] Fuchs, Kedem and Naylor, On Visible Surface Generation by A Priori Tree Structures, SIGGRAPH '80, pp124-133

[6] Chugh, An Object-oriented Approach to Physically-based Human Tissue Modeling for Virtual Reality Applications, Dissertation, SUNY at Buffalo, Diss C58 2001 C48

[7] Mayrose, A Physically-based Deformable Model for Real-time Haptic Simulation of Soft Tissue Palpation, Dissertation, SUNY at Buffalo, Diss M4 2000 M39

Medicine Meets Virtual Reality 02/10
J.D. Westwood et al. (Eds.)
IOS Press, 2002

Visible Korean Human: Another Trial for Making Serially-Sectioned Images

Jin Yong Kim, Min Suk Chung, Woo Sup Hwang, Jin Seo Park, Hyung-Seon Park*
Department of Anatomy, Ajou University School of Medicine, Suwon, Korea
**Factual Database Department, Korea Institute of Science and Technology Information,*
Daejeon, Korea

Abstract. In this ongoing study, we are trying to make Visible Korean Human (Mar 2000 - Feb 2005). The complete MRIs and CTs of the Korean cadaver's entire body are scanned. The cadaver is serially-sectioned at 0.2 mm thickness without any missing images. The anatomical structures in the sectioned images are segmented. The Visible Korean Human is expected to be more helpful than Visible Human in the following ways. First, the Korean data will be more helpful in diagnosing and treating the patients belonging to the yellow race. Second, MRIs and CTs of the entire body at 1 mm thickness will be more helpful in studying the MRIs and CTs. Third, sectioned images without any missing images will be more helpful in making the complete 3D images. Fifth, small pixel size (0.2 mm X 0.2 mm) and thin thickness (0.2 mm) of sectioned images will be more helpful in showing the small anatomical structures greater than 0.2 mm. Sixth, the additional segmented images will be more helpful in making the 3D image and virtual dissection software. The Visible Korean Human will be the basis for making better 3D image and virtual dissection software which will be more helpful in medical education.
Keywords: Visible Korean Human, Serially-sectioned images, MRIs, CTs

1. Introduction

In the United States, serially-sectioned images of the entire body, namely Visible Human, were made with male and female cadavers consisting of magnetic resonance images (MRIs), computed tomographs (CTs), and sectioned images [1,2]. The Visible Human made it possible to reconstruct three-dimensional (3D) images using the computer, and to section and rotate them at free angles. The Visible Human and 3D images have been helpful in medical education [3,4].

However, there are several problems with the Visible Human. First, it is difficult to be adapted to the yellow or black races because the shape and size of human organs differ according to race. Second, it does not include the MRIs of trunk and limbs because only MRIs of head were scanned, and it does not include complete CTs because the lateral parts of upper limbs' CTs were cut off (Figure 1). Third, it has missing sectioned images between four blocks because the cadavers were divided into four blocks using a saw before serial-sectioning (Figure 1). Fourth, it cannot show the anatomical structures which are smaller than 1 mm (male) and 0.33 mm (female) because thickness of sectioned images was greater than 1 mm (male) and 0.33 mm (female). Fifth, it does not include the segmented images, which are helpful in making 3D images and virtual dissection software [1,5].

Thus, to solve the problems encountered with the Visible Human, we decided to use the entire body of a Korean cadaver to scan complete MRIs and CTs and to make complete sectioned images and segmented images at 0.2 mm thickness. This study is called the Visible Korean Human.

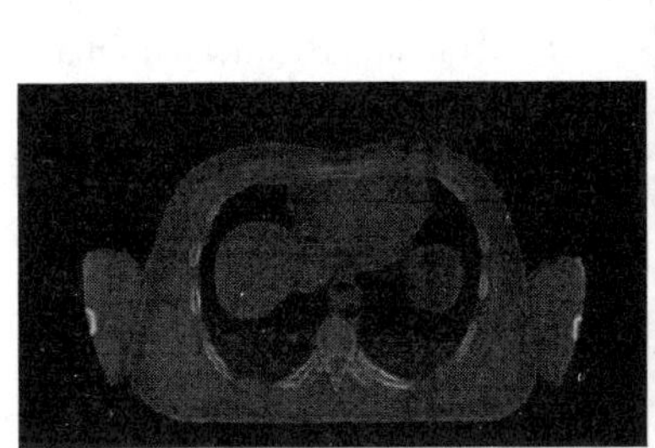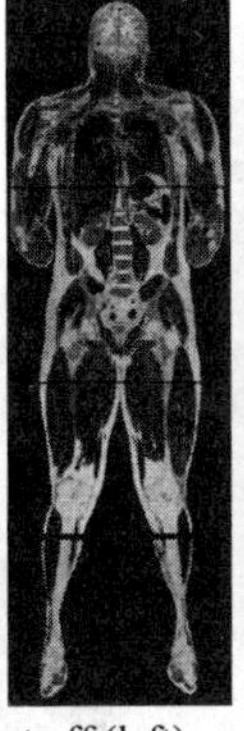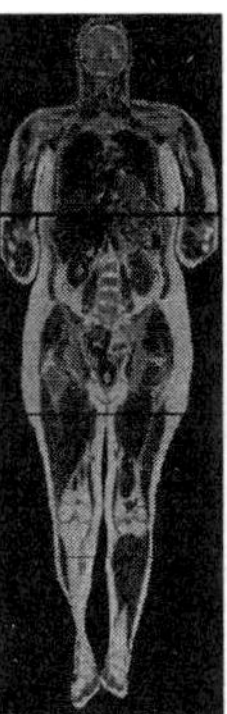

Figure 1. Visible Human in which the lateral parts of CTs are cut off (left) and sectioned images between four blocks are missed (center and right).

2. Materials, Method, and Result

To make the Visible Korean Human, a preliminary experiment was performed as follows. First, the cadaver was received. A donated Korean cadaver was used. His age, body size, and pathological findings were not suitable for the main experiment, but for the preliminary experiment (Table 1).

Table 1. Cadavers used for the preliminary and main experiments

	Sex	Age	Height (mm)	Weight (kg)	Cause of death	Period of experiment
Preliminary experiments	Male (first)	65	1,789	53	Brain tumor	Jan 2001 - Mar 2001
	Male (second)	60	1,720	65	Traffic accident	Apr 2001 - May 2001
Main experiments	Male (third)	33	1,745	55	Leukemia	Nov 2001 - Mar 2003
	Female		(to be donated)			Nov 2003 - Mar 2005

Second, MRIs and CTs of the cadaver were scanned. Two tubes containing both MRI and CT contrast media, which are helpful in aligning MRIs and CTs, were attached to the cadaver from head to foot (Figure 2). The cadaver was put into an immobilizing box, and the cadaver's posture was fixed with immobilizing agent (Mev-Green^{TM}) for making MRIs and CTs correspondent (Figure 2). MRIs of the entire body were scanned at 1 mm thickness. CTs of the entire body were also scanned at 1 mm thickness. Then, MRIs and CTs were inputted into the personal computer (pixel size 1 mm X 1 mm).

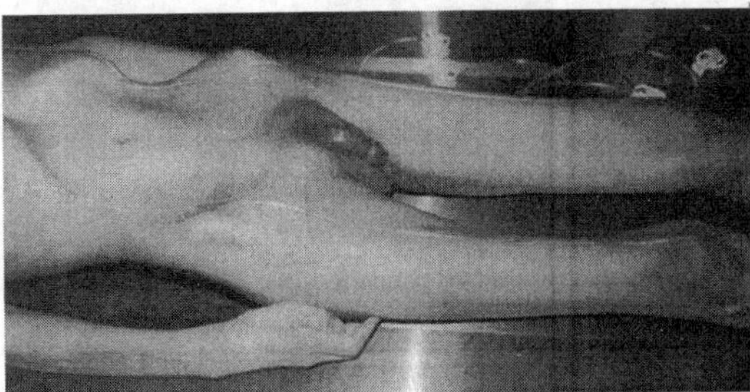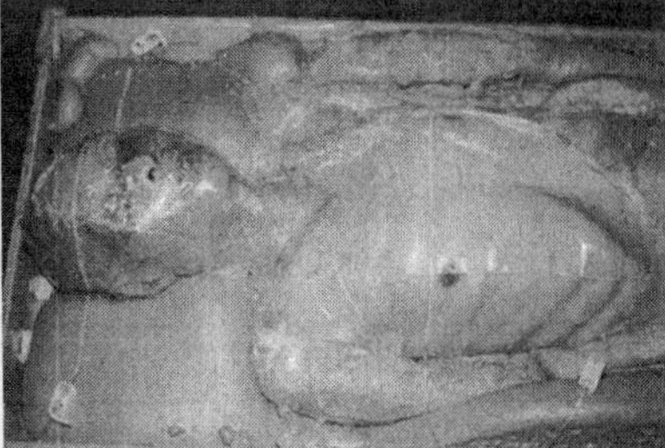

Figure 2. Cadaver to which tubes containing contrast media were attached (left) and cadaver whose posture was fixed with immobilizing agent (right).

Third, MRIs and CTs were processed. All bones of CTs were segmented. By stacking two-dimensional images, 3D images were reconstructed. The 3D images were similar to the photographs of the cadaver. The 3D images were sectioned coronally and sagittally. In the sectioned planes, correspondence of MRIs, CTs, and segmented images were verified (Figure 3). The 3D images were rotated at free angles. At this time, only skin could be displayed, only bone could be displayed, or both skin and bone could be displayed together (Figure 4). In addition, 3D images which looked like plain radiographs were rotated (Figure 5).

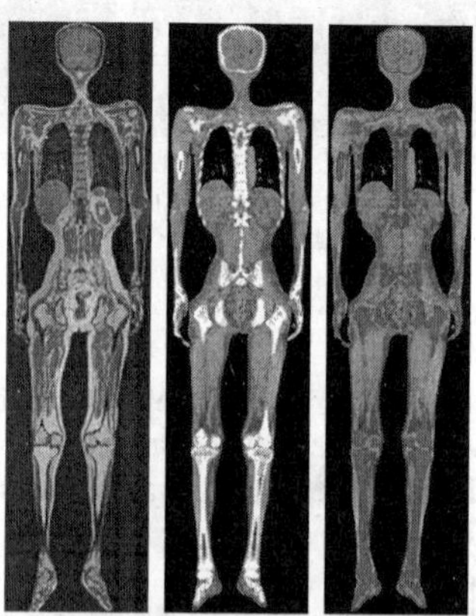

Figure 3. Sectioned planes in which MRI (left), CT (center), and segmented image (right) are correspondent.

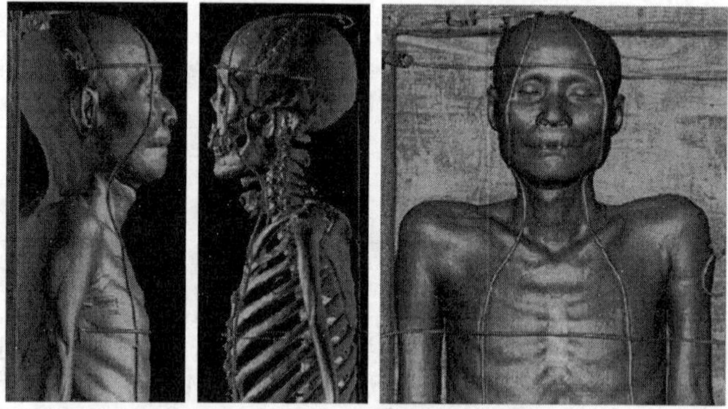

Figure 4. Rotated 3D images in which only skin (left), only bone (center), or both skin and bone (right) could be displayed.

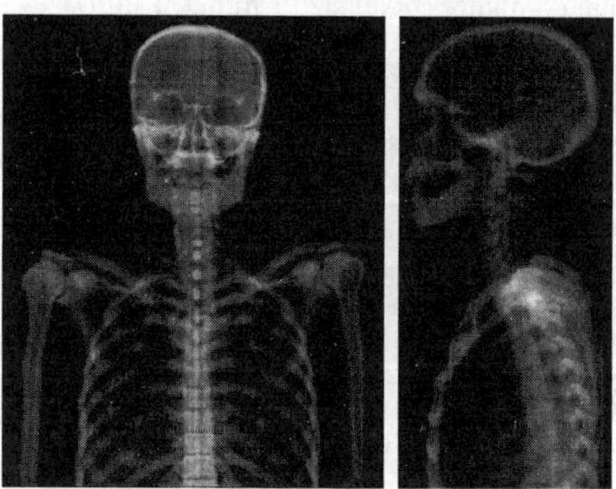

Figure 5. Rotated 3D images which look like plain radiographs.

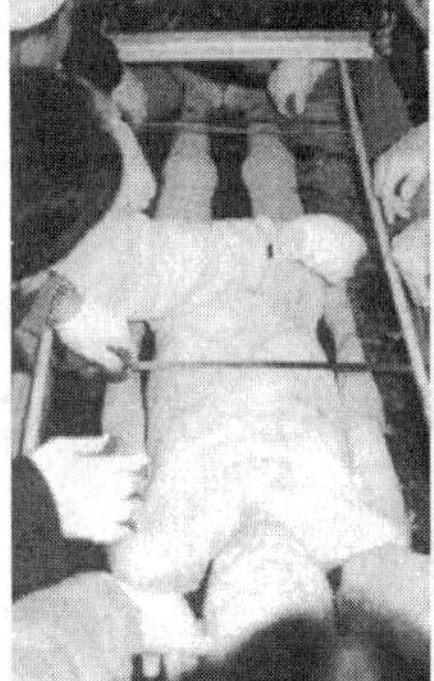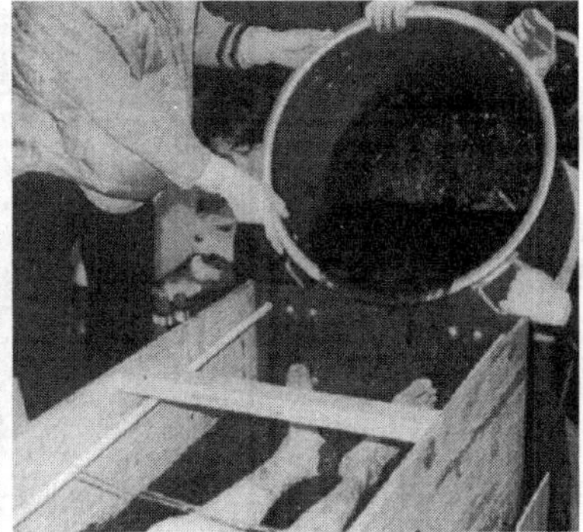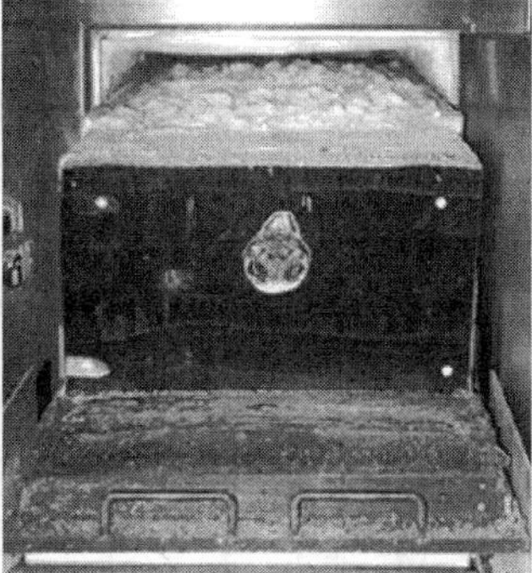

Figure 6. Putting the cadaver (left) and embedding media (center) into an embedding box and putting the embedding box into a freezer (right).

Fourth, the cadaver was embedded and frozen because the cadaver could be serially-sectioned only after embedding and freezing. The cadaver was put into an embedding box into which alignment rods were already inserted. Embedding media, made of 3% gelatin solution and blue dye, was poured into the embedding box and frozen in a freezer (Figure 6).

Fifth, the embedding box was serially-sectioned. A cryomacrotome for serial-sectioning of the entire body was made (Figure 7). An embedding box was so heavy (1 ton) that cart and crane were used to transfer the embedding box between freezer and cryomacrotome. Dry ice was sprayed on the embedding box, and liquid nitrogen was sprayed on the sectioned surfaces to prevent the embedding box from melting. When the embedding box fixed on the cryomacrotome was moved at serially-sectioned thickness (1 mm), it was moved towards the sectioning disk. And when the embedding box was serially-sectioned, it was moved parallel with the sectioning disk (Figure 7). During serial-sectioning of the embedding box, the sectioning disk, which had 20 grinding teeth, was rotated. If a cavity appeared on the sectioned surfaces, embedding media was poured into the cavity and frozen by liquid nitrogen or dry ice.

Sixth, sectioned surfaces were inputted into the computer. The curtains were hanged on the laboratory windows and black plates were placed around the sectioned surface to create a darkroom. Then, strobe lights were flashed on the sectioned surface. Consistent brightness of the sectioned surfaces was verified using the exposure meter. After serial-sectioning, dense connective tissue, protruding from the sectioned surface, was cut out manually. The frost on the sectioned surfaces was removed with ethyl alcohol. The sectioned surfaces were photographed using a digital camera (DSC560 Kodak™, resolution 3,040 X 2,008) and inputted into the personal computer (pixel size 0.2 mm X 0.2 mm).

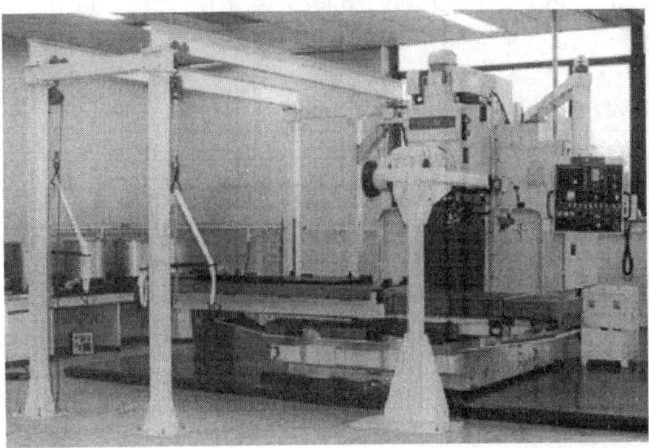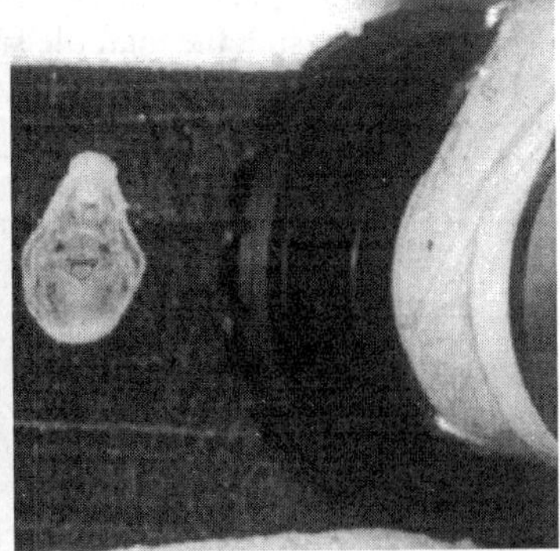

Figure 7. Cryomacrotome (left) and serial-sectioning of embedding box (right).

                    J.Y. Kim et al. / Visible Korean Human

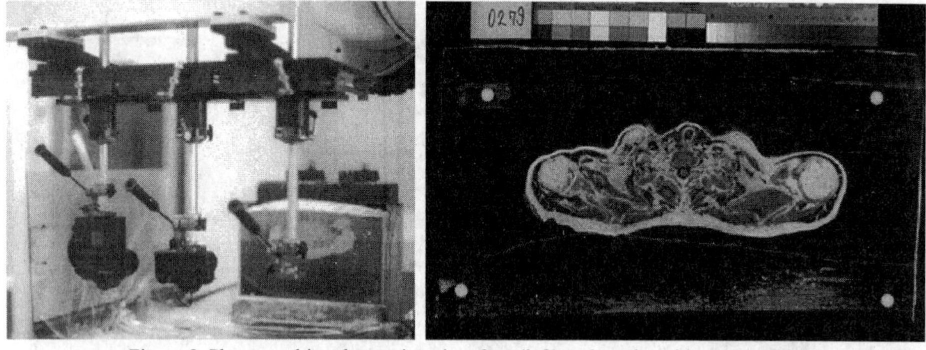

Figure 8. Photographing the sectioned surface (left) and sectioned image (right).

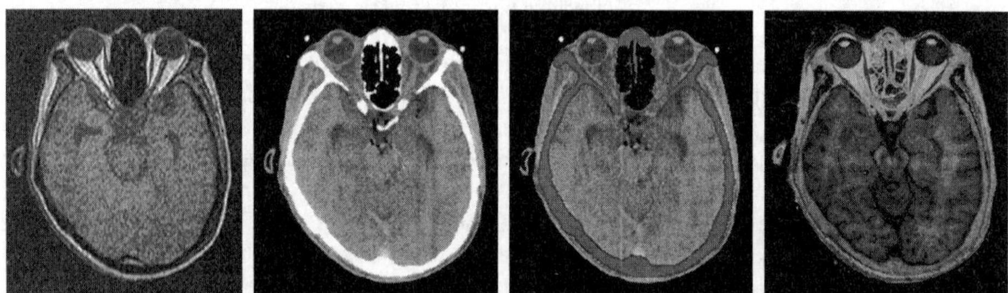

Figure 9. Corresponding MRI, CT, segmented image, and sectioned image (left to right).

The camera was mounted to maintain consistent position and direction of the camera (Figure 8). Alignment of sectioned images was verified using the alignment rods. Consistent brightness of sectioned images was verified using the color patch and grey scale (Figure 8). Corresponding MRIs, CTs, segmented images, and sectioned images were acquired (Figure 9). The length of the cadaver was 1,798 mm and the thickness of images was 1 mm, so that 1,798 sets of serially-sectioned images were acquired. In the main experiments, sectioned images will be used for making better segmented images.

3. Discussion

The second preliminary experiment was also performed with another male cadaver. The main-experiment will be performed with a male cadaver and a female cadaver. We recently received a male cadaver, whose age, body size, and pathological findings would be suitable for the main experiment (Table 1). In the main experiment, MRIs and CTs will be scanned at 1 mm thickness, and sectioned images and segmented images will be made at 0.2 mm thickness. As a result, the total file size of each sex will be 216.4 GB (Table 2).

Table 2. File size of MRIs, CTs, sectioned images and segmented images

	Thickness (mm)	Number	File size (GB)
MRI	1.0	1,800	1.4
CT	1.0	1,800	1.4
Sectioned images	0.2	9,000	160.0
Segmented images	0.2	9,000	53.6
Total		21,600	216.4

The Visible Korean Human, which is being made in this study, is expected to be more useful than Visible Human in the following ways. First, the Korean data will be more helpful in diagnosing and treating the patients belonging to the yellow races. Second, complete MRIs and CTs of the entire body at 1 mm thickness will be more helpful in studying the MRIs and CTs. Third, sectioned images without any missing images will be more helpful in making the complete 3D images. Fourth, small pixel size (0.2 mm X 0.2 mm) and thin thickness (0.2 mm) of sectioned images will be more helpful in showing the small anatomical structures greater than 0.2 mm. Sixth, the additional segmented images will be more helpful in making the 3D image and virtual dissection software [1].

4. Conclusion

In this ongoing study, we are trying to make the Visible Korean Human, which can compensate for the problems with the Visible Human. The Visible Korean Human will be the basis for making better 3D images and virtual dissection software which will be more helpful in medical education. Like the Visible Human, The Visible Korean Human will be distributed worldwidely free of charge.

References

[1]   V.M. Spitzer *et al*, The visible human male. Technical report. *J Am Med Inform Assoc* 3 (1996) 118-130.
[2]   V.M. Spitzer and D.G. Whitlock, The Visible Human dataset. The anatomical platform for human simulation, *Anat Rec* 253 (1998) 49-57.
[3]   M.J. Ackerman, The Visible Human Project, *Proceeding on IEEE* 86 (1998) 504-511.
[4]   M.J. Ackerman, The Visible Human Project. A resource for education, *Acad Med* 74 (1999) 667-670.
[5]   MS Chung and SY Kim, Three-dimensional image and virtual dissection program of the brain made of Korean cadaver, *Yonsei Med J* 41 (2000) 299-303.

Medicine Meets Virtual Reality 02/10
J.D. Westwood et al. (Eds.)
IOS Press, 2002

High Performance Bilateral Telerobot Control

Robert Kline-Schoder, William Finger
Creare Incorporated, Hanover, NH, USA 03755

Neville Hogan
Massachusetts Institute of Technology, Cambridge, MA, USA 02135

Abstract. Telerobotic systems are used when the environment that requires manipulation is not easily accessible to humans, as in space, remote, hazardous, or microscopic applications or to extend the capabilities of an operator by scaling motions and forces. The Creare control algorithm and software is an enabling technology that makes possible guaranteed stability and high performance for force-feedback telerobots. We have developed the necessary theory, structure, and software design required to implement high performance telerobot systems with time delay. This includes controllers for the master and slave manipulators, the manipulator servo levels, the communication link, and impedance shaping modules. We verified the performance using both bench top hardware as well as a commercial microsurgery system.

1. BACKGROUND

Clinicians are currently working on techniques and procedures to enable telerobot-assisted, minimally invasive surgeries. The advantages of using telerobots for clinical applications are that the robot can be used to de-amplify the hand motions of the surgeon; the robot can filter out operator tremor; and the surgeon does not need to be in the same room as the patient.

However, to achieve their full potential, telerobotic systems require the development of new control system design concepts for improved tactile and force feedback. Force feedback is important for telerobot control because it: (1) provides important sense information to the operator; (2) facilitates completion of some assembly tasks; (3) improves safety; and (4) greatly reduces the risk of overstressing the robot hardware. The major limitation in force feedback telesurgery systems is the presence of time delays between the master and slave manipulators which can cause instability.

2. METHODS AND TOOLS

Bilateral telerobot control systems can be designed to guarantee stability in the presence of long, unstructured time delays by combining impedance control for the manipulators with a passive communication link achieved using wave variables instead of kinematic variables [1, 2]. Our control algorithm and software combines this impedance-based control methodology for stability with impedance shaping [3] to achieve high performance. The essence of impedance shaping is to add model-based feedback to the sensor-based feedback that is normally used for force-reflecting systems. Our technique combines passivity concepts to guarantee stability and impedance shaping to achieve high performance.

As shown in Figure 1, the control system is based on an impedance shaping algorithm that implements real-time estimation that augments the physical environment, is used by the master controller to achieve realistic perception of touch, and is employed by the slave controller to achieve perfect impedance matching to the transmission line. The system is augmented with an environment impedance estimator and master and slave impedance shapers. The environment klnt impedance estimator uses the time history of the control force and the slave motion to estimate the impedance of the environment. The slave impedance shaper uses the estimate of the environment impedance to modify its controlled impedance to ensure perfect impedance matching to the transmission line. The master impedance shaper uses the estimate of the environment impedance to match to the transmission line/slave impedance and to provide an estimate of the environment interaction force immediately to the operator.

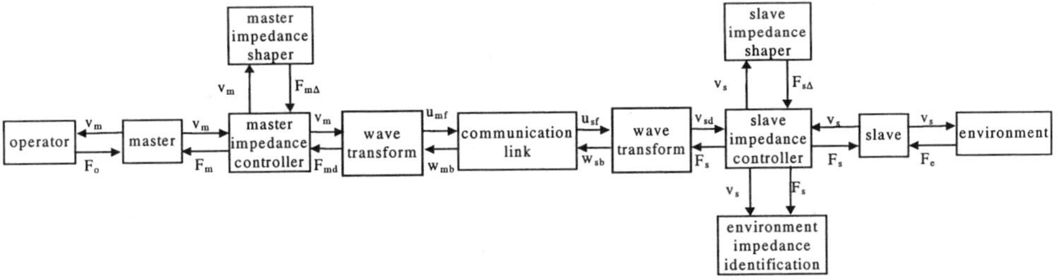

Figure 1. Impedance Control and Wave Variable-Based Telerobot Control System Architecture

3.　RESULTS

During this research, we have: (1) defined the specifications for the control system; (2) developed a telerobot control system architecture for guaranteed stability and high performance; (3) demonstrated the telerobot control system using computer simulation; (4) implemented the control system in real-time using three-degree-of-freedom master and slave robots; and (5) measured the stability margin and performance as a function of communication link time delay.

We have defined performance to be the damping felt by the master when the slave is in free motion and the stiffness felt by the master when the slave is constrained. Our analysis and laboratory experiments show that we can significantly increase the constrained-slave stiffness without affecting the free-slave damping as compared to standard wave variable communication link implementations.

Figure 2 shows a comparison of the measured free- and constrained-slave data for two different time delays: 0 msec (Figure 2a) and 50 msec round-trip (Figure 2b). These data show that the system behaves very similarly, maintaining stability, with a reduction in the amount of constrained-slave stiffness. For the free-slave portion, the damping can be shown to be approximately 2 N/m/sec for the free-slave without time delay and between 1 and 2 N/m/sec for the free-slave case with a 50 msec round-trip delay time. The stiffness for no delay is approximately 200 N/m, while for the 50 msec delay time, the stiffness can be shown to be approximately 10 N/m. As described above, this result is consistent with the underlying theory of our bilateral telerobot control system. Further, this points out the fact that our controller maintains stability and can be used, even though there are significant time delays in the system. Our controller allows optimum performance for the given time delay without the need for making changes to the software or implementation that depends on the time delay.

We also measured data from the same hardware using a standard position controller for both the master and slave robots. We used this controller configuration to serve as a comparison to the Creare controller. The data show that the position controller can achieve higher constrained-slave stiffness for no time delay at the expense of significantly greater damping for the free-slave case and at the risk of instability for moderate time delays. The free-slave damping can be shown to be approximately 5 N/m/sec (over a factor of 2 greater than that experienced with the Creare controller). The constrained-slave damping for this case can be shown to be approximately 500 N/m, which is approximately a factor of

2 greater than that achieved with the Creare controller. When there is time delay, however, the position controller shows signs of impending instability. For the free-slave data with a 50 msec round-trip time delay, the velocity data shows severe oscillations that are only very lightly damped. Any additional time delay and the system has been shown to go unstable. This is a severe limitation to the existing technology, especially when combined with the additional effort required to overcome the much higher level of free-slave damping.

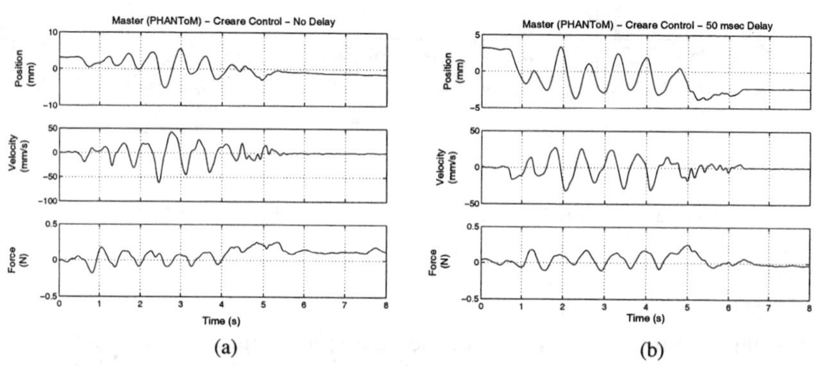

Figure 2. Comparison of Creare Controller Performance for 50 msec Time Delay

4. CONCLUSIONS

Our research findings have demonstrated our telerobot control system. We developed the necessary theory, structure, and software design required to implement high performance telerobot systems. We have demonstrated the control system in simulation, implemented the control system on bench-top hardware, and have measured stability and performance of the hardware implementation both with and without time delays.

We expect that the Creare telerobot control software will find applications in the government as well as in commercial industry. For NASA, telerobots operated from space or from the ground will be necessary to support future human space missions. They will reduce reliance on astronaut extravehicular activity, decrease the time required to complete tasks, improve dexterity, and enhance astronaut safety. Also, telerobots will be used on Earth for telesurgery, delicate vascular microsurgery, minimally-invasive surgery, manipulation of individual cells, the interrogation of atomic surfaces, and the inspection and repair of micro-mechanical or electrical devices.

5. ACKNOWLEDGEMENTS

This research has been supported by both the U.S. Army Research Office and NASA Small Business Innovation Research (SBIR) Program.

REFERENCES

[1]   Anderson, R. and Spong, M., "Bilateral Control of Teleoperators with Time Delay," *IEEE Transactions on Automatic Control*, V34, N5, pp. 494-501.

[2]   Colgate, J.E., "Robust Impedance Shaping Telemanipulation," *IEEE Transactions on Robotics and Automation*, V9, N4, 1993, pp. 494-501.

[3]   Niemeyer, G. and Slotine, J-J., "Stable Adaptive Teleoperation," *IEEE Journal of Oceanic Engineering*, V16, N1, pp. 152-162.

Medicine Meets Virtual Reality 02/10
J.D. Westwood et al. (Eds.)
IOS Press, 2002

Daily patient set-up control in radiation therapy by coded light projection

*R. Krempien, **S. Daeuber, **H. Hoppe, *M. Treiber, *W. Harms, ** J. Raczkowsky,
*J. Brief, *J. Debus, **H. Woern, *M. Wannenmacher

*University of Heidelberg, Department of Clinical Radiology
**University of Karlsruhe (TH), Institute for Process Control and Robotics, Germany*

Abstract:

Advances in conformal radiation therapy to control disease via dose escalation are challenged by set-up uncertainties. Recently, techniques have been developed to use surface features to evaluate the patient's position and correct it where necessary. The aim of this study was to use the patient's surface as a tool for daily set-up control and monitoring. We use a surface scanner based on the projection of coded light to receive -in a daily routine- a large amount of surface points which enables us to register the CT-based planning data with the patient's current position. By superimposing current and planned volumes, a volume of congruency was obtained. An error below 1 mm was considered acceptable. In cases where set-up was not satisfactory a map of the surface comparison was evaluated showing the areas of missing alignment. According to this information a manual repositioning was performed. This procedure was repeated until the error was acceptable. No more then 3 repetitions where necessary to obtain an acceptable result. The whole procedure including registration, calculation and visualization took about 20 sec for one repetition. The use of structured light projection in the daily set-up control and monitoring proved to be a noninvasive, easy, quick, inexpensive and reliable solution.

1. Background/Problem

Advances in conformal radiation therapy to control disease via dose escalation are challenged by set-up uncertainties [Killoran]. Recently, techniques have been developed to use surface features to evaluate the patient's position and correct it where necessary [Milliken, Berry]. The aim of this study was to use the patient's surface as a tool for daily set-up control and monitoring.

2. Method and Tools Used

We use a surface scanner based on the projection of coded light to receive -in a daily routine- a large amount of surface points which enables us to register the CT-based planning data with the patient's current position [Hoppe]. The presented system consists of a ordinary video projector, two CCD-cameras and a state-of-the-art PC (800 MHz CPU, 256 Mbytes RAM). The system generates a set of three-dimensional coordinates, i.e. points, which all are located on the surface of the patient. The first step is to project a set of lines varying in width, the so-called coded light. data. The cameras gather the deformation of the lines on the surface. As their widths correspond approximately to the lattice parameter of the CCD matrix, moiré patterns emerge.

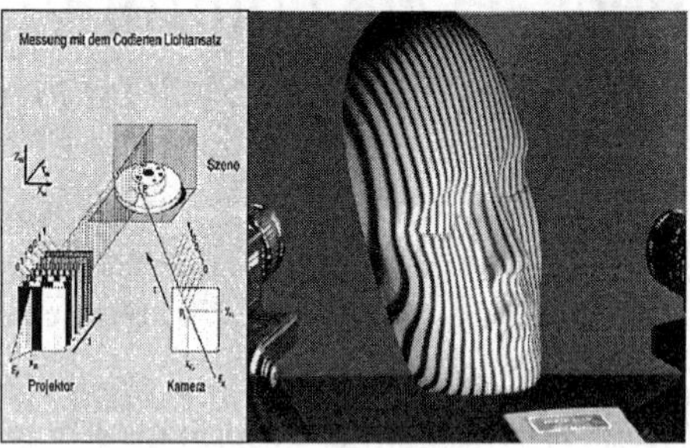

Fig. 1:   Surface reconstruction using coded light projection.

The software is able to analyze the patterns and decode the body's surface, represented then by a three-dimensional point cloud. The error of a single point is below 1 mm. The density of the point cloud is approx. 4 per mm^2. After the initial scanning of the patient's present position, the data must be registered with the planning CT-data. The CT-images are transformed to a distance tomogram. An arbitrary matching algorithm served to minimize the sum over all distances from the CT-surface to the point cloud. The result of this process is the information of the patients present position compared to the CT-based planning data, i.e. a 4x4-transformation matrix describing postponement and rotation. With this information it is possible to iteratively scan and correct the patient's position to find the optimal set-up according to the predefined planning

Fig. 2: Initially the patient is scanned in planing position in the CT. Based on these data a radiation treatment plan is defined. The position of the patient in the planing CT defines the ideal position while the surface of the

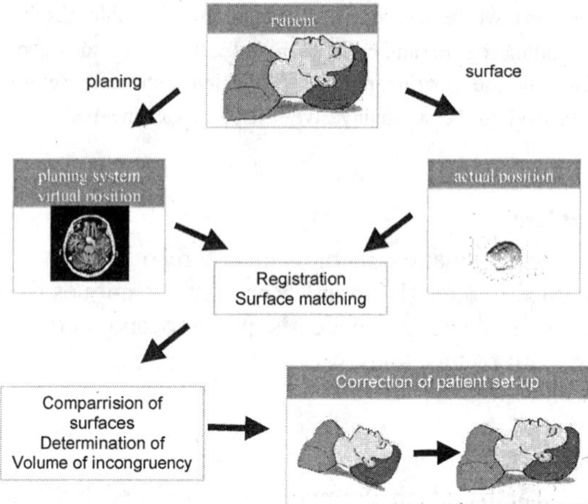

patient is used as a virtual shell. In the treatment room the surface of the patient is scanned using coded light projection. The point cloud of the patient representing the actual position of the patient is registered with the CT-defined virtual shell using a surface matching. The differences in the set-up of the patients are used to define volumes of incongruency using vector analysis. After calculation of color codes and reprojection onto the patients surface a repositioning of the patient is performed. To ensure a correct positioning this process is repeated until a satisfying alignment of the virtual set-up and the actual set-up of the patient could be achieved.

3. Results

Daily after positioning, a point cloud of an anthropomorphic phantom was acquired using the coded light projector. The CT-rendered body surface in planing position was then registered with the surface data of the phantom. By superimposing current and planned volumes, a volume of congruency was obtained. An error below 1 mm was considered acceptable. In cases where set-up was not satisfactory a map of the surface comparison was evaluated showing the areas of missing alignment. According to this information a manual repositioning was performed. This procedure was repeated until the error was acceptable. No more then 3 repetitions where necessary to obtain an acceptable result. The whole procedure including registration, calculation and visualization took about 20 sec for one repetition.

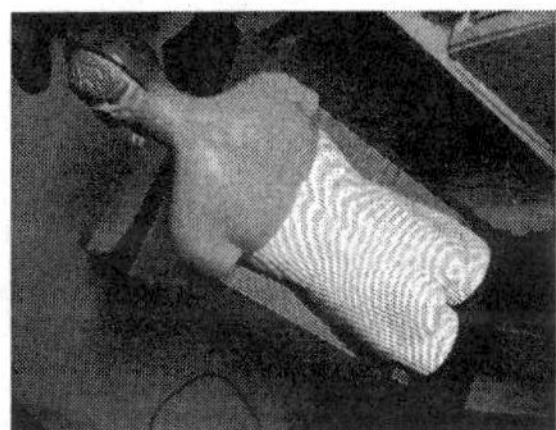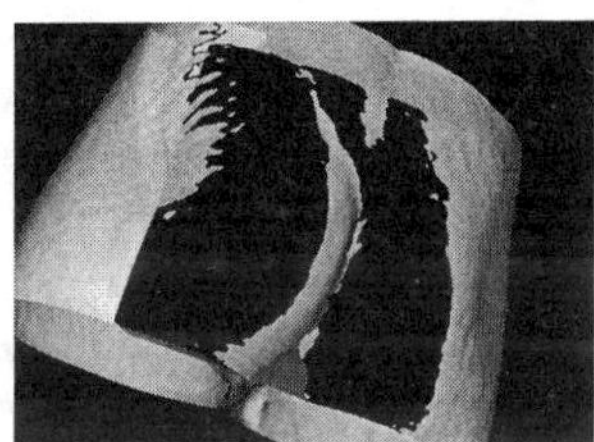

Fig. 3: Projection of coded light onto the phantom (left). Surface reconstruction of the phantom and registration with the virtual shell obtained through the planing-CT data (right). The dark grey areas resemble surface parts of missing aligment between the virtual CT-shell and the actual patient position.

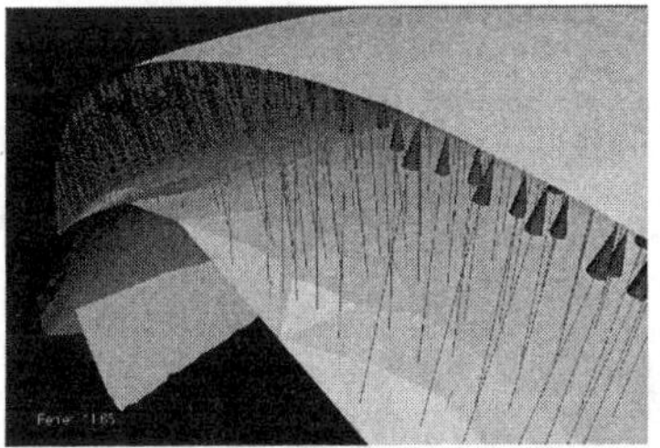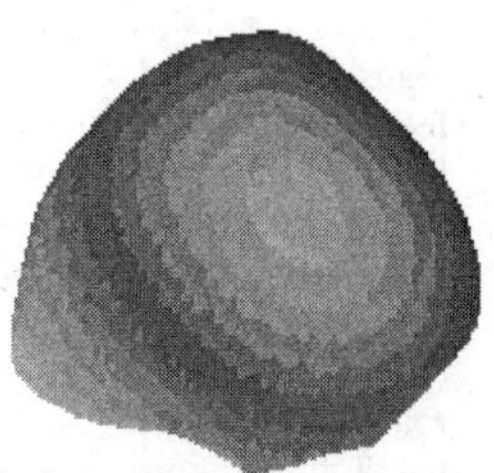

Fig. 4: Calculation of a volume of incongruency by vector analysis of multiple surface points (left). Projection of the differences as color maps onto the phantoms surface using the video projector. This color maps were used to determine the necessities of changes in the patient set-up.

4. Conclusions

The use of structured light projection in the daily set-up control and monitoring proved to be a noninvasive, easy, quick, inexpensive and reliable solution.

5. References

Harald Hoppe, Sascha Däuber, Jörg Raczkowsky, Heinz Wörn, Jose Luis Moctezuma: *Intraoperative Visualization of Surgical Planning Data Using Video Projectors*, In: Medicine Meets Virtual Reality 2001, J.D. Westwood et al. (Eds.), IOS Press, 2001

Berry JA, Aldrich JE *Surface topography for patient repositioning*. Medical Dosimetry 1991;16:71-77

Milliken B, Rubin S, Hamilton R, Johnson L, Chen G *Performance of a video-image-substraction-based patient positioning system*. Int J Radiat Oncol Biol Phys 1997;38:855-866

Killoran J, Kooy H, Gladstone D, Welte F, Beard C *A numerical simulation of organ motion and daily set-up uncertainties: implications for radiation therapy*. Int J Radiat Oncol Biol Phys 1997;37:213-221

Medicine Meets Virtual Reality 02/10
J.D. Westwood et al. (Eds.)
IOS Press, 2002

The Development and Clinical Trial of a Driving Simulator for the Handicapped

Jeonghun Ku[1], Dongpyo Jang[1], Heebum Ahn[1], Jaemin Lee[1], Jeong A Kim[2], Bumseok Lee[2], In Y. Kim[1], Sun I. Kim[1]

[1]Department of Biomedical Engineering, Hanyang University, Seoul, Korea
[2]National Rehabilitation Center, Seoul Korea

Abstract. We developed a Virtual Reality Driving Simulator in order to safely evaluate and improve the driving ability of the handicapped. The Virtual Environment consists of 18 sections (e.g. a speed limited road, a strait road, a curved road, a left turn course, etc) and each section is linked naturally. For the interface of our driving simulator, an actual car was adapted for realism and then connected to a computer. We also equipped it with hand control driving devices especially adapted for the handicapped. A beam projector was used so that the subjects could see the virtual scene on a large screen which was set in front of them. The subjects selected for this trial were 10 normal drivers with valid driving licenses and 15 patients with thoracicor lumber cord injuries who had prior driving experience. For evaluation, 5 driving skills were measured including average speed, steering stability, centerline violations, traffic signal violations, and driving time in various road conditions such as strait and curved roads. The normal subjects manipulated the gas pedal and the brake with their feet while the patients manipulated a hand control with their hands. After they finished driving the whole course, the participants answered the questions such as "How realistic did the Virtual Reality Driving Simulator seeme to you?" and "How much was your fear reduced". The five driving skills measured between the two groups (normal vs. handicapped) did not show any significant differences ($p > 0.05$). And in the three kinds of road conditions (a speed limited road and roads with a sharp curve and left-hand turn), the average speed of the handicapped group was 45.6 Km, less than 61.2 Km ($p<0.05$) of the normal group. In all, 11 patients (73%) reported that their fear of driving was reduced. Furthermore, their average score on the degree of realism question was 51.5%.

1. Introduction

Cars have become necessities of life and their importance has increased as a form of locomotion and transportation. Driving is especially important to the handicapped because it extends the range of their activity and makes it possible for them to participate in social life. Cars are also necessary for the daily life of people who have difficulties in using public transportation. Therefore driving is essential for many handicapped people to maintain independent lifestyles. And assessment and improvement of their driving ability has become an important part of rehabilitation therapy.

In many rehabilitation hospitals and centers including the National Rehabilitation Center in Korea, movie-based driving simulators have been deployed for driver training and skill improvement because "on road" tests are considered to be too dangerous to the handicapped who don't have sufficient skills to control a car[1-6]. Such simulators have some shortcomings in driver training because they are non-interactive.

Virtual Reality (VR) is a technique which constitutes a three-dimensional environment that puts the subject in a condition of active exchange with a virtual world created by a computer. The ability to not limit the paradigm of interaction in a unidirectional sense represents a strong advantage of the new technology: the subject is not merely an external observer of pictures or one who passively experiences the reality created by the computer. On the contrary, in VR the subject can actively modify the three-dimensional world in which he or she is acting, in a condition of complete sensorial immersion[7].

Applying a virtual reality technique to the field driver training can create a realistic and interactive situation in the eye of the participant. A virtual reality driving simulator can overcome the disadvantages of "on road" tests and movie-based simulators because it provides a more safe and efficient training method, which can create diverse and interactive driving situations[8, 9].

The goal of this study is to implement a virtual driving simulator and use it to assess and improve the driving skills of the handicapped.

2. Virtual Reality System Architecture

A virtual driving simulator is mainly composed of a hardware system and a virtual environment scenario. The hardware for the driving simulator consisted of: an actual car which is adapted for the handicapped, interfaces between components of the car (steering wheel, brake and accelerator, directional ramp and gear) and a computer, a beam projector and screen (3m X 4m) and a sound system. See Figure 1 below.

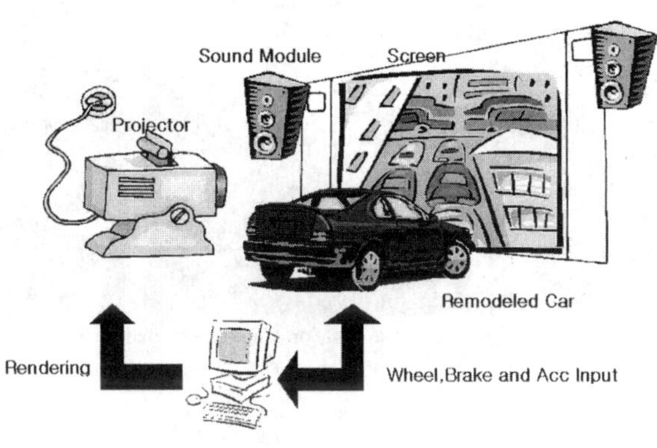

Figure 1. System Diagram for Virtual Driving Simulator

We used an actual car connected to a personal computer for realism and attached the hand control device for subjects afflicted with lower limb palsy. A beam projector displayed virtual situations on a screen in front of the car and sound were generated as appropriate for the vehicle's speed to increase realism for the participant.

The virtual environment scenario for assessing and improving basic driving ability is based on an actual driver examination in Korea. The virtual environment for these scenarios was runs with Rhinoceros and 3D Studio Max and was developed with DirectX 7.0 and Visual C++ for real time rendering. A city scene was created for the simulator, which included: S and T courses, building, park, and tunnel road sections (amongst others), 4 right turns, 4 left turns, 5 traffic signals, 4 stop signs, 2 lane changes and other scenarios. The roads in the virtual city were divided into 18 sections. See Figures 2 and 3 below.

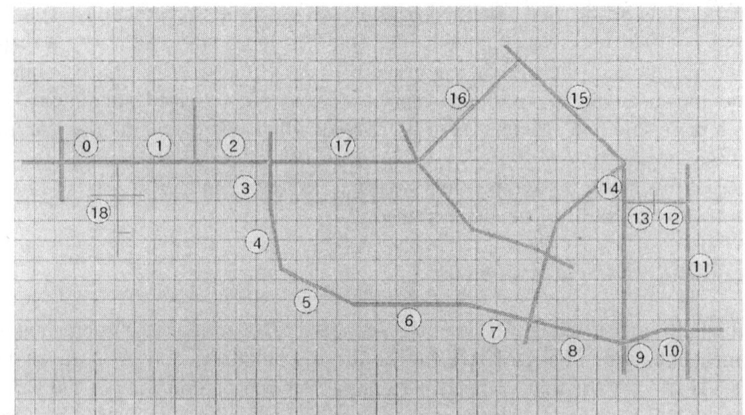

Figure 2. Road Sections of Driving Simulator

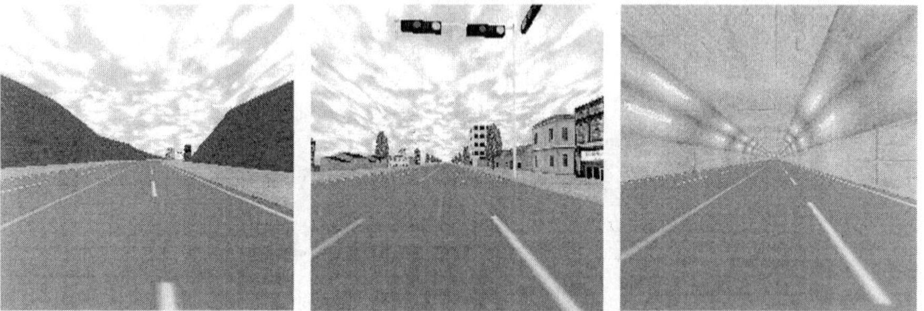

Figure 3. Scene of Virtual Environment (on a mountain road, in a town, in a tunnel)

3. Materials

The subjects were 10 normal drivers (9 were male and 1 was female) with driving licenses and 15 patients (all male) who were in the National Rehabilitation Center in Korea for treatment of thoracic or lumber cord injuries. The patient group all had prior driving experience. The ages and driving histories of the normal drivers are shown in Table 1.

Table 1.   General Characteristics of Normal Subjects

Normal subjects(n=10)	Mean (SD)
Age(years)	31.4 (1.3)
Driving history(years)	8.9 (3.4)

Among spine injury patients, 13 had thoratic cord injuries and 2 had lumber cord injuries. Also, 12 members of the patient group had driving licenses and 3 did not. (See Table 2).

Table 2.   General Characteristics of Spinal Cord Injured Subjects

		Number of cases (%)
Age	20-29	5(33)
	30-39	2(13)
	40-49	6(40)
	50-59	2(13)
License	+	12(80)
	-	3(20)
Level	Thoracic	13(87)
	Lumber	2(13)
Sex	Male	15(100)
	Female	0 (0)

4. Method

Patients manipulated the break and accelerator pedal of the simulator by manipulating the hand control device, whereas the normal drivers did so with their foot. Subjects filled out a questionnaire which asks their age, clinical history, period of driving absence, etc. The subjects were familiar with the road which they should drive, and they have were given enough time (about 5 minutes) in order to be accustomed to the virtual environment (See Figures 4, 5 and 6).

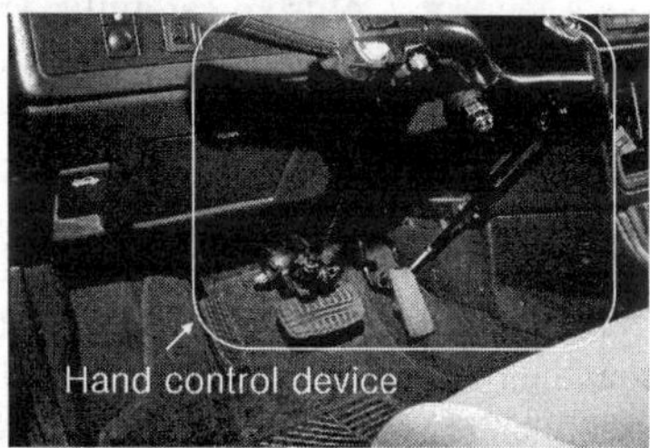

Figure 4. The hand control device for the handicapped

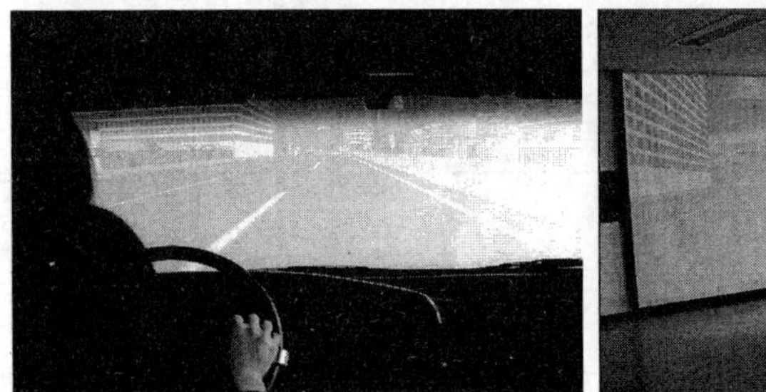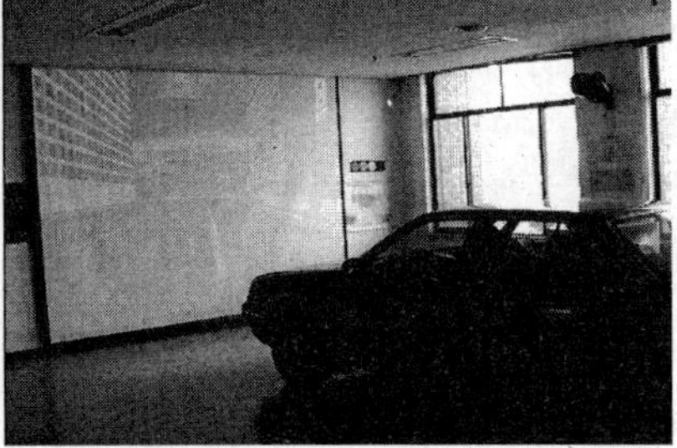

Figure 5. Driving in the simulator (left is an interior view, right is an exterior view of the car)

During each simulation (which takes approximately 20 minutes), driving data was recorded by the computer. We analyzed this data and obtained evaluation parameters. For evaluation purposes, 5 driving skills were measured in various road conditions (e.g., such as straight road, curved road, etc.) including : average speed, steering stability, centerline violations, traffic signal violations, and driving time. Measurements were taken all along a road which was divided by 18 sections. After subjects finished driving the whole course, they answered the following questions two questions:

1."How realistic the Virtual Reality Driving Simulator seemed to you?"
2."How much your fear reduced in driving?"

5. Results

In the patients group, the average period of driving abstinence after an accident was 14.5 months and 14 member of the patient group (93.3%) manipulated hand-control device for the first time.

The measurements of the 5 driving skills measured between the two groups (normal vs. handicapped) were not significantly different ($p > 0.05$). It indicates that their driving skills were not influenced significantly by the driving manipulating methods (i.e., hand or foot control) (See Table 3).

Among the 18 road sections, the average speed of the patients group was 45.6 Km/h, less than the 61.2 Km ($p < 0.05$) of the normal group in sections 1, 2, 3, 4, 8, 10, 11, 12 and 13. It indicates that the patients have a tendency to drive carefully. This may also be due to the fact that these were more challenging road sections: sections1 and 8 were road entrances, section 2 is a speed limited road and sections 3 and 4 have sharp curves. The patient group also drove carefully in the T course and left turn sections: 10, 11, 12 and 13. It indicates that there are no differences between the patients group and the normal group in simple road conditions, whereas there are significant differences (i.e., the patients group drove with much lower speed) in roads conditions which require high driving skills.

11 patients (73%) reported that their fear of driving was reduced when they drive with their hands and their average score on the realism question was 51.5%. This suggests that in future trials it is necessary to enhance the degree of realism in the driving simulator.

Table 3.   Speeds in each section (km/h)

Sections	Normal(Mean	SD)	Patient(Mean	SD)	p-value
1	36.8	12.1	22.6	7.1	0.005*
2	47.6	13.7	31.1	11.5	0.017*
3	53.4	9.9	33.4	16.5	0.021*
4	70.6	9.6	50.0	20.4	0.046*
5	57.0	10.5	52.5	20.7	0.652
6	85.0	11.6	62.3	23.1	0.052
7	58.8	22.8	46.8	20.4	0.285
8	57.6	9.3	52.8	10.5	0.213
9	52.2	15.3	39.9	14.5	0.123
10	44.2	9.3	26.4	8.8	0.001*
11	61.2	5.6	45.6	13.6	0.024*
12	30.8	7.9	21.8	6.2	0.017*
13	26.8	7.8	21.8	6.7	0.001*
14	52.2	9.9	51.8	6.8	0.184
15	52.6	5.2	52.8	15.6	0.978
16	63.0	9.3	48.8	16.9	0.095
17	71.2	12.9	58.1	19.4	0.181
18	31.8	13.3	22.0	4.3	0.019*

*p< 0.05

6. Discussion

The act of driving involves the interaction of cognitive abilities, sensory perception, and physical exertion with various environmental factors. Therefore methods to investigate driving ability broadly are needed including physical, psychiatric (i.e., cognitive and attention ability) and driving assessment (i.e., written exam, driving simulator and behind the wheel road test)[2].

A driving simulator using virtual reality techniques is very helpful in driving rehabilitation because it can provide objective data on the participant's driving ability and skill as a screening process as to whether a participant should drive or not[8, 9]. Although it is possible to assess the ability to control a vehicle including steering and gas and break pedal control, there are shortcomings in not investigating the interaction between the subject and other drivers objectively.

In spite of these deficiencies, there are reports that virtual driving simulators are helpful in developing a minimum standard for driving fitness "on-road"[10].

Until now, there have been many studies mainly to determine whether cognitive and perceptual ability are impaired rather than to assess the driving skills of the handicapped on the road due to economic considerations, the time required and road safety issues. However, these studies in 1980-1990 were inconsistently, inconclusive and lacked validity and practicality in their methods[3]. Interestingly, the Glaski, et. al. study on the assessment of driving ability focused extensively on the Cybernatic Model of Driving in 1992[1, 5-6]. He also assessed how much driving ability and technique differed according to road conditions, road type and weather conditions, etc. using a movie-based driving simulator[4].

In this study, the difference in manipulation method (i.e., the patient group's hand control vs. the normal driver's foot controls) does not seem influence relative performance in virtual driving simulator. It shows that the method of assessment with the virtual driving simulator is reliable. The patients' tendency to decelerate while driving in some specific conditions reflects their tendency to drive more carefully in difficult conditions. Training to improve the use of hand controls in the virtual driving simulator would be useful to reduce the fear that the patients feel while driving. Furthermore, 73% of the patients reported that their fear of driving dissipated after finishing their drive in the virtual city.

7. Conclusion

In this study, a virtual driving simulator which interacts with participants for assessing and improving the driving skills of the handicapped was developed and validated by clinical trial. This demonstrated the driving abilities of patients with spinal cord injuries and helped to reduce their fear of driving with their hands. In future research, it is necessary to enhance the realism of the simulation and increase the variety of training situations.

Acknowledgments

This study was funded by the National Research Laboratory(NRL) Program at Korea Institute of Science & Technology Evaluation and Planning

8. References

1.　　T. Galski, H.T. Ehle and J.B. Williams, *Off-road Driving Evaluations for Persons with Cerebral Injury: A Factor Analytic Study of Predriver and Simulator Testing,* The American Journal of Occupational Therapy (1997) **51**(5), pp. 352-359.

2.　　R.T. Katz et al., *Driving Safety after Brain Damage: Follow-up of Twenty-two Patients with Matched Controls,* Arch. Phys. Med. Rehabil. (1990) **71**, pp. 133-137.

3.　　T. Galski, R.L. Bruno and H.T. Ehle, *Prediction of Behind the Wheel Driving Performance in Patients with Cerebral Brain Damage: A Discriminant Function Analysis,* The American Journal of Occupational Therapy (1992) **47**, pp. 391-396.

4.　　T. Galski, H.T. Ehle and J.B. Williams, *Estimates of Driving Abilities and Skills in Different Conditions,* American Journal of Occupational Therapy (1998) **52**, pp. 268-275.

5.　　T. Galski, R.L. Bruno and H.T. Ehle, *Driving after Cerebral Damage: A Model with Implications for Evaluation,* The American Journal of Occupational Therapy (1991) **46**(4), pp. 324-332.

6.　　T. Galski, H.T. Ehle and R.L. Bruno, *An Assessment of Measures to Predict the Outcome of Driving Evaluations in Patients with Cerebral Damage,* The American Journal of Occupational Therapy (1990) **44**(8), pp. 709-713.

7.　　G. Riva, *Virtual Reality as Assessment Tool in Psychology,* in: Virtual Reality in Neuro-Psycho-Physiology, G. Riva (Ed.) (IOS Press, Amsterdam, 1997).

8.　　L. Liu, M. Miyazaki and B. Watson, *Norms and Validity of the DriVR: A Virtual Reality Driving Assessment for Persons with Head Injuries,* CyberPsychology & Behavior (1999) **2**(1), pp. 53-67.

9.　　J. Wald et al., *The Use of Virtual Reality in the Assessment of Driving Performance in Persons with Brain Injury, in:* Medicine Meets Virtual Reality 2000 (IOS Press, Amsterdam, 2000) pp. 365-367.

10.　　G.K. Fox, S.C. Bowden and D.S. Smith, *On-Road Assessment of Driving Competence After Brain Impairment: Review of Current Practice and Recommendations for a Standardized Examination,* Arch. Phys. Med. Rehabil. (1998) **79**, pp. 1288-1296.

Medicine Meets Virtual Reality 02/10
J.D. Westwood et al. (Eds.)
IOS Press, 2002

Realtime Textured 3D-Models for Medical Applications

Carsten Kübler, Lars Bauer, Peter Heinze, Jörg Raczkowsky, Heinz Wörn
Universität Karlsruhe (TH), Institute for Process Control and Robotics,
Kaiserstr. 12, D-76128 Karlsruhe, Germany, e-mail: kuebler@ira.uka.de

Abstract. Realistic visualisation becomes more and more important in medicine. Whenever a patient individual 3D-model was generated the aim is to visualise the model as realistic as possible. We use 3D-models in our diagnostic and therapeutic tools for intraoperative visualisation of e.g. CT-scans. Most medical tools uses surface-rendering or volume-rendering for virtual visualisation. The coloration of a visualised model is normally done by using a convenient colour for each surface resp. volume. Our approach for 3D-models generated from motion in image series (e.g. videoendoscopes) is to add textures to the 3D-model. The main problem is, to handle the huge amount of videoimage-data (20Mb/sec.) and render the model in realtime.

1. Background

The use of patient individual 3D-models in medicine is limited through the power of actual computer hardware and their graphics accelerators. Simple surface-rendering is state of the art for most 3D-models because of the model's complexity. Volume-rendering is a second possibility with much higher requirements of computer and graphic power. These 3D-models have almost all in common that they base on CT-, MRI-scans or other methods which reconstructs only 3D-geometry. To improve quality of a virtual reconstructed 3D-model, one possibility is to add the patient individual look of the surface. A lot of medical simulators and virtual training systems use a common look for the surface. This approach has no relevance for diagnostic nor medical planing applications. Instead a patient individual look of the surface increases the significance of the 3D-model. Today in most applications there is no way to determine the look of the surface. To add an individual look to a 3D geometric model, we use images taken with a standard colour camera. In our approach the camera's image-sequences are used to determine the geometry of the 3D-model (see fig. 1).

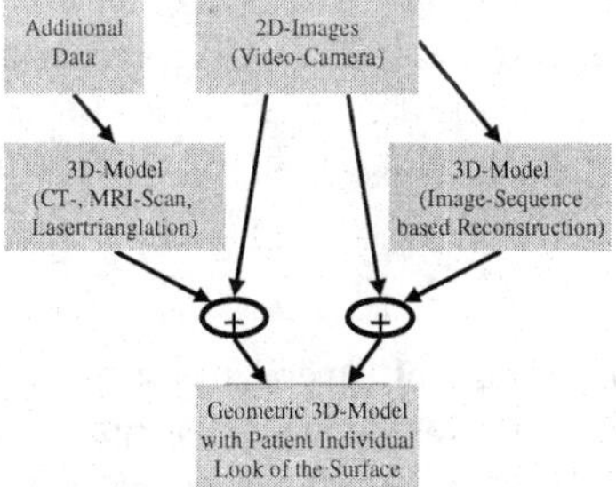

Figure 1: Two different ways to generate patient individual 3D-models and look.

2. Preliminary Investigation

We use OpenGL and VTK (the visualisation toolkit) [1] to visualise our 3D-models. For this application we had to add an object factory which adds some features to use lots of textures in one 3D-model. After this extension we made a wide investigation about rendering 3D-models with simple (24kbyte) and complex (768kbyte) textures. This tests were performed on standard PCs with "high-end"-graphic-accelerators for gamers and "mid-end"-workstations from SGI. We used a standardised 3D-model to measure the performance of both platforms. The test consisted of a tube with 300-layers. Every layer had a surface of 100 triangles and one individual texture with a size of 128x64x3 resp. 256x1024x3 (see fig. 2). To visualise this model we couldn't bind all texture at the same time (225Mbyte textures and 30000 triangles) so we extend VTK to determine the minimal distance between a texture and the camera to use only nearest textures (active textures). Remaining triangles were assigned with colours which were derived from corresponding areas in the texture. The second restriction was to visualise only textures, which could be seen from the camera. This reduced about one-fifth of applied textures (see fig. 3).

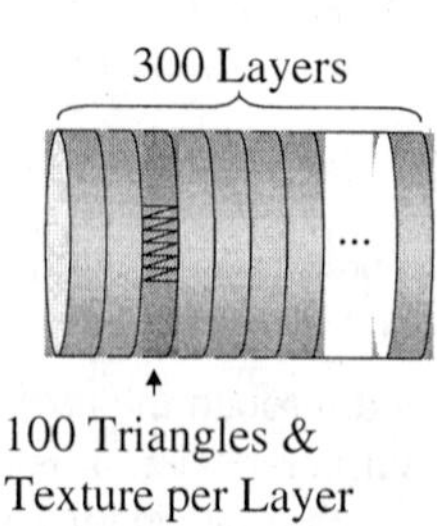

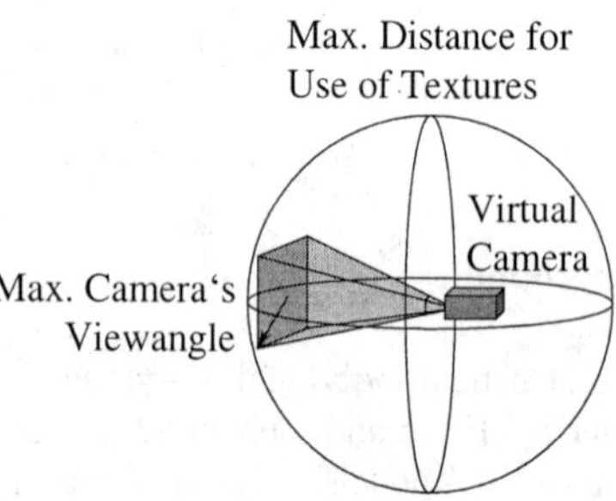

Figure 2: Standardised test for complex 3D-models with textures.

Figure 3: Restricted area for use of textures

On some computers was a second possibility for increasing the performance to use mipmapping. For mipmapping the same texture is offered in different sizes and OpenGL chooses the necessary size [2]. This feature in combination with trilinear interpolation results in highest quality. Different sizes of a texture were calculated at the moment when the texture got active. The use of mipmapping demands 33% more memory.

We measure the time to fly through the 3D-model in 315 steps. The amazing result was the slight difference of performance between an Octane2 with V12 graphic-accelerator (more than $25.000) and a low cost PC Athlon 1333 with GeForce2Ultra (for less than $2.500). The fastest flight through the tube was done in 23.4 sec (13.5 frames per sec.) on a PC. We measured the performance by using mipmapping (textures with different level of details – LOD – for every texture) and standard texture mapping (only one level of detail with highest resolution).

The following results are an average of several measurements. Bilinear (one LOD) resp. triangular sampling (mipmappind) was applied to textures because of less difference to simple point sampling. The difference in performance between mipmapping and one LOD come from calculating the different texture sizes. If this calculation was performed at beginning, mipmapping normally results in better results as one LOD textures.

Platform	Mipmapping		One LOD	
PC (AMD 1333 Gforce2 Ultra)	30.5 sec.	10.3 frames/sec.	23.6 sec.	13.3 frames/sec.
PC (Intel PIII 800 Quadro2)	46.6 sec.	6.8 frames/sec.	37.5 sec.	8.4 frames/sec.
SGI (Octane2 R12000 1x400MHz V12)	33.7 sec.	9.3 frames/sec.	33.4 sec.	9.4 frames/sec.
SGI (Octane R12000 2x270MHz V6)	532.5 sec.	0.6 frames/sec.	119.7 sec.	2.6 frames/sec.

We used only five different images for the first test to reduce memory problems on all system. Every fifth layer had the same image for texture but all active layers had its own texture mapped. 65 layers had been detected to be visualised at the same time (65 active layers). The requirements during the test are about 64Mb texture memory and 4Mb system memory for the images.

The second test used 300 images (225Mb of image data). Every layer had its individual image. The test requires additionally more system memory as the first.

Platform	Available System Memory	One LOD	
PC (AMD 1333 Gforce2 Ultra)	512Mb	23.7 sec.	13.3 frames/sec.
PC (Intel PIII 800 Quadro2)	320Mb	43.3 sec.	7.3 frames/sec.
SGI (Octane2 R12000 1x400MHz V12)	512Mb	478.2 sec.	0.7 frames/sec.

The SGI-workstations weren't able to handle the huge system memory requirements for image data which were loaded before timemeassurement. The system memory requirement was less than available system memory. On the other side performance of PCs didn't break in.

The performance of new graphic-accelerators is enough to render 3D-models with individual textures in realtime. There is no need to prefer high-end-workstations for this task. Instead the visualisation of eight times cheaper standard PCs with "high-end" graphic-accelerators for $500 are more powerful as our SGI-workstations. The next improvement is to use a scheduling strategy for texture-management to handle huge models with more than 10Gb of image-data. To handle a video-image-stream with 21Mb/sec. in realtime assume a fast access to required image-data.

3. Fast access to image-data

Our next step was to introduce a textureproxy, which schedules the necessary images and subimages for a texture. The proxy determines automatically which LODs are necessary and reload the images from extern cache. The proxy reloads missing LODs if there are unused system resources (see fig. 4). It also deallocates textures which aren't in use. Figure 5 demonstrates the strategy of the textureproxy. The desired minimum LODs for textures depends on one the hand on the angle between the camara-normal (camera-plane) and every vertex (of the surfaces) and on the other hand on the distance of every vertex to the camera-center.

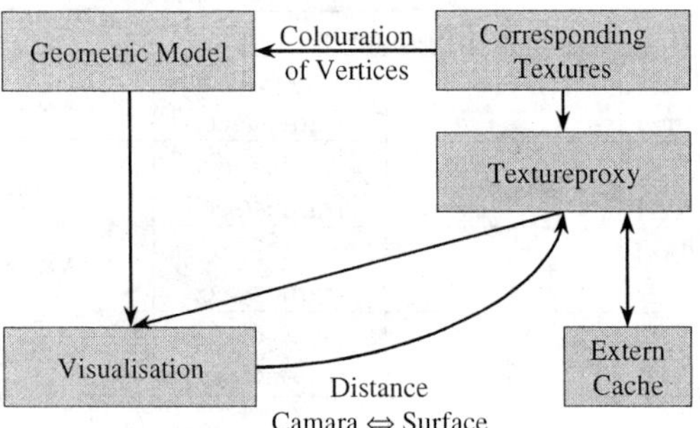

Figure 4: Introduction of a textureproxy for lots of textures

The texture-proxy requires more texture memory as our first extension of VTK, but the performance of visualisation varies less on the number of new active textures. With the utilisation of OpenGL 1.2 it's possible to reload missing LODs during the use of a texture. It's also possible to omit small LODs of a textures and we doesn't need this LODs because we are colouring the vertices of the 3D-model depending on the corresponding texture.

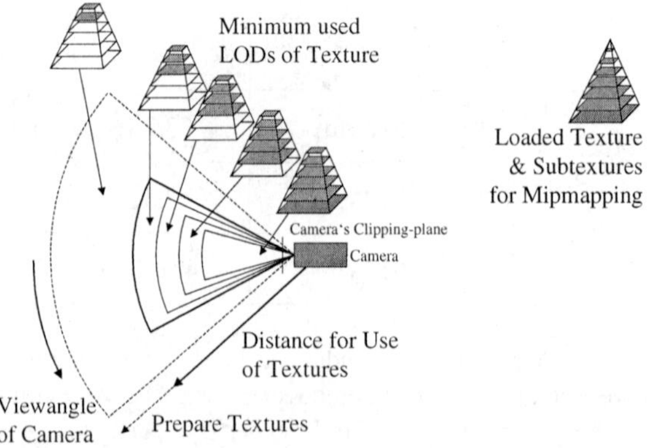

Figure 5: Minimum loaded LODs of an texture, depending on
distance and angle between surface and camera

Figure 6 shows a reconstructed view of our 3D-test-model. This model uses maximal 6 LODs for all textures with a size of 1024x256x3 Pixels. The smallest four LODs are omitted.

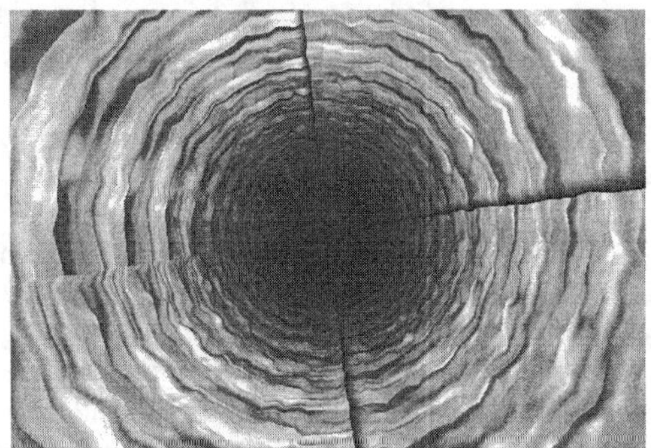

Figure 6: Reconstructed view of our 3D-test-model

4. Reconstruction of small 3D-models

The small 3D-models are reconstructed by triangulation of corresponding local unique patterns in two images. To reconstruct a new small 3D-model, the previous small 3D-model is translated with the measured rotation and translation of the tracking system. The local unique patterns, which were used to reconstruct the previous model, are now used to register the exact rotation and translation between the two images (see fig. 7 outer ring of the images). The second ring, neighbouring to the first, include new local unique patterns, which haven't actual a correspondence in an previous image. These local unique patterns are matched in the new image by using epipolar lines. These two areas are used to reconstruct an new small 3D-model. The third ring in the new image includes new local unique patterns, which are used for triangulation in the next step. The inner ring hasn't local unique patterns, because this area is to far away for reconstruction.

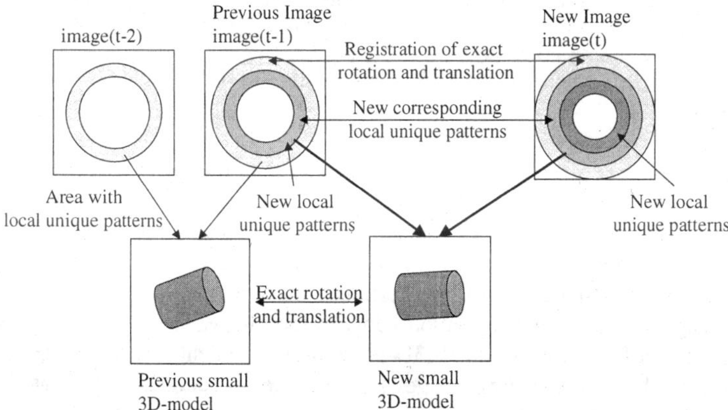

Figure 7: Step by step reconstruction of small 3D-models

5. Conclusions

Using patient individual textures on patient individual 3D-models lead to meaningful virtual reconstructed images and allow new diagnostics in medicine. It's also possible to view this 3D-model in different perspectives. The physician is able to see the 3D-model, using an head-mounted-display, in stereo whereas the input information was only 2D-videoimages-series from one camera. An other possibility is to unroll tubular like 3D-models to see the whole surface in a plan view.

This study points out that textured 3D-models can be used in realtime for medical applications.

6. Acknowledgement

This work is performed at the IPR, Prof. H. Wörn. The research is being funded by the Ministry for Science, Research and Arts of Baden-Württemberg.

References

[1]   Will Schroeder, Ken Martin, Bill Lorensen: "The Visualization Toolkit", Prentice Hall PRT 1998
[2]   Mark Segal, Kurt Akeley, Chris Frazier, Jon Leech: "The OpenGL Graphics System: A Specification (Version 1.3)", 2001 Silicon Graphics, Inc.

Medicine Meets Virtual Reality 02/10
J.D. Westwood et al. (Eds.)
IOS Press, 2002

3D Structure from Endoscopic Images

Carsten Kübler, Peter Heinze, Jörg Raczkowsky, Heinz Wörn
*Universität Karlsruhe (TH), Institute for Process Control and Robotics,
Kaiserstr. 12, D-76128 Karlsruhe, Germany, e-mail: kuebler@ira.uka.de*

Abstract. Endoscopy is an important procedure for the diagnostic and therapy of various pathologies. In 2000, the Institute for Process Control and Robotics/Universität Karlsruhe (TH) has developed a basic framework for reconstructing 3D models from image sequences. The framework is able to realise automatic navigation for new colonoscopes with own driving system and on the other hand to offer a virtual 3D endoscopic view during bad visibility conditions caused by e.g. abrupt bleeding. This method generates a 3D-model intraoperatively compared to preoperatively generated 3D-models in virtual endoscopy.

1. Framework

3D-models for endoscopy are almost all generated through preoperative taken CT-scans. We use a non-linear approach to reconstruct small 3D-models from successional taken endoscopic video-images. For fast reconstruction, an electromagnetic tracking system supplies the algorithm with an initial translation and rotation (see fig. 1). The size of the reconstructed small 3D-model can't be determined from point correspondence [1] so we use the electromagnetic measured translation between the images to get the correct size of the 3D-model. The surface of every small 3D-model uses a patient individual texture which is calculated from the corresponding images [2]. We join all successive generated small 3D-models to one global virtual 3D-model.

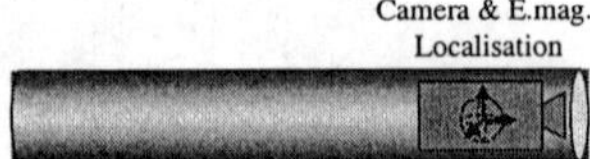

Figure 1: Standard endoscope with an electromagnetic tracking sensor
at the tip of the endoscope

To get relations between the small 3D-models we introduce an relational model. The relational model is used to describe the correspondence between small 3D-models. At beginning all small 3D-models have only an temporal and geometric relation with the two neighbouring small 3D-models (see fig. 2). After basic image recognition and geometric analysis of the tracking information, some additional relations are added (see fig. 3).

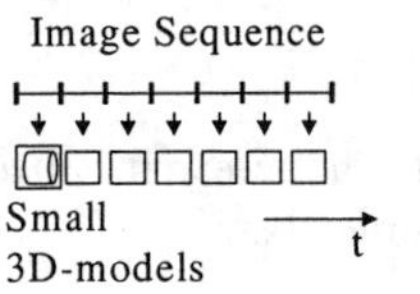

Figure 2: Temporal relation between
all small 3D-models

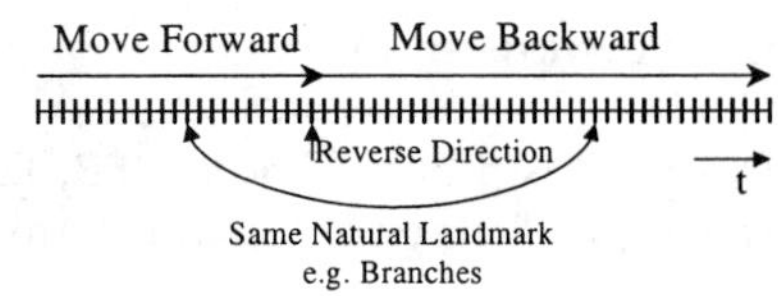

Figure 3: Basic relations between some
images

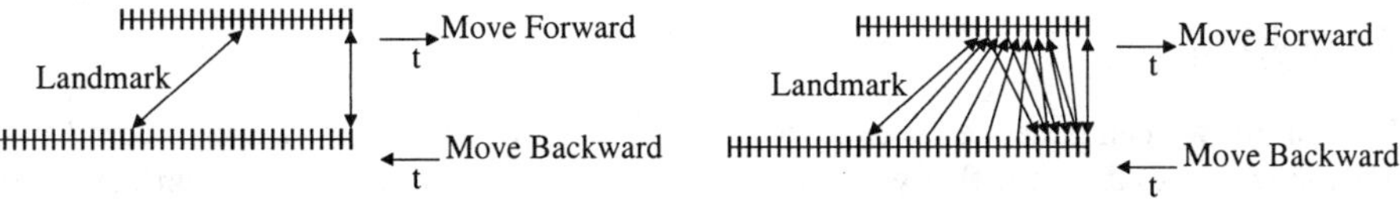

Figure 4: Reorganised coarse relation　　**Figure 5:** Basic extension of relation

The whole image sequence is divided in small image sequences which are related (see fig. 4) concerning to the position in the organ. Motion can additionally be analysed, because an endoscope can normally moved only in one direction (in and out of the tube). At this moment the relation is very coarse. To analyse two small image sequences, we analyse the geometric motion of the tracking system and extend the coarse relation basically (see fig. 5). We use temporal operators for this analysis (see fig. 6)[3]. After analyse of related images, the relation becomes improved. The result is an exact correspondence between all related images resp. all small 3D-models (see fig. 7). Every exact relation consists of a rotation and translation which describe precise how to transform one small 3D-model to the second (see fig. 8).

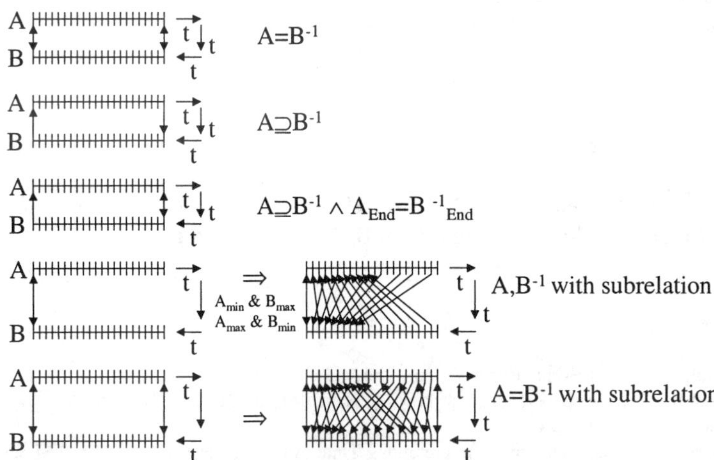

Figure 6: Relation between image sequences resp. small 3D-models

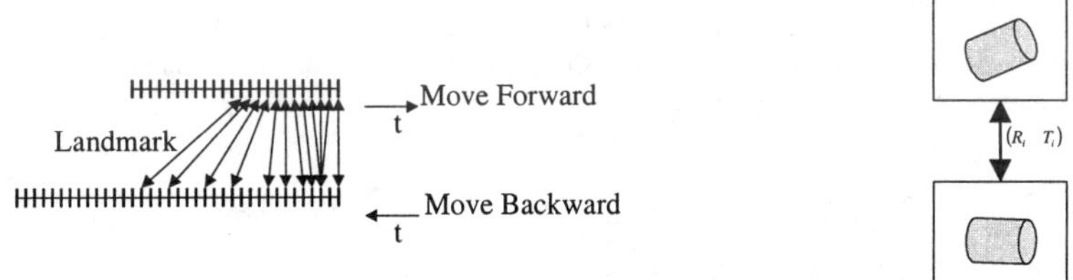

Figure 7: Exact relation between models　　**Figure 8:** Transformation between small models

After a precise analyse of all relations, the small 3D-models can be brought together to one global 3D-model. The physician is now able to visualise the actual position of the endoscopic tip with most exactness in an virtual view of the reconstructed organ. The precision and accuracy of the virtual view depends on the flexibility of the organ and the possibility to register corresponding natural landmarks in two corresponding images.

2. Results

First of all, we can generate an endoscopic 3D-model without preoperatively taken CT- or MRI-scans. Also it results that we can use standard techniques to match the surfaces of our 3D-model with a corresponding preoperative reconstructed virtual endoscopic 3D-model to localise the exact position of the endoscopic tip in a CT-scan. Our approach copes with the motion problem of flexible structures like bronchial tree and the colon. The third advantage is that we are able to virtualised the resulting 3D-model in different views e.g. to unroll tubular like 3D-models to see the whole surface in a plan view.

3. Conclusions

New colonoscopes with an own driving system require a navigation system to automate the diagnostic. These work is predestined to navigate these new flexible endoscopes. The registration of real and virtual endoscopy is improved. Temporal bad visibility conditions caused by e.g. abrupt bleeding can be overcome with this work.

We have developed a method to generate 3D-models for endoscopy independent from preoperative taken CT- or MRI-scans. As far as we know, the concept is new and yet unpublished. Furthermore, This work is the first which uses textures to generate an authentic virtual 3D-model of a endoscopic examination.

4. Acknowledgement

This work is performed at the IPR, Prof. H. Wörn. The research is being funded by the Ministry for Science, Research and Arts of Baden-Württemberg.

References

[1]   Berthold Klaus Paul Horn: "Robot Vision", The MIT-Press, 1986.
[2]   Carsten Kübler, Lars Bauer, Jörg Raczkowsky, Heinz Wörn: "Realtime Textured 3D-Models for Medical Applications", MMVR 2002
[3]   Thomas Wahl, Kurt Rothermel: "Representing Time in Multimedia Systems". Proceedings IEEE 1st Intl. Conference on Multimedia Computing and Systems, Boston, May 1994, Page 538-543.
[4]   Markus Kukuk, Bernhard Geiger: "Registration of real and virtual endoscopy - a model and image based approach", MMVR 2000, pp. 168-174
[5]   Krishnan S.M., Kumar S. Yap C.J., Kassim M.I., Goh P.M.Y., "Computer-Assisted Intelligent Endoscopy". Proceedings of the 13th International Congress and Exhibition for Computer Assisted Radiology and Surgery - CARS'99, Page 156-160.

Visualization and Attributation
of Vascular Structures
for Diagnostics and Therapy Planning

Tobias KUNERT, Matthias THORN, Hans-Peter MEINZER
Deutsches Krebsforschungszentrum, Medical and Biological Informatics,
Im Neuenheimer Feld 280, 69120 Heidelberg, Germany

Abstract. In various medical fields vascular structures have to be examined with usually two-dimensional views which present imaging techniques produce. The interpretation of the data can be supported by 3-dimensional visualization techniques. The further analysis requires often the attribution of the particular functional or anatomical entities. To attribute these interactively we developed two different visualization strategies. In the first one the shape of the structures is modelled with OpenGL achieving very fast response times, most notably during the navigation. The second strategy, the direct rendering of the volume, benefits from the accurate reproduction of the vascular structures. Although the rendering needs much more time, the strategy provides similar response times for the attribution. Thus, the strategies complement one another.

1. Introduction

The examination of vascular structures plays a central role in the medical fields of neurology, cardiology and surgery. Imaging techniques like angiography, contrast enhanced CT, contrast enhanced MRT and ultrasound are commonly used. Because they give only two dimensional views of the structures of interest, the interpretation of such images requires a high degree of expertise. Three-dimensional visualization techniques simplify this task and lead to a quality improvement in diagnostics and therapy planning, e.g. [1]. They provide images which give the physician a more realistic impression and they facilitate the orientation in the volume of interest, because the viewpoint can be arbitrarily chosen. But for further analysis there is often a mechanism needed for attributing functional or anatomical entities interactively.

Two different 3-dimensional visualization strategies are compared in respect of these requirements. Possible applications are the interactive classification of vessels in the liver operation planning [2] or the interactive flow measurement in the heart coronaries.

2. Material and Methods

For the visualization of vascular structures contrast agent is applied. The images acquired by CT or MRI are automatically segmented by thresholding. Based on the skeletonization [3], a symbolic description of the segmented vessel system is generated in the next step. This description is used to attribute the vessels and to color them in a particular way.

The first strategy uses a surface model of the vessels, which is derived from the symbolic description, and is then rendered with the OpenGL graphics library. The second strategy follows the more direct way by volume rendering. In both cases, the navigation within the volume as well as the interaction with individual vessels is possible.

2.1. Model-Based Visualization (Strategy 1)

For the visualization the surface model provides a simplified representation of the vessel structures. The vessels are assembled with cylinders whose diameters are varying. These diameters are calculated during the skeletonization of the volume data. Vessel branches are directly linked with the symbolic description by identifiers which are implemented by OpenGL display lists. For interactions like selecting or attributing vessels, the picking mechanism of OpenGL is used. The identifiers provide direct access to the associated part of the symbolic description such that attributes of the vessel branches can be modified individually. The altered branches are then rendered once more by OpenGL.

2.2. Voxel-Based Visualization (Strategy 2)

The Heidelberg Raytracing Method [4], a specific volume rendering technique for medical data, is used for rendering the vessels directly. Instead of compositing the reflected light along the casted rays, only the surfaces of the vessels are shaded. This simplification is acceptable, because we are not interested in the interior of the vessels. Since there is usually only a small part of the volume occupied, further optimizations like octree data structures are possible. For interactions the shaded image is colored additionally. Besides the shaded image, the renderer generates a second image which links each pixel with a particular vessel branch. This image makes it possible to determine the vessels the user has picked or

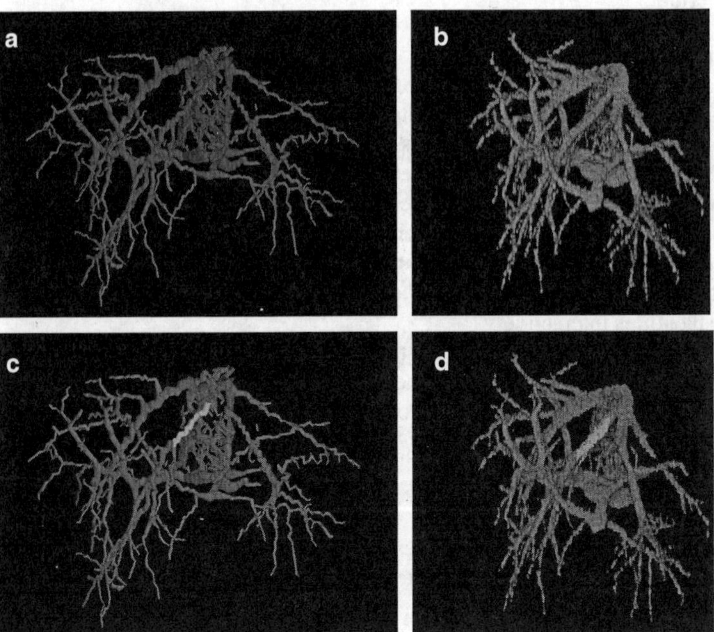

Figure 1: Vessels within the liver. The vessels are rendered based on the symbolic description (a) and on the volume data (b). After picking a vessel branch, the view is immediately updated by both strategies (c-d) such that the selected branch is highlighted.

to color the branches in different ways depending on the attributes. Furthermore, the view can be very efficiently updated with these images when the attributes have changed.

3. Results

The two visualization strategies are demonstrated for liver surgery planning (Figure 1). For the surface model, it is remarkable that the diameters of the vessels are incorrect. This is caused by the assumption that the vessels are circular. Contrary, the volume rendering provides a much more detailed view including shadows such that the user can place complete reliance on the visualization result.

The first strategy achieves very fast response times, which is very important for interactive navigation, but a pre-processing step for creating display lists is necessary. The second one is able to viualize the vessel structures which are not represented by the symbolic description. That is an additional advantage, because the content of the symbolic description can be validated and corrected in case of errors. Furthermore, the surface rendering needs a costly processing for transfering the attributation results to the volume data, whereas the volume rendering directly transfers the data.

4. Conclusion

Applications in diagnostics and therapy planning need a satisfying compromise between an accurate visualization and an interactive usability. Neither the surface rendering nor the volume rendering meet these requirements at present. But both visualization techniques complement one another and lead in a compound way to the most promising approach for the future.

5. Acknowledgement

This work is being funded by the Sonderforschungsbereich 414 "Information Technology in Medicine – Computer and Sensor Supported Surgery" of the Deutsche Forschungsgemeinschaft and furthermore by the project "Navigation in the Liver Surgery" of the Tumorzentrum Heidelberg/Mannheim.

References

[1] W. Lamadé, G. Glombitza, L. Fischer, P. Chiu, C.E. Cardenas, M. Thorn, H.P. Meinzer, L. Grenacher, H. Bauer, Th. Lehnert, C. Herfarth, The Impact of 3-Dimensional Reconstructions on Operation Planning in Liver Surgery. *Arch Surg*, 135: 11 (2000) 1256-1261.
[2] M. Thorn, M. Vetter, C. Cardenas, P. Hassenpflug, L. Fischer, L. Grenacher, G.M. Richter, W. Lamadé, H.P. Meinzer, Interaktives Trennen von Gefäßbäumen am Beispiel der Leber. In: H. Handels, A. Horsch, T. Lehmann, H.P. Meinzer (ed.), Informatik Aktuell - Bildverarbeitung für die Medizin 2001 - Algorithmen, Systeme, Anwendungen, Springer, Heidelberg, 2001, pp. 147-151.
[3] C. Zahlten, H. Jürgens, H.O. Peitgen, Reconstruction of Branching Blood Vessels from CT-Data, In: M. Göbel, H. Müller, B. Urban (ed.), Visualization in Scientific Computing, Springer, Wien, 1995, pp. 41-52.
[4] H.P. Meinzer, K. Meetz, D. Scheppelmann, U. Engelmann, H. Baur, The Heidelberg Raytracing Model, *IEEE Computer Graphics & Applications*, 11: 6 (1991) 34-43.

Medicine Meets Virtual Reality 02/10
J.D. Westwood et al. (Eds.)
IOS Press, 2002

Development of a Virtual Speaking Simulator Using Image Based Rendering

J. M. Lee, H. Kim, M. J. Oh, J. H. Ku, D. P. Jang, I. Y. Kim, S. I. Kim
Department of Biomedical Engineering, Hanyang University, Seoul, Korea

Abstract. The fear of speaking is often cited as the world's most common social phobia. The rapid growth of computer technology has enabled the use of virtual reality (VR) for the treatment of the fear of public speaking. There are two techniques for building virtual environments for the treatment of this fear: a model-based and a movie-based method. Both methods have the weakness that they are unrealistic and not controllable individually. To understand these disadvantages, this paper presents a virtual environment produced with Image Based Rendering (IBR) and a chroma-key simultaneously. IBR enables the creation of realistic virtual environments where the images are stitched panoramically with the photos taken from a digital camera. And the use of chroma-keys puts virtual audience members under individual control in the environment. In addition, real time capture technique is used in constructing the virtual environments enabling spoken interaction between the subject and a therapist or another subject.

1. Introduction

The fear of speaking is often cited as the world's most common social phobia. Public speaking anxiety is the fear of social situations and the associated interpersonal interactions that can automatically bring on self-consciousness, judgment, evaluation, and criticism that often occurs when a person speaks in front of the general public. People having such a fear often manifest symptoms like shame and timidity in everyday personal relationships. They also fear that they will be ridiculed for their mistakes [1].

Even though there are many treatment methods, VR therapy (VRT) has been used in the treatment of psychological disorders including the fear of public speaking. Research has shown that VRT can be successful in reducing the fear of public speaking [1][2].

There are two techniques to develop VR systems for the treatment of the fear of public speaking: a model-based and a movie-based technique. Model-based technique has a disadvantage in that the virtual environment and audiences designed with it appear unreal with unnatural features and motions [1]. In the case of movie-based technique employing movies shot with real audiences, there is a disadvantage in that the virtual audiences can't be controlled individually since they are all included in one movie file [3][4].

In order to overcome these problems, this paper presents a virtual environment developed using IBR and chroma-keys together. In addition, real time capture technique is employed to give the subject more interaction through speaking with other subjects.

2. Image Based Rendering (IBR)

IBR is a popular way to produce a VR experience using a collection of images. A number of techniques have been developed for capturing panoramic images of real world scenes. In this paper, the method to stitch all images was employed [5].

In order to capture a full 360 degree (horizontal) by 180 degree (vertical) view of a scene such as Figure 1(d), many images must be captured in rows. Figure 1(a) and (b) show a panorama that consists of five rows of images where each row consists of 12 shots. The images in each row are captured at 30 degree increments:

After stitching the images by row as shown in Figure 1(c), all of the rows are stitched together to produce the final image. Two images taken straight up and down are added to the top and bottom of the panorama since the final image would not otherwise include those regions.

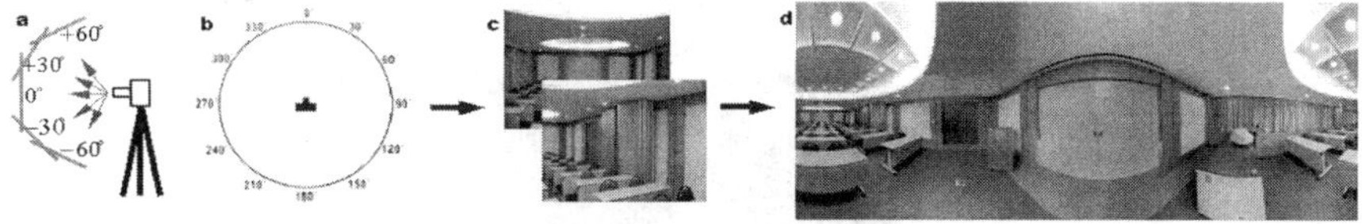

Figure 1. Image Stitching. (a) 5 rows are captured vertically. (b) Each row consists of 12 shots horizontally. (c) Stitching the images by row. (d) Stitching all of the rows together to produce the final image.

3. Movie-making & Chroma-keys

The movie-based methods developed to treat anthrophobia in earlier studies have a disadvantage in that the therapist cannot control each virtual audience member individually [3][4]. But if each audience member is shot individually, then it is possible to flexibly control virtual audiences and compose many more situations.

Figure 2(a) shows how virtual audiences can be produced using film with a blue screen and a digital camcorder. Next, the outer frames of the original scene shot with the camcorder are clipped and the images are scaled down. In order to render the regions other than the actor's body transparently as shown in Figure 2(b), pixels with an intensity over a specific threshold value are made transparent. This is the key-point of chroma-key.

Each audience member has 9 possible actions consisting of a neutral (handclapping), 4 positive actions (laughing, interested, understanding, acclaiming) and 4 negative actions (indifference, chatting, dozing, yawning).

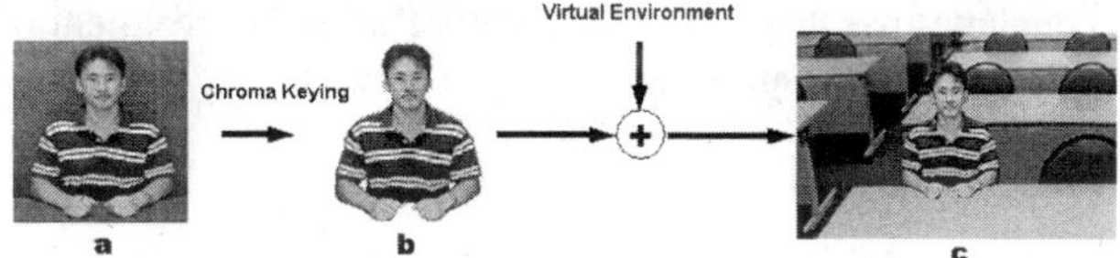

Figure 2. Chroma-key technology (a) with a blue screen. (b) Application of chroma-key (c) Rendering as a virtual audience member in a virtual environment

4. Real-Time Capture

So far, most studies have included animated avatars as virtual audience members. The avatars acted only as previously arranged. These methods cannot, however, show a suitable and diverse set of actions except those made previously. For solving this problem, the real time capture technique using a PC camera was applied to the virtual environment. This technique can be especially beneficial by giving subjects more presence and interaction with other subjects or a therapist in real-time.

The Intel Computer Vision Library was used to capture images in memory. And then captured AVI sequences are mapped as a texture into the surface designated previously.

5. The implementation of Virtual Reality System

Figure 3 shows 12 virtual audience members sitting at their desks on initialization of the VR system. A subject can see another person being captured by PC camera in real time. A therapist can also give a subject instructions and reassurance during treatment. Further, the therapist instructs virtual audience members to act positively or negatively in accordance with the speech.

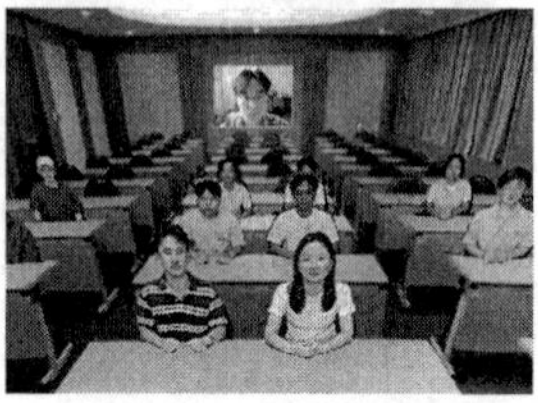

Figure 3. The implementation scene of VR system

6. Conclusions

In this research, a VR simulator was developed to treat the fear of public speaking by using IBR, moving pictures and real-time capture.

In comparison with previous studies, the VR public speaking simulator developed has many advantages. First, the public speaking virtual environment presented is more realistic than existing systems using many graphical textures as real photos were stitched using IBR technology. Second, an operator can select a specific action for each virtual audience member during a subject's speech. It is possible to flexibly control the virtual audiences and compose many diverse situations. Finally, the display of another person interacting in real-time through with a PC camera enables a subject to feel more presence and interaction than when they merely see animated avatars.

Therefore, we conclude that this system will be useful in the treatment of many subjects suffering from the fear of public speaking.

References

[1] M. Slater, D. P. Pertaub, A. Steed. Public Speaking in Virtual Reality: Facing an Audience of Avatars. *IEEE Computer Graphics & Application* March/April 1999; Vol.19 No.2 pp6-9.

[2] M. M. North, S. M. North, and J. R. Coble. Virtual Reality Therapy: An Effective Treatment for the Fear of Public Speaking. *Int'l J. of Virtual Reality* 1998; Vol.3, No.2, pp.2-6.

[3] Anderson, P., Rothbaum, B. O., & Hodges, L. F. Social phobia: Virtual reality exposure therapy for fear of public speaking. Paper presented at *the Annual Meeting of the American Psychological Association* 2000; Washington, DC.

[4] H. J. Jo, J.H. Ku, D. P. Jang, B. H. Cho, H. B. Ahn, J. M. Lee, Y. H. Choi, I. Y. Kim, S. I. Kim. Movie-Based VR Therapy system for Treatment of Anthropophobia. *23rd Annual International Conference of the IEEE Engineering in Medicine and Biology Society* 2001.

[5] Richard Szeliski, Heung-Yeung Shum. Creating full view panoramic image mosaics and environment maps. *Proceedings of the 24th annual conference on Computer graphics & interactive techniques* 1997, Pages 251 - 258.

Medicine Meets Virtual Reality 02/10
J.D. Westwood et al. (Eds.)
IOS Press, 2002

Real-time Soft Tissue Modelling for Web-based Surgical Simulation: SurfaceChainMail

Ying Li[1] , Ken Brodlie[1], Nicholas Phillips[2]
[1]*School of Computing, University of Leeds, Leeds LS2 9JT UK*
[2]*Department of Neurosurgery, Leeds General Infirmary, Leeds, UK*
E-mail: {ying,kwb}@comp.leeds.ac.uk
nickp@ulth.northy.nhs.uk

Abstract. The Web provides a useful environment for simple surgical training simulations. A combination of VRML for 3D rendering, and Java code for the simulation engine, has been used for a range of simple neurosurgical demonstrators. However the elements in these simulators are rigid, to avoid the computational complexity of deformable modelling. In this paper we describe a variation of the ChainMail technique that allows us to provide real-time deformable modelling, even in a Web browser environment on a PC. Our new algorithm, SurfaceChainMail, has been used to develop a simulator for the cutting of two layers of tissue, and separating the layers by pulling them apart.

1. Introduction

There is increasing interest in the use of the Web to deliver simple surgical training simulators. These use a combination of VRML for 3D rendering, and Java code for the simulation engine [5, 6]. A major advantage is their simplicity, available for use at any time, anywhere, with the only requirement being a PC and Web browser. This technology has proved sufficient to create simple neurosurgery demonstrators, where all the elements can be treated as rigid bodies and no deformations occur.

However there are many cases in which soft tissue is involved, and this requires the use of deformable modelling. The challenge we address in this paper is to provide an approach to soft tissue modelling that can be used in a Web-based simulation environment. The work is motivated again by a neurosurgical application; it involves the separation of two layers of tissue, by progressively cutting the material which links the layers, and gradually pulling on the layers to separate them. This requires real-time deformable modelling – which typically requires high performance computing facilities in order to provide an accurate solution. The challenge in our context is to find a feasible solution for simple PC-based computers, trading a degree of accuracy in return for greater speed.

The two principle approaches to soft-tissue modelling over the past decade have been the mass-spring approach, and the Finite Element Method (FEM). Mass-spring models [7] comprise a set of nodes connected by springs, with point masses attached at each node. Real time performance can be achieved with a limited number of nodes, but the behaviour is often unrealistic and can be unstable.

The FEM approach [1,8] produces more accurate results. However, a major problem for real-time modelling is the high computational cost, since the true elastic behaviour of soft tissue is nonlinear, and for large meshes, a large system of equations have to be solved. To counter this, Bro-Nielson *et al* [1] propose a simplified approach: the elastic deformation is assumed to be linear (so only small deformations are accurately modelled); a condensation procedure and pre-processing are included. This condensation step effectively focuses only on the surface nodes of the mesh, reducing the size of the linear system of equations. However, interactive topology changes, such as cutting of soft tissues, are not possible since the pre-processing assumes a certain topology.

A different approach to soft tissue modelling has been proposed by Gibson in a series of papers [2,3,4]. 3D ChainMail is a simple technique but is able to handle in real-time large datasets and large deformations. An object is modelled as a set of point elements, linked in a uniform rectilinear mesh. In contrast to FEM, where complex calculation is carried out on a (relatively) small number of mesh elements, ChainMail carries out simple calculations on a (potentially) large number of elements. There are two steps involved: the ChainMail process itself which imposes simple geometric constraints on movement, similar to chainmail armour; and a relaxation process where energy minimization is applied to refine the shape. An important advantage is that a change in position of one element is typically propagated only to a small number of neighbouring elements. In addition, changes in topology are easily accommodated by breaking links – so cutting is readily simulated.

For our application, speed is of the essence. The Gibson ChainMail is designed for volumetric objects, in which deformations, not only on the outer surface, but also in the interior, are modelled. We study a rather different approach, still using the ChainMail idea, but where we only consider surface elements and do not attempt to model interior behaviour. The result is a promising approach to soft tissue modelling that can be used for Web-based simulation on low-cost PCs.

2.   *3D ChainMail on Uniform Meshes*

In the ChainMail algorithm [2], the deformation of an object is determined by two processes. In the first process, a deformation step, one element is moved to a new position, potentially causing each of its neighbours, and their neighbours, and so on, to move to new positions, in a chain reaction. Neighbours only move if they fail to satisfy proximity constraints which determine the softness of an object. The raw positions of this deformation step are then adjusted by a second process, a relaxation step, which aims to minimize the energy of the configuration.

We illustrate the method in more detail in Figure 1 – which shows the technique in 2D for ease of understanding. Suppose element A has been moved to the new position shown. Then its right neighbour, E, is a candidate for movement in the chain reaction. E is constrained to be greater than *MinDist*, and less than *MaxDist*, in its horizontal separation from A; and to be less than *MaxShear* in its vertical separation. If any of these constraints are violated, then E moves the minimum distance to be within the marked region in Figure 1, and therefore within the constraints. Next the right neighbour of E has to be checked, and so on for all right neighbours. If an element is moved, its left, top and bottom neighbours also have to be checked, and the algorithm builds up lists of elements that need to be checked later. Once the right neighbours are processed, the list of left neighbours is dealt with; then the top neighbours; and finally the bottom neighbours. The top and bottom neighbours are constrained in a similar way to Figure 1, except that the movement is constrained relative to vertical position. The key point however is that any element is moved no more than once. Softness is controlled by the values of the constraints: clearly if *MinDist* is very close to *MaxDist*, then the object is nearly rigid, and all elements move in concert.

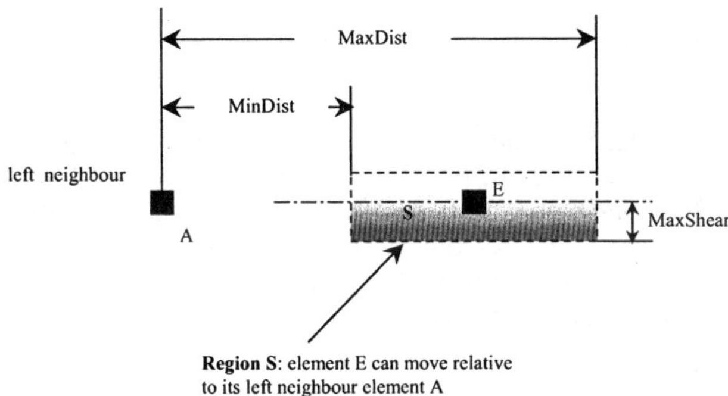

Region S: element E can move relative
to its left neighbour element A

Figure 1 The moved element **E** is limited by the constraints of its left neighbour **A**.

The 3D ChainMail algorithm works in exactly the same way as the 2D version just described, except we now have front and back neighbours as well, and the constraints define a cuboid rather than the rectangle of Figure 1.

In the relaxation process, the system energy (defined in terms of the distance between elements) is iteratively reduced to a minimum. The positions of the elements are locally adjusted so that the distances between these elements are within an optimal range.

3. *Extension to Non-uniform Grids*

The Gibson ChainMail algorithm is defined only for uniform meshes. However it is straightforward to handle non-uniform meshes by replacing the absolute constraints of Figure 1 by constraints expressed relative to the separation. This generalisation to non-uniform meshes will enable us to use the ChainMail technique in a wider class of modelling applications. By non-uniform we mean any mesh topologically equivalent to a uniform rectilinear mesh – that is, a mesh with connections from each interior element to left, right, top, bottom, front and back elements. The mesh can be rectilinear or curvilinear.

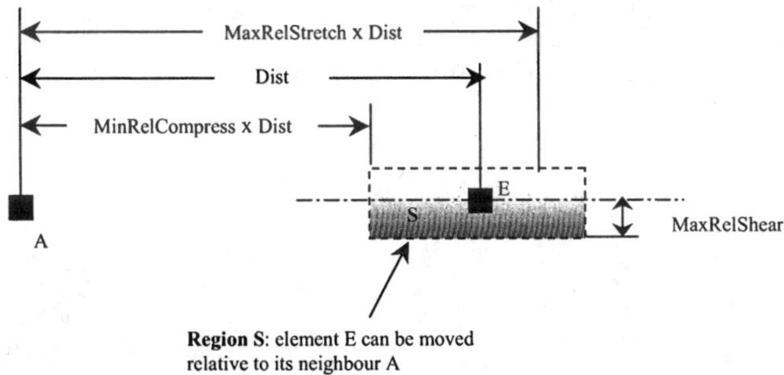

Region S: element E can be moved
relative to its neighbour A

Figure 2. The constraints between element A and its neighbour E

The modification is to separate each geometric constraint into two parts: first, a material parameter which controls the softness, and second, the distance between the linked elements.

Again suppose A has been moved to a new position, and its right neighbour, E, has become a candidate for movement in the chain reaction. Suppose Dist is the distance between A and E. The valid region for E is shown in Figure 2, and is expressed by material parameters, *MaxRelStretch*, *MinRelCompress* and *MaxRelShear*, relative to the separation, *Dist*. With this modification, we can apply ChainMail to non-uniform grids. By tuning the values of the material parameters, objects with different elasticity can be modelled in an efficient way.

4. *Extending to Surfaces in 3D : SurfaceChainMail*

The Gibson ChainMail algorithm was designed for 3D volume modelling where the elements are on a regular, rectilinear mesh – the usual voxel-type structure. Many objects, however, are perfectly well modelled as surfaces. In this section we describe a new variation of ChainMail designed specifically for surfaces: we decompose the deformation proess into two steps – first, a deformation in the plane of the surface (using the extension to non-uniform grids just described), and second, a deformation in the direction of the surface normal.

In the first process, a 2D mesh is mapped onto the surface of the 3D object (as we do with texture mapping in graphics). Thus we first define a 2D non-uniform mesh, S, in the (u,v) – plane. The mesh is then mapped onto the target 3D surface object T(x, y, z), where x, y and z are the co-ordinates in the 3D surface domain. The transformation can be specified by three functions: x = X(u, v), y = Y(u, v) and z = Z(u, v). The 2D ChainMail technique is performed on the 2D mesh and the updated positions are then transformed onto the 3D surface.

In the second process, the surface normal at an element is obtained by the local average of the normals of surrounding facets. If the displacement of the moved element in the normal direction is less than *MaxRelShear*Dist*, then its neighbour is unchanged; but if the displacement is greater than this, the neighbour is moved in its normal direction so that the separation in that direction between the two elements is *MaxRelShear*Dist*.

At the end, the updated results from these two processes are combined together to produce a deformed new shape of the 3D surface. Figure 3 shows the examples of using these techniques. In the three pictures to the left, a cut cylinder is pulled and pushed; to the right, a cut sphere is deformed. We term the new technique: SurfaceChainMail.

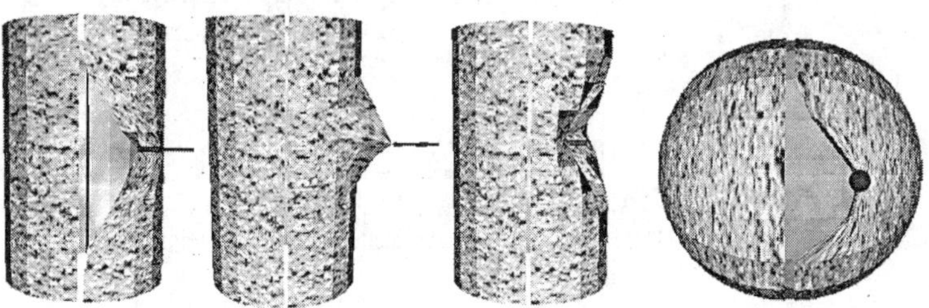

Figure 3. Examples of deformable surface using surface based ChainMail

5. *Implementation in Web-based Environment*

SurfaceChainMail has been implemented as a Web-based application so that it can be used as a surgical training simulator in the collection of such tools being developed [9]. It uses a combination of VRML and Java: VRML to provide the visual display and Java code to provide the real-time soft tissue modelling using SurfaceChainMail. The Java External Authoring Interface provides the link between the two. The system structure is shown in Figure 4.

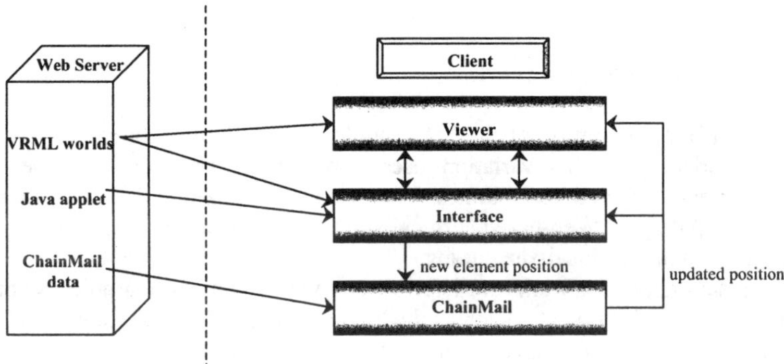

Figure 4 – System Structure

The system has three main components: the view, the interface and the ChainMail engine. When the simulator Web page is loaded from the server, the VRML world is downloaded into the view component and into the interface component, a Java applet is downloaded into the interface, and the mesh structure into the ChainMail engine. When the user alters a position of an element, this is transmitted from the interface to the ChainMail engine which then computes the resulting new mesh positions. These are transmitted back to the view and interface components. The Java EAI for VRML provides the 'glue' which allows the components to communicate with each other.

SurfaceChainMail has been applied to the cylindrical and spherical objects as shown in Figure 3, and also to a box-shaped object as described below (see Figure 5).

6. Surgical Training Application

One of the advantages of the ChainMail approach is that it supports topological changes in the interactive modelling : links between an element and its neighbours can be easily disconnected when needed. This applies in exactly the same way to SurfaceChainMail. This has allowed us to build a general simulator for the cutting and separation of layers of soft tissue. This models a very fundamental technique in surgery of all types for dissecting out structures as part of a more complex operation. In neurosurgery a common start to many operations involves the dissection of the covering layers of the brain (- the meninges) to allow access to deeper structures such as blood vessels.

Figure 5 shows a screenshot of the simulator. There are two linked VRML worlds: the trainee manipulates the cutting instrument in the lower left browser window, while a view of the resulting deformation is provided for the trainee, and observers, in the upper window.

Cutting is simulated when the user defines a 'cut path' using a mouse as virtual instrument. Elements close to the cut path are identified, and any links with their neighbours which are crossed by the cut path are removed from the data structure. Deformation is simulated when the virtual instrument pulls or pushes the object: an element is moved to a new position by the instrument and SurfaceChainMail calculates the resulting effect. In Figure 5, we see two layers of tissue that have been cut, and teased apart using the instrument.

7.   Conclusions and Future Work

We have described a variation of the 3D ChainMail algorithm introduced by Gibson for volumetric modelling. This variation uses non-uniform grids and can be used for modelling surfaces as well as volumes. Its simplicity makes it suitable for real-time deformable modelling in Web-based surgical simulators, and we have used it to develop a simple training simulator for tissue cutting.

The present approach works well for objects where there is a simple mapping from the (u,v) mesh to the 3D object – such as the box, cylinder and sphere described here. We are currently working on a further development in which the surface may be defined as a general unstructured mesh: this mesh is triangulated, and the sides of the triangles become the mesh links. This will extend to 3D tetrahedral meshes to give a chainmail-type method for volumetric modelling on unstructured meshes.

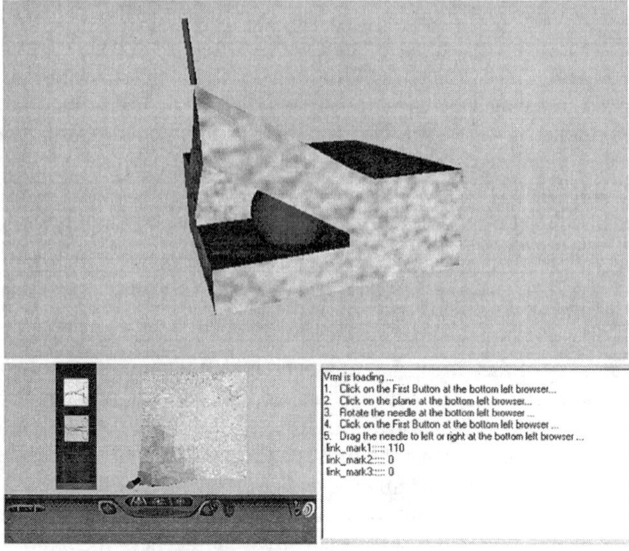

Figure 5. Surface based deformable modelling and cutting with web-based environment. The browser window at the bottom left is the controller, where the user manipulates the instrument and performing deformation and cutting process. The instrument can be selected at the left bar of the window and rotated as well as inserted. The window at the top displays the results from the controller. The applet viewer at the bottom right is the monitor.

References:

[1] Morten Bro-Nielsen and Stephane Cotin, Real-time Volumetric Deformable Models for Surgery Simulation using Finite Elements and Condensation. Computer Graphics Forum, 15(3) 57-66 (Eurographics'96), 1996.

[2] Sarah F. F. Gibson, 3D chainmail: a fast algorithm for deforming volumetric objects. In Michael Cohen and David Zeltzer, editors, 1997 Symposium on Interactive 3D Graphics, pages 149-154. ACM SIGGRAPH, April 1997. ISBN 0-89791-884-3.

[3] Markus A. Schill, Sarah F. F. Gibson, H. J. Bender, and R. Manner, Biomechanical Simulation of the Vitreous Humor in the Eye Using an Enhanced ChainMail Algorithm. Proceedings Medical Image Computation and Computer Assisted Interventions, MICCAI'98, October, 1998, pp. 679-687.

[4] Sarah F. Frisken-Gibson, Using Linked Volumes to Model Object Collisions, Deformation, Cutting, Carving, and Joining. IEEE Transactions On Visualization And Computer Graphic, Vol. 5. No. 4. 1999.

[5] Ying Li, Ken Brodlie and Nicholas Phillips, Web-based VR Training Simulator for Percutaneous Rhizotomy, in Medicine Meets Virtual Reality 2000, edited by JD Westwood, HM Hoffman, GT Mogel, RA Robb and D Stredney, IOS Press, pp175-181.

[6] Nigel W. John and Nicholas Phillips, Surgical Simulators Using the WWW, in Medicine Meets Virtual Reality 2000, edited by JD Westwood, HM Hoffman, GT Mogel, RA Robb and D Stredney, IOS Press, pp146-152.

[7] Kühnapfel U., Çakmak H. K. and Maass H, Endoscopic Surgery Training using Virtual Reality and deformable Tissue Simulation. Computers & Graphics 24(2000) 671-682, Elsevier (2000)

[8] Morten Bro-Nielson, Finite Element Modeling in Surgery Simulation. Proceedings of the IEEE. Vol. 86. No. 3. March 1998.

[9] Web-Based Surgical Simulators and Medical Education Tools. http://synaptic.mvc.mcc.ac.uk/simulators.html

Medicine Meets Virtual Reality 02/10
J.D. Westwood et al. (Eds.)
IOS Press, 2002

Virtual Food in Virtual Environments for the Treatment of Eating Disorders

José A. LOZANO, Mariano ALCAÑIZ, José A. GIL, Carlos MOSERRAT, Mari C. JUÁN,
Vicente GRAU, Hugo VARVARÓ
*MedICLab (Medical Image Computing Laboratory) - DEGI / UPV, Camino de Vera s/n,
46022 Valencia, Spain*

Abstract. Eating disorders (Eds) are one of the problems with higher social repercussion in the last years. Sometimes, these clinical syndromes, which are characterized by an altered eating behavior, can have dramatic consequences. In eating disorders, one of the more critical situations, in addition to other of equal or more importance, is the patient's confrontation with food: the visual confrontation, the eating process and the repercussion on his weight. Virtual Reality (VR) technology has been used in psychology, as a therapeutic help tool for the treatment of different psychological problems, for several years now. Their helpfulness is increasingly being recognized. Some developed virtual environments (VE) and their corresponding published studies endorse the efficiency of this tool. Nevertheless, in order to increase the possibilities of success, it is very important to obtain a complete patient immersion in the VE: visual, auditory and interactive. Sometimes there are processes or actions of reality, which are difficult to simulate virtually, and simulating them coarsely would result in the patient lack of immersion in the VE, thus seriously decreasing the possibilities of success. The eating process is an example, since it consists of several steps, some of which (biting, chewing, etc.) don't have an evident virtual solution. This article shows how food and eating process have been simulated virtually in the development of a virtual environment for the treatment of eating disorders.

1. Introduction

Eating disorders are clinical conditions involving severe alterations of eating behaviour, the most representative cases being anorexia and bulimia nervosa. These clinical syndromes have become sort of an epidemic at the end of the millennium, at least in western societies. The condition affects mainly pre- and post-pubertal adolescent females [1].

Considering that eating disorders can directly lead to death, the efforts being carried out in order to find more effective therapeutic methods are not surprising. A number of studies have been published supporting the efficacy of VR as a therapeutic tool for different psychological problems: acrophobia [2], agoraphobia [3], and arachnophobia [4]. Our group - MedICLab (UPV – Universidad Politécnica de Valencia), together with the Psychology Department of UJI (Universidad Jaime I) and UV (Universidad de Valencia), has also contributed to this pioneering field, designing and validating VR applications for the treatment of claustrophobia [5] [6] [10] and flying phobia [7] [8] [9] - with very good results among the clinical population suffering from these problems.

In VE development for the treatment of psychological phobias, one of the main objectives is to obtain the patient's immersion. For this purpose, it is very important to simulate with realism the conditions that cause his/her problems. The more real the VE looks, the higher is the immersion degree and thus the possibilities of success. In eating disorders, one of the most critical situations is coping with food and eating processes.

For the treatment of eating disorders, MedICLab, together with the Psychology Department of UJI and UV, has developed a VE which has six rooms; in each of them, the patient will cope with some problematic situations. One of these rooms is a kitchen. The idea is that the patient deals with food, the eating process and their consequences (the alteration of their weight). To do this, different *virtual foods* have been incorporated and, interacting with them, the patient will simulate the eating process. A *virtual scale* has also been used so that patients can see what their *real weight* is, enter their *subjective weight* (the weight that they think they have put on after eating food), enter their *desired weight* (the weight that they would like to have) and see what their *healthy weight* is (the weight that they really should have). In order to obtain a realistic eating process, tried to have the patient cope with food, not only in a visual way, but also including all other steps necessary in the eating process: taking the food to his/her own mouth, eating step by step (biting and chewing) and to listening to the sounds related to this process. The problem to solve was how to simulate all these steps.

2. Method and tools used

The following method was carried out. A detailed research of the more important aspects of the eating process was performed: movements, sounds, etc.

The first conclusion of this research was that the eating process is constituted by these steps: selecting the food, moving it close to the mouth, biting it and chewing it –in the case of solid food (apple, pizza, etc.)-, sipping it –in the case of liquid food (water, wine, etc.)- and swallowing it. Therefore, the first objective was to incorporate, in our virtual environment, a virtual eating process as similar as possible to the real eating process, and subsequently design a virtual eating process inclosing all these steps (Figure 1).

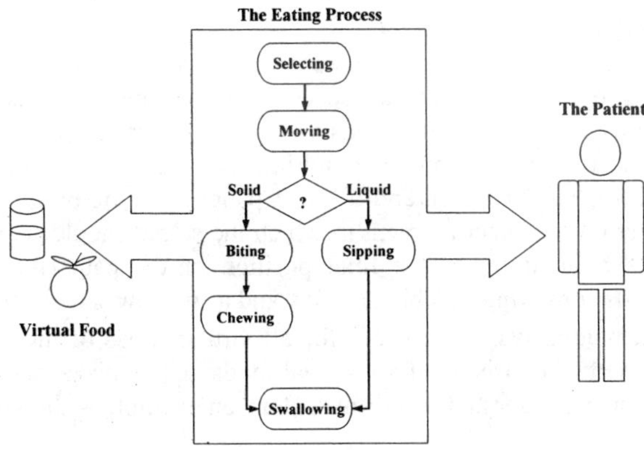

Figure 1

The second conclusion was that, the most normal way of eating or drinking food is step by step (bites or sips). Therefore, the second objective was to incorporate, in our virtual environment, virtual foods with a shape (3D geometry) and an appearance (2D textures) as similar as possible to reality. Modelling certain types of food as a whole was not enough. It was also necessary to model particular pieces of food. That is to say, it was necessary to make a 3D modelling with a high level of detail. However, in the virtual environments, incorporating 3D objects with many polygons can considerably reduce the displacement speed of the user in the environment.

The third conclusion was the importance of listening to the sounds related to the eating process (biting, spitting, chewing and swallowing) in order to increase its realism. Therefore, the third objective was to incorporate, in our virtual environment, sounds as similar as possible to those emitted in reality.

Next, the technical viability to carry out these aspects with the software tools used for making our virtual environments (WorldToolKit , 3D Studio MAX, PhotoShop, Cool Edit, etc.) was studied.

- Food selection:

Food selection was simulated by programming the interaction objects (using WorldToolKit). With this, when the patient placed the mouse pointer over a virtual food, the icon changed its appearance. In this way, the patient deduced that he could interact with this virtual food.

- Food movement:

Food movement towards the patient´s mouth was simulated in a similar way, by programming the object´s motion trajectories. A motion path was incorporated in every virtual food. The initial path position was the one that virtual food had in the kitchen and the final path position was the one that simulated the patient´s mouth and that was located slightly beneath the camera spot (the patient´s point of view). When the patient was interacting with virtual food, it moved towards him. But, when he stopped the interaction with the virtual food, it moved back to its initial position.

- Biting:

Food bites were simulated by modelling (3D Studio MAX) several geometries for every kind of food and each given bite. The realism increased by means of the use of appropriate textures, which were perfectly adapted (PhotoShop). Later, it was programmed that every time the patient approached virtual food to the mouth, the food changed its appearance to show the bite given.

- Chewing, sipping and swallowing:

The simulation of biting, sipping, chewing and swallowing was enhanced by incorporating the appropriate sounds in the virtual environment. It was impossible to use a sound library, since these kinds of sounds were very specific. Therefore, all sounds were recorded using a microphone, a complete multitrack digital audio recorder, editor and mixer software tool (Cool Edit Pro 1.2), and a lot of patience in the process. Moreover, it was necessary to program the exact moment in which the sound should be played. Whenever a virtual food was brought up to the final position of the path (the patient's mouth) a sequence of sounds consisting of a bite, a chew and a swallow sound effect was played.

This implementation was carried out for all virtual foods of the virtual environment. Specifically, our virtual consisted of six virtual foods: apple, pizza, salad (tomatoes, carrot, lettuce and cucumber), water and soft drinks. Next, an example is shown: the apple.

When the patient approaches the apple (Figure 2) and positions the mouse icon on top of it, it changes its appearance (Figure 3). This will indicate to the patient that he can interact with this virtual apple.

Next, if the patient right-clicks on it and holds it down, the virtual apple will move towards him (Figure 4). When it reaches his mouth, it changes its shape (Figure 5), to look like a bite has been taken out of it. This will go along with the characteristic sound heard when biting, chewing and swallowing an apple, which increases the realism of the situation. After biting it, if the user decides to release the button being held down, the virtual apple will return to its original position.

The patient can repeat this process until the virtual apple has been completely eaten. In this case, the process can be carried out up to 7 times, and each time a bite will be taken, and a smaller amount of apple will be left to eat. In the end, the apple will completely disappear. Moreover, all virtual foods have been programmed in order to follow this same path. If after eating the whole apple, the psychologist decides to give the patient an opportunity to eat another one, he will press a specific key and another virtual apple, just like the previous one, will appear in the same place.

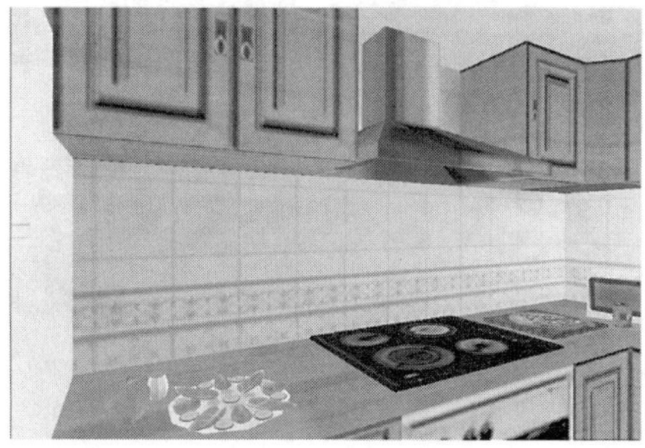

Figure 2

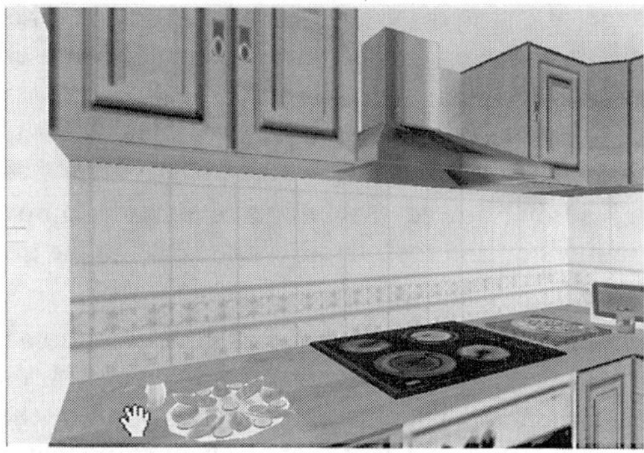

Figure 3

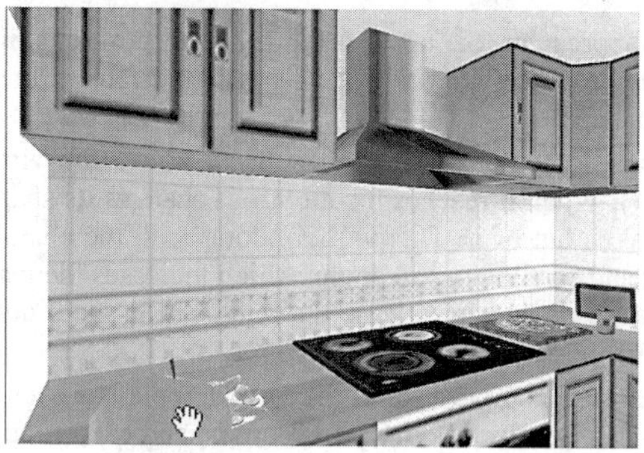

Figure 4

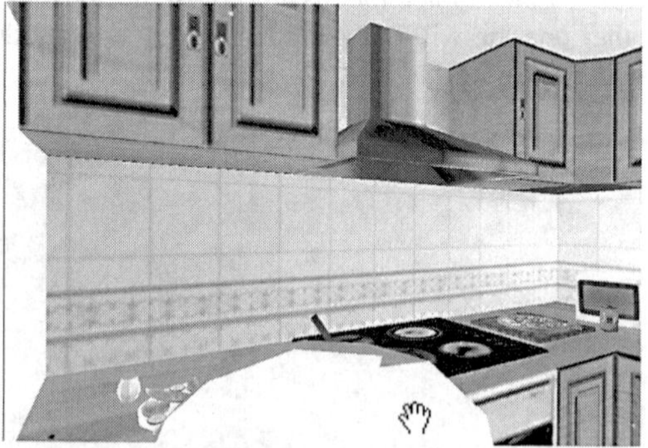

Figure 5

3. Results

The Department of UJI and UV conducted a study with the aim of evaluating whether this improvement in the interaction process with virtual food was useful or not and whether it improved the treatment of eating disorders with virtual reality. This research satisfied the following requirements: it was a controlled study, conducted in a clinical population, and allowing a comparison of the efficacy of our virtual eating process versus other simpler processes (the patient selected the virtual food, interacted with it, and the virtual food disappeared), which were nevertheless incorporated to our virtual environment.

The results of this study showed that all patients had improved significantly their sensation of realism, immersion and motivation with respect to the treatment.

- Sensation of realism and immersion:

Despite the "virtual" nature of the situation, patients gave credit to a high degree of realism in the virtual kitchen: visual, auditory and interactive realism with the virtual food. In fact, in the kitchen setting, when the patients "ate" virtually, they chewed, swallowed and became very nervous - even though they were eating something that did not really exist.

- Increase of treatment motivation:

One of the difficulties arisen by eating disorders treatment is the low patient motivation towards therapeutic procedures. In this new therapeutic scenario, however, these resistances decrease and the motivation for therapy increases. Offering the possibility to interact with several kinds of food and presenting a very realistic interaction process constitute a great help.

4. Conclusions

Although the eating process is a relatively complex process that consists of several steps, it is possible to obtain a realistic enough simulation to increase the level of immersion in the process of interaction with the virtual objects. This considerably improves the patient's therapeutic results.

We have had patients who had not eaten a piece of pizza or put on certain clothes for years, until they did so virtually - followed shortly after by corresponding genuine practice and integration in their daily lives.

All this leads us to the following conclusion: increasing the realism of the patient's interaction process with the virtual objects, greatly improves the therapeutic results of virtual environments usage for the treatment of eating disorders.

References

[1]　C.Perpiña *et al.*, Imagen Corporal en los Trastornos Alimentarios. Evaluación y Tratamiento mediante Realidad Virtual. Editorial Promolibro, Valencia, 2000.

[2]　M. North and S. North, Virtual Reality Psychotherapy. *The Journal of Medicine and Virtual Reality* 1 (1996) 28-32.

[3]　M. North *et al.*, Virtual Reality Theraphy, I.P.I Press, Michigan, 1997.

[4]　A. Carlin *et al.*, Virtual Reality and Tactile Augmentation int the Treatment of Spider Phobia: a case report. *Behaviour Research and Therapy* 35 (1997) 153-158.

[5]　C. Botella *et al.*. Virtual Reality Treatment of Claustrophobia: a case report. *Behaviour Research and Therapy* 36 (1998) 239-246.

[6]　C. Botella *et al.*, Virtual Environments for the Treatment of Claustrophobia. *International Journal of Virtual Reality* 3 (1998) 8-12.

[7]　R. M. Baños *et al.*, El Tratamiento de la Fobia a Volar por medio de Realidad Virtual. Ponencia presentada en XXX *Congress of the European Association for Behavioural and Cognitive Therapies*, 2000.

[8]　C. Botella, El Diseño de Escenarios Clinicamente Significativos para el Tratamiento de la Fobia a Volar. *1° Congreso Virtual de Psiquiatría*, 2000

[9]　R. M. Baños *et al.*, Fobia a Volar. Tratamiento Mediante Realidad Virtual. Editorial Promolibro, 2000.

[10]　C. Botella *et al.*, Claustrofobia. Manual de Tratamiento Mediante Realidad Virtual. Editorial Promolibro, 2001.

Medicine Meets Virtual Reality 02/10
J.D. Westwood et al. (Eds.)
IOS Press, 2002

Advancements in Immersive VR as a Tool for Preoperative Planning for Laparoscopic Surgery

Michael J Mastrangelo Jr, Jeremy Stich, James D Hoskins, Wayne Witzke, Ivan George, Jason Garrison, Mathew Nichols and Adrian E Park

Department of Surgery
Center for Minimally Invasive Surgery (UKCMIS)
University of Kentucky College of Medicine

Abstract

The utility of three-dimensional (3D) models for planning laparoscopic surgery and surgical training has been demonstrated. (1) Computed tomography (CT) scans with oral and intravenous contrast medium are frequently used for preoperative evaluation of patients undergoing complex laparoscopic surgery. Immersive 3D VR overcomes many of the conceptual limitations encountered when conveying or teaching 3D relationships via 2D images traditionally produced by these scans. Over the past year we have made advancements in several areas. First, we have improved the quality of our datasets by utilizing higher resolution multi-detector scans and altering the protocols used. Second, we now register multiple isosurface views with standard axial views and volume textured views to provide additional information and perspective. Third, we now routinely use auto-segmentation techniques to visualize individual structures.

Introduction:

Unlike traditional open surgery, laparoscopic or minimally invasive surgery is performed through small "key-hole" incisions, utilizing a videoscope for visualization. Therefore, the ability to manipulate 3D models of the patients' anatomy and to view anatomy from different perspectives is especially useful in laparoscopic surgery where preoperative planning and port placement dictate the angle of approach to the surgical site. Computed tomography (CT) scans with intravenous contrast media are widely available for preoperative evaluation. Automated software packages are now available that produce accurate useful models on standard desktop PCs. Most accomplish this by constructing surfaces from areas with similar threshold values and thus avoid the bias of a technician manually selecting areas to represent. Multiple models constructed at varying threshold windows can be colorized, combined in a single image (registered) and displayed in a 3-D immersive environment. This allows groups of physicians and students to navigate through and orient themselves in an "uncluttered" model with fewer surfaces represented, before advancing to greater detail. Navigation through structure walls to view the inner-space of organs or vessels is also possible. Over the past year we have made advancements in several areas. First, we have improved the quality of our datasets by utilizing higher resolution multi-detector scans and altering the protocols used. Second, we now register multiple isosurface views with standard axial views and volume textured views to provide additional information and perspective. Third, we now routinely use auto-segmentation techniques to visualize individual structures.

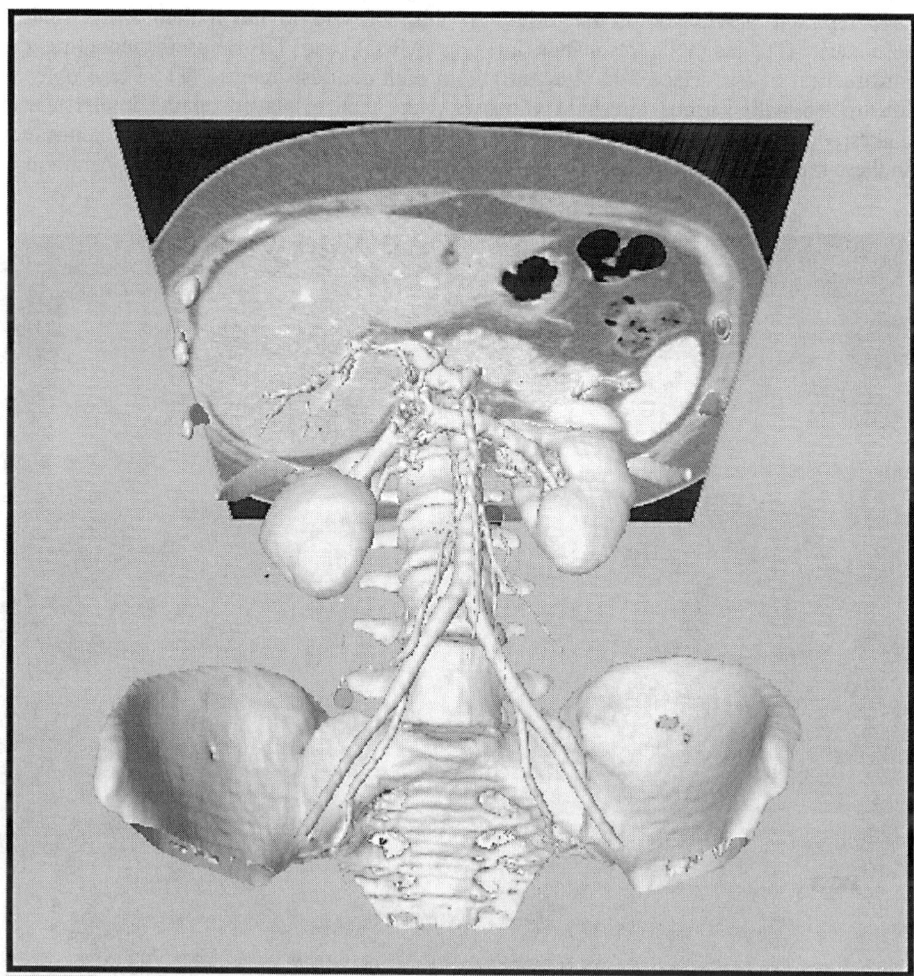

Figure 1 The correlation of a standard 2-D axial CT image with a 3-D isosurface is shown. The isosurface can be cropped, manipulated or navigated to demonstrate relationships from any perspective and the appropriate axial image can be represented instantly at any level of the model.

Methods & Tools:

The industry standard DICOM (Digital Imaging and Communications in Medicine) format CT datasets were viewed utilizing Amira Software version 2.3 (Template Graphics Software Inc.), a commercially available automated package that renders accurate and useful 3D visualizations in seconds to minutes. The software accomplished this by constructing isosurfaces and other objects based on radiodensity threshold values. We have reported previously on the utility of this software to manipulate and visualize volumetric CT, magnetic resonance imaging (MRIs), and TIF datasets, including the construction of isosurface 3-D structures from high contrast images. (1) These objects, constructed with various threshold windows, were then displayed on the ImmersaDesk (Fakespace). Physicians and students were able to navigate through and orient themselves on these models prior to performing procedures. We have continued to research Amira in

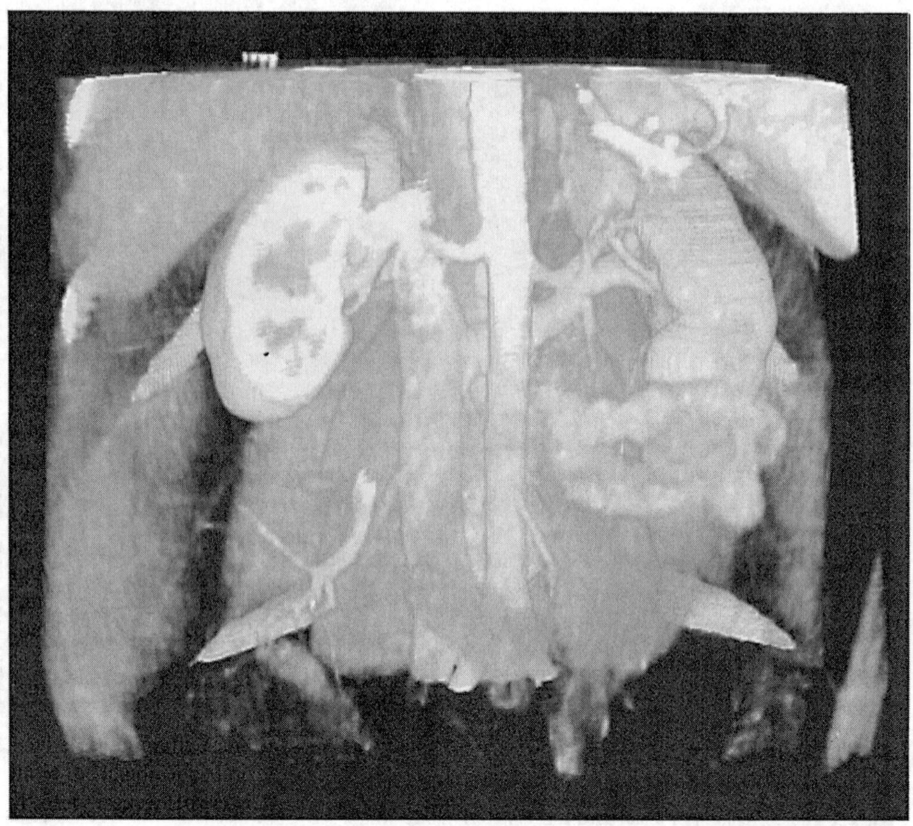

Figure 2 A volume textured (voltex) view of the abdomen is shown. This environment can be navigated and viewed from any level or position. Attaching a clipping plane to a voltex environment allows for a virtual dissection through the patient's anatomy. This view is especially useful for assessing the association of an organ to surrounding structures.

conjunction with our immersive 3-D display in order to overcome the limitations of standard 2D viewing environments.

In addition to the polygonal surfaces created from these datasets, we now include volume texturing and auto-segmentation in the construction of our visualizations. Most visualizations are converted to VRML (Virtual Reality Modeling Language) worlds and subsequently transferred to the ImmersaDesk, where they are viewed stereoscopically and manipulated in real-time. Stereoscopic views from any necessary angle at any required position, and navigation through structure walls to view the inner-space of organs or vessels are possible.

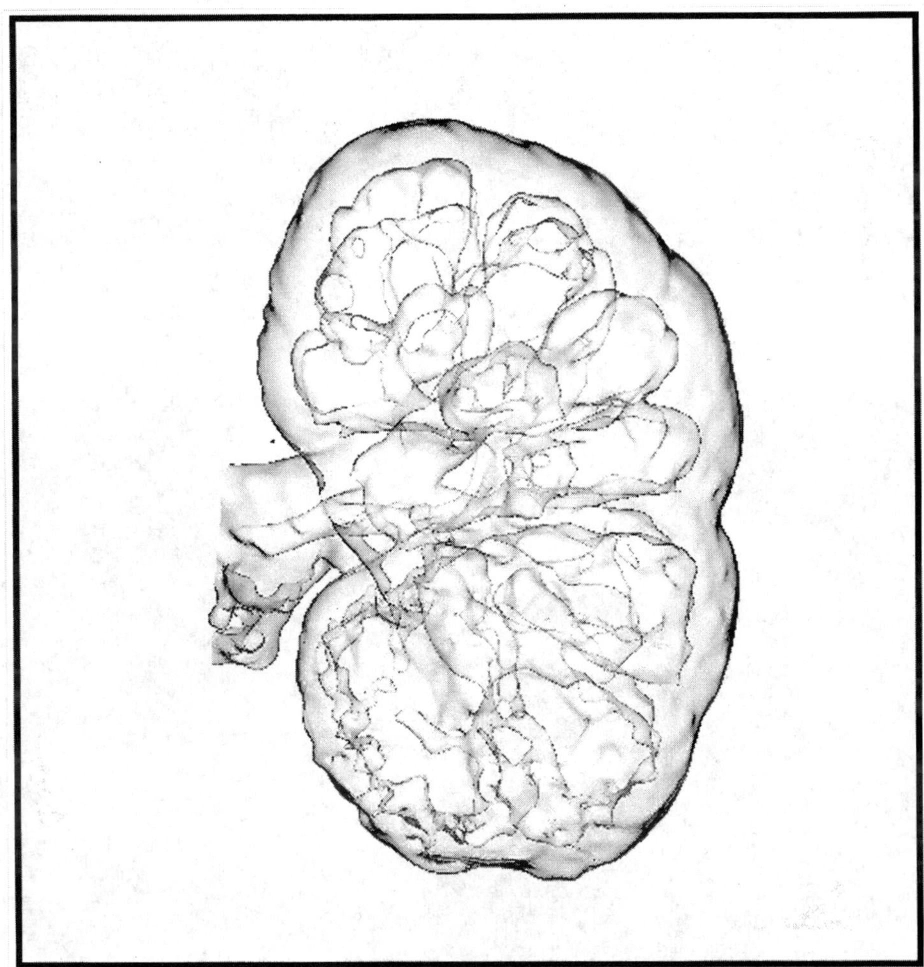

Figure 3 A surface model of a kidney with a semi-transparent surface that allows visualization of internal organ structures.

Results:

Complete CT datasets from a broad range of surgical cases were processed by Amira. The resulting visualizations were transferred to the ImmersaDesk and viewed by surgeons involved in each patient's care. In all cases the surgeons felt that the 3-D images provided additional complementary information when compared to the standard axial CT images and reports alone. Datasets from high resolution, multi-detector CT scanners with finer cuts (.5 mm) produced 3D models that were sharper and more detailed. The diagnostic quality of visualizations was also improved by combining multiple scans, such as arterial and venous phases.

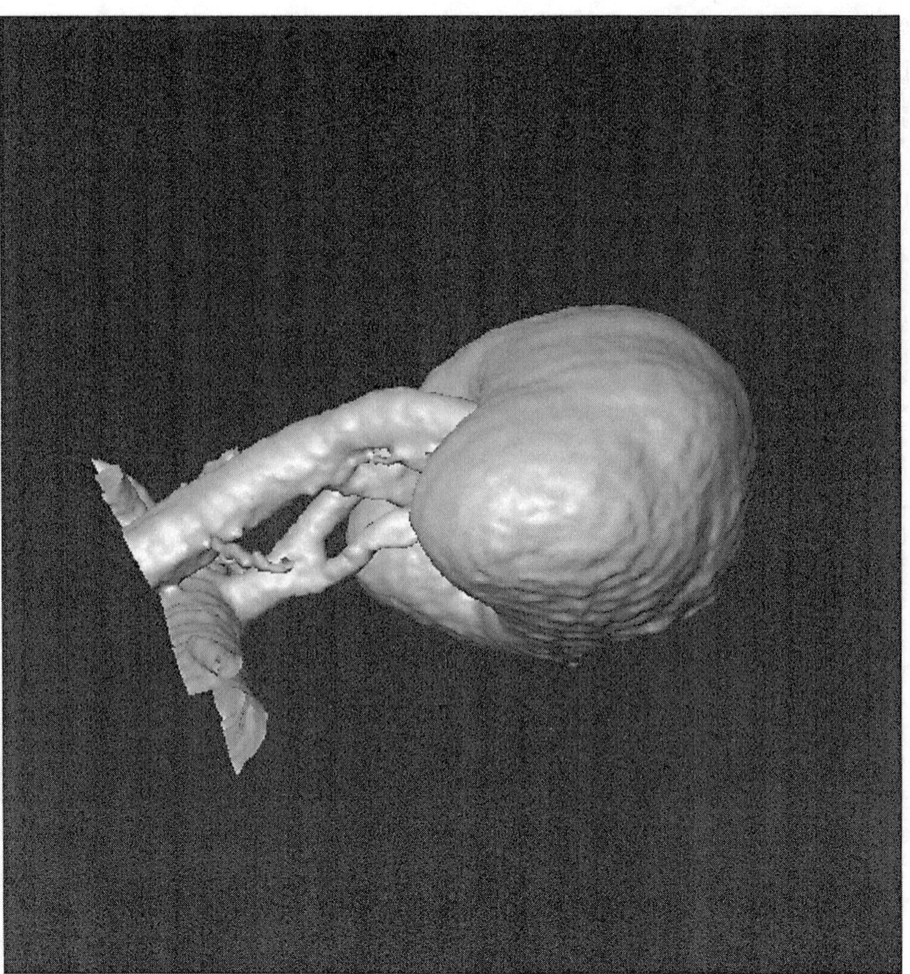

Figure 4 An isosurface of the left kidney from an axial perspective is shown. These simplified models delineate key anatomy and are useful in planning surgical approaches.

Conclusions:

We were able to create level II models that incorporate transparent surfaces, allowing the internal structure of organs to be visualized. (2) We were also able to overlay and register accurately multiple datasets in the same visualization. This allowed us to selectively colorize structures and have specific parts of the scene disappear and reappear as needed. We have refined and improved our auto-segmentation techniques improving quality and production time for the organ models we are using in our educational simulations. This allows our simulations to incorporate data from actual patients that physicians and physicians in training interact with. As a result, we are able to efficiently receive scan data from our radiology department, create specific organ models, create translucent shells of patient's outer body, and reassemble the models on the ImmersaDesk to allow the residents to navigate through an immersive representation of the actual patient's anatomy.

Initial results suggest that this is an effective combination for evaluation and teaching. The combination of the Amira software and the ImmersaDesk provides a useful, accurate platform for evaluating CT datasets prior to laparoscopic surgery. Physicians now have access to an accurate and flexible system for visualizing the anatomy of their patients in 3D. This provides a potentially valuable tool for diagnosis, training and preoperative planning. Improvements in CT imaging, software and end user familiarity with these tools will further improve the utility of this modality in the future.

References:

(1) Mastrangelo MJ Jr, Hoskins JD, Nichols M, Munch LC, Johnston TD, Reddy KS, Ranjan D, Witzke WO, Park A. Using Immersive VR as a Tool for Preoperative Planning for Minimally Invasive Donor Nephrectomy. Student Health Technology Information. 2001;81:298-304.
(2) Robb, RA, Biomedical Imaging, Visualization and Analysis. New York, NY USA: VCH Press 2000326-328.

Medicine Meets Virtual Reality 02/10
J.D. Westwood et al. (Eds.)
IOS Press, 2002

Quantitative Methodology of Evaluating Surgeon Performance in Laparoscopic Surgery

Paul B. McBeth[1], Antony J. Hodgson[1], PhD, Alex G. Nagy[2], MD, Karim Qayumi[2], MD PhD

*Departments of [1]Mechanical Engineering and [2]Surgery,
University of British Columbia, Vancouver, BC, Canada V6T 1Z4*

Abstract

Quantitative performance and skill assessments are critical for evaluating the progress of surgical residents and the efficacy of different training programs. Current evaluation methods are subjective and potentially unreliable, so there is a need for objective methods to evaluate surgical performance. We identify a feasible method to measure kinematic data in the live operating room setting and to assess the repeatability of an analysis method based on a hierarchical decomposition of surgical tasks. We used an optoelectronic motion analysis system to acquire postural data and tool tip trajectories of one expert surgeon over a period of four months. To assess repeatability of performance measures, we created a hierarchical decomposition diagram describing the procedure in terms of surgical tasks, tool sequences and fundamental tool actions. From the kinematic data, we extracted characteristic measures of individual tool actions and compared these measured distributions using the Kolmogorov-Smirnov statistic. The comparisons of distributions show consistent performance over time by a trained surgeon and little effect from patient variability, and so are likely reliable measures of performance. An expanded set of reliable kinematic measures will form the basis for quantifying surgical skill and should be useful in validating surgical simulations for use in training, certifying surgeons and designing and evaluating new surgical tools.

1. Introduction

Although minimally invasive techniques have been rapidly adopted into mainstream surgery over the last decade, developments in teaching and evaluation methods have not kept pace. Quantitative performance and skill assessments are critical for evaluating the progress of surgical residents and the efficacy of different training programs. They are also important in assessing new surgical tool sets and techniques. Current evaluation methods are subjective and potentially unreliable [1], so there is a need for objective methods to evaluate surgical performance. One valuable approach, which was recently demonstrated on a porcine model, is based on an analysis of tool-tip force/torque signatures [2]. In this paper, we discuss a complementary approach which incorporates kinematic features of both tool motion and surgeon posture. The purposes of this study were to identify a feasible method to measure kinematic data in the live operating room setting and to assess the repeatability of an analysis method based on a hierarchical decomposition of surgical tasks. An abbreviated sample of the kinematic data results is presented due to limited space.

2. Methods

2.1 Equipment

An optoelectronic motion analysis system and video recordings were used to acquire postural data and tool tip trajectories at frequencies of ~20 Hz. For this study, we used a Northern Digital Polaris Hybrid Optical Tracking System capable of tracking the 3D position of both active infra-red light emitting diodes (IREDs) and passive retro-reflective markers with an accuracy of ~0.2-0.3 mm. The Polaris system was connected to a standard PC (800 MHz AMD Duron) running custom-designed data acquisition software written in Matlab.

In addition to the optoelectronic system, we recorded video images of the surgery using both a laparoscope and an external camera focused on the surgeon. The images from these two sources were time stamped and recorded onto standard VHS tape; from these images, we could later determine the stage of the operation and correlate it with the detailed motion measurements. All equipment used in the operating room was tested and approved by Vancouver Hospital's Biomedical Engineering Dept. and sterilized with ethylene oxide when appropriate.

2.2 Experimental Protocol

One expert surgeon was evaluated in seven clinical laparoscopic cholecystectomies over a period of four months at Vancouver Hospital. We attached sterilized marker arrays to the surgeon's torso and dominant arm (on the proximal and distal forearm and on the hand), as shown in Figure 1(L,C). This set of marker arrays enabled us to track and record the surgeon's joint angles at the shoulder, elbow, and wrist. Arrays were secured to the surgeon using elastic and Velcro® harnesses. Custom-designed Multi-Directional Marker Arrays (MDMArray) were attached to the each laparoscopic tool handle used by the dominant hand, as shown in Figure 1(R). A planar marker array was attached to the non-dominant hand tool. The MDMArrays were equipped with a quick release clip to allow easy attachment and removal. The Polaris system is capable of tracking six different laparoscopic tools.

One researcher scrubbed into the surgery and attached the sterilized marker arrays to the surgeon's hands, lower arms and torso and laparoscopic tools. This researcher remained to assist the surgeon with any adjustments to the marker arrays or support cuffs. Immediately postoperatively, the surgeon's joint center locations were calibrated using a set of standard isolated joint motions. The tip position of each surgical tool was found using a sphere-fitting calibration procedure in which the tip was placed in a small depression on a fixed surface while the tool was manipulated about that point.

2.3 Missing Data

Optoelectronic systems have inherent line-of-sight limitations causing segments of missing data. Custom-designed tool marker arrays with multiple faces visible from several directions (the MDMArrays mentioned above) were developed to minimize these problems. To establish the feasibility of using an optoelectronic system for tool tip and posture tracking in the operating room, we measured the frequency of marker occlusions and estimated the errors associated with interpolating missing data.

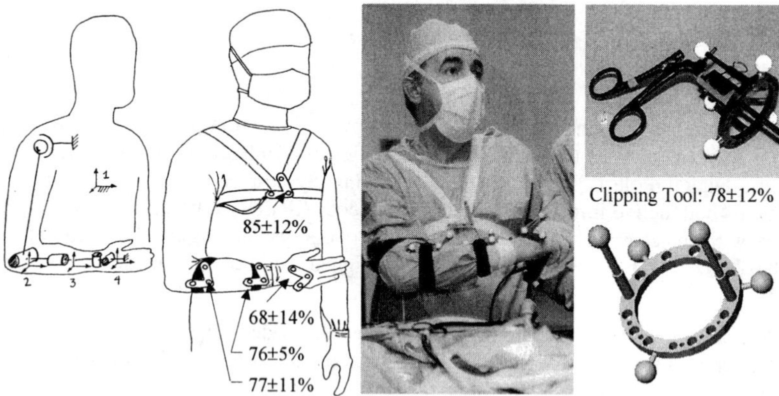

Figure 1 - *Model of the surgeon's arm (L). Marker array mounting (schematic and as mounted in the operating room (C)). Multi-Directional-Marker-Array (MDMA) (schematic and as mounted on a laparoscopic surgical tool (R). The values labeled on each marker represent the percentage of time it was visible during manipulation segments (%).*

2.4 Hierarchical Decomposition

Many performance measures (e.g., distance for a tool tip relocation maneuver) can only be defined for low-level movement segments. To assess repeatability of such performance measures, we therefore created a hierarchical decomposition describing the procedure in terms of surgical phases and stages, tool tasks and subtasks, and fundamental tool actions (see Figure 2). This five-level hierarchical decomposition provides the foundation for a quantitative analysis of surgeon performance since it allows us to identify related tool actions performed at different points during the procedure and consolidate the associated performance measures for analysis.

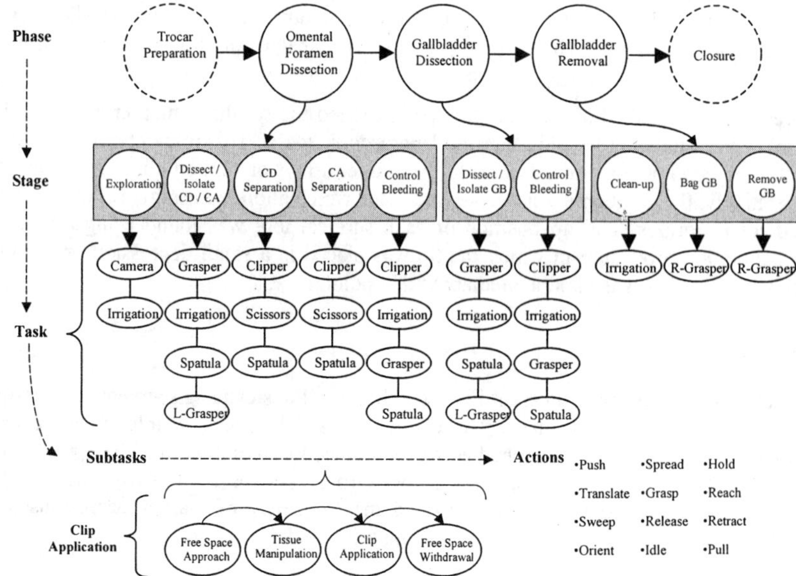

Figure 2 - *Laparoscopic Cholecystectomy Hierarchical Decomposition*

2.5 Performance Measures

From the kinematic data associated with each subtask, we extracted characteristic measures of individual tool movements; for example: duration, mean and peak tool-tip velocity, peak acceleration, jerk cost, straight-line deviations. In additional to the kinematic performance measures we also investigated mean membership values throughout a subtask in each of 12 prototypical actions (e.g., reach, sweep, idle, etc.); membership is expressed using fuzzy membership functions based on instantaneous tool tip position. We selected an example task (applying a clip) which is performed comparatively frequently (at least 6 times per procedure) and compared the characteristic measures associated with its component actions across the 35 clipping segments recorded.

2.6 Comparative Analysis (KS Statistic)

To demonstrate the reliability of the proposed analysis procedure, we must show the performance measures are comparatively unaffected by variations between patients yet sensitive to real differences such as training effects. We assess similarity by comparing distributions of performance measures obtained from multiple executions of particular subtasks in two different contexts (e.g., comparing clip application times from the first three procedures to those from the last three could reveal a learning effect). To compare distributions, we use the Kolmogorov-Smirnov (KS) statistic (d), which represents the maximum vertical difference between cumulative distribution functions (see Figure 3); this measure ranges from 0 (similar) to 1 (different). The associated p value expresses the probability that the two measured distributions arise from the same underlying distribution.

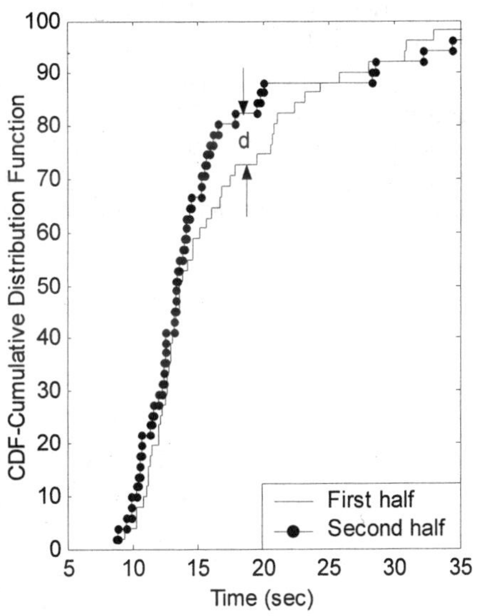

Figure 3 – Application of the Kolmogorov-Smirnov Statistic to the cumulative distribution functions of task completion times

We performed several comparative analyses related to the clip application subtask. Most commonly, clips are used in the vessel separation (CD and CA) stage of the procedure; however, they are also occasionally used to control bleeding throughout the procedure. We would expect that there would be no significant difference between performance measures taken from alternate clip applications, as both patient variability and any learning effects will be equally represented in the two data sets. Since the surgeon is fully trained, we would hope for little variation between the first four and the last three procedures studied; any differences will be primarily due to patient variability and the results will represent the reliability of our analysis procedure. Finally, we prospectively investigated several other divisions of the data set in hopes of demonstrating the existence of significant and interesting differences; for example, we considered whether there might be differences between clips applied for: vessel separation vs. control of bleeding; separating the cystic duct vs. the cystic artery; first placement vs. subsequent placement on the same vessel.

3. Results

3.1 Missing Data

A certain amount of position data is lost during the course of the surgery due to marker occlusion or internal localization errors. Figure 1(L) illustrates the marker array visibility averaged over the seven procedures multiple trials for individual markers. Using video analysis to separate manipulation from non-manipulation tasks, we found that the majority of missing data could be attributed to marker occlusions during segments not directly related to performing a surgical task (e.g. changing instruments). During tissue manipulation tasks, we had complete joint angle data 80% (SD: 10%) of the time and at least one sample per second 92% (SD: 4%) of the time. The trackability of the dominant hand tool depends on which tool is being used (we tracked the tool 78% (SD: 12%) of the time during the clipping task; 12 of the 45 tasks had no lost data and 20 successfully recorded more than 90% of the samples).

We used a generalized cross validation (GCV) filtering technique [3] to find an optimal smoothing parameter for fitting a quintic spline to position data. The data was resampled at constant intervals and missing data segments interpolated. The error associated with interpolating across varying gap sizes was calculated and shown in Figure 4. An RMS error of 1mm was chosen as an acceptable error which suggests that a maximum gap size of 0.5 sec (10 samples) can be interpolated. We were able to reduce the amount of missing joint angle data by 20% (SD: 2%) using our interpolation technique with a maximum 1mm RMS error. Using the same interpolation, we reduced the amount of missing data for the right and left hand tool data by 6% (SD: 2%) and 14% (SD: 3%) respectively.

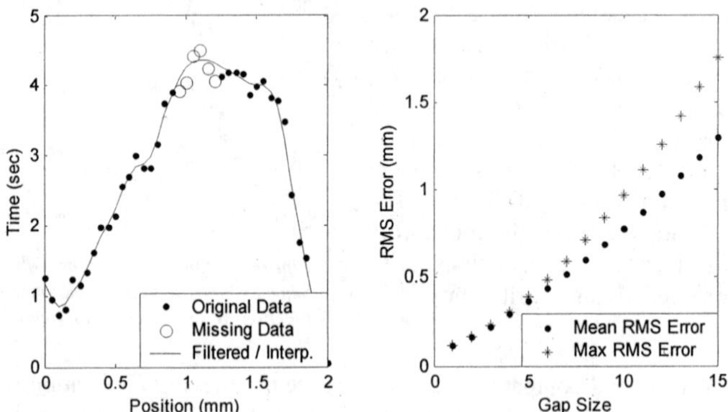

Figure 4 - *Graphical representation of missing data interpolation (L). RMS error associated with missing data gap size (R).*

3.2 Hierarchical Decomposition

The hierarchical decomposition of the procedure provides an organizational framework for the kinematic and event sequencing analysis of different surgical tasks. The decomposition design was based on the standard elements of laparoscopic cholecystectomies and was developed in consultation with two expert surgeons; the decomposition approach can be readily adapted to other laparoscopic procedures. The decomposition has five levels, each containing more specific details than the previous. The phase level (1) outlines the global goals of the procedure. The stage level (2) outlines local goals required to complete each phase. The task level (3) involves the use of a single tool. The subtask level (4) describes how the surgical tool is moving inside the patient. Finally, actions (5) describe kinematic features of stereotyped fundamental movements such as reaching or sweeping. Figure 2 shows the various levels of the hierarchical framework.

3.3 Performance Measures

Performance measures and mean action membership values were evaluated at the task and subtasks levels for the clip application task. Figure 5 Illustrates a limited collection of performance measures and their respective difference scores for clipping tasks.

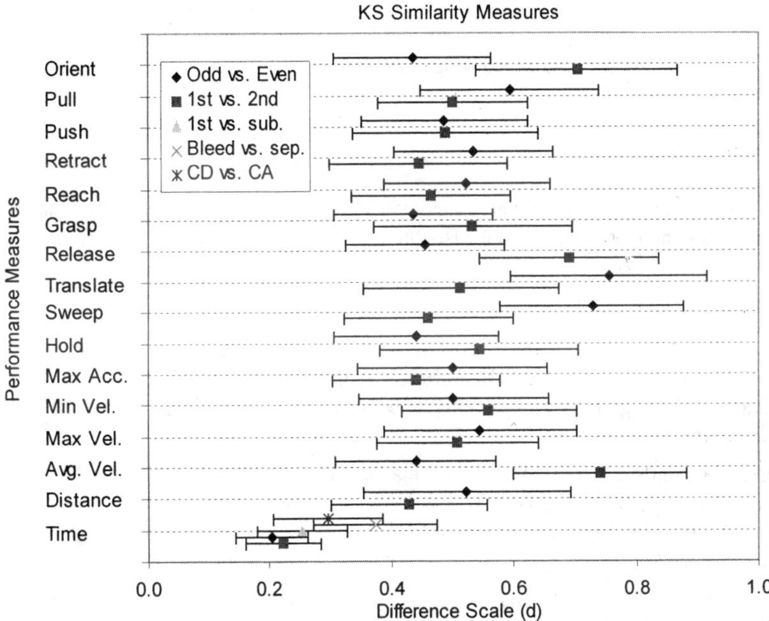

Figure 5 – Kolmogorov-Smirnov difference statistic of performance measures and mean membership action variables .

4. Discussion

We successfully recorded tool tip position 82% (SD: 22%) of the time the surgeon was performing tissue manipulation tasks and posture data at least once per second 92% (SD: 4) of the time. Using a generalized cross validation interpolation technique, we were able to interpolate one second gaps with estimated RMS errors less than 0.64 mm. Using the KS statistic the small difference between the time measures in the odd and even trials and 1st half / 2nd half trials suggests there are no obvious learning effects and no significant effect of patient variability. This is confirmed by the kinematic measures, although the difference measures are higher in large part because of the limited sample size. In addition, there appears to a significant difference between clips applied to control bleeding and clips applied for vessel separation.

5. Conclusion

We used an automated high-frequency tool tracking and postural measurement system to identify kinematic features of specific surgical actions of laparoscopic cholecystectomies as defined in a hierarchical decomposition diagram. The results demonstrate that an optoelectronic and video motion analysis, particularly in conjunction with a missing data interpolation technique, is a reasonable method for recording kinematic data in the operating room, despite occasional periods of missing data. Additional data is required to decrease the confidence intervals of the reported difference measures. The comparisons of distributions of those performance characteristics of surgical actions which we evaluated show consistent performance over time by a trained surgeon, and so are likely reliable measures of performance. An expanded set of reliable kinematic measures and data will form the basis for quantifying surgical skill and should be useful in validating surgical simulations for use in training, certifying surgeons and designing and evaluating new surgical tools.

6. Acknowledgements

We thank the operating room staff at Vancouver Hospital and Health Sciences Center for their cooperation and assistance. We also thank the Natural Sciences and Engineering Research Council of Canada (NSERC).

7. References

[1] Rosser JC, Rosser LE. Savalgi RS. (1998). Objective Evaluation of a Laparoscopic Surgical Skill Program for Residents and Senior Surgeons. Archives of Surgery. 133(2):657-661.

[2] Rosen J., Hannaford B., Richards C.G. Sinanan M.N., Markov Modeling of Minimally Invasive Surgery Based on Tool/Tissue Interaction and Force/Torque Signatures for Evaluating Surgical Skill, IEEE Transactions on Biomedical Engineering, 2001, Vol. 48, No. 5, 579-91.

[3] Woltring H.J., A Fortran Package for Generalized, Cross-validatory Spline Smoothing and Differentiation., Advances in Engineering Software, 1986, Vol. 8, No. 2, 142-51.

Anesthesiology Point of Care Project

John S. McDonald, M.D.
Carl R. Noback, M.D.
Drew Cheng, M.D.
T.K. Lee, M.D.
Val Nenov, PhD.

Department of Anesthesiology, Harbor-UCLA Medical Center
Department of Neurosurgery, UCLA Medical Center

We are developing a dynamic prototype visual communication system for the operating room environs. This has classically been viewed as an isolated and impenetrable workplace. All medical experiences and all teaching remain in a one to one closed loop with no recall or subsequent sharing for the training and education of other colleagues. The "Anesthesia Point of Care" (APOC) concept embraces the sharing of, recording of, and presentation of various physiological and pharmacological events so that real time memory can be shared at a later time for the edification of other colleagues who were not present at the time of the primary learning event. In addition it also provides a remarkably rapid tool for fellow faculty to respond to obvious stress and crisis events that can be broadcast instantly at the time of happening. Finally, it also serves as an efficient and effective means of paging and general communication throughout the daily routines among various healthcare providers in anesthesiology who work as a team unit; these include the staff, residents, CRNAs, physician assistants, and technicians. This system offers a unique opportunity to eventually develop future advanced ideas that can include training exercises, presurgical evaluations, surgical scheduling and improvements in efficiency based upon earlier than expected case completion or conversely later than expected case completion and even as a unique window to development of improved billing itemization and coordination.

1. Introduction

The department of anesthesiology of Harbor-UCLA Medical Center believes that acquisition and database storage of certain pertinent physiological and medical data may be a crucial part of effective and smooth management of patients in the operating room environment of a busy academic training center hospital. This environment has been viewed as relatively hostile from the viewpoint of capture, presentation, and movement of data. This is due to its relative isolation, i.e. operating rooms are usually located on one of the ground floors, often encased in solid concrete and sometimes lead walls. The "point of care" project uses a basic interactive platform (PDAs) to capture, view, and move information of physiological status on patients in the operative area, the preparation area, and the recovery area. Certain pertinent data that guides the anesthetic course such as blood pressure, heart rate, and saturation values plotted against a time coordinate are the current values shared. The sharing of this data for the first time will allow viewing from many different vantage points other than just the one where the data is being generated. This can allow one faculty who may be responsible for a given room to view the progress and actively interact with the resident physician who is managing the case in situ by first viewing the active data and then by contact with the resident by quick memo formats that can be received and viewed seconds after being generated. Since the data will be sampled intermittently by the central server for storage, this will also provide a storage source for later retrieval. The latter is important because that information can be used in a multitude of training or teaching scenarios post ipso facto.

2. Purpose

Over the entire teaching history of anesthesiology the experience has been a single one that is isolated in a single room with a single resident monitored by a single staff physician. Furthermore, no other staff or residents have any idea what has transpired in that room due to its isolation by geography and location. Teaching experiences are shared only on a weekly basis at scheduled case management sessions where the "mistakes" or difficult to manage cases are discussed. This is an excellent teaching and learning experience but it is not augmented by any "real time" data for supplemental information and accuracy. In addition, physicians are not inclined to ask for help in crisis situations that may occur in a spontaneous, instantaneous, and unexpected manner; thus, there may be times when extra staff help could be not only an appreciated effort but also a lifesaving one for the patient.

3. Methods

Client/Server Hardware

The Intel CPU based server, running a Microsoft Windows operating system, is located centrally within the operating suite. Each active anesthetizing location is connected to the central server through a standard Ethernet wired network.

All faculty staff, residents, and CRNAs have individual personal digital assistants (PDAs) that are identical and networked to the server via a 802.11b standard wireless Ethernet network. All participants will complete initial questionnaire forms that will identify their position in relation to use of such equipment. The system as designed has multiple nodes placed throughout the hospital as not all anesthetizing locations are within the operating room module.

Data Recording

While multiple systems exist for recording intra-operative anesthetic data, this is the first system to combine at least nine operating room vital signs/variables. In addition to the standard measurement of heart rate, systolic and diastolic blood pressure, and plethysmographic oxygen saturation, this system collects and stores data on end-tidal CO_2 and anesthetic agent identification and concentration, EKG waveform with ST segment analysis, neuromuscular function (train-of-four and percentage of depression), and the bispectral index (BIS – a process EEG which correlates with anesthetic depth/hypnosis). The data is available for real-time viewing by the appropriately authorized party as well as for later analysis in chart review, quality improvement, critical event analysis, and research.

Security

Security and integrity of data transmissions and confidentiality of patient data are the most critical issues to the use of wireless technologies in health care. The US government has sought to address security and privacy issues regarding the use of information technology and telecommunications in the health sector through legislation under the Health Insurance Portability and Accountability Act (HIPAA). The HIPAA regulations cover all administrative transactions, medical data transfers, and all formats of data transfer including electronic and written, and apply to all organizations, providers and third parties with access to personal health information (PHI). We are taking steps to ensure compliance with HIPAA standards.

HIPAA's stringent security requirements provide the IT architecture necessary to protect PHI. In the same manner, the privacy rules clearly outline procedures and conditions for obtaining and disclosing PHI, and patient rights with regard to the information. Since HIPAA rules are technology neutral, the security and privacy standards apply equally to wired and wireless systems; we do not anticipate separate legislation specific to mobile communications in health care.

Data Utilization

The anesthesiology faculty is able to observe the data regarding the care of a patient at the bedside as well as at remote locations. This allows the faculty more effective interchange of instruction with trainees by utilizing instant messaging to instruct residents and CRNAs in clinical actions to be taken as the conditions as documented by the data flow to the PDA warrant. Earlier interventions in response to clinical events are therefore possible because the transit time of the human body from one location to the next is eliminated. Faculty, for instance, may be teaching in one room while simultaneously observing the care and clinical situation of a patient in a remote location. In addition to the direct benefits in facilitating patient care, there are benefits in terms of data collection and recovery for quality improvement analysis, billing of goods and supplies, and billing of professional services. With this system there is easy documentation with compliance with HICFA supervisory requirements. Attribution and utilization of controlled substances can also be more effectively tracked to prevent misutilization and possible diversion. Retrospective clinical research can be swiftly and efficiently performed utilizing a central repository of data as opposed to manual search of individual patient charts.

4. Discussion

All system users complete follow-up forms on a regular basis to plot their experience and impression of this method of following and managing a patient. Problems in use of the equipment and its addition to clinical management will be carefully assessed after all the data is collected. We anticipate completing some 500-1,000 cases during this years project, i.e., the July 1, 2001 to June 30, 2002 academic year. Interval analyses are performed every 500 cases or when accumulation of sentinel events dictates.

An ongoing statistical analysis of the function of the system is an integral part of the process. Specific attention will be paid to the cost effectiveness of the system as measured by statistical and quality-of-care analysis. An APOC system such as this is certainly within reasonable fiscal reach for many academic centers, but only time will tell if such a system is really cost effective and worthy of the time and effort necessary to keep it going.

This project may well set a new standard in patient data recording, monitoring, and management in the specialty of Anesthesiology. The APOC system may become standard of care for anesthesia delivery.

5. References

Metnitz, P.G. and K. Lenz, *Patient data management systems in intensive care--the situation in Europe.* Intensive Care Med, 1995. **21**(9): p. 703-15.

Metnitz, P.G., et al., *Computer assisted data analysis in intensive care: the ICDEV project-- development of a scientific database system for intensive care (Intensive Care Data Evaluation Project).* Int J Clin Monit Comput, 1995. **12**(3): p. 147-59.

Nenov, V., T. Atanassov, and J. Klopp. *Take a Java Break: Critical Care Trending in the Web Age.* in *Medicine Meets Virtual Reality V.* 1997. San Diego, CA.

Pangalos, G.J., *Medical database security policies.* Methods Inf Med, 1993. **32**(5): p. 349-56; discussion 357.

Gagliano, D., *Wireless ambulance telemedicine may lessen stroke morbidity.* Telemed Today, 1998. **6**(1): p. 22.

Kops, S.R., *The Health Insurance Portability and Accountability Act of 1996 (P.L. 104-191).* Benefits Q, 1997. **13**(2): p. 8-13.

Medicine Meets Virtual Reality 02/10
J.D. Westwood et al. (Eds.)
IOS Press, 2002

CT, MRI and Video Based Analysis of Knee Kinematics - A Basis for CT based Simulation

*Dietmar Meister, **Peter Heinze, *Martin Gonser, *Rudolf Kober, **Heinz Wörn
*URS Ortho GmbH & Co. KG, Kehler Str. 31, D-76437 Rastatt, Germany
**University of Karlsruhe (TH), Institute for Process Control and Robotics,
Kaiserstraße 12, D-76128 Karlsruhe, Germany*

Abstract. With the new computer aided surgery techniques a surgery can be split in two phases, which are pre-operative planning and intervention. The planning is frequently based on three dimensional image data and takes place in the office of the surgeon. Using this approach the surgical feeling, the physical feedback of the patient, is not available during the planning phase. However, this feedback yields information, which is helpful or necessary for the planning. This lack of information can be compensated by a simulation module, which simulates kinematic data from image volume data. To develop such a module first both image volume data and kinematic data have to be captured from a wide range of patients. In this work a new approach for kinematic analysis of the knee is presented which yields an accuracy which is necessary for such simulation. Because the analysis has to be done for many patients the degree of invasiveness is emphasized. This contactless and non invasive approach is based on external fixations, anatomical skin markers, video sequences and computer tomograms. Position tracking of femur and tibia for any motion pattern is possible. Because the individual anatomic structures extracted from the tomogram are tracked, an analysis of any point or coordinate system can be done later using the originally captured data. This gives a new degree of freedom for analysis.

1 Introduction

In orthopaedic surgery many computer assisted planing systems are in frequent clinical use. The importance of pre-operative planning increased with these systems. As a lack of this off-line approach a direct feedback of the patient specific physical behaviour is not available. However, this information has a significant impact on the planning. In knee surgery the individual biomechanics of the lower limb is important. For the reconstruction of the anterior cruciate ligament (ACL) the knowledge of kinematic of the knee joint is necessary to determine the change in length of the implant while flexing the leg. An isometric ligament is the aim of the reconstruction. It is also important to avoid an impingement between bone and ligament. A violation of one of both constraints can yield a laxity of the joint or a rupture of the ligament. In total knee reconstruction (TKR) the aims of the surgery are a sufficient range of motion, stability of the joint and the load balanced in the right way over the prosthesis area. To get these values the geometrical relation between the involved bones is needed for the entire flexion process and not only for one position, which is captured during the computer tomogram (CT) or magnet resonance tomogram (MRT). A solution to extend the pre-operative planning with kinematic information is to simulate the movement from the image data, which is given by CT or MRT anyway. To build this simulation, a sufficient number of patient data containing the volume image data and the individual kinematic data is necessary. It is the aim of this work to develop a new approach for kinematic recording and analysis, which is suitable to gain the data needed for the simulation model.

In the past several approaches have been developed to analyze the kinematics of the lower limb [1]. A feature to classify these methods is the degree of invasiveness. The first group of methods uses markers fixed to each bone [2]. Another possibility to estimate the bone positions is to use radiographs, either with stereo radiography (RSA) [3] or with planar radiographs [4]. Because all these approaches are more or less invasive they are not suitable for this study. There are other approaches using optical or magnetic markers which are either glued to the skin [5] or mounted on a fixation unit, which is clamped externally to skin and bone [6, 7]. For these approaches the error in estimation of the bone positions is more than 4 mm [7, 8] and therefore the level of accuracy is to low for this study. The last technique for motion capture comes from computer animation and virtual reality. It uses video sequences from one or more views and fits skeletal models to entire persons or body parts [9]. However, this technique yields an error measure which is much higher than the other approaches.

2 Materials and methods

In this work a new approach for kinematic analysis of the lower limb should be presented, which can be used to examine about 100 patients. The procedure combines the advantages of skin mounted markers, external fixation units, video sequence analysis and CT/MRT volumes, in order to estimate the movement of the tibia relative to the femur with an error of less than 4 mm.

2.1 Individual anatomy

In this study the MRT is used because it enables a tuning of the scanning parameters which is necessary to identify cortical bone, cartilages and ligaments in a single image volume. In CT volumes the identification of the cartilages is not possible though these structures are important for the kinematics. We use a 1.5 T scanner (Magnetom Harmony (TM), Siemens AG) and capture 6 turbo-spin-echo sequences with emphasis on proton density (T_R=3205 ms, T_E=14 ms). Each sequence consists of images using a 256x256 matrix. The read direction is anterior to posterior. The scanning starts with the leg in extension capturing a transversal series (S_1) and a sagittal series (S_2) from the knee area. The slice distance (SD) and slice thickness (ST) is 3 mm and the field of view (FOV) was 200 mm. In order to define the mechanical axis of the leg the hip center (S_3) and the ankle center (S_4) is scanned with transversal orientation (SD=10 mm, ST=5 mm). To estimate the relative bone positions in flexion two further series of the knee are captured flexing it about 20° (S_5) respectively 40° (S_6) using the parameters T_R=301 ms, SD=3 mm, ST=6 mm. Because the signal-noise ratio limits ST and SD to 3 mm the resolution of the image volume in proximal-distal direction is not sufficient for 3D segmentation of the gliding surfaces at the knee. To increase this resolution the series S_1 and S_2 were combined to a new image volume which had a voxel size of 0.8 mm.

The segmentation of cortical bone and cartilage in S_1 to S_4 is done manually with an editor for medical volume data sets (Analyze (TM), AnalyzeDirect Inc.). For further processing the segmented image volumes are triangulated. To estimate the bone position in the flexed positions S_5 and S_6 the retrieved triangulated surfaces of femur, tibia and patella are transformed

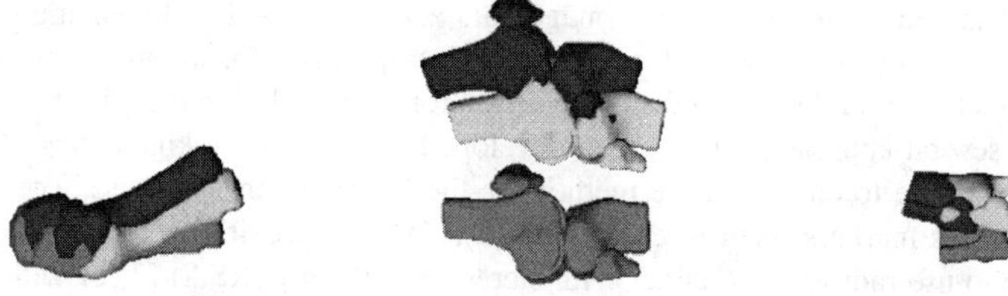

Figure 1: Femur, tibia and patella in 3 flexions

to the bone structures of the image volumes using a surface-volume-matching. The resulting surface models in 3 different flexions can be seen in figure 1.

2.2 Motion capture using marker tracking

To reduce the skin-bone shift during flexion 2 belts are strapped to each segment of the leg. To each belt 2 reflective balls are mounted. These balls can be tracked by the 3D camera system (Polaris (TM), Northern Digital Inc.). Additionally reflective discs are glued to the skin in order to mark some anatomical landmarks (trochanter major, femur epicondyle, fibula head, distal fibula). Over all 12 markers are fixed to the leg. In a first step a single capture of the extended leg is done. In this scene all markers are manually identified ($\vec{P}_{Ref}$). Using the relation between all markers and their anatomical position the coordinate system of the MRT can manually transformed to the camera coordinate system.

For the different motion sequences the position of all visible markers is determined with a frame rate of 20 Hz. Because of the skin shift the relation between the markers of a single leg segment changes. Therefore the position estimation of a segment using a rigid matching is not possible. Some basic constraints from biomechanics are applied, which identify each marker even if not all markers are visible. In the next step the transformation for femur and tibia has to be determined. A frequently used technique uses a rigid matching for each segment where the involved markers have individual weights. For large flexion angles with a high degree of segment distortion this method yields an error of several millimeters. At this step the flexion positions gained from the MRT are useful. They are used as key-frames for the flexion process. For these frames both the anatomically correct transformation from the MRT $\vec{K}$ and the in real-time measured marker positions including skin-bone shift $\vec{P}_{Flex}$ are known. With these values for each key-frame k and each marker m an offset value $\vec{C}_{k,m}$ can be estimated.

$$\vec{C}_{k,m} = \vec{K}_k * \vec{P}_{Ref,m} - \vec{P}_{Flex,m} \qquad (1)$$

Using an adequate interpolation between the three key-frames an offset value for each flexion angle and each marker can be estimated. With this offset applied to each marker a rigid matching as described in [10] is possible. In figure 2 the coordinates of some markers with and without the correcting offset are given.

2.3 Video overlay

In the gait analysis laboratory 4 video cameras are used additionally to the 3D camera system. These cameras capture the scene with 50 Hz from different view points. To render the bones

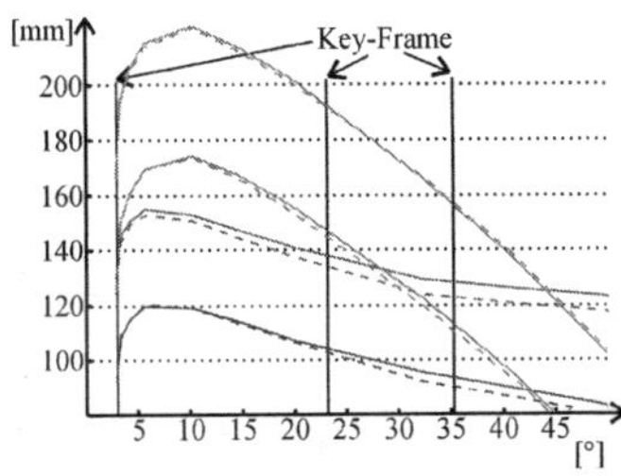

Figure 2: Key-frame based correction of the marker positions

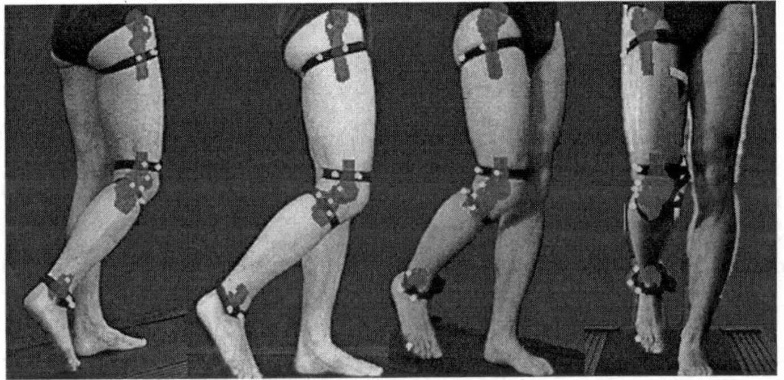

Figure 3: Overlay of bones and markers over video sequences

into the video sequences, it is necessary to know the projection function. This function transforms a point from the 3D camera system (world coordinate system) $\vec{P}_w$ into a point inside the video bitmap $\vec{P}_b$. As projection model for the video cameras a ideal pin-hole camera is assumed. The transformation defined by this model can be described by a $4{\times}4$ matrix $\mathbf{A}$.

$$\vec{P}_b = \mathbf{A} * \vec{P}_w = \mathbf{C} * \mathbf{S} * \mathbf{P} * \mathbf{T} * \mathbf{R} * \vec{P}_w \tag{2}$$

The intrinsic camera parameters as center of the bitmap, scale and perspective projection (focal length) are described by the matrices $\mathbf{C}$, $\mathbf{S}$ and $\mathbf{P}$. The extrinsic camera parameters as translation and rotation which define the position of the camera are coded in the matrices $\mathbf{T}$ and $\mathbf{R}$. To estimate the 10 independent parameters composing matrix $\mathbf{A}$ a set of calibration points is used, which can be identified in the bitmap of the video sequence and in the 3D camera system. The optimization process, which yields the 10 parameters, is described in [11]. For each video camera 40 calibration points are used. The points are spread over the entire volume of interest. The projection error was 0.4 mm $\pm$ 0.2 mm. Additionally to this spatial calibration the video sequences have to be synchronized to the capture of the 3D camera. This is done with oscillating markers, which can be identified in both modalities. In figure 3 a snapshot from a walking pattern can be seen from all 4 video cameras. Femur, tibia and the markers are rendered into each video bitmap.

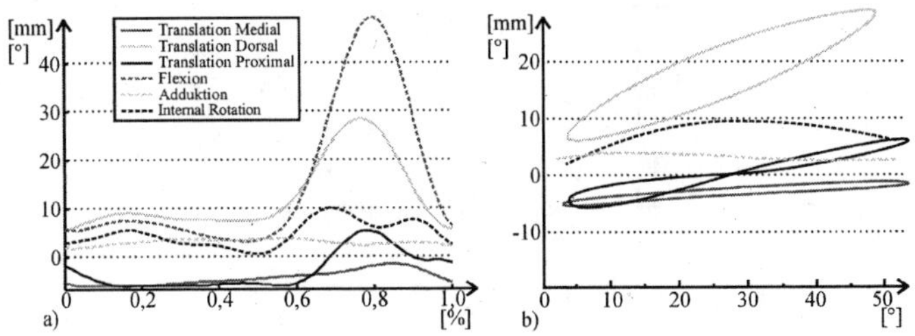

Figure 4: Position of tibia coordinate system relative to femur coordinate system over gait cycle (a) and knee flexion angle (b)

3   Results

For one patient several motion patterns as standing up from a chair, walking, running, flexing the knee or cycling were captured and analyzed. An important result is the position of tibia relative to femur for the entire motion. For a better analysis of the resulting transformation matrix first an individual coordinate system was applied to femur and tibia according to the guidelines from the CASPAR(TM) system (URS Ortho GmbH) for TKR. Several motion cycles were captured, normalized and compressed to a mean cycle. The maximum of the standard deviation was 1,6 mm for the translation components and 3,2° for the rotation components. In figure 4a the translation and rotation components of the tibia over the normalized gait cycle are given. The gait cycle starts and ends with the heel strike. In figure 4b the transformation components are given over the flexion angle. Here the maximum of the tibial internal rotation of about 10° can be seen at 25° flexion. The dorsal translation shows a hysteresis of about 10 mm using the values from start and end of the swing phase.

4   Discussion

A new approach for kinematic recording and analysis of the knee joint, which is based on MRT data, optical marker tracking and video overlay, was presented. One patient was examined and analyzed. The error for the repeatability was less than 2 mm and 4° and the optical check of the bones rendered to the video images was successful. A major advantage of this volume image based approach is the possibility to define all coordinate systems and landmarks in the volume data. This is more precise than using only some landmarks which can be seen on the skin. Using this approach the position of the coordinate systems can be defined after the motion capture, which enables an optimization for these positions.
The proposed procedure can be improved in several ways. One way is to use an additional distortion for the camera model, which models the lens of the video camera. This will reduce the error for projecting the bones into the video images. The presented error for repeatability was estimated from a set of cycles which were just overlaid. This does not take into account the change of the walking velocity and the amplitude. A better normalization of each gait cycle would yield a more realistic value for the repeatability. A further improvement of accuracy can be achieved if the overlaid video sequences are not only used for plausibility. A corrective measure could use the error determined from the overlaid images. For a better automatic procedure a simple model consisting of muscle, fat, and skin extracted from the MRT

could be used. In order to extract further information from the motion capture the trajectory of the patella could be estimated. Its position at fixed flexion angles is already given in the key-frame MRTs. For interpolation the position of the patella could be tracked in the video images. This should be possible, because it is not covered with thick tissue layers.

The presented approach can be used as the basis to examine many patients in the way which is needed to build a model for CT based simulation of knee kinematics.

References

[1] Andriacchi, T.P., Alexander, E.J.: Studies of human locomotion: past, present and future. Journal of Biomechanics **33** (2000) 1217–1224

[2] La Fortune, M.A., Cavanagh, P.R., Sommer, H.J., Kalenak, A.: Three dimensional kinematics of the human knee during walking. Journal of Biomechanics **25** (1992) 347–357

[3] Jonsson, K., Karrholm, J.: Three-dimensional knee joint movements during a step-up: evaluation after cruciate ligament rupture. Journal of Orthopedic Research **12** (1994) 769–779

[4] Banks, S.A., Hodge, W.A.: Accurate measurement of three-dimensional knee replacement kinematics using single-plane fluoroscopy. IEEE Transactions on Biomedical Engineering **46** (1996) 638–649

[5] Lu, T.W., O'Connor, J.J.: Bone position estimation from skin marker co-ordinates using global optimization with joint constrains. Journal of Biomechanics **32** (1999) 129–134

[6] Sati, M., de Guise, J.A., Larouche, S., Drouin, G.: Improving in vivo knee kinematic measurements: application to prosthetic ligament analysis. The Knee **3** (1996) 179–190

[7] Ganjika, S., Duval, N., Yahia, L'H., de Guise, J.: Three-dimensional knee analyzer validation by simple fluoroscopic study. The Knee **7** (2000) 221–231

[8] Cappozzo, A., Catani, F., Leardini, A., Benedetti, M.G., Della Groce, U.: Position and orientation in space of bones during movement: experimental artefacts. Clinical Biomechanics **11** (1996) 90–100

[9] Lugné, P.C., Alizon, J., Collange, F., Van Praagh, E.: Motion analysis of an articulated locomotion model by video and telemetric data. Journal of Biomechanics **32** (1999) 977–981

[10] Veldpaus, F.E., Woltring, H.J., Dortmans, L.J.M.G.: A least squares algorithm for the equiform transformation from spatial marker co-ordinates. Journal of Biomechanics **21** (1988) 45–54

[11] Heikkilä, J.: Geometric camera calibration using circular control points. IEEE Transactions on Pattern Analysis and Machine Intelligence **22** (2000) 1066–1077

Medicine Meets Virtual Reality 02/10
J.D. Westwood et al. (Eds.)
IOS Press, 2002

Spring: A General Framework for Collaborative, Real-time Surgical Simulation

Kevin Montgomery, Cynthia Bruyns, Joel Brown, Stephen Sorkin, Frederic Mazzella,
Guillaume Thonier, Arnaud Tellier, Benjamin Lerman, Anil Menon
National Biocomputation Center, 701A Welch Rd, Suite 1128 Stanford, CA 94305

Abstract: We describe the implementation details of a real-time surgical simulation system with soft-tissue modeling and multi-user, multi-instrument, networked haptics. The simulator is cross-platform and runs on various Unix and Windows platforms. It is written in C++ with OpenGL for graphics; GLUT, GLUI, and MUI for user interface; and supports parallel processing. It allows for the relatively easy introduction of patient-specific anatomy and supports many common file formats. It performs soft-tissue modeling, some limited rigid-body dynamics, and suture modeling. The simulator interfaces to many different interaction devices and provides for multi-user, multi-instrument collaboration over the Internet. Many virtual tools have been created and their interactions with tissue have been implemented. In addition, a number of extra features, such as voice input/output, real-time texture-mapped video input, stereo and head-mounted display support, and replicated display facilities are presented.

1. Introduction

The benefits of computer-based surgical simulation have been widely discussed and quantitatively demonstrated by many researchers[1]. The benefits include the ability to broaden surgical training by easily providing different training scenarios, including anatomical variations (gender, size), pathologies (diseases, trauma), and operating environment conditions (emergency room, microgravity, battlefield). In addition to these benefits, the ability to objectively quantify surgical performance[2] and perhaps simulate the result of an intervention has been cited as a major benefit and drawn the attention of surgical societies as a future means of precertification. Besides these benefits, the potential to accelerate the acquisition of baseline surgical skills through the use of computer-based simulation has also been identified[3]. Perhaps the most important feature of all is that computer-based simulation can realize all these benefits without risk to any real patients.

Because of these benefits, many research groups in academia, government, and industry have been developing simulators for some time[4-13]. Each group must instill the clinical knowledge of the surgeon through the engineering technology of the computer scientist in order to realize a working and usable system. However, the technical knowledge required to produce such a simulator spans many subdisciplines including graphics, algorithm design, numerical integration methods, collision detection, networking, user interface design, and mechanical engineering. Replicating this wide breadth of technical knowledge is difficult and, for many clinical groups, represents an insurmountable obstacle to the production of a complete, functioning, useful simulator. Moreover, within other groups with broad engineering skills, achieving expertise in each of the areas required and developing their own software for each of these tasks can also increase costs and the time before the realization of a working simulator.

If the surgical simulation community instead had a common framework of shared code, then the time to realization of a working simulator would be shortened, and the barrier to entry for clinical groups of more limited engineering resources would be lessened. In essence, the entire surgical simulation community would work together on a common platform, sharing their individual expertise, and thereby accelerate the production, and ultimately adoption, of computer-based surgical simulators.

However, the challenges of building one simulator that could be used for many applications are great. Such a simulator would run the risk of trying to be *everything to everyone* and perhaps end up providing *nothing to anyone*. Beyond these factors, the technical challenge of producing a real-time, haptic-rate simulator is extraordinarily difficult in itself.

We have developed a surgical simulation framework named *Spring*. This evolving framework was designed to be a general simulator with a broad base of technological features and a broad range of potential applications, with the emphasis on real-time performance. During its production, we have developed a number of applications to ensure that the system is usable and useful for application. It is our goal to release this code to the surgical simulation community in open source form to, at the least, provide a useful example code to compare implementation details with others. At most, we hope that other groups may use it as a common framework in which to insert their expertise and enable the sharing of all our talents with the wider community.

2. Methods

The *Spring* surgical simulator code is cross-platform and runs on Unix (Sun Solaris, SGI Irix, and Linux) and Windows (98, NT, 2000) platforms. It is written in C++ and uses OpenGL for graphics; GLUT[14], GLUI[15], and MUI[16] for user interface; and supports parallel processing using the pthreads facility of POSIX. It allows for the relatively easy introduction of patient-specific anatomy and supports many common file formats, including SMF[17], Wavefront OBJ, VRML, Mesh, and Cyberware formats. It performs soft-tissue modeling[18], some limited rigid-body dynamics, and suture modeling[18]. The simulator interfaces to many different interaction devices and provides for multi-user, multi-instrument collaboration over the Internet in latency-dependent or latency-moderated modes. Many surgical and non-surgical virtual tools have been created and their interactions with tissue have been implemented. Collision detection is provided through an enhanced[19] bounding-sphere algorithm[20]. In addition, extra features such as voice input/output, real-time texture-mapped video input, stereo and head-mounted display support, and replicated display facilities are implemented.

2.1 Architecture

An overview of the architecture is provided in Figure 1. It consists of a main program (Spring), an object representation structure (ObjectArray class, with individual Objects comprising arrays of Nodes (vertices), Edges (springs), Faces (triangles), and Tetra (tetrahedral) elements that are cross-linked), an abstraction of tracking/haptic devices (Sensor class) with the individual interface subclasses including networked devices, a collision detection subsystem (BoundingSphere), and other features (Voice I/O, DisplayReplicator, etc).

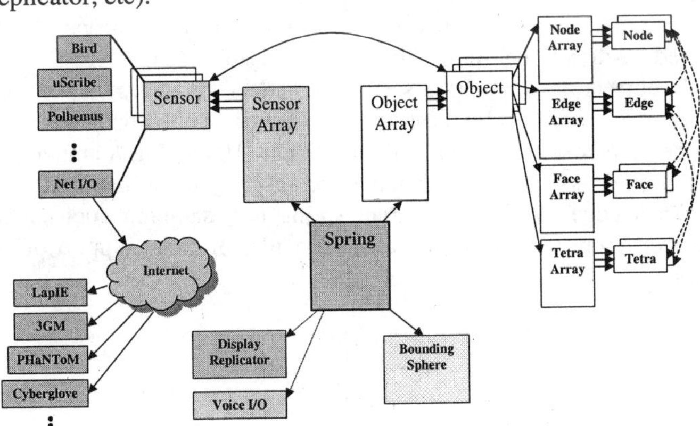

2.2 Main Program

The main program (Spring) contains code for interfacing to the operating system (through GLUT, GLUI, MUI, Posix) and contains callback functions for keyboard, mouse, and other input. In addition, it contains the main display and simulation functions and all menu creation routines. Finally, it also has the ability to create objects and interface to the (optional) voice I/O and DisplayReplication subsystems. In essence, it contains the main thread(s) of control, data structures, and interface routines.

2.3 Anatomy Acquisition

Anatomy can be introduced from many sources and is provided by reading in world description files, containing lists of objects and their attributes. These data could be acquired from serial-section, volumetric (CT, MR), or surface scans (Cyberware), segmented using any tools[21], followed by mesh generation and reduction (Qslim[17], or others). Once the geometry is built using these tools, the world description file is produced, which allows one to specify all the individual objects in the world to be created, as well as their attributes. The attributes for each object consist of the geometry information itself, graphical attributes (textures, material properties, etc), simulation properties (dynamics, numerical method, spring constants, etc), collision detection and resolution attributes (detection method, faces to consider, etc), and other attributes. In this way, a single file can be used to set all parameters for a particular simulation and points to other files, in standard, industry-wide formats (where available), for the individual information.

2.4 Object Representation

The world description information is used to create objects with the given properties. Each object contains attributes as listed above and also contains arrays of Nodes, Edges, Faces, and Tetras. Note that, for a particular object, it may not contain all of these elements. Blood could be modeled as a particle system and represented as an object consisting only of Nodes. A suture is modeled as an object with only Nodes and Edges. Most 3D objects can be modeled with Nodes, Edges, and Faces, while Tetras are presently only required for some forms of cutting and volume preservation. An extrusion algorithm is also implemented to provide some 3D structural dynamics from a surface-only mesh.

2.5 Simulation Core

The core simulation code within each object processes the dynamics of each object (deformable, rigid-body, or suture dynamics) at every simulation timestep. Providing rigid-body kinematics within a dynamic solver is an open area of research, therefore limited support is currently provided. Suture dynamics are modeled by considering the suture to be comprised of short, linear segments (edges), forming an articulating object. This articulating object has constraints imposed by its contact with other objects (virtual instruments, tissue, other points of collision) and computes the locations of intermediate nodes as a weighted, bi-directional follow-the-leader algorithm[18].

For deformable objects the simulation system considers the nodes as point masses and edges as spring/dampers to form a 3D mesh for mass-spring simulation. These edges can be considered as linear, piece-wise linear, or non-linear 1D springs/dampers. While we currently do not provide support for torsional springs[22], their introduction would be straightforward. Each edge can have different spring and damping coefficients and the nodes can provide different mass distributions to provide for some support of anisotropic, heterogeneous tissues.

For deformable objects, a number of numerical methods have been implemented. The traditional Euler and Runge-Kutta (2nd and 4th order) have been implemented. In addition, a quasi-static method, appropriate for heavily damped tissues and low interaction velocities, assumes the tissue to always be in static equilibrium and ignores dynamic inertial and damping forces for a corresponding increase in simulation performance. Other simulation methods are also under development. Relative performance numbers for each method is given in Table 1.

Numerical Method	Node updates per second	Edge updates per second
Euler	178,000	530,000
Runge-Kutta 2nd order	97,000	288,000
Runge-Kutta 4th order	46,000	136,000
Quasistatic	220,000	651,000

Table 1: Performance of Numerical Integration Techniques (5000 node, 15000 edge, 10000 face object)

An open area of research in soft tissue deformation concerns taking as large an integration step size as possible[23], while maintaining stability of the numerical method. To address this issue, we have produced an antidivergence feature that, when numerical divergence is detected, continues to halve the step size of the numerical method until stability is acheived. While this violates the time-accurate goal of the simulation, it was judged more important to maintain stability under such degenerate conditions.

Other features include tracking the region of deformation and only processing within this region in order to provide a significant (possibly order of magnitude) increase in performance[18]. This is accomplished by breadth-first ordering the nodes from a point of interaction into levels, processing the nodes in this level-based order, then ceasing computation when a level has no nodes that move more than a threshold. These regions may increase to include other levels as the deformation increases, or decrease in size as the nodes of the object at a particular level return to rest.

This scheme allows for many objects, each with large geometries, to be on the screen with high resolution graphical display, while the simulation is only processing what is needed. In addition, the simulation can use the information of the extent of the deformed region for other purposes, such as to indicate to the collision detection system to update its structures for those nodes.

Volume preservation code is also provided for each object. Based on this attribute, the object can decide to disable volume preservation or perform global volume preservation (compute object volume at each timestep and induce a corresponding force on each node in the direction of its normal), or to preserve volume within the deformed region alone.

Finally, it is also possible to produce links between objects. In this way, for example, an object with deformable dynamics (skin) could be linked to an object with rigid-body kinematics (bone). This is accomplished through the use of *tie-nodes*: the skin has a node which exists in the same position as a node in the bone and the two nodes can thereby pass forces between their respective objects.

2.6 Sensors

A Sensor is an abstraction of a 6D tracking and/or haptic device. It contains a position in 3D space, along with orientation information (rotation matrix) and contains an array of floating-point activation values to store information from any buttons, handles, or other controllers associated with the device. A sensor can be linked to a particular object (typically a virtual instrument) and, when that object is updated, it will be transformed by the sensor data. In addition, the activation values can be used to specify hinge angles (for example, to indicate and display how opened or closed the scissors are) or telescoping/plunger depth (for a syringe or resectoscope handle) for the object's subparts (the subpart id is denoted by a field in each Node).

We functionally classify instruments into a number of different categories, based upon their methods of operation. Instruments are single pieced (e.g., scalpel, dilator, probe), hinged (scissors, endoscopic scissors, graspers), multihinged (3-prong grasper- where we specify each hinge's location, axis of rotation, and activation value upon which it depends), dependent-hinged (hand, multiaxis endoscopic grasper- where the location of one hinge is dependent upon another), telescoping (resectoscope, syringe- with one part that slides in relation to another), lasso (resection loop- with a part that constricts based upon the activation value) and multitools (with working channels for the insertion of tools of the kinds stated above). Note that these classifications merely define how the instrument articulates based upon its activation values. We will later discuss the interactions of these tools with other objects.

The Sensor superclass is inherited by subclasses that communicate with their individual devices. These include non-haptic devices such as electromagnetic trackers (Ascension Flock-of-Birds and pcBird, Polhemus FasTrak), inertial trackers (Intersense InterTrax), armature-based trackers (Immersion Microscribe), composite devices (Virtual Technologies/Immersion CyberGlove) or a computer mouse. Haptic devices supported include devices from Immersion (3GM, Laparoscopic Impulse Engine, Bimanual Laparoscopic Device) and SensAble Technologies (Phantom).

Because many devices can only be interfaced through methods available only on PC platforms, and due to the desire to have the simulation capable of running on the most appropriate (perhaps non-PC) hardware, the system also provides for a network-based module that communicates with a sensor or *hapticserver* program running on a different, perhaps dedicated computer over the network. In this way, we can decouple the interfacing restrictions of these devices from the simulation itself.

In either case, this method of network-based sensor- and hapticservers inherently provides for multi-user and multi-instrument interaction and supports collaborative procedures. However, when performing a collaboration at some distance, it is necessary to also replicate the display of the simulation, as described in section 2.10 below.

2.7 Collision Detection

Over time, a number of collision detection methods were implemented. First, a node-node force-sphere model was introduced. Later, static partition methods, Axis-Aligned Bounding Boxes[24], and Oriented Bounding Boxes[25] were implemented. While these methods worked well in many cases, a more general scheme that better supported deformable objects was sought. For this reason, we moved to a Bounding Sphere algorithm[20], with enhancements for deformable objects[19]. The generality of this method, and its fast update capability, provided a reasonable tradeoff for many cases. As with any hierarchical method, ultimately the detection method decomposes to testing collisions between primitive elements, such as face-face (surface collisions), edge-face (suture wrapping over vessel), edge-edge (suture wrapping onto itself), etc.

To further increase performance, a number of other enhancements were made. First, each node within the bounding sphere tree can be individually enabled. In this way, large portions of the tree can effectively be ignored when appropriate. In order to easily support this, a world description file can identify the list of faces to be used for collision detection. Moreover, objects (virtual instruments) can be created to have internal faces which are invisible to the user, but upon whom the collision detection system relies. In this way, virtual instruments can be very detailed graphically, but a dramatic decrease in the number of collision detection tests can be realized, leading to large performance increases[26]. Finally, a fast path within the collision detection subsystem was created to provide a quick rejection test for appropriate applications.

When a collision is detected, the collision detection subsystem places, in each colliding object, a collision pair list denoting the details of the collision (which primitive elements collided, the intersection point if available). In this way, the collision detection subsystem merely provides a general service of detection and enables a more general system for collision response.

2.8 Collision Resolution/Interactions

As each object is processed by the simulation and any collisions noted, each object's collision handling routine is called. A probing interaction (pick, dilator, hand) induces an instantaneous displacement of the deformable faces to resolve the collision (relying on the antidivergence algorithm to ensure stability in degenerate cases). Grasping tools (forceps, endoscopic graspers) attract nodes of the surface to the tool tip when that tool is active, with the rest of the object is processed as a probing interaction as above. Piercing (needle, syringe) subdivides the surface at the point of entry of the tool tip, with the rest of the object considered as a probing interaction (hence, the tip of the syringe is "sharp" and pierces into tissue, while the rest of the syringe merely bumps the tissue upon interaction). Cutting interactions[28] (scalpel, scissors, endoscopic scissors) have edges that are denoted as sharp. When one of these edges comes in contact with the tissue, the tissue is cut and the mesh subdivided. If a non-sharp edge or face comes in contact with the tissue, then a probing interaction is produced (the back of a scalpel can be used to probe, while the cutting edge can be used to slice the tissue). A cauterizing interaction (roller ablator, loop cautery), when active and in contact with tissue, progressively yellows, browns, then blackens the area of contact by changing the color of the contacted faces and using blended textures to achieve the desired graphical result.

In each case, the collision resolution algorithm processes each of the elements of the collision pair list, performs their interaction function, and computes the resulting haptic force of that interaction upon the tool. Then, the interaction forces are averaged to calculate the overall force vector that should be realized upon the virtual instrument.

2.9 Display

A number of display devices are supported. Traditional CRT-based displays in monoscopic or stereoscopic (using CrystalEyes or NuVision glasses) modes are supported. In addition, projection displays, such as the Immersive WorkBench (FakeSpace), as well as custom displays such as the Surgical WorkBench[29] are supported. Head-mounted displays are also supported, where user-based tracking is achieved by tying the viewing position to one of the Sensors. In this way, we can integrate user-based tracking into the environment as easily as we integrate other tracking and haptic devices. In addition, by attaching the viewing location to a sensor linked to an instrument, we can trivially obtain an endoscopic view from any given instrument

2.10 Other features

As briefly stated above, the system also supports a number of other features. Voice input and output is achieved by *Spring* connecting to a *voiceserver* computer over the network. In this way, the user can select surgical instruments by speaking their name and indicating other commands in an easy, hands-free manner.

A mechanism for replicating the display of the simulation is required for collaborative viewing. A DisplayReplicator class can, at each screen refresh, copy the data from the screen (in stereo or monoscopic modes), compress it, and send it to a remote client to view the live (possibly stereo) video imagery of the simulation at real-time rates.

In other applications, it is sometimes necessary to receive live video and texture map this video data in real-time within the environment. Therefore, Spring can also connect to a videoserver to receive live video and texture map that data live onto an object.

Finally, in surgical simulation, sometimes other senses besides vision and tactile are necessary in order to reproduce the experience of a particular surgical procedure. For this reason, limited support for audio output is also provided.

3.0 Applications

A number of applications have been developed during the production of this simulator, including a microsurgery simulator[30,31]; a clinically evaluated, haptic-rate hysteroscopy simulator[26,27] simulating cervical dilation, endometrial ablation, and resection of intrauterine polyps; an intraoperative assistance environment with an advanced system for surgical assistance with voice input and output and virtual "hanging windows" for the live display of CT data, vital signs, and live endoscopic video; a surgical simulator for rat dissection and astronaut training system[32] with hand-based interaction with objects in the virtual environment; and its use for patient-specific surgical planning[33,34]. New applications under development include a colonoscopy simulator[35], a stent placement simulator), as well as a cleft-lip surgery simulator.

4.0 Conclusion

We have sought to develop a generalized framework for surgical simulation that can support the requirements of many surgical simulation applications. The simulator has been refined and enhanced during the development of a number of applications and supports multi-instrument, generalized interactions with networked haptics within a collaborative, multi-user environment. We hope that the description presented here enhances the discussion of the technical details of simulation and leads to the greater proliferation of surgical simulation applications.

5.0 Acknowledgements

The authors would like to thank the numerous other individuals that have contributed to the production of this system. Other developers (Michael Madison, Bharath Beedu, Jeremie Roux, CJ Slyfield, Yanto Muliadi, and Tyler Kohn), together with clinical collaborators (Simon Wildermuth, Michael Stephanides, Stephen Schendel, Leroy Heinrichs, Parvati Dev) have greatly contributed to this work. In addition, other technical collaborators (Jean-Claude Latombe, Richard Boyle, and Alexander Twombly) also contributed to this effort. This work was supported by grants from NASA (NCC2-1010), NIH (NLM-3506, HD38223), NSF (IIS-9907060), and a generous donation from Sun Microsystems.

References

1.   Satava, R; "Robotics, Telepresence, and virtual reality: a Critical Analysis of the future of surgery", Minimally Invasive Therapy v1:357-363, 1992.

2.   P. Gorman, J. Lieser, W Murray, R Haluck, and T. Krummel, "Evaluation of Skill Acquisition Using a Force-Feedback, Virtual Reality-based Surgical Trainer", Medicine Meets Virtual Reality 1999, Ed: J Westwood, IOS Press, 1999, pp. 121-123.

3.   R., O'Toole, Playter, R, Krummel, T, Blank, W, Cornelius, H; Roberts, W; Bell, W; Raibert, M; "Measuring and developing suturing technique with a virtual reality surgical simulator", J. Amer Coll Surgeons, v189(1), 1999, pp 114-127.

4. D. Baraff and A. Witkin. Dynamic simulation of nonpenetrating flexible bodies. *Computer Graphics*, 26(2):303– 308, 1992.

5. E. Keeve, S. Girod, and B. Girod. Craniofacial surgery simulation. In *Proceedings of the 4th International Conference on Visualization in Biomedical Computing (VBC '96)*, pages 541–546, Sept. 1996.

6. U. G. K¨uhnapfel, H. K. C¸ akmak, and H. Maaß. Endoscopic surgery training using virtual reality and deformable tissue simulation. *Computers & Graphics*, 24:671–682, 2000.

7. G. Picinbono, H. Delingette, and N. Ayache. Non-linear and anisotropic elastic soft tissue models for medical simulation. In *Proceedings of the IEEE International Conference on Robotics and Automation*, May 2001.

8. D. Terzopoulos and K.Waters. Physically-based facial modelling, analysis, and animation. *The Journal of Visualization and Computer Animation*, 1:73–80, 1990.

9. N. Ayache, S. Cotin, and H. Delingette. Surgery Simulation with Visual and Haptic Feedback. In *Robotics Research*, Springer, 1998, pp. 311-316.

10. J. Berkley, S. Weghorst, H. Gladstone, G. Raugi, D. Berg, and M. Ganter. Fast Finite Element Modeling for Surgical Simulation. *Proc. Medicine Meets Virtual Reality (MMVR'99)*, ISO Press, 1999, pp. 55- 61.

11. C. Bosdogan, C. Ho, M.A. Srinivasan, S.D. Small, and S.L. Dawson. Force Interaction in Laparoscopic Simulation: Haptics Rendering of Soft Tissues. *Proc. Medicine Meets Virtual reality (MMVR'98)*, Jan. 1998, pp. 28-31.

12. M. Bro-Nielsen and S. Cotin. Real-Time Volumetric Deformable Models for Surgery Simulation Using Finite Elements and Condensation. *Proc. Eurographics'96*, Vol. 15, 1996, pp. 57-66.

13. G. Szekely; M. Bajka; C. Brechbuhler; J. Dual; R. Enzler; U. Haller; J. Hug; R. Hutter, N. Ironmonger; M Kauer; V. Meier; P. Niederer; A. Rhomberg, P. Schmid; G. Schweitzer; M. Thaler; V. Vuskovic; G. Troster; "Virtual Reality-Based Surgery Simulation for Endoscopic Gynecology", *Proc. Medicine Meets Virtual reality (MMVR'99)*, Jan. 1999, pp. 351-357.

14. N. Robins, GL Utility Toolkit (GLUT)- http://www.opengl.org/developers/documentation/glut

15. P. Rademacher, GL User Interface (GLUI) Library- http://www.cs.unc.edu/~rademach/glui

16. T. Davis, Micro User Interface (MUI) library- http://www.opengl.org/developers/code/mjktips/mui

17. M. Garland and P. Heckbert, "Surface Simplification Using Quadratic Error Metrics", In *ACM SIGGRAPH 97 Conference Proceedings*, pages 43–52, 1997.

18. Brown, J; Sorkin, S; Bruyns, C; Latombe, JC, Montgomery, K; Stephanides, M; "Real-Time Simulation of Deformable Objects: Tools and Application", Computer Animation 2001, Seoul, Korea, November 6-8, 2001.

19. Sorkin, S; "Distance Computation Between Deformable Objects", Honors Thesis, Computer Science Department, Stanford University, June 2000.

20. Quinlan, S, "Efficient Distance Computation Between Nonconvex Objects", Proc. IEEE Int Conf on Robotics and Automation, pp. 3324-3329, 1994.

21. 3D Reconstruction Web Site: http://biocomp.stanford.edu/3dreconstruction

22. H. Delingette. Towards realistic soft tissue modeling in medical simulation. In *Proceedings of the IEEE : Special Issue on Surgery Simulation*, pages 512–523, Apr. 1998.

23. D. Baraff and A. Witkin. Large steps in cloth simulation. In *ACM SIGGRAPH 98 Conference Proceedings*, pages 43–52, 1998.

24. G. van den Bergen. Efficient collision detection of complex deformable models using AABB trees. *Journal of Graphics Tools*, 2(4):1–13, 1997.

25. S. Gottschalk, M. C. Lin, and D. Manocha. OBB-tree: A hierarchical structure for rapid interference detection. In *ACM SIGGRAPH 96 Conference Proceedings*, pages 171– 180, 1996.

26. Montgomery, K; Bruyns, C; Wildermuth, S; Hasser, C; Ozenne, S; Bailey, D; Heinrichs, L; "Surgical Simulator for Hysteroscopy: A Case Study of Visualization in Surgical Training", IEEE Visualization 2001, San Diego, California, October 21-26, 2001.

27. Montgomery, K; Heinrichs, L; Bruyns, C; Wildermuth, S; Hasser, C; Ozenne, S; Bailey, D; "Surgical Simulator for Operative Hysteroscopy and Endometrial Ablation", International Society for Computer-Aided Surgery (ISCAS), Computer-Aided Radiology and Surgery (CARS 2001), Berlin, Germany, June 27, 2001.

28. Bruyns, C; Senger, S; Montgomery, K; Wildermuth, S; "Real-Time Interactive Cutting Using Virtual Surgical Instruments", Medical Image Computing and Computer-Assisted Interventions (MICCAI 2001), Utrecht, The Netherlands, October 14-17, 2001.

29. Montgomery, K; Mazzella, F; Stephanides, M; Schendel, S; "A High-Resolution Stereoscopic Computer Projection Display for Surgical Planning", Society for Information Display 2001 International Symposium Digest of Technical Papers, Vol. 32, pp. 359-361, June 2001.

30. Montgomery, K; Stephanides, M; Brown, J; Latombe, JC; Schendel, S; "A Virtual Environment for Training in Microsurgery", SPIE- The Optical Engineering Society, v3639(1), pp. 398-403, Jan 1999.

31. Brown, J; Montgomery, K; Latombe, JC; Stephanides, M; "A Microsurgery Simulation System", Medical Image Computing and Computer-Assisted Interventions (MICCAI 2001), Utrecht, The Netherlands, October 14-17, 2001.

32. Bruyns, C; Montgomery, K; Wildermuth, S; "A Virtual Environment for Simulated Rat Dissection: A Case Study of Visualization for AstronautTraining", IEEE Visualization 2001, San Diego, California, October 21-26, 2001.

33. Montgomery, K; Stephanides, M; Schendel, S; "Development and application of a virtual environment for reconstructive surgery", Journal of Computer-Aided Surgery, v5(2), ISSN: 1092-9088, 2000, pp:90-97.

34. Montgomery, K; Stephanides, M; Schendel, S; Ross, M; "A Case Study Using the Virtual Environment for Reconstructive Surgery", IEEE Visualization, Research Triangle Park, NC, October, 1998

35. Wildermuth, S; Bruyns, C; Montgomery, K; Beedu, B; Marincek, B; "Patient Specific Surgical Simulation System for Procedures in Colonoscopy", Vision, Modeling, and Visualization (VMV01), Stuttgart, Germany, November 21-23, 2001.

Medicine Meets Virtual Reality 02/10
J.D. Westwood et al. (Eds.)
IOS Press, 2002

Objective Surgical Performance Evaluation based on Haptic Feedback

Louise Moody, Chris Baber, Theodoros N. Arvanitis
Electronic, Electrical and Computer Engineering,
The University of Birmingham,
Edgbaston,
UK
B15 2TT

Abstract. In order to develop effective virtual reality training systems for surgery there is a need to provide appropriate sensory and performance feedback to the user. This paper aims to demonstrate a method by which performance data can be collected. This is used to investigate the effect of haptic feedback on performance.

A PHANTOM desktop device was used in conjunction with a suturing simulation. A pair of needle-holders was instrumented with strain gauges and attached to the stylus of the PHANTOM allowing the measurement of force application and time. Suturing performance was evaluated in terms of stitch completion time, peak force application, and the length and straightness of the stitch. The effect of the level of force feedback provided by the simulation and performance over time was considered.

The results indicate that the presence of force feedback affected task completion time, peak force application and the straightness of the stitch. Task completion time was shown to increase with the level of force feedback provided. Performance was seen to improve over time in terms of task completion time and the accuracy of the stitch.

The work has examined how the presence and level of force feedback affects performance of a simple task. The accuracy of haptic feedback is important in the design of surgical simulation systems to ensure effective training transfer. A data collection method by which objective performance evaluation can be made is demonstrated. The method can be applied to training using bench models, simulations and potentially in the operating theatre.

1. Introduction

Good surgical performance can be characterised by minimal tissue damage, efficient task completion and accuracy [1], [2], [3]. In conventional open surgery the surgeon is able to detect tissue properties through direct contact using their hands and tools. The precise forces necessary to manipulate tissues are developed through experience. They are hard to teach, explain or quantify. But they are essential to avoid tissue trauma [4], reduce operational time, and limit fatigue to the surgeon due to poor manipulation techniques [5]. In an effective training simulation virtual tissue should feel realistic by providing accurate haptic feedback thus ensuring appropriate transfer of skills.

The objective evaluation of task performance during surgical manipulation can be used for the provision of informative feedback on performance [6], the determination of competence, and as a useful tool for the design and validation of simulated environments.

In this paper the objective metrics of time, peak force application and accuracy are applied to the evaluation of performance in a virtual suturing task. Time is taken as an indication of the efficiency and coordination with which actions are combined during a surgical task [2], [7], [8]. Accuracy is considered necessary to achieve task efficiency and to avoid tissue damage [3], [9], [10], [11]. Accuracy is partly determined by appropriate grip force application. The measurement of grip force is important not only as a performance metric but in the development of accurate tissue models and the provision of haptic feedback [6], [12].

The aim of this paper is to demonstrate the importance of accurate haptic feedback in the design of virtual reality surgical training systems. The effects of varying degrees of haptic feedback are related to performance in a suturing task. A method by which performance data can be collected in terms of time, force application and accuracy is demonstrated.

2. Method

2.1 Equipment

The experimental design made use of a PHANTOM desktop device [13] and a suturing simulation of a skin excision [14] (figure 1). The simulation allowed the production of sutures across a virtual wound using a virtual needle and thread. Manipulation of the end effector of the PHANTOM allowed orientation of the virtual needle and provided resistance to movement as the virtual tissue was contacted.

A pair of surgical needle-holders was attached to the end effector. The needle-holders were instrumented with four strain gauges (2mm, 120Ω from Radiospares) on the arms of the instruments. The strain gauges were arranged in a Wheatstone bridge and wired to a strain gauge amplifier (Applied Weighing SGA (A). As pressure was applied to the instruments the resulting forces were automatically recorded. Output from the strain gauge amplifier was fed into an A: D board (Computer Boards Inc. DAS 801*).* Using Das Wizard, the data were fed into Excel '97 and processed.

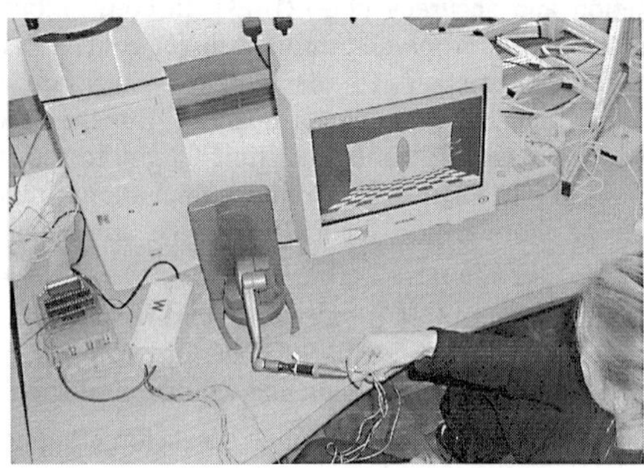

Figure 1. The experimental setting

2.2 Study 1

Twenty right-handed engineering students took part in the experiment. Each undertook a total of ten trials. They were assigned to one of two conditions. In the first, the PHANTOM device provided force feedback to the user during the task and in the second force feedback was withheld.

Following standardised task explanation and familiarisation the participants were asked to form one suture across the skin excision. It was specified that the suture should be approximately 4cm long (as marked on the simulation) and orthogonal to the direction of the wound. The wound edges were to be bought together with minimum overlap and tissue distortion. The experimental time allowed for each trial was limited to 40 seconds.

2.3 Study 2

The suturing simulation allowed variation in the material properties of the wound. The level of force feedback provided by the virtual tissue could be varied on a scale from 0 to 10. The levels of 0, 2, 4, and 6 were applied. A further ten right-handed students took part in this study. Each participant produced sutures to the same requirements as previously. 20 trials were completed, five at each level of force feedback. The levels of force feedback were presented to the participants in a randomised order. The available task completion time was increased to 60 seconds.

2.4 Metrics

Performance was measured in terms of:

1. The time to complete each stitch. This was recorded from the first movement of the needle until the suture was completed.

2. The peak force exerted in each trial.

3. The accuracy of the suture. Each suture produced was traced onto acetate for analysis. They were then measured in length (cm) and scored from 0 to 6 for straightness (i.e. being at right angles to the direction of the wound).

3. Results

3.1 Study 1

The results were analysed to compare the effect of force feedback on task performance (table 1).

Table 1. The effect of force feedback on performance

Condition	Time (s)		Peak force (N)		Length (cm)		Straightness (x/6)	
	Mean	SD	Mean	SD	Mean	SD	Mean	SD
Force feedback	20.17	12.48	5.67	2.14	2.52	1.19	5	1.49
No force feedback	20.53	10.49	4.16	1.87	2.8	1.47	5.15	1.46

Independent samples t-tests revealed that the presence of force feedback significantly increased the peak force applied during suture production [t (198) =2.88 p=0.004]. The time to complete the stitch was reduced [t (198)= -2.69 p=0.008] and the straightness was found to improve [t (198) = 2.38 p=0.018].

Results were averaged across all of the participants and comparisons made between the first and last trials.

Table 2. The effect of trial on performance

Trial	Time (s)		Peak force (N)		Length (cm)		Straightness (x/6)	
	Mean	SD	Mean	SD	Mean	SD	Mean	SD
1	25.51	11.46	4.77	2.13	2.23	1.4	4.6	1.85
10	15.18	8.84	5.07	2.17	3.09	1.12	5.55	0.69

Table 2. shows the mean values across conditions and participants for each metric for the first and last stitch. A paired sample t-test revealed that over the trials the time to complete a stitch was significantly reduced [t (19) = 3.10p=0.001] (see figure 2) and the

length of the stitches became more accurate (i.e. closer to the 4 cm target) [t (19) =-2.14, p=0.04].

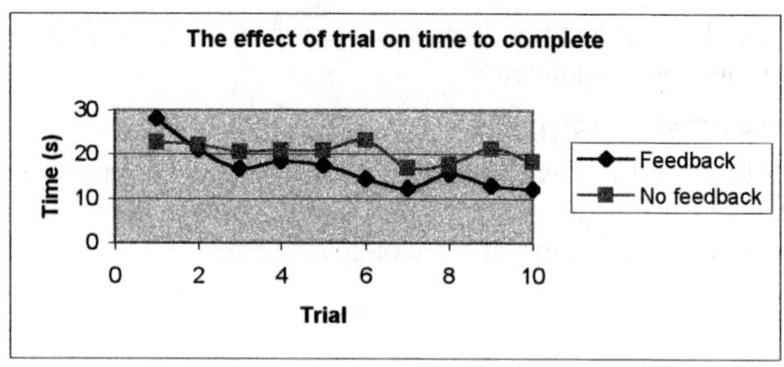

Figure 2. The effect of trial number on task completion time

3.2 Study 2

Table 3. The effect of force feedback level on performance

Force feedback condition	Time (s)		Peak force (N)		Length (cm)		Straightness (x/6)	
	Mean	SD	Mean	SD	Mean	SD	Mean	SD
1 (level 0)	14.5	9.5	6.0	1.4	2.8	1.4	4.9	1.8
2 (level 2)	18.1	10.9	5.7	1.6	2.7	1.6	5.1	1.4
3 (level 4)	20.0	12.9	5.8	1.4	2.9	1.5	5.4	1.1
4 (level 6)	25.9	15.9	6.0	1.4	3.0	1.6	4.8	1.7

Table 3. shows the effect of the level of force feedback on performance. Using repeated measures ANOVA the results from the four levels of force intensity were compared. A significant effect of force feedback intensity was found on task completion time [F (3, 147) = 11.3, p < 0.001].

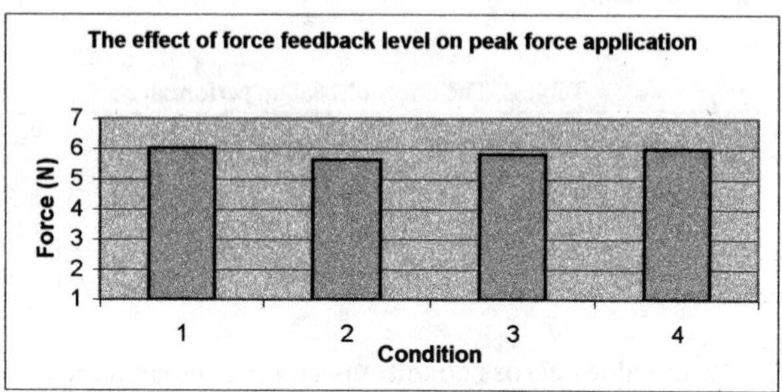

Figure 3. The effect of force feedback level on peak force application

While a significant difference was not found, it can be seen in figure 3 that the level of force feedback provided by the virtual tissue has had some effect on the force application to the tools.

Table 4. The effect of trial number on performance

Trial	Time (s)		Peak force (N)		Length (cm)		Straightness (x/6)	
	Mean	SD	Mean	SD	Mean	SD	Mean	SD
1	26.9	18	5.9	1.6	3.0	1.6	4.3	1.9
5	16.7	8.2	5.7	1.6	3.0	1.5	5.4	1.1

Table 4. shows the mean values across force feedback conditions and participants for each metric for the first and last stitch. Paired sample t-tests were used to compare the results from the first and last trial. A significant effect of trial was found on task completion time [t (39) = 3.4, p< 0.005] and on the straightness of the stitch [t (39) = -2.8 p< 0.01].

4. Discussion and Conclusions

In the first study the results show that the presence of force feedback reduced the time taken to complete the suturing task, increased the peak force application and improved the straightness of the stitch. The peak force application is greater in order to overcome the haptic effects provided. The provision of force feedback enables the user to judge the level of force required to insert the needle hence performance becomes more efficient. Attention can then be directed to the accuracy of the task and hence the stitches produced were straighter.

In the second study it can be seen that with increased levels of force feedback the time taken to perform the task increased. Higher levels of resistance provided by the tissue required more time and appeared to require a greater force application to overcome the haptic effects to insert the needle.

In both studies comparison between task performance in the first and last trial indicated an improvement. In the first study this was shown in terms of task completion time and accuracy of stitch length. In the second in terms of task completion time and the straightness score. This suggests that familiarisation with the task is rapid. Although caution should be taken in the assumptions made regarding a training effect after a limited number of trials, performance has been shown to improve.

The work has demonstrated how the presence and level of force feedback in a simulation affects performance in a simple task and the rate of task familiarisation. This has important repercussions for the design of virtual training systems. The provision of accurate feedback is necessary to ensure positive skill transfer to real tissue and to maximise learning rates.

Research in simulator design tends to lack validation. Robust methods to determine the validity of both the training environment and the proposed metrics are required. The instrumented surgical tools as a data collection technique allow the tracking of performance in a practice environment that is potentially transferable across media. The current study has demonstrated the use of time, force and accuracy as performance metrics.

There are a number of problems with the level of fidelity in the experiment, such as the realism of the simulation and the use of uni-manual action in a typically bi-manual task. The simulation was created in order to demonstrate the potential of Fast Finite Element Modelling not. as a training package. However it is argued that the aim to demonstrate the importance of accurate force feedback for a simple task and data collection techniques has been achieved.

References

[1] Hamdorf, J. M. and J. C. Hall (2000). Acquiring surgical skills. British Journal of Surgery **87**: 28-37.

[2] Kaufman, H. H., R. L. Wiegand, et al. (1987). Teaching surgeons to operate- principles of psychomotor skills training. Acta Neurochirurgica **87**: 1-7.

[3] O'Toole, R. V., R. R. Playter, et al. (1999). Measuring and developing suturing technique with a virtual reality surgical simulator. Journal of American College of Surgeons **189**(1): 114-27.

[4] Caraugh, J. H., M. Martin, et al. (1999). Modelling surgical expertise for motor skill acquisition. American Journal of Surgery **177**: 331-6.

[5] Gupta, V., N. P. Reddy, et al. (1997). Forces in laparoscopic surgical tools. Presence **6**(2): 218-28.

[6] Chen, E. and B. Marcus (1998). Force feedback for surgical simulation. Proceedings of the IEEE **86**(3): 524-30.

[7] Kopta, J. A. (1971). An approach to the evaluation of operative skills. Surgery **70**(2): 297-303.

[8] Macmillan, A. I. and A. Cuschieri (1999). Assessment of innate ability and skills for endoscopic manipulations by the Advanced Dundee Endoscopic Psychomotor Tester: Predictive and concurrent validity. American Journal of Surgery **177**: 274-7.

[9] Platt, A. J., G. Holt, et al. (1997). A new method for the assessment of suturing ability. Journal of the Royal College of Surgeons, Edinburgh **42**: 383-5.

[10] Rosser, J. C., L. E. Rosser, et al. (1997). Skill acquisition and assessment for laparoscopic surgery. Archives of Surgery **132**: 200-4.

[11] Torkington, J., S. G. T. Smith, et al. (2000). The role of simulation in surgical training. Annals of the Royal College of Surgeons England **82**: 88-94.

[12] Rosen, J., M. MacFarlane, et al. (1999). Surgeon-tool force/ torque signatures - evaluation of surgical skills in minimally invasive surgery. Studies in Health Technology and Informatics, San Francisco, CA, IOS Press.

[13] SensAble Technologies *www.sensable.com*

[14] Berkley, J. Weghorst, S. et al. (1999) Fast finite element based deformation and force-feedback: Suture demo/version 1.0 alpha, SensAble Technologies.
www.hitl.washington.edu.people/jberkley.download.htm

Nasal Airflow Diagnosis -
Comparison of experimental Studies and Computer simulations

Wolfgang MÜLLER-WITTIG[1], Gunter MLYNSKI[2], Ivo WEINHOLD[2],
Uli BOCKHOLT[3], Gerrit VOSS[1]

[1]Centre for Advanced Media Technology (CAMTech)
Nanyang Technological University (NTU)
Nanyang Avenue, Singapore 639798
Phone: (65) 790-6988, Fax: (65) 792-8123
Email: mueller@camtech.ntu.edu.sg
[2] ENT-Clinic, Ernst-Moritz-Arndt University Greifswald
Rathenaustrasse 43-45, 17487 Greifswald, Germany
[3] Fraunhofer Institute for Computer Graphics (Fraunhofer-IGD)
Department Visualization & Virtual Reality

Abstract

The lack of suited diagnostic tools providing insight into patient specific flow
characteristics of the nasal airflow is one of the main problems in functional
diagnosis. Diagnostic methods currently used do not provide the necessary
information for flow analysis. But the flow distribution is essential for a
physiological respiration, in particular for cleaning, moistening and tempering of the
inhaled air as well as for the olfactory function of the nose. To overcome this current
situation a cooperation project of the ENT surgeons and computer graphic engineers
was established to develop the computer assisted planning system STAN (Simulation
Tool for Airflow in the human Nose) combining Computer Fluid Dynamics (CFD)
with advanced Computer Graphic Technology. The idea of the STAN system is to
perform patient specific airflow simulations in the patient's nasal cavities. Therefore a
geometrical model of the nasal airways is derived from the patient's tomography
scans. A discretization of the surrounded flow volume is made by a computational
grid. To establish the flow simulation Finite Element Methods are performed on the
grid. A tailored visualization is offered to the surgeon that overlaps the flow pattern to
the patient's tomography data shown in the coronal, sagittal and transversal plane.
The surgeon can not only analyze the patient's current respiratory situation he has
also the possibility to describe the planned surgical intervention. The goal is to
simulate the flow distribution that can be expected after the surgical intervention and
to offer a possibility to validate various surgical strategies. To verify the simulation
results experimental investigations and measurements are made in nasal models.
Silicon Models of patient's nose channels are made to analyze flow characteristics.
The CT or MR scans of the same patients are used as input data for the simulation.
The experimental outcome is compared to the simulation results to validate this
diagnostic approach.

1. Background

"Léssentiel est invisible pour les yeux" the fox said to little prince, but it is not for
sure that he meant a rhinologist looking at patient's tomography slices and trying to

understand the reasons of his pathologic endonasal airflow. However, the lack of suited diagnostic tools providing insight into patient specific flow characteristics of the endonasal airflow is one of the main problems in functional diagnosis. Diagnostic methods currently used, like acoustic rhinometry, do not provide the necessary information for flow analysis, because only the diameters but not the 3-D geometry of the nose cavities are considered [1]. But the flow pattern in the nose plays an important part in respiration. The nose inhales the air at a speed up to 20 m/s. The air is warmed, moistened and cleaned. The endonasla mucosa, which lines the cavum, is responsable for this respiratory function. The turbulent kinetic energy of the flowing air has to be balanced to contact the mucosa in an appropriate proportion. In laminar case, the air is flowing parallel to the surface of the nose cavities. In this case only particles nearby the surface get in contact with the mucosa. In the turbulent case air contact of the mucosa can be too intensive and cause desiccation [2]. This is the reason, why a cooperation project between ENT surgeons and computer graphic was started trying to use Finite Element Methods (FEM) for the simulation of patient specific endonasal airflows. FEM made big progress within the last years and the use has become standard procedure in the area of engineering for example for the optimization and verification of aerodynamic properties. Also in the medical domain FEM simulations are used. In biomechanics detailed exemplary FEM studies foster profound insight into physiological functions of anatomic structures. An algorithm to derive FEM models from CT data was first introduced by Finnigan et al [3]. Biomechanical simulations on patient specific data are performed to analyse the load distribution in the human spine. The simulations will be integrated into a complex planning system designed to support the surgeon to specify type and positioning of pedicle screws in computer assisted pedicle screw insertion [4]. Taylor et al. use FEM in vascular medicine for the simulation of blood flow in arteries. With this system a bypass operation can be planned. Not only patient arterial flow but also the resulting flow after the bypass insertion can be simulated [5].

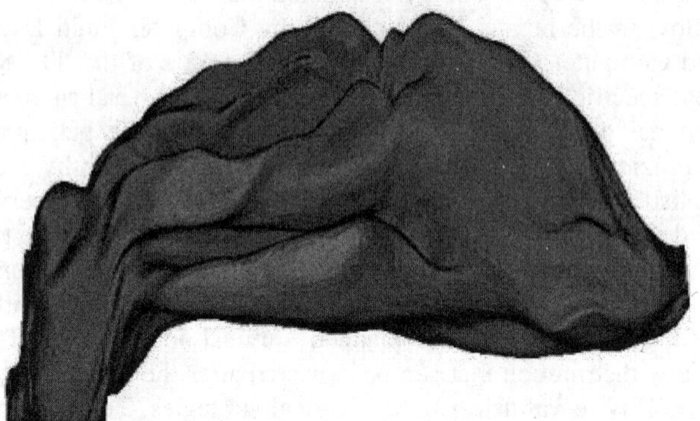

Figure 1: Representation of the Freeform Surface of the nose channel

2. Simulation Tool for Airflow in the human Nose

Input data for the STAN (Simulation Tool for Airflow in the human Nose) system are the patient's tomography scans. Based on a computational model describing the flow volume can be derived from the tomography data. Now Finite Volume Methods are used for the simulation. The simulation results are overlapped to the patient's tomography scans. The surgeon now has the possibility to describe a planned surgical intervention. The STAN system now tries to predict the surgical outcome and to give a possibility to validate several planned approaches. To verify the simulation system

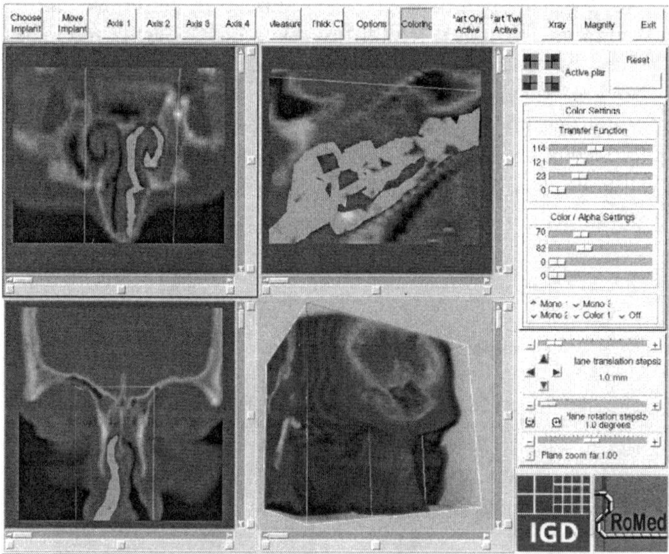

experimental investigations are performed that can be compared with the simulation results.

Figure 2: STAN User Interface

2.1. Generation of the Computational Grid

The generation of the Computational Grid can be divided into two necessary steps. The first one is the 3-D Reconstruction of a surface model describing the nose channel the second one is the discretization of the contained flow volume with Finte Elements, e.g. tetraeder or hexaeder elements. For the 3-D Reconstruction of the surface model different approaches have been tested out. Input data for the 3-D Reconstruction pipeline are 20-30 CT/MRI slices from the nasal region. The CT/MRI slices are segmented using the so called hystheresis threshold method [6] . The first approach for the 3-D Reconstruction was a volume based method derived from the marching cubes algorithm, where polygonized models of the nasal cavities have been generated. This method is easy to implement but it generates often a somehow blocky representation of the anatomical structures. As basis for the FEM these models are often not well suited because the rough edges of the surface can cause artifacts in the flow simulation. Even attached smoothing operations, like e.g. Laplacian smoothing, could not compensate these artifacts.

That was the reason why a contour based approach has been chosen for the 3-D Reconstruction. Via mouse clicks the surgeon is marking contours on the binariesized images slice by slice. At first the contours have been interpolated to the surface model using Delaunay Triangulation. The result of the Delaunay Triangulation is also a polygonized surface model but it is much smoother than the volume based generated. The best way to create the geometry of the nasal airways is the use of freeform surfaces. To generate a freeform surface the contours on the tomography slices are described using 2D freeform curves. The number of interpolation points as well as the curve order have do be specified for the 2D curves. The next step is the interpolation of these 2D freeform curves to obtain a 3-D freeform surface representation (c.f. Figure 1). The tessellation of this freeform surface is performed during the grid generation algorithm. The use of freeform surfaces guaranties the smoothest possible definition of the boundary walls and the optimal basis for the generation of the numerical grid. For grid generation either tetraeder or hexaeder elements can be used. Input data for the algorithm is the surface model of nasal airways. The grid has to fill out the flow volume. Commercial grid generators designed for structured CAD models are not usable for the irregularly shaped surfaces generated in the 3-D reconstruction.

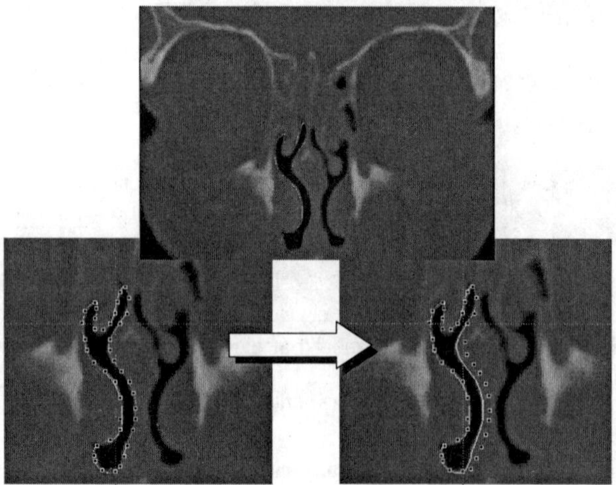

Figure 3: Description of the planned anatomical correction via contours

2.2.   Flow Simulation

To perform the simulation the following boundary conditions have to be specified:
- Inlet/Outflow
  The areas forming inlet and outflow on the surface model have to be marked via mouse click.
- Fluid definition
  The simulation can be done for the fluids air and water. The simulation with water is necessary for comparability with the experimental results.
- Inlet flowrate
  As inlet velocity flowrates from 100 cm^3/s up to 500 cm^3/s can be chosen. Only the speed (volume per second) has to be defined at the inlet, the flow direction is assumed to be normal to the inlet surfaces. The speed can either be constant (stationary flow) or a function describing the respiration cycle (instationary flow).

For the simulation the Finite Volume Method is used. The nasal flow is assumed to be incompressible and it can be laminar or turbulent. The solving is essentially based on the integration of the Navier-Stokes equations, which are in general analytically not solvable. In this case the RNG (Renormalization Group) k-eps model is used for the solution. The distribution of the velocity, temperature and the turbulent kinetic energy are most interesting results of the simulation.

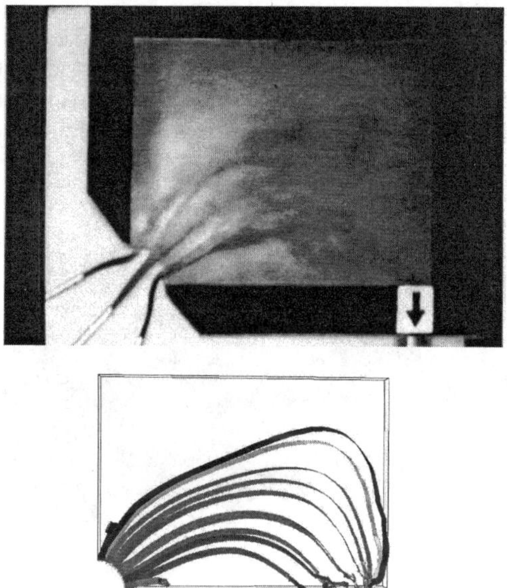

Figure 4: Modeling of nasal flow characteristics using Mink Boxes

2.3.   The STAN User Interface

An important feature for the interpretability of the simulation result is an intuitive and tailored visualization software that allows the physician to analyze the huge and complex data sets. With the tomography as well as the simulation data there are two different sources of volume data that have to be considered. To visualize this large amount of data, a volume render is developed, that uses the volume slicing technique [7]. The data is stored as a set of parallel cutting planes. Textures holding the gray values (in the case of tomography data) or the color values (e.g. representing the air speed) are mapped onto these cutting planes. The STAN User Interface consists of a display area including three orthogonal and a 3-D view and functional areas to query status information or to control the diagnosis session (c.f. Figure 2). It shows the tomography as well as the simulation data in the sagittal, coronal and transversal cut. The forth quadrant offers the possibility to render vectorplots, steamlines, isosurfaces or volume-rendered views. Slices can be inserted into the flow channel illustrating speed distribution on the 2-D plane. Another possibility to display the simulation result is the use of equipotential contours showing airspeed or turbulent kinetic energy on the surface of the nose cavity.

2.4.   Description of the planned intervention

The STAN system can also be used to describe the planned interventions that may be necessary to optimize a pathologic respiration. Thereby the contour-based 3-D Reconstruction method can be reused for the description. The contours have been used to mark slice-by-slice the nose geometry on the tomographic scans. They have been defined with freeform curves that can easily be modeled via control points as it is the case in standard image processing tools. The surgeon now defines his planned intervention by modeling of the contours using the control points (c.f. Figure 3). Based on these modeled contours a changed geometric model of the nose channel can be generated via a reiterated 3-D Reconstruction. This model is used to perform a further simulation. The changed flow pattern can be examined with the visualization component. The goal of this approach is to predict the surgical outcome and to validate the change functionality that can be expected after the surgical intervention.

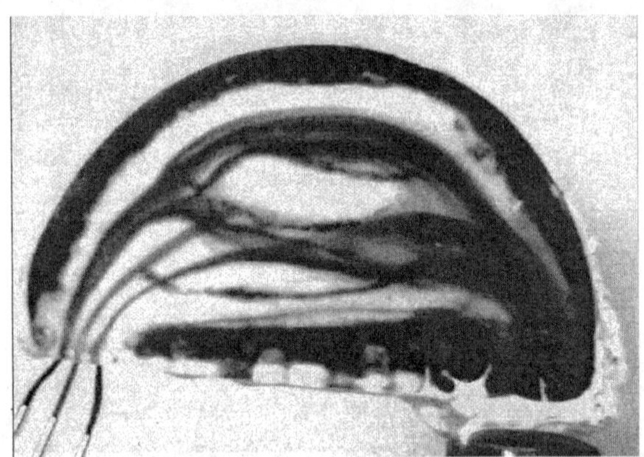

Figure 5: Experimental Studies of patient specific respiratory flow using silicon models of the nose channel

2.5. Validation

The most important topic for the usability of the system is the possibility to validate the simulation results. Therefore different validation concepts have been established. The first approach was to use the so called Mink Boxes for the validation(c.f. Figure 4). The Mink Boxes are brick formed boxes that have been used to explore basic functional properties of the nose like the diffusion behavior [8]. They show similar flow characteristics as the nasal flow and they can be digitized exactly and easily.

In the next validation step silicon models of patient's nose channels are made to analyze flow characteristics [9]. The CT or MR scans of the same patients are used as input data for a simulation. As fluid water is used for the experimental simulations (c.f. Figure 5). In the simulation the fluids air and water (for comparison) can be chosen. Experiment and simulation show similar characteristics in distribution of velocity field and turbulence. To have a consistence as high as possible these silicon models are also scanned by a tomograph and the scans are used as input for a simulation. So geometrical inaccuracies caused by the difficult generation of the patient specific silicon model can be avoided.

3. Conclusions

Experiment and simulation show similar characteristics in distribution of velocity field and turbulence but some parameters remain still unconsidered. Studies are made to measure the variation of the nose's hydraulic diameter during a respiratory cycle. The first validation results are motivating further investigations. So far only physiologic cases are considered, the next step will be the validation based on pathologic cases.

4. Acknowledgments

Part of this research was founded by the German Research Society (Deutsche Forschungsgemeinschaft) DFG under grant ML/2-1. We thank Prof. Dr. h.c. Dr.-Ing. José L. Encarnação for providing the environment in which this work was possible. We also thank all our colleagues and students at our laboratory, especially Albert Schäffer, Mario Becker and Siegfried Bauer without their contribution we would not have been able to achieve the results presented herein.

[1] Mlynski G., Loew J. *Die Rhinoresistometrie - eine Weiterentwicklung der Rhinomanometrie.* Laryngorhinootologie. 1993; 72(12): 608-610.

[2] Grützenmacher S, Mlynski G, Zacek G., Mlynski *Correlation of nasal mprphology and respiratory functionof the nose,* 17th European Rhinologic Society & International Symposium on Infection and Allergy of the Nose, Vienna *1998*

[3] Finnigan, P., Hathaway A., Lorensen W., (1990), *Merging CAT and FEM, Mechanical Engineering,* vol. 112, no. 7, pp. 32-38

[4] Voss G., Bisler A., Bockholt U., Müller-Wittig W., Schäffer A. *ICAPS –An Integrative Computer-Assisted Planning System for Pedicle Screw Insertion* In: Proceedings of Medicine Meets Virtual Reality 2001, pp. 561-563, IOS Press, 2001

[5] Taylor C.A., Hughes T.J.R. Zarins C.K., *Finite element modeling of blood flow in arteries,* Computer Methods in Applied Mechanics and Engineering,Vol. 158, 158-196 (1998).

[6] Koller T., (1996) From Data to Information: Segmentation, Description and Analysis of Cebral Vascularity, M. Sc. Dissertation, Swiss federal institute of technology Zurich

[7] Grzeszczuk R, Henn C, Yagel R, *Advanced Geometric Techniques for Ray Casting Volumes,* SIGGRAPH 1998

[8] Mink, P. J. Physiologie der oberen Luftwege, Leipzig, Vogel, 1920

[9] Mlynksi, G., Grützenmacher S., Mlynski B. *The Flow in the anterior part of cavum nasi* European Archives of Oto- Rhino- Laryngology, 1998

Medicine Meets Virtual Reality 02/10
J.D. Westwood et al. (Eds.)
IOS Press, 2002

Virtual Reality Therapy: Case Study of Fear of Public Speaking

Max M. North, Curt M. Schoeneman and James R. Mathis
Virtual Reality Technology Laboratory
Computer Science and Information Systems
Kennesaw State University
URL: www.vrt1.com E-mail: Max@acm.org

Abstract. The major goal of this research case study was to investigate the effectiveness of Virtual Reality Therapy (VRT) in the treatment of the fear of public speaking. A twenty-eight-year-old Caucasian male was selected from questionnaires distributed to a class of undergraduate students enrolled at Kennesaw State University. Two assessment measures were used in this study. The first measure used was the Attitude Towards Public Speaking (ATPS) Questionnaire. The second measure used was the eleven-point Subjective Units of Disturbance (SUD) scale. These measurements assessed the anxiety, avoidance, attitudes and disturbance associated with the subject's fear of public speaking before and after each VRT treatment session. This case study of public speaking fear indicates that VRT may be used as an effective treatment method for reducing self-reported anxiety.

1. Introduction

The fear of public speaking is often reported as the most common social phobia. This communication disorder is frequently identified among the top five most prevalent phobias. It does not appear to be limited by age, gender, economic or educational variables. Until recently, traditional treatment has included systematic desensitization, cognitive restructuring and skill building [1],[2]. Current advances made through the use of computer display technology and the work of researchers is responsible for the creation of virtual reality technology used for treating the fear of public speaking and other psychological disorders [3], [4], [5]. This case study was conducted in the Virtual Reality Technology Laboratory at Kennesaw State University, Kennesaw, Georgia.

This disorder is related to and shares the panic-like symptoms (dizziness, dry mouth, rapid heart rate, etc.) of agoraphobia, fear of being in open or public places. The public speaking disorder frequently limits opportunities and denies success to many people, especially professionals. Its successful treatment by VRT would be a significant addition to traditional therapies.

2. Methodology

A twenty-eight-year-old Caucasian male was selected from questionnaires distributed to a class of undergraduate students enrolled at Kennesaw State University. The screening process ensured that the subject was suffering from a fear of public speaking and had no other serious physical or psychological conditions. The subject's participation was voluntary and informed.

Prior to VRT treatment, the subject completed a modified ATPSQ (Attitude Toward Public Speaking Questionnaire), and during treatment the subject was exposed to four situations:

(1) speaking in an empty auditorium;
(2) speaking in an auditorium with an audience;
(3) speaking to an audience in which members talked to each other and paid no attention to the speaker; and
(4) speaking to an audience whose members laughed at him.

In these situations, the number of people in the audience varied from zero to 100. The subject rated each situation for discomfort.

As a simple measure of anxiety, a modified version of the SUD (Subjective Units of Disturbance) scale was used every few minutes during exposure on a 0 (no discomfort) to 10 (panic-level anxiety) scale [1], [6]. This SUD method has been shown to correlate with objective physiological measures of anxiety.

The treatment schedule consisted of eight weekly sessions. The length of each session ranged from 10 to 15 minutes. In the first session, the subject talked about himself and his issues relating to public speaking. Next, the subject had to read aloud eleven ideas or values that are irrational and counterproductive. The ideas of value were taken from Ellis' Rational-Emotive Psychotherapy. Each session ended with the subject completing the modified Attitude Toward Public Speaking Questionnaire.

Apparatus for this case study consisted of a Pentium based computer, and a head-mounted display with head-tracker (Virtual – I/O). The VRT software program used was VREAM™ Virtual Reality Development Software Package and Libraries (VRCreator™) to create a virtual reality scene of an auditorium located in a university science building. The virtual auditorium, seats 100 people, is 100 feet deep, 48 feet wide, and 55 feet high.

3. Results

Although the mean for self-reported discomfort fluctuated over the eight sessions (a normal phenomenon in VRT research), the mean SUD (mean=1.42) and ATPSQ (mean=2.33) for the post-test was significantly lower than the mean SUD (mean=5.80) and ATPSQ (mean=8.50) for the pre-test. Also, the subject reported that he felt more comfortable in public speaking situations after the VRT sessions.

4. Conclusion

Symptoms experienced by the subject during VRT sessions were just as real to the subject as they were in actual speaking situations. The symptoms included a dry mouth, increased heart rate, and general dizziness. Anxiety experienced during VRT sessions attested to the sense of virtual presence. This case study of public speaking fear indicates that VRT is an effective treatment method for reducing self-reported anxiety. The VRT sessions resulted in both a significant reduction of anxiety symptoms (SUD and ATPSQ measurements) and increased self-confidence in speaking in front of his classmates when called upon to make class presentations.

5. Discussion

Based on the authors' initial VRT research and several case studies for combating fear of public speaking and other psychological disorders, they have consistently observed and collected comments from the subjects. These comments positively correlate with the SUDs and ATPSQs data collected after each VRT session. The following comments are from the subject after the VRT treatment. "I didn't believe it when people would tell me that the more I spoke in public, the easier it would become, but I now agree. The main thing was getting over my fears. The virtual reality lab was a place I could go to practice speaking in public, when I was actually only speaking in front of one other person. At first, when the simulated audience started saying things such as 'we can't hear you, speak up.' It made me nervous and it was hard to recover, but after more and more sessions, it didn't bother me as bad and it became easier to recover. As a result of participating in the Virtual Reality Therapy and making a few presentations in my classes last semester, I have overcome my fear of public speaking. I still get a little nervous when speaking in public; however, it is now easier because I have more self-confidence and realize that it is impossible to please everyone. I use to get nervous in some class when the instructor would ask us to introduce ourselves to the class. Now, that does not bother me. I would recommend Virtual Reality Therapy to any one who has a fear of public speaking."

Acknowledgement

The current case study research was conducted in the Virtual Reality Technology Laboratory under the auspices of the Computer Science and Information Systems Department at Kennesaw State University, Kennesaw, Georgia. The initial hardware, software configuration and pilot study projects were sponsored by a grant from Boeing Computer Services (Virtual Systems Department), partially supported by the U.S. Army Center for Excellence in Information Science under contract number DAAL03-92-6-0377 and The Speech Improvement Company. The views contained in this document are those of the authors and should not be interpreted as representing the official policies of the U.S. Government, either expressed or implied.

References

[1] J. Wolpe, The Practice of Behavior Therapy. Pergamon Press, New York, 1969.
[2] American Psychiatric Association: Diagnostic and Statistical Manual of Mental Disorders, 4th Edition. Washington, D.C., American Psychiatric Association, 1994.
[3] M. North and S. North, Virtual environment and psychological disorders. *Electronic Journal of Virtual Culture*, 2(4), 1994, pp. 37-42.
[4] M. North, S. North and J. Coble, Effectiveness of virtual environment desensitization in the treatment of agoraphobia. *International Journal of Virtual Reality*, 1(2), 1995a, pp. 28-32.
[5] North, M.M., North, S.M. and Coble, J.R.(). A virtual reality application in the treatment of psychological disorders. *Journal of Medicine and Virtual Reality*, 1(2), 1995b, pp. 28-32.
[6] B. Thyer, J. Papsdorf, R. Davis and S. Vallecorsa, Autonomic correlates of the subjective anxiety scale. *Journal of Behavior Therapy and Experimental Psychiatry*, 15, 1984, pp. 13-17.

Medicine Meets Virtual Reality 02/10
J.D. Westwood et al. (Eds.)
IOS Press, 2002

Virtual Image Grafting:
Image Based Generation and Visualization of Virtual Skin Defects

Peter Oppenheimer, Jeffrey Berkley, Suzanne Weghorst
Human Interface Technology Lab
University of Washington,
Seattle, WA 98195

Dan Berg, MD
Division of Dermatology
University of Washington Medical Center
Seattle, WA 98195

Abstract We have developed methods for rapidly generating 3d dermatologic datasets for use in education, training simulations and procedure planning. By compositing local surface features of cutaneous wounds onto patient images and 3d models, one can flexibly generate large patient variability from a small initial 3d library. The wound database is generated from clinically captured photographic images. The wound image is extracted from the image of the surrounding tissue. The 3d anatomy database is generated from MRI scans and from multiple photographic views. Extracted wound images can be moved rotated and scaled and blended in the final composite.

1. Background Problem

Over 1 million new skin cancers are diagnosed in the US each year [1]. Removal of skin cancers results in the creation of wounds that require surgical reconstruction. Options for repair of the wounds include side-to-side closure, skin grafts and local tissue transfer. Choice of repair method depends in part on the size, depth and site of the wound. Training techniques are limited to traditional apprenticeship as well as use of animal, mechanical or cadaver models all of which have significant drawbacks [2]

There are no efficient means to expose trainees to the large variety of wound sizes and locations that they will encounter in clinical practice. The surgeon preparing to treat a new case must be able to visualize the resulting wound and closure options. Although digital images of previous cancer excisions can serve as a useful archive for teaching, retrieving the appropriate case study requires searching through databases that are limited by archiving practices and privacy issues. In addition to viewing case study imagery, there is also the need for hands-on interaction.

2. Proposed Solution

We have developed methods for rapidly generating 3d dermatologic datasets for use in education training simulations and procedure planning. By compositing local surface features of cutaneous wounds onto patient images and models, one can flexibly generate large patient variability from a small initial 3d library.

For example, a close up image of the defect created by the excision of a cancer from one patient's cheek can be "virtually grafted" onto the chin of a model of another patient to create a new data set. By scaling, rotating and positioning the wound image, the modeler can design the desired result.

The processes for generating these composited datasets is image-based [3] that is we begin with anatomy and wound images captured by digital camera. Along the way to generating the final composites we generated several intermediate libraries. Figure 1 illustrates the various library components and the general process flow.

3. Image and Model Libraries

The database for our approach contains five components

1) Defect Image Library: Close-ups digital images of surface defects
2) Extracted Defect Library   Defects separated from surrounding tissue
3) Regional Anatomy Image Library Baseline images of anatomy (e.g. arm, head)
4) Regional Anatomy 3D Models   Generated 3d models of anatomy (e.g. arm, head)
5) Composite Library: Composites of elements of 1) onto elements of 2)

The Defect Image Library consists of clinically captured images. Using Photoshop and other processing tools, these images are segmented to extract the defect from the surrounding skin. Depending on the nature of the wound the defect can be extracted with either a hard edge or a soft edge that is blended with the surrounding target tissue.

The elements of the resulting Extracted Defect Library can then be scaled, oriented, positioned and composited onto target Regional Anatomy Library images and models of other patients.

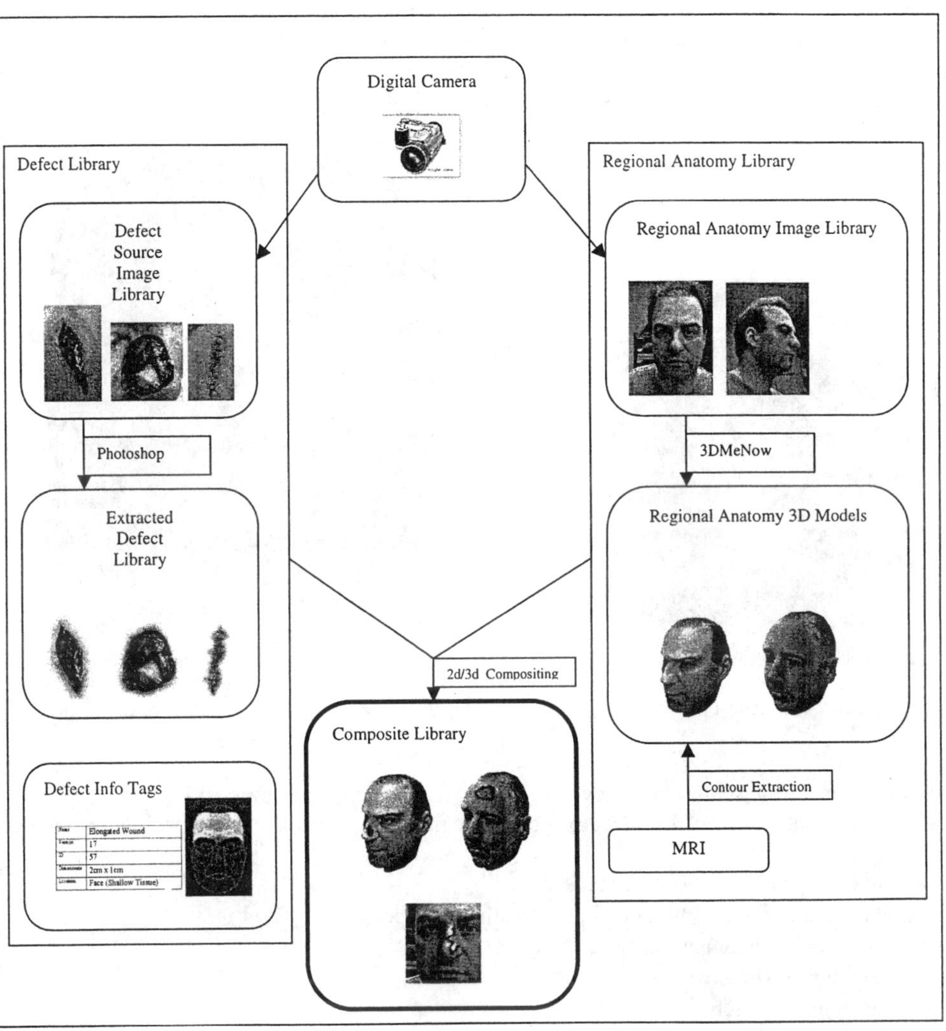

Figure 1) Databases and Process Flow

A single wound can be adapted to fit various anatomical locations on a variety of patients. However, there are limits on how and where a wound can be transferred. For example, the wound in figure 2a) extracted from a nose reveals cartilage that wouldn't be found on a forehead. The forehead composite in figure 2b) is therefore anatomically inappropriate -- the nose composite is more feasible.

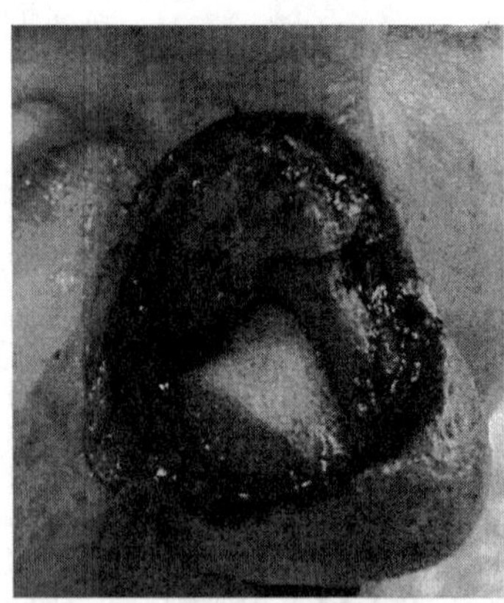

Fig 2a)　Nose Defect

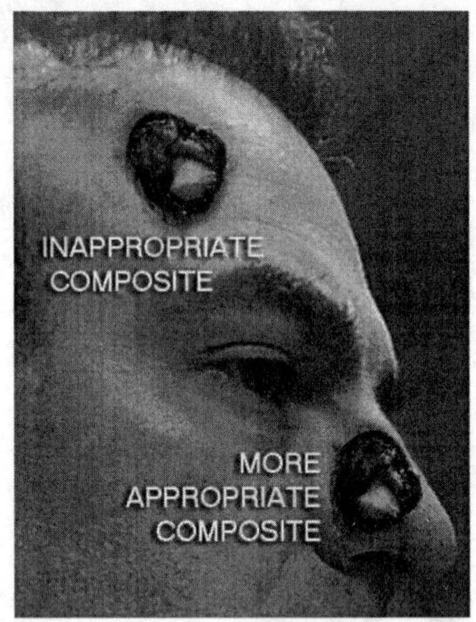

Fig 2b)　Appropriate and Inappropriate Composites

For this reason, a rule set has been developed which governs wound compositing.
Composing can be performed subject to certain integration parameters. These parameters include:

- Skin variability between patients
- Range limits of scaling of defect in the final composite
- Anatomical Incompatibility
- Lighting Variations.
- Shading Variation
- Model Curvature

These parameters form the compositing guideline tag associated with each extracted defect.
See figure 3

Elements of the Extracted Defect Library are classified to correspond to localized areas of the target anatomical region (e.g. "This defect can only be placed on the cheek"). Unique parameters are also defined for image processing tools, such as brightness, contrast, color, and wound edge blending of defect boundary.

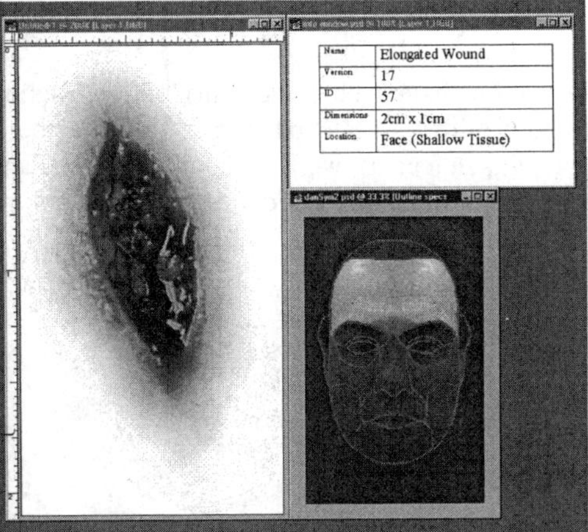

(Figure 3) Extracted Defect with Guideline Tag and Location Guideline Image

The regional anatomy libraries contain images and 3d models of anatomical regions onto which the extracted defects are to be composited. The 3d models are generated by several methods. Some models are based on surface reconstructions from MRI scans with draped photographic surface texture maps [4] Head models were generated from front and side view photographs. 3DMeNow software tool allows attachment of control points to the two photographs and generates the resulting model. Figure 4 shows the 3DMeNow Interface.

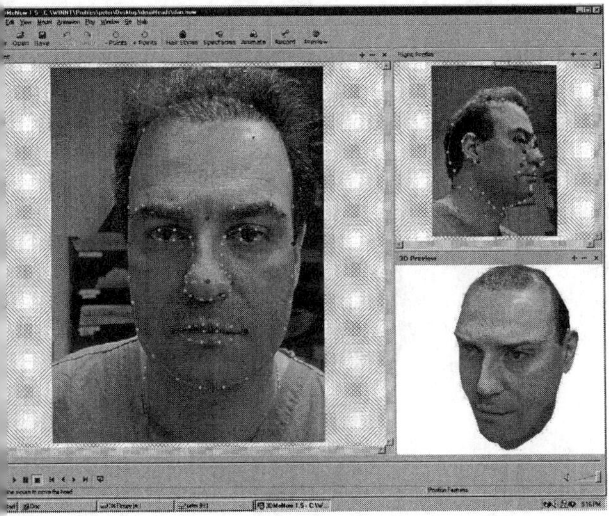

Figure 4)   Interface for generating 3D Head model from front and side views   (3DMeNow)

4. Composing Extracted Defects onto Regional Anatomy

Elements from the Extracted Defect Library are composited onto elements of the Region Anatomy Library using "Deep Paint 3D". This tool allows one to paste directly onto the 3 models or 2D images, translate, rotate and scale the defect as well as adjust color balanc brightness and contrast. Figure 5 and 6 shows examples of composited wounds as well as suturi composites.

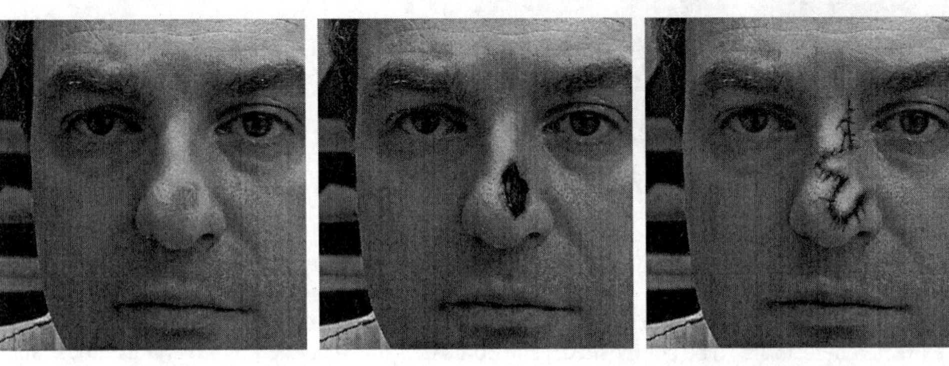

Figure 5) Composited cancer, and subsequent excision wound, and closure

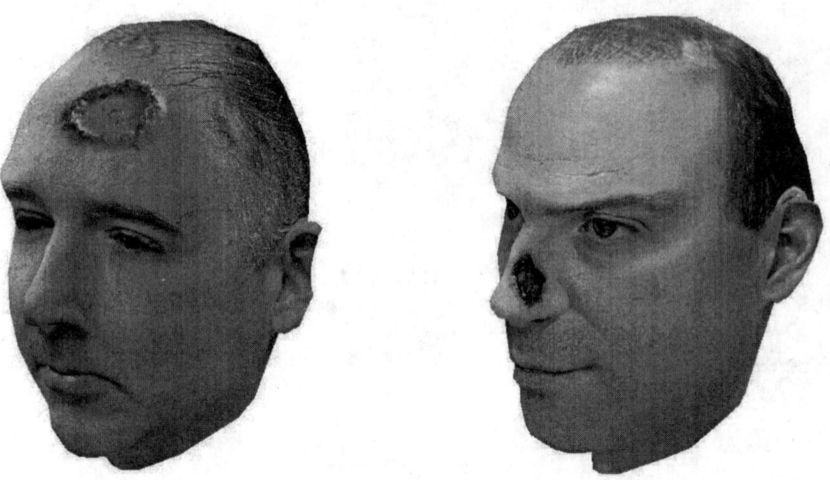

Figure 6) Defects composited onto 3D head models

Using Composite Models for Training and Pre-Operative Planning

Ve plan to use the composite datasets to allow easy access to a library of composited wounds of
arying sizes and locations. These wounds will be used in teaching sessions with residents to
aluate the options for wound reconstruction. Off the shelf programs like Microsoft Power Point®
n be used to import the images and allow trainees to draw the proposed incision lines of their reconstruction (see figure 7)

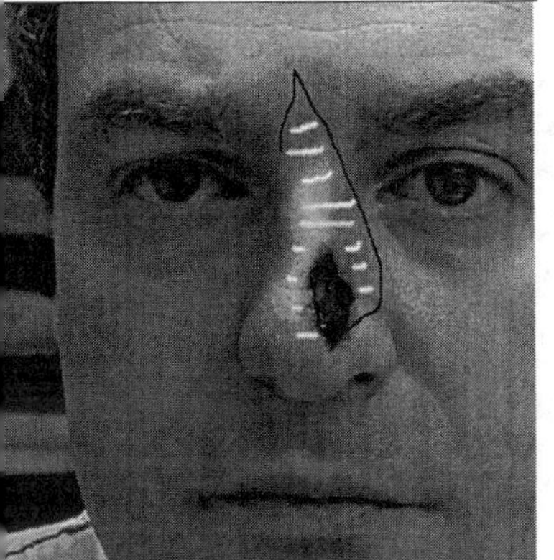

After a patient's wound is closed a scar remains along the edge of the closure. The shape of the scar is a function of how the wound is excised and how the wound edges are sutured together. The choice of closure also determines how the surrounding skin stretches and the overall quality of the reconstruction. To pre-visualize the reconstruction outcome, during surgical planning, the surgeon can draw possible closure shapes directly on the 3d model and see the resulting scar rendered as composited photographic suture edge textures.

gure 7) Composite wound with proposed incision line (black) and area of undermining (white)
awn by trainee.

Ongoing Research

Ve plan to import the composite datasets into our dermatological surgery simulator [5], which
es deformable finite element models and a haptic display to train students in dermatologic wound
osure.
Ve will be conducting ongoing evaluation by experienced dermatologic surgeons as to the
parent realism of the composites, appropriate modifications, and organization of the libraries.

eferences

] Garner KL, Rodney WM. Basal and squamous cell carcinoma. Prim Care 2000;27(2):447-58.
] Gladstone HB, Raugi GJ, Berg D, Berkley J, Weghorst S, Ganter M. Virtual reality for
   dermatologic surgery: virtually a reality in the 21st century. J Am Acad Dermatol 2000;42(1 Pt
   1):106-12.
] Oppenheimer P., Sweet R., Weghorst S., Porter J., Gupta A. The Representation of Blood Flow
   in Endourologic Surgical Simulations. Meets Virtual Reality 9 Proceedings. 2001. Newport
   Beach, CA: IOS Press, Amsterdam, 2001, pp. 365-371.
] Berkley J., et al. Creating Fast Finite Element Models from Medical Images. Medicine Meets
   Virtual Reality 8 Proceedings. 2000. Newport Beach, CA: IOS Press, Amsterdam, 2000
] Berkley J., et al., Banded Matrix Approach to Finite Element Modeling for Soft Tissue
   Simulation. Virtual Reality: Research, Development and Applications, 1999. 4: p. 203-212.

Medicine Meets Virtual Reality 02/10
J.D. Westwood et al. (Eds.)
IOS Press, 2002

In vivo measurement of solid organ visco-elastic properties

Mark P. Ottensmeyer, Ph.D.
Simulation Group, CIMIT, 65 Landsdowne St., rm 147, Cambridge, MA, 02139
mpo@alum.mit.edu

To support the ongoing development of software-based surgical simulation systems, work is underway to acquire the mechanical properties of living tissue. When such simulations include force feedback, visco-elastic properties must be evaluated over a range of frequencies relevant to human perception and motor control. A minimally invasive instrument has been developed which can perform normal indentation on solid organs, and apply and measure deformations over a frequency range from DC to approximately 100Hz. Measurement performance was validated on a series of objects and materials with known properties, and the device was subsequently used in *in vivo* tests on porcine liver. Results of these validation tests as well as the data extracted from the *in vivo* experiments are presented. Testing in ongoing, and will be expanded to more completely characterize liver, as well as porcine spleen and other solid organ tissues. While these animal tissue property tests are valuable in and of themselves, they pave the way for the development of instruments and experimental protocols suitable for the measurement of human tissue properties.

1. Introduction

One of the difficulties in developing realistic computer-based simulators for surgery is the scarcity of material properties for living tissue. Models which capture the mechanical behavior of tissues typically use estimates or *in vitro* measurements of the model parameters for given types of healthy or diseased tissues.

While estimates from experts may be suitable for surgical training, new instrument and new procedure prototyping will require more precise property values to closely match real organs. *In vitro* testing is useful as a place to begin, but because of changes like absence of blood perfusion and oxygenation, changes in boundary conditions, temperature, etc., one must also pursue *in vivo* acquisition to get accurate tissue property data.

Researchers are pursuing non-invasive [1, 2], minimally invasive [3, 4] and open surgical techniques [5, 6, 7]. Among the non-invasive techniques, are ultrasound [1] and MRI elastography [2], which make use of static or dynamic deformations at the surface of the body, and observations of the strain field imposed within the body. By performing inverse calculations, elasticities of tissues relative to each other can be determined. This is, however, a complex process, and is highly dependent on knowledge of the relevant boundary conditions. The minimally invasive and open surgical techniques impose local deformations on tissue, and examine relatively local responses. [3] and [4] employ surgical instruments equipped with sensors to measure the local force-displacement response. [5], [6] and [7] use larger instruments to impose tensile loads, indentation or suction to tissues. By comparing the force-displacement responses with either simplified or finite element models of the tissue, again the inverse problem is solved to extract the tissue properties. These latter techniques can be computationally less expensive, and can impose larger deformations on tissue than the non-invasive techniques. However, they suffer limitations in that local measurements must be repeated at numerous locations over a given organ to yield a complete set of data. In addition, for organs with capsules (e.g. liver, spleen, or kidney), it may be difficult to differentiate the contributions to the measured stiffness of the parenchyma versus the capsule, since both structures are deformed simultaneously. For liver and spleen, which have relatively thinner/weaker capsules than kidney, this effect might be negligible, but further experiments will be necessary to find out what those contributions are.

In vivo tissue property measurement is still a young field, and the broad range of tissue types, the number of parameters needed to describe them, and the issues of age, type of disease and individual differences mean that there is still a need for additional data. No single technique will likely provide all of the data necessary, so all reliable data is a welcome contribution.

2. Methods and instruments

This research makes use of a single axis indentation device called the Tissue Material Property Sampling Tool (TeMPeST 1-D) [8, 9, 10]. It can pass through a 12mm surgical cannula or be used in open surgery, and generates small amplitude oscillations up to approximately 100Hz. Range of motion is +/-500μm, and the maximum force that can be applied with a 5mm right circular punch is 300mN. Oscillations are generated by driving a voice-coil motor with a voltage controlled current amplifier.

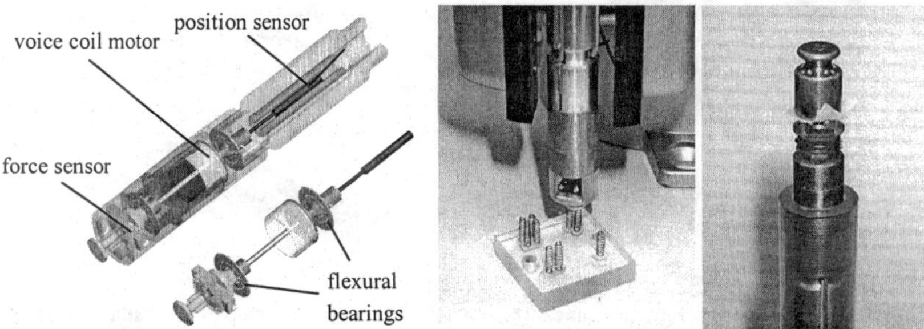

Figure 1. (left) Detail of sensor/actuator tip of TeMPeST 1-D and moving core elements. 12mm overall diameter. Force sensor is compression-only, suitable for indentation testing. Flexural bearings provide friction free support for voice-coil motor-driven core elements. Non-contact position sensing performed with LVDT sensor. (center & right) TeMPeST 1-D in validation tests on springs and inertial loads.

2.1.   Validation Tests

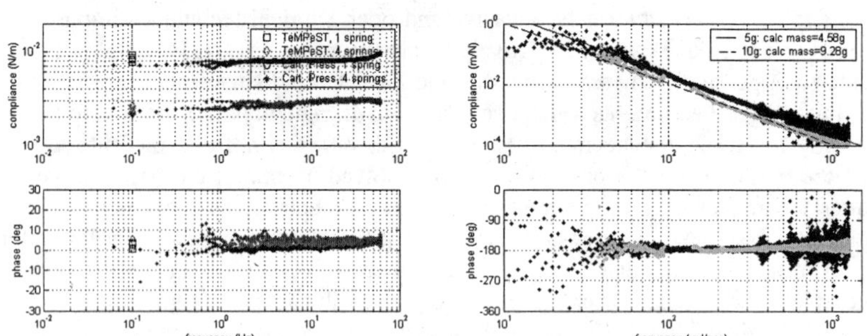

Figure 2. Frequency dependent compliance tests on springs and masses. For springs, TeMPeST 1-D frequency sweep data agree well with 0.1Hz fixed frequency (quasi-static) data, also with cartilage press instrument. For masses, fitting inertial load characteristic to data, yields good measurements of mass.

To verify that the instrument could be relied upon to provide accurate data, and to determin measurement limitations, a series of tests on mechanical springs (compliant loads), known masses (inertial loads) and silicone gels (visco-elastic materials) were performed. When tested over a range of frequencies, springs should exhibit a constant compliance, while for masses, the compliance should fall by two orders of magnitude while frequency increases by one order. As shown in Figure 2, both of these results are observed. Further, for the springs, the TeMPeST 1-D measurements agree with those made using a small compression testing device (cartilage press). Similarly, the masses calculated are close to the masses employed during testing.

Springs and masses have simple dynamic characteristics, so a series of silicone gels exhibiting visco-elastic responses within the bandwidth of the TeMPeST 1-D were created and tested. The gels were independently tested using a parallel plate rheometer, and again good agreement was obtained (see Figure 3).

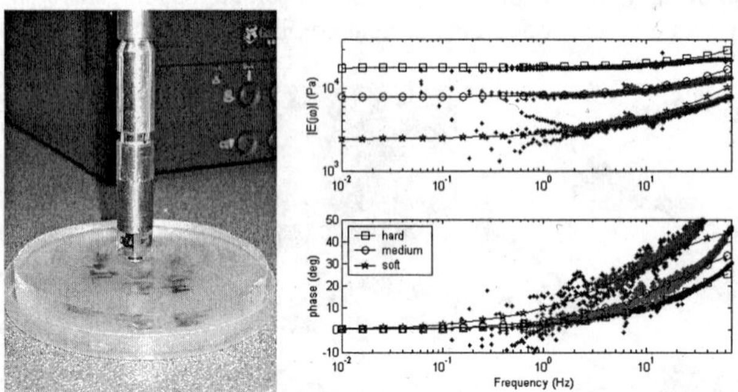

Figure 3. Visco-elastic material testing. Three different mixtures of two-part RTV silicone rubber were made and tested using a parallel plate rheometer (symbols) and compared with chirp data (point clouds) taken with the TeMPeST 1-D. For softest gel, force sensor signal to noise ratio is too small to obtain reliable data, providing lower limit of tissue stiffness that can be measured without modifications to the instrument.

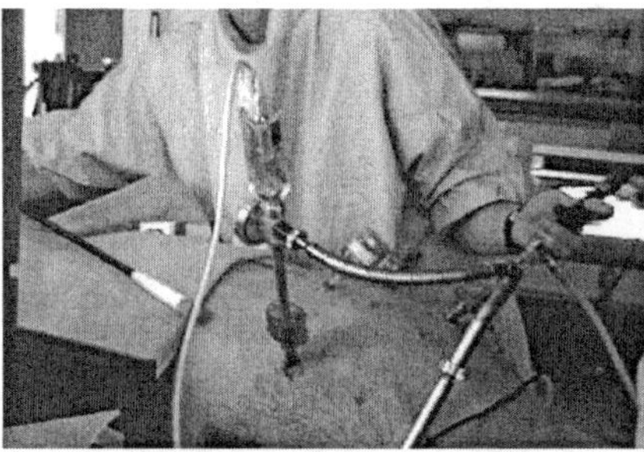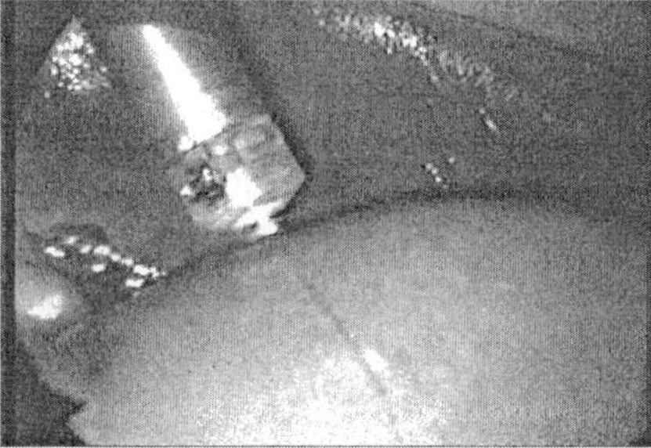

Figure 4. TeMPeST 1-D instrument in use measuring porcine liver *in vivo*. TeMPeST 1-D visible in foreground (left), mounted on flexible laparoscope holder arm. Testing guided under laparoscopic camera guidance (handheld, background, and view shown at right).

The TeMPeST 1-D is being used in ongoing *in vivo* testing on porcine solid organs[1] to investigate viscous and non-linear elastic behaviors over the range relevant for haptics in surgical simulation. Figure 4 is an image from early, proof-of-concept testing, confirming that the instrument could be successfully employed in a minimally invasive environment. One disadvantage of this particular prototype, however, is that given the convex shape of most of the desirable internal organ surfaces, it is possible to make normal contact at at most one location on a given organ. To obtain data over the surface of the organ, one would require numerous insertion points, at least when used minimally invasively.

A series of tests was begun in conjunction with other researchers performing open surgical testing, which afforded access to large regions of the porcine liver. Anesthesia was achieved using an initial injection, and was maintained using an inhaled anesthetic throughout the testing. The pig was placed on pure oxygen ventilation, which could be suspended for periods of approximately 20 seconds. During this time, the TeMPeST 1-D was brought into contact with the surface of the organ with a predetermined pre-load force; the indentation waveform was generated with the voice-coil motor and imposed on the tissue for approximately 16.5 seconds; the TeMPeST 1-D was removed from the tissue and ventilation resumed. Blood oxygen saturation was monitored and was not observed to fall below 95% during testing.

3. Results

Tests on porcine liver have been performed using both sinusoidal and chirp signals, covering the frequency range of 0.01 to 100Hz, and preloads from 8 to 75mN. Within this range, the elastic modulus, calculated from the measured stiffness and the assumption of a semi-infinite, incompressible elastic medium, has been shown to be a non-linear function of mean applied stress (and therefore with strain) and frequency. A preliminary fit to the fixed frequency sinusoidal data takes the form:

$$\log_{10} E = 3.31 + 0.161 \log_{10} f + 2.15\,\text{E-}4\sigma^{*}_{med}$$

Equation 1

---

[1] All *in vivo* testing was performed under protocols approved by the animal use committees of all of the institutions involved. To minimize the number of animals used, testing was performed either as an addendum to a pre-existing protocol, or was performed together with other researchers conducting similar tests.

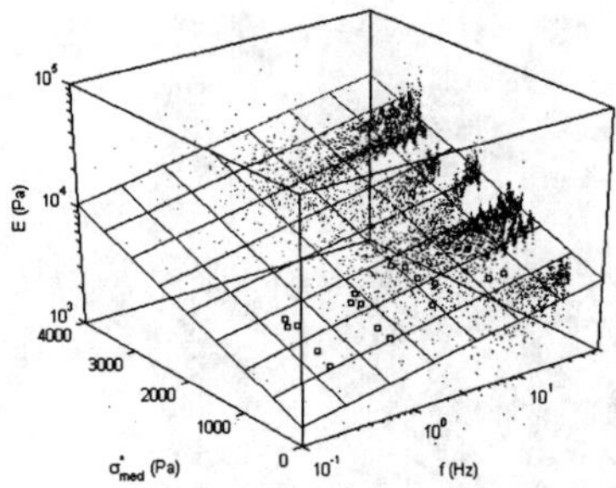

Figure 5. Chirp and fixed frequency sinusoidal data obtained *in vivo* from porcine liver.

where E is the elastic modulus in Pa, f is frequency in Hz, and σ^*_{med} is the median applied stress (median force/punch area). These data, and the fit are shown in Figure 5. What is clear from the testing performed to date is that the chirp tests, while convenient in terms of acquiring a range of frequency dependent data in one trial, have poor accuracy, so further testing will likely be performed using fixed frequency sinusoids.

Recognizing that the elastic modulus is the derivative of stress with respect to strain, this expression can be rewritten as:

$$\sigma = -2020\ln(1 - 0.0005e^{7.62+0.161\ln f}\varepsilon)$$

Equation 2

This fit is based only on the form exhibited by the data, rather than necessarily having a physical basis. As more data become available, parameters for more traditional models will be extracted.

4. Conclusions and ongoing work

The TeMPeST 1-D instrument for measuring visco-elastic properties of solid organ tissues has been completed. Validation testing on known materials was performed to verify the device's performance, and it has been used to gather frequency and stress dependent elasticity data for porcine liver.

Testing is ongoing, and tests planned for the remainder of 2001 and early 2002 include investigations of variation between individuals, inhomogeneity across organ surfaces, and tests of porcine spleen.

Based on the learning experience of these tests, the testing system will be further developed to be sensitive to a wider range of tissue stiffnesses; be less sensitive to disturbances caused by cardiac action; and eventually be modified for use on human organs. Ultimately, such properties will be used in creating surgical simulation systems, which would provide realistic force-feedback to end users from surgical students learning the basic skill required, to experienced surgeons refreshing their skills or developing new procedures.

Acknowledgements

This work was supported in part by the Department of the Army, under contract number DAMD17-99-2-9001. The views and opinions expressed do not necessary reflect the position or the policy of the government, and no official endorsement should be inferred.

References

[1]   Maass, H., Kuhnapfel, U.G.: Noninvasive measurement of elastic properties of living tissue, Computer Assisted Radiology and Surgery (CARS '99): proceedings of the 13th international congress and exhibition (1999) pp. 23–6.

[2]   Suga, M., Matsuda T., Okamoto, J., Takizawa, O., Oshiro, O., Minato, K., Tsutsumi, S., Nagata, I., Sakai, N., Takahashi, T.: Sensible Human Projects: Haptic Modeling and Surgical Simulation Based on Measurements of Practical Patients with MR Elastography–Measurement of Elastic Modulus, Medicine Meets Virtual Reality 2000, Studies in Health Technology and Informatics, 70, Newport Beach, CA (27-30 Jan 2000) pp. 334–40.

[3]   Rosen, J., Hannaford, B., MacFarlane, M.P., Sinanan, M.N.: Force Controlled and Teleoperated Endoscopic Grasper for Minimally Invasive Surgery-Experimental Performance Evaluation, IEEE Transactions on Biomedical Engineering, 46(10) (1999) pp. 1212–1221.

[4]   Scilingo, E.P., DeRossi, D., Bicchi, A., Iacconi, P.: Haptic display for replication of rheological behavior of surgical tissues: modelling, control, and experiments, Proceedings of the ASME Dynamics, Systems and Control Division, Dallas, TX (16-21 Nov 1997) pp. 173–176.

[5]   Brower, I., Ustin, J., Bentley, L., Sherman, A., Dhruv, N., Tendick, F.: Measuring In Vivo Animal Soft Tissue Properties for Haptic Modeling in Surgical Simulation, Medicine Meets Virtual Reality 2001, Studies in Health Technology and Informatics, 81, Newport Beach, CA (24-27 Jan 2001) pp. 69–74.

[6]   Miller, K., Chinzei, K., Orssengo, G., Bednarz, P.: Mechanical properties of brain tissue in-vivo: experiment and computer simulation. Journal of Biomechanics 33 (2000) pp. 1369–76.

[7]   Kauer, M., Vuskovic, V., Dual, J., Szekely, G., Bajka, M.: Inverse Finite Element Characterization of Soft Tissues, Proceedings of Medical Image Computing and Computer-Assisted Intervention, MICCAI 2001, Utrecht, Netherlands, (15-17 Oct 2001), pp. 128-136.

[8]   Ottensmeyer, M.P., Ben-Ur, E., Salisbury, J.K.: Input and Output for Surgical Simulation: Devices to Measure Tissue Properties in vivo and a Haptic Interface for Laparoscopy Simulators, Proceedings of Medicine Meets Virtual Reality 2000, Studies in Health Technology and Informatics, 70, Newport Beach, CA (27-30 Jan 2000) pp. 236–242.

[9]   Ottensmeyer, M.P., Salisbury, J.K.: In vivo mechanical tissue property measurement for improved simulations, Proceedings of Digitization of the Battlespace V and Battlefield Biomedical Technologies II, R. Suresh and H.H. Pien, Eds., Proc. SPIE 4037, Orlando, FL (24-28 Apr 2000) pp. 286–293.

[10]   Ottensmeyer, M.P., Salisbury, J.K.: *In Vivo* Data Acquisition Instrument For Solid Organ Mechanical Property Measurement, Proceedings of MICCAI 2001, Utrecht, Netherlands (15-17 Oct 2001) pp. 975-982.

Medicine Meets Virtual Reality 02/10
J.D. Westwood et al. (Eds.)
IOS Press, 2002

On Defining Metrics for Assessing Laparoscopic Surgical Skills in a Virtual Training Environment

Shahram Payandeh, Alan J. Lomax, John Dill, Christine L. Mackenzie and

Caroline G. L. Cao

Schools of Engineering Science and Kinesiology
Simon Fraser University
Burnaby, British Columbia
CANADA, V5A 1S6

Abstract. One of the key components of any training environment for surgical education is a method that can be used for assessing surgical skills. Traditionally, defining such a method has been difficult and based mainly on observations. However, through advances in modeling techniques and computer hardware and software, such methods can now be developed using combined visual and haptic rendering of a training scene. This paper presents some ideas on how metrics may be defined and used in the assessment of surgical skills in a virtual laparoscopic training environment.

1. Introduction

Since the advent of laparoscopic surgery it has become apparent that new methods of training surgeons are required. Researchers in this field [1,2,3,4,5] have developed a number of virtual training systems; although they have gained some acceptance in the research community none have been fully accepted by surgeons. Many current training environments try to mimic the feel and look of the actual surgical environment, however a simpler intermediate training environment can offer an incremental training process [6,7,8]. One of the key requirements of any virtual training system is methods or metrics that can be used to measure the task performance of the trainee during various training sessions [9]. The metrics can then be used in the skill evaluation modules of such training systems for performance evaluation.

Based on an initial task and motion study of laparoscopic surgical training, various tasks and subtasks were defined [11]. For each subtask, a number of motion and force primitives can be defined. These definitions can then be used as a guideline for modeling and development of components or modules of a virtual training environment. In this initial study the performance of expert and novice surgeons was analyzed and a number of key parameters were identified that can be used to compare the surgical skills of novice and expert surgeons.

In the following section illustrative results from the task analysis study are presented and in the third section examples of the Simon Fraser University Laparoscopic Training Environment (SFU-LTE) are outlined. The fourth section of the paper includes a summary and suggestions for future research directions.

2. Task Analysis of Laparoscopic Surgery

Training sessions in laparoscopic surgery conducted for University of British Columbia surgical residents at the Jack Bell Research Institute's animal laboratory facilities were video taped and the performance of participants analyzed [11]. A video camera recorded the surgeon's hand movements. In addition the image of the operative site in a pig abdomen, including the end-effectors of the manipulators, from the endoscopic camera was combined with the view of the surgeon's hands using a digital mixer and recorded on the same videotape. These two images were displayed on the monitor as a split-screen view. (See Figure 1). In this way we were able to conduct time-line studies of tool movements during various surgical tasks.

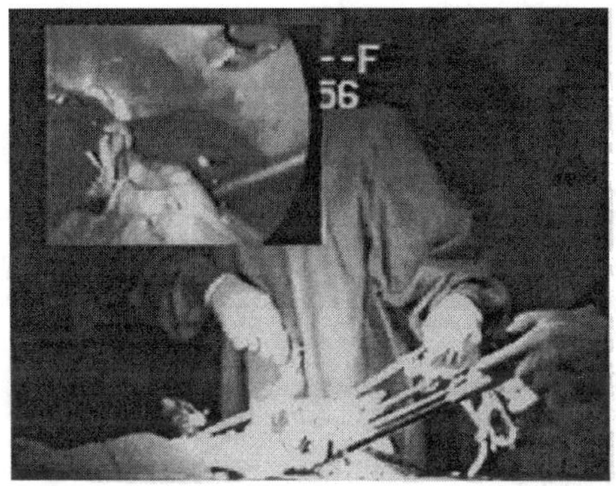

Figure 1 split-screen view of an actual training session.

Evaluation of the videotaped training sessions identified five basic motions that the surgeon/tool performed: reach and orient; grasp and hold/cut; push; pull; and release. Four surgical tasks were evaluated in detail, suturing, tying knots [10], cutting suture and dissecting tissue. Through time-line analysis of the tasks performed by the novice and expert surgeons, the time duration of these basic tasks was used as an independent parameter for comparing various subtasks. For example, Figure 2 shows the breakdown of the dissecting tissue task into two sub-tasks namely pull taut tissue and snip tissue. It also shows the average time for novice surgeons compared to expert surgeons. It can be concluded from this analysis that a measure of performance differences between novices and experts is the length of time taken to complete the pull taut tissue subtask.

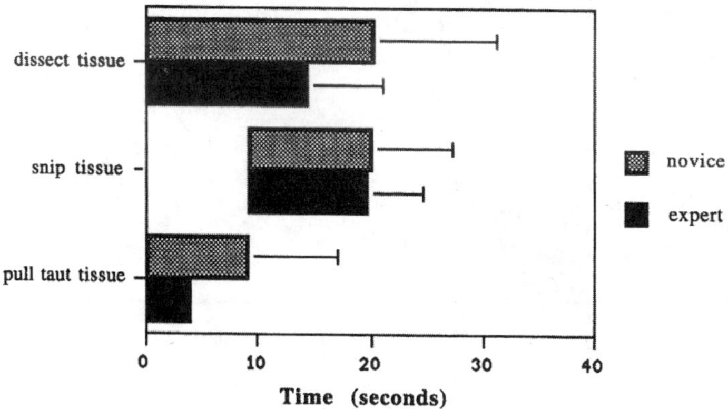

Figure 2 Timeline for the dissecting tissue task, with two subtasks.

Figure 3 shows a breakdown of the suture task into seven subtasks. These subtasks are: position needle; bite tissue; pull needle through tissue; reposition; re-bite tissue; re-pull needle; and pull suture through. Figure 4 shows the average time obtained through time-line analysis of videotapes of these subtasks. It can be seen that compared with expert surgeons, novices took longer, on average, during all the subtasks. Hence, any training system should have components that train novices in these subtasks with the aim of reducing the time taken during the subtasks.

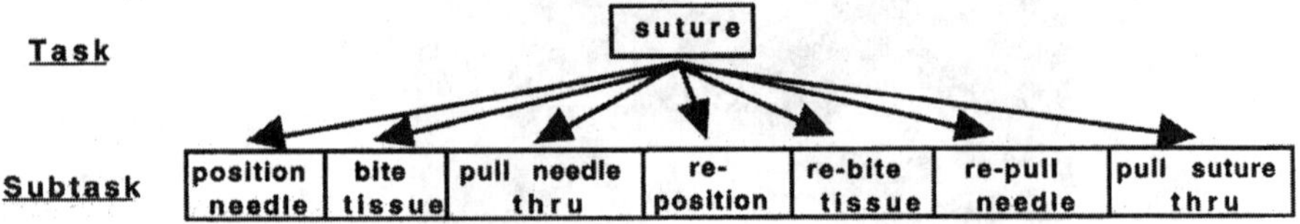

Figure 3 Decomposition of suturing into seven subtasks.

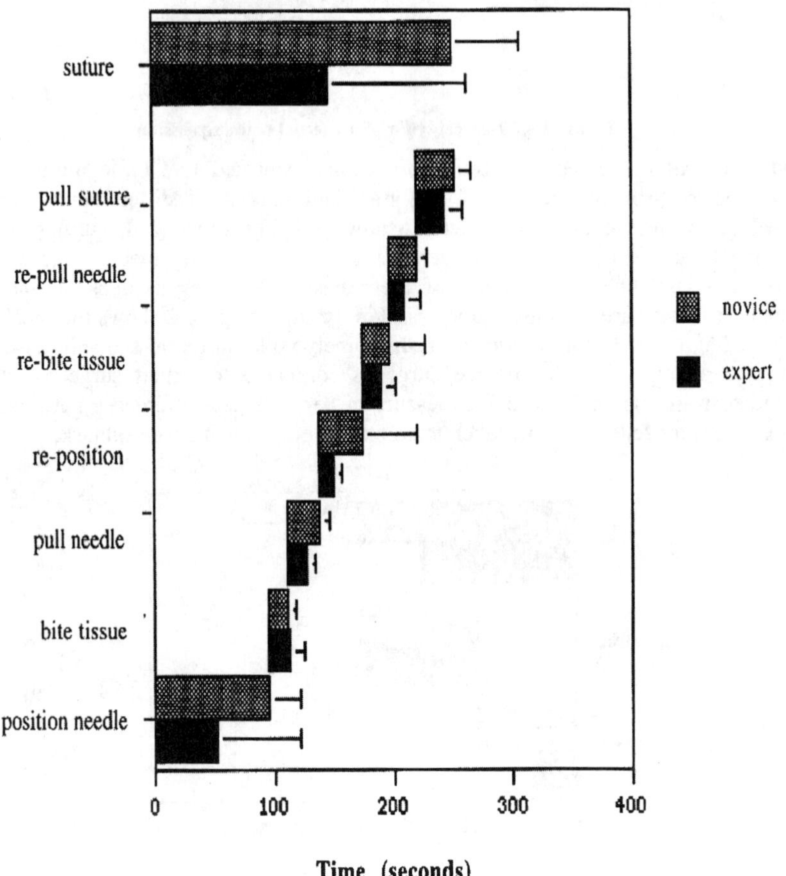

Figure 4 Timeline for the suturing task, and the subtask components.

3. Simon Fraser University Virtual Training Environment

Our task and motion analysis study confirmed that hand-eye coordination tasks are important in the design of laparoscopic surgery training systems and time is a key measure or metric of performance. Figure 5 shows a training exercise where at the beginning of the session, a red flag appears at various locations on one of the three compliant objects [13]. The objective is for the user to reach and touch the flag with the tip of the tool. At the end of the session, a window appears which shows the net distance traveled and the time of flight.

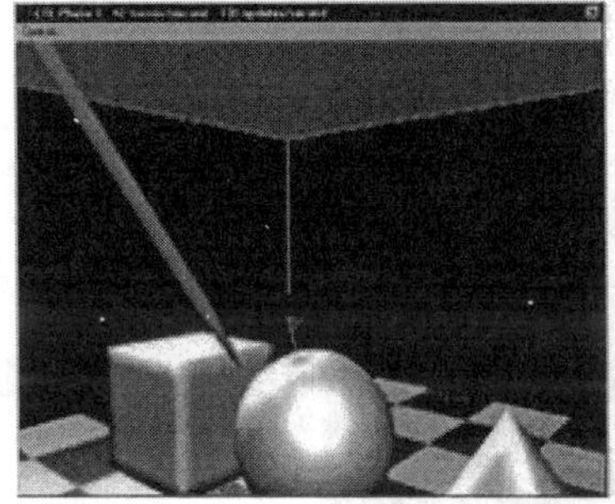
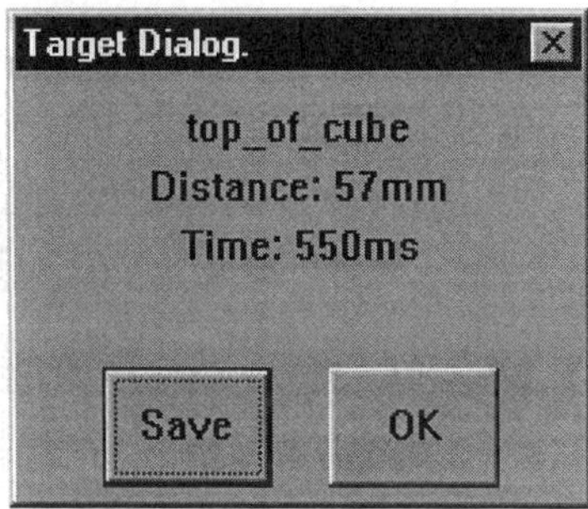

Figure 5 Example of a training session where the user attempts to make contact with the flag and the two metrics used to assess the performance of the user.

Figure 6 shows a virtual training scenario designed to develop the skill required in performing one of the five elemental motions of laparoscopic surgery, the grasping movement. Here the user can initialize a timer by pressing on a virtual button in the scene. The objective is for the user to grasp and pluck a marked flag from a compliant object in the scene.

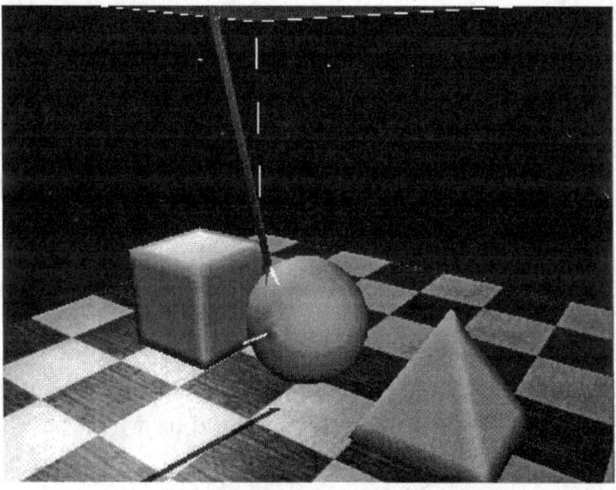

Figure 6 Example of the training session where the task performance is measured by measuring the time that it will take the user to pluck a flag post from a compliant object.

Dissection was studied as one of the four basic tasks, and figure 7 shows the virtual environment initially designed to train this skill. The goal is to dissect the small cylinder from the large one. As shown in the Figure 2, subtasks are pull-taut tissue and snip tissue.

Several measures of user performance were defined. These range from the time between the contacts until the time the object is dissected, to the impedance of the tasks: namely the ratio between the overall force generated during the dissection task and the overall speed of the tip during its trajectory. This latter measure is important since it can give an indication of how fast or slow the user is dissecting the tissue as opposed to ripping the tissue. Another measure is the trajectory of the tip in relation to the direction of the effective pulling of the tissue. Figure 7 shows an example of one of the training sessions where two laparoscopic graspers were used for the dissection task.

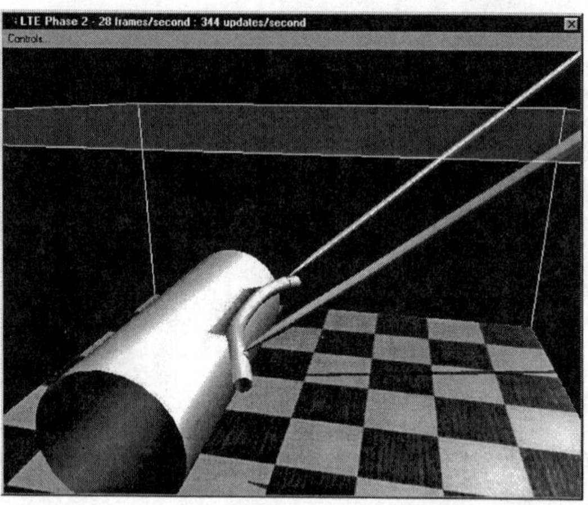

Figure 7 A training session for the dissection task. The small deformable cylinder is dissected from the larger one.

Another training example; we have developed; can be regarded as a metric of tracking dexterity and precision. Here a deformable object is presented in the scene. A nominal trajectory on the object is then generated by the expert or through a lookup library of the paths associated with a certain procedure. The objective of this training phase is for the user to track this nominal path on the deformable object. Figure 8 shows an example of this session. The figure on the left shows the nominal path generated by the expert using a laparoscopic probe while the figure on the right also shows the path generated by the novice. The measures during this phase are, a) the total amount of deviation of the path from the nominal trajectory, b) the force profile on the object created by the novice and c) the total number of contact discontinuities created by a novice when tracing the nominal path. These measures can be the basis for further training of dexterity and precision in this tracking task.

The final example of a training session we have developed is an attempt to simulate organ contact and manipulation. An example would be when the surgeon elevates the right lobe of the liver to examine the under-surface of the lobe. Here the purpose is to identify a specific marker that is hidden under a deformable object. In this example, the object is modeled such that it is resting on a surface in a gravity environment. The trainee then manipulates the object by lifting it with the simulated tool. Markers (here a random letter of the alphabet) are hidden under the compliant object. The variable used for measuring the performance of the trainee is the amount of time it takes for the user to lift and identify the letter under the object. Figure 9 shows the wire-frame view of this training session. Here a letter P is hidden under the compliant sphere. The object can also be constrained or attached to other objects in the scene. Our goal is to incrementally enhance the scene to increasingly resemble the actual surgical environment.

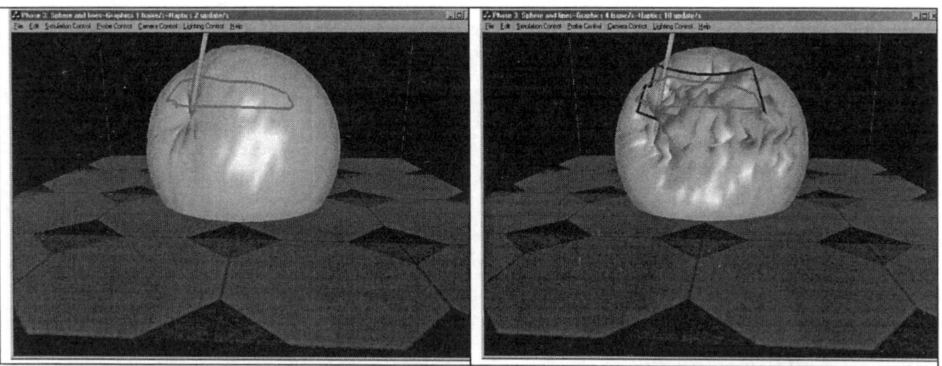

Figure 8 is an example of a training session where the nominal tracing path on a deformable object is generated by an expert surgeon. The trainee then has to trace this path. The metrics of assessment are number of errors, contact discontinuities and excess force

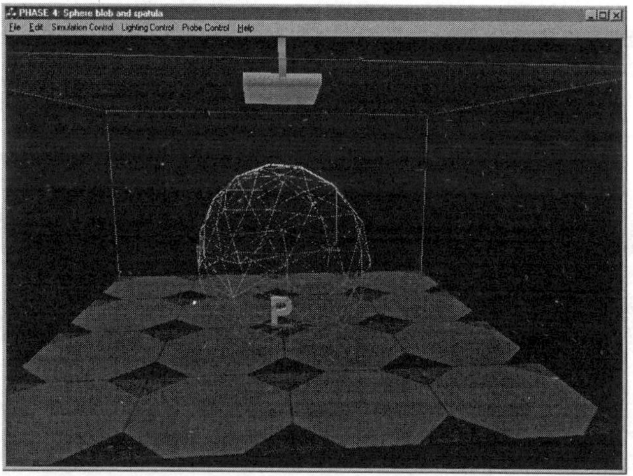

Figure 9. Training session involving a compliant object that is resting on a surface in a gravity environment and a laparoscopic tool. The goal is to identify the hidden letter by lifting the object. The metric of performance is time.

4. Conclusion

The purpose of this paper is to demonstrate the value of task and motion studies in determining the components of basic laparoscopic surgical skills and that these components should be the basis on which virtual training environments are designed. Eventually for virtual surgical simulation to progress standard measures or metrics of laparoscopic surgical skills will be required. At present highly realistic virtual surgical simulations that also have good interactivity are not possible; we are therefore developing the SFU-VTE using simple objects but with good interactivity. We believe that the models we have designed to date can train basic laparoscopic skills and we will in the near future carry out controlled empirical studies to evaluate this. Progress in the design of simulators for the training of laparoscopic surgical skills will require three parallel approaches: increasingly realistic simulations of surgical environments, the study of human interactivity in real-time systems with minimal lag [12], and content based on empirical studies of surgeons' cognitive processes and visuomotor skills.

References

1. U. Kuhnapfel, H.K. Cakmak, H. Maab, Endoscopic Surgery Training using Virtual Reality and Deformable Tissue Simulation, Computer & Graphics, Vol. 24, 671-682 2000.
2. Lapsim simulation, "Surgical Science", www.surgical-science.com
3. R.V. O'Toole et al, Measuring and Developing Suturing Technique with a Virtual Reality Surgical Simulator. J Am Coll Surg, 189: 114-128, 1999.
4. XiTact SA, www.xitact.com
5. MIST-VR: A virtual reality trainer for laparoscopic surgery assesses performance. Ann R Coll Surg Engl 79: 403-404, 1997
6. R.M.Satava, Accomplishments and challenges of surgical simulation dawning of the next generation surgical education. Surg Endosc *15*: 232-241, 2001
7. N.J. Avis , Virtual environment technologies. Min Invas Ther&Allied Technol: 9(5) 333-340, 2000
8. P.J. Gorman et al, The Future of Medical Education Is No longer Blood and Guts, It Is Bits and Bytes. Am J Surg. 180 ; 353-355 , 2000
9. S. Smith et al, The objective assessment of surgical skill. Min Invas & Allied Technol 9(5) 315-320, 2000
10. S. Payandeh and A. Lomax, A Knotting theory and knotting mechanisms. Proceedings of ASME 25th Biennial Mechanisms Conference, 1998
11. C. G. L. Cao, C. L. MacKenzie and .S. Payandeh, Task and Motion Analysis in Endoscopic Surgery. Proceedings of ASME Dynamic Systems, 5th Annual Symposium on Haptic Interface for Virtual Environment and Teleoperation. 1996
12. Z. Stanisic, E. Jackson and S. Payandeh, Virtual Fixtures as an Aid for Teleoperation. Proceedings of 9th Canadian Aeronautic and Space Institute Conference, 1996
13. Z. Cai, J. Dill and S. Payandeh, Haptic Rendering: Toward Deformation Modelling with Haptic Feedback. Proceedings of ASME Dynamic Systems, 9th Annual Symposium on Haptic Interface for Virtual Environment and Teleoperation, 2000.

Medicine Meets Virtual Reality 02/10
J.D. Westwood et al. (Eds.)
IOS Press, 2002

A Virtual Fluoroscopy System and its use for Image Guidance in Unicompartmental Knee Surgery

R Phillips[1], PhD, V Peter[1,2], G-E Faure[1], Q Li[1], PhD, KP Sherman[1,2], PhD, FRCS,
WJ Viant[1], M Bielby[1], AMMA Mohsen[1,2], PhD, FRCS(Orth).

1. Department of Computer Science, University of Hull, UK HU6 7RX.
*2. Department of Orthopaedics and Traumatology, Hull Royal Infirmary, Hull and
East Yorkshire Hospitals NHS Trust, Hull, UK HU3 2JZ.*

Abstract. The C-arm fluoroscope is an indispensable intraoperative 2D imaging device for orthopaedic surgery. However, its frequent use in an operation presents a significant radiation hazard to the theatre staff and patient. A recent technique known as virtual fluoroscopy (VF) enhances the fluoroscope's capability for image guided surgery by tracking optically the position of the C-arm, surgical instruments and the patient. Virtuality is achieved by overlay of surgical instruments onto one or more previously captured fluoroscopic images. A key benefit of VF is that it reduces considerably the radiation hazard. This paper reports on a new VF technique for tracking and calibration of the fluoroscopic C-arm. Also reported is the use of our VF system to provide a new image guided technique for the accurate placement of the femoral component of unicompartmental knee prosthesis.

1. Introduction

The C-arm fluoroscope is an indispensable intraoperative 2D imaging device for orthopaedic surgery. Its frequent use in an operation presents a significant radiation hazard to the theatre staff and patient. A recent technique known as virtual fluoroscopy (VF) enhances the fluoroscope's capability by producing virtual images of the patient and surgical instruments. This is achieved by tracking during surgery the position of the C-arm, surgical instruments and the patient. As these virtual images are produced without radiation, VF is particularly well suited to image guided surgical interventions.

In VF appropriate actual fluoroscopic images of the bones being operated upon are taken using a C-arm fluoroscope; the C-arm may then be removed from the operation field. The position of surgical instruments is then tracked optically through attached reference frames and this allows the computer to overlay a real time projection of the instrument onto previously captured images. By attaching an optically tracked frame (known as a dynamic reference frame - DRF) to the bone, surgical instruments can be overlaid onto these virtual images even when the bone moves. The surgical application of VF include insertion of pedicle screws, insertion of hip screws and distal locking of intramedullary nails [1].

Available VF systems include Medtronic Sofamor Danek's Fluoronav[TM] and Medivision's SurgiGATE. In these systems an optically tracked grid is permanently attached to the C-arm's x-ray receptor. This grid both tracks the position of the C-arm and calibrates the image distortion inherent in fluoroscopic images. This paper reports on a new technique for tracking the position and calibrating the distortion for a C-arm fluoroscope. This technique is based on a small registration phantom that is placed close to the operation site whilst imaging.

This paper also reports on a new image guided technique, namely the accurate placement of the femoral component for an Oxford unicompartmental knee prosthesis.

2. A Phantom-based Approach to Virtual Fluoroscopy

To overlay the position of surgical instuments onto previously captured fluoroscopic images requires, firstly, accurate 2D calibration of fluoroscopic images and, secondly, accurate registration of the fluoroscopic image cone space with the coordinate space of the optical tracking system.

2.1 Preoperative Calibration of X-ray Images

Fluoroscopic images suffer from a number of distortion effects, such as pincushion, S shaped distortion, etc [2, 3]. This image distortion is dynamic both in terms of time and with the position of the C-arm. A major factor of this dynamic variation of distortion is the strength and orientation of the magnetic fields surrounding the C-arm.

Calibration in our VF system involves preoperative imaging of an x-ray translucent plate containing an evenly spaced grid of 64 x 64 balls. This plate is placed on the x-ray receptor cover of the C-arm and an image taken. Software automatically detects the grid and calculates and then files a distortion-undistortion map. Intraoperatively, distortion from each fluoroscopic image is subsequently removed before displaying it to the surgeon as a virtual fluoroscopic image.

We have found that sufficient image accuracy for the placement of surgical instruments is obtained by calibrating in just two positions, i.e. with the axis of fluoroscopic image cone vertical and horizontal. Furthermore, we have found that calibration is only required infrequently, typically once a month and it is undertaken as a maintenance task.

2.2 Intraoperative Registration of fluoroscopic image space

Registration of the fluoroscope's image space involves accurate localisation of the position (in the coordinate space of the optical tracking system) of the x-ray source and the virtual image plane (i.e. the grid plane of the calibration plate) of the C-arm. This registration occurs for each actual fluoroscopic image taken.

Registration involves placing a small registration phantom (Fig. 1) in the image space of the C-arm and, where possible, close to the patient operating site. To assist positioning of the phantom, a laser cross showing the centre of the image beam can be projected onto the patient.

The phantom consists of an H arrangement of 21 metal balls that measures approximately 2" x 2" by ½". The projection of these balls appears in a fluoroscopic image. The phantom is held by an end-effector and a lockable passive arm (Fig 2). The position of the phantom is tracked by an NDI Polaris optical tracking system. When a patient is actually imaged, software undistorts the image and then automatically detects the position of the phantom in the image. Then knowing the position of the phantom, a registration algorithm (based on a pinhole camera model) calculates the position of the C-arm in the coordinate space of the optical tracking system. Significant obscuration of the phantom frequently occurs in the image due to shadow of muscles, bone edges, retractors, etc, but the phantom extraction software has considerable robustness to such obscuration.

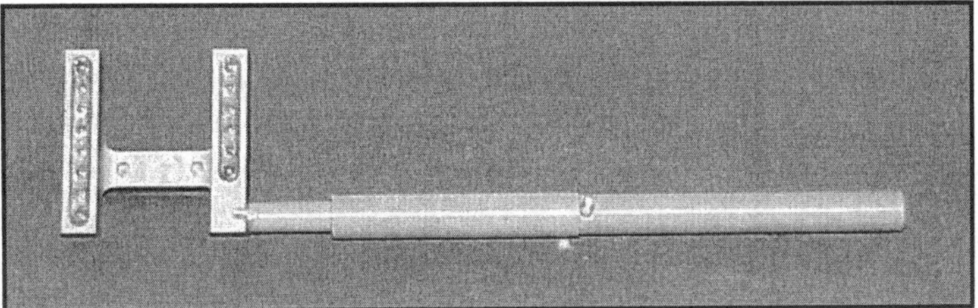

Fig. 1 The registration phantom.

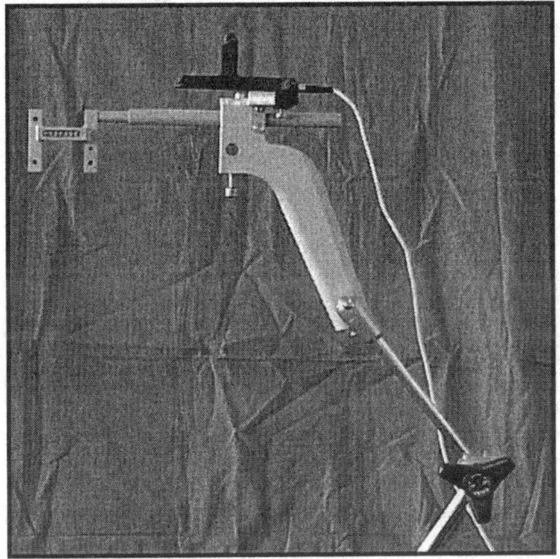

Fig. 2 Registration phantom in end-effector with optically tracked reference frame; end-effector is held by a lockable passive arm.

The registration technique compensates for C-arm flex and the linear elements of dynamic distortion. It is worth noting that a typical C-arm span can flex between 1 and 5 mm and this also changes the orientation between the x-ray source and the x-ray receptor. In fact the registration algorithm also compensates for the rotational and translation parameters of image distortion and this reduces considerably the effects of the dynamic distortion of images that occur.

The design of the registration phantom was developed using extensive computer simulation that modelled the fluoroscopic image intensifier and the propagation of errors. The design simulation was used to determine the best trade-off between optimising reconstruction performance and the clinical requirements of being as unobtrusive in fluoroscopic images and as small as possible. Practical validation tests have shown that an image has a maximum calibration error of 0.5 mm [4].

3. Protocol for Unicompartmental Knee Surgery

3.1 Unicompartmental Knee Replacement

Unicondylar total knee replacements have come a long way since their introduction some fifteen years ago. It was first designed as a simple surface replacement device for unicompartmental osteoarthritis when just one compartment of the knee was involved. Today it is also used in medial compartment osteoarthritis and has largely replaced high tibial osteotomy as the treatment of choice for this condition.

Since its initial introduction the implant design, instrumentation and surgical technique has been refined a great deal. The extent of the surgical exposure has progressively been reduced and greater attention is being paid towards getting the alignment of the implant correct. Currently the approach to the knee is through a 5-8 cm incision. The advantage of this is that there is less postoperative pain, it decreases the incidence of postoperative adhesions and joint stiffness and therefore recovery is much faster. In fact there are several centres where patients are having unicondylar knee replacements done as day cases.

A disadvantage of the minimally invasive approach is that it limits the visualisation of the structures within the knee and thus can make selection of anatomical reference points for aligning the components of the implant more difficult. A potential advantage of an image guided surgery approach would be to assist in selection of these reference points and in positioning surgical guides, thus reducing implant alignment error and improve consistency of outcome.

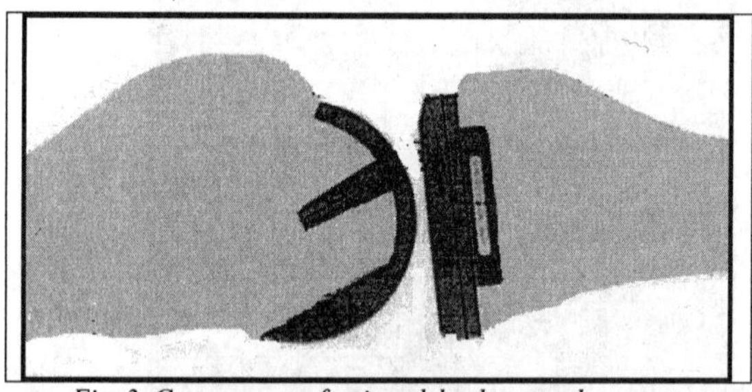

Fig. 3 Components of unicondylar knee replacement

A unicondylar total knee replacement replaces the joint surfaces of the medial compartment of the knee joint (Fig 3). The prosthesis comprises a tibial and a femoral component. The tibial component replaces the joint surface of the tibia plateau. Similarly, the femoral component replaces the joint surface of the medial condyle of the distal femur. A polyethylene bearing completes the prosthetic joint.

The goal of unicompartmental knee arthroplasty is to create a mechanical axis that is neutral. Over correction will result in accelerated degeneration of the opposite compartment. Under correction will cause early wear and loosening of the prosthesis. The joint line of the replaced component should be parallel to the floor and perpendicular to the mechanical axis. To achieve this the femoral and tibial components are aligned to be perpendicular to the mechanical axis. A well-designed instrumentation set greatly assists accurate cut placement and thus hopefully assure stable component fixation. An image guided surgery approach offers the opportunity to provide simpler instrumentation and reduce the complexity of the procedure.

This paper will focus on using virtual fluoroscopy for the accurate placement of the femoral component of the uncompartmental prosthesis. This placement fits well a basic principle of orthopaedic surgery [5] which is the "placement of an object (guide wire, saw, screw, tube, scope, etc) at a specific site within a region, via a trajectory which is planned from x-ray based 2D images and governed by 3D anatomical constraints".

3.2 Existing Protocol for Unicompartmental Knee Replacement Surgery

Prior to surgery the size of the femoral component is chosen preoperatively using an x-ray templates applied to the x-ray image of the medial femoral. The template of the component should lie about 2 mm outside the radiographic image of the condyle to allow for the thickness of the articular cartilage.

With the patient in the supine position and with the hip flexed and leg dependent, a small (5-8 cm) incision is made on the medial side of the knee. Osteophytes are then removed from the condyle and the intercondylar notch.

To prepare the tibia for its tibial component a tibial saw guide is attached to the tibia. This guide is positioned so that it is parallel in both planes to the long axis of the tibia and at the right resection level. A vertical and horizontal saw cut is then made in the tibial plateau. While making the vertical cut the saw is directed towards the head of the femur so that the attachments of the cruciate ligaments are not accidentally removed. Making this vertical cut could also be assisted by virtual fluoroscopy, but this is not discussed further in this paper.

Preparing for the femoral component is a complex procedure. It starts by making a femoral drill hole 1 cm anterior to the anteromedial corner of the inter condylar notch. This is the point where the anatomical and mechanical axis intersects in almost all knees and it is important that this drill hole is correctly located. An intramedullary rod is then inserted into the femoral intramedullary canal using this starter hole. The axis of the rod represents the anatomical axis of the femur and the intramedullary rod should thus be parallel to the shaft in both AP and lateral planes.

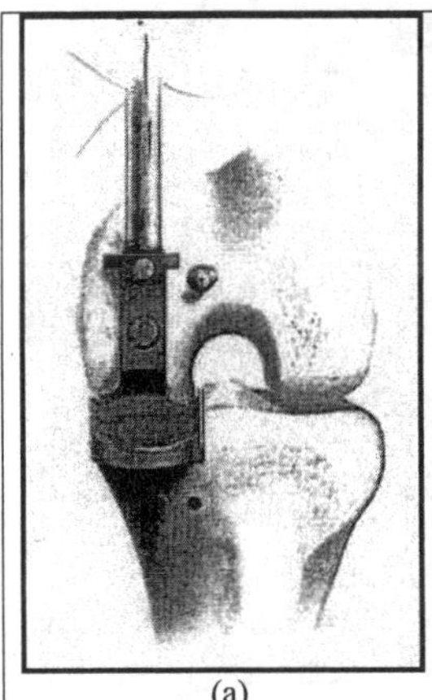 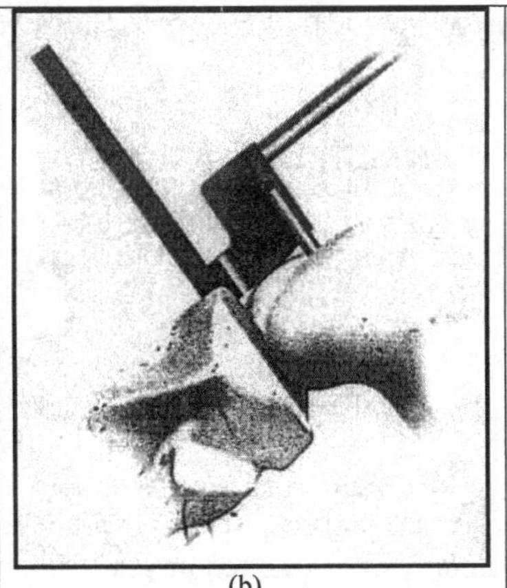 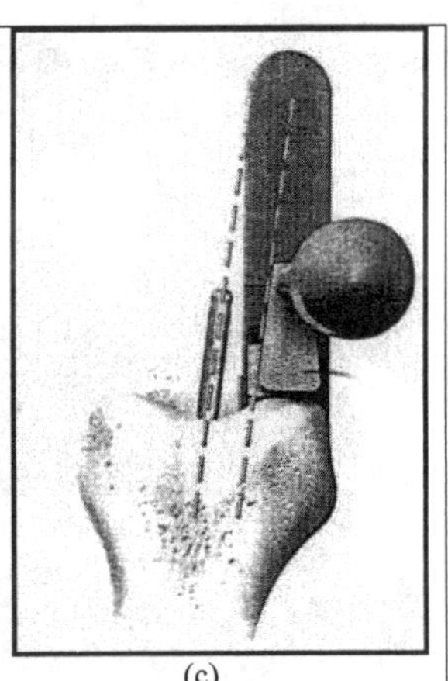

(a) (b) (c)

Fig.4 Alignment of the femoral drill guide

The femoral drill guide is now positioned in the knee joint using a tibial template and a feeler gauge of suitable width (Fig 4). The alignment criterion for the femoral drill guide are as follows.
1. From the front the femoral guide is in the middle of the condyle (Fig 4 a).
2. The handle of the femoral guide is parallel with the long axis of the tibia (Fig 4a).
3. The upper surface of the guide should be parallel with the intramedullary rod (Fig 4b)
4. The 7° angled fin must be parallel with the intramedullary rod when viewed from above (Fig 4c). The purpose of this is to achieve alignment with the mechanical axis of the femur.

When all these criterion are met, two holes are drilled into the femur through the appropriate holes in the femoral drill guide and a femoral saw block inserted into the drill holes. The placement of these two drill holes with the femoral drill guide is the critical steps in the accurate placement of the femoral component. (It is for this positioning of the femoral drill guide that we shall use virtual fluoroscopy.) A flat cut is then made to remove the posterior part of the condyle. Finally a spigot is inserted into the larger of these two holes and a mill is used to remove the necessary amount of bone from the distal end of the femur. Using trial components the flexion and extension gaps of the knee joint are checked and if necessary more bone is milled from the femur.

The operation is completed by equalization of the flexion and extension gaps, final preparation of the tibial plateau, checking for tissue impingement, insertion and then cementing of the components.

3.3 A Virtual Fluoroscopy-Based Protocol

As mentioned above we are investigating the effectiveness of using virtual fluoroscopy to site the drill holes in the femoral condyle in preparation for fitting the femoral component. Thus the revised procedure using virtual fluoroscopy is as follows.

In the operating theatre a Polaris optical tracking system is used to track both patient anatomy and surgical instruments. More specifically dynamic reference frames are attached both to the femur and the tibia. This allows the overlay of surgical instruments onto fluoroscopic images to take account of movements of both femur and tibia. A reference frame is attached to the femoral guide (Fig 5) so that its position may be tracked.

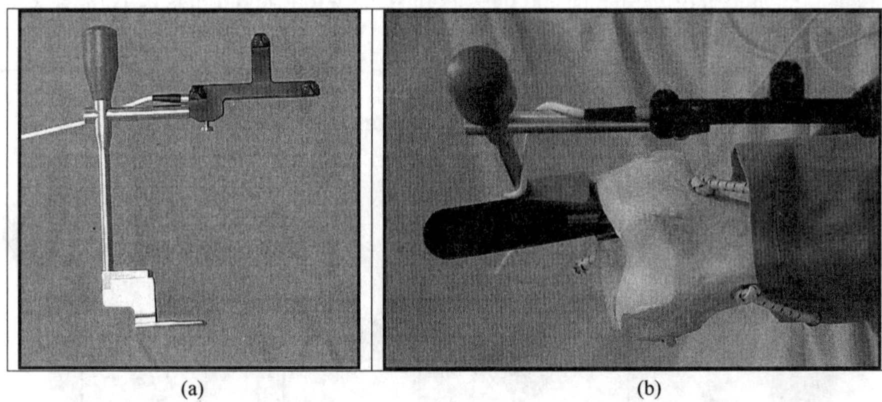

(a)   (b)

Fig.5 (a) Femoral guide with reference frame (b)Alignment of the femoral drill guide

The following intraoperative fluoroscopic images are taken of the patient: AP view of the femur head, AP and lateral view of the femur shaft, AP and lateral view of the tibia and an AP of the knee in 40° of flexion with a beam view 30° off vertical. Our VF system allows the surgeon to locate and view in a convenient way 3D points, lines and planes on these images. Thus the surgeon locates on these images the anatomy features of interest, namely: the head of the femur, the anatomical and mechanical axis of the femur and the axis of the tibia. These are used later to help position the femoral drill guide.

In preparing the femoral component with VF there is no need for the initial intramedullary locating hole or no need to implant the intramedullary rod. This is because the anatomical axis can be determined directly from virtual fluoroscopic images.

As before the femoral drill guide is now positioned in the knee joint using a tibial template and a feeler gauge of suitable width (Fig 4). To meet the guide's alignment criterion the surgeon uses the 7 virtual fluoroscopic images upon which appears the outline of the surgical instrument as it moved by the surgeon. To assist guide positioning some axis of the drill guide are extended on the virtual fluoroscopic views. The use of virtual fluoroscopy for positioning the guide is as follows.

1. *Femoral guide is in the middle of the condyle* – this is checked both visually and on the various virtual fluoroscopy views.
2. *Handle of the femoral guide parallel with the long axis of the tibia* – this is checked by viewing the guide's handle on the AP and lateral virtual views of the tibia.

3. *Upper surface of the guide parallel with the anatomical femur axis* (in conventional approach this is given by the intramedullary rod) – this is checked in the lateral virtual view of the femur.
4. *Femoral guide is aligned with anatomical axis of femur* (in conventional approach this is checked using the angled fin and the intramedullary rod) – this can be check in the AP virtual view of the femur where the fin should be parallel to the anatomical axis and the centre line of the guide should pass through the centre of femoral head.

Once all these alignment criterion have been met, then the two locating holes for the femoral saw block are drilled. After drilling the first hole, the position of the guide is checked and adjusted using again the virtual fluoroscopic views. The main drill hole is then made and the rest of the procedure then continues as described previously.

4. Results

The registration and calibration technique described has already been proven clinically in our other existing computer assisted orthopaedic system (CAOS) projects [6]. A laboratory-based VF system is being evaluated for effectiveness and efficacy for unicompartmental knee surgery as described in this paper. This evaluation is using a configuration of plastic bones. A modular design approach has been used and we can use our VF system also with a Flashpoint optical tracking system.

5. Conclusions

We have developed a new registration technique for virtual fluoroscopy. The potential for VF is being evaluated for unicompartmental knee surgery. It should lead to a simpler, more precise and less demanding surgical technique. Our approach to virtual fluoroscopy has advantages over existing VF systems. Our approach reduces very significantly the optically tracked volume during surgery; it interferes less with existing clinical practice; and the image obscuration is significantly reduced. These benefits arise from using a small registration phantom that is placed close to the operating site whereas most other VF systems track a much larger grid phantom attached to the C-arm.

6. References

1. R Hofstetter, M Slomyczykowski, M Sati, *et al.*, Fluoroscopy as an imaging means for computer-assisted surgical intervention. *Computer Aided Surgery*, **4** (1999), 65-76.
2. JM Boone, JA Seibert and W Blood, Analysis and correction of imperfections in the image intensifier TV-digitiser imaging chain. *Medical Physics*, **18** (1991), 236-242.
3. E Pietka and HK Huang. Correction of aberration in image intensifier systems. *Computer Medical Imaging Graphics*, **16** (1992), 253-58.
4. WJ Viant, R Phillips, MS Bielby, *et al.*, A Technique for a Very High Accuracy Image Intensifier Calibration, Medicine Meets Virtual Reality '7 Conference Proceedings, pp 379-380, January 20-23 1999, IOS Press.
5. AMMA Mohsen, KP Sherman, TJ Cain, *et al.*, End user issues for a surgical computer - robotic assisted systems. *Transactions of Institute of Measurement and Control*, **17** (1995), 265-71.
6. WJ Viant, R Phillips, JG Griffiths, *et al.*, A Computer Assisted Orthopaedic Surgical System for Distal Locking of Intramedullary Nails, *Proc of the Institute of Mechanical Engineers* Part H, **211** (1997), pp 293-300.

Medicine Meets Virtual Reality 02/10
J.D. Westwood et al. (Eds.)
IOS Press, 2002

Neuropsychological Performance and Integrated Evaluation for Disabled People using Virtual Reality: Integrated VR Profile

PierAntonio Piccini
Centro Sistemi Virtual Reality-CSVR
Opera Diocesana Assistenza
95030 Catania, Italy
E-mail: csvr.oda@tiscalinet.it

Abstract. This chapter describes a Virtual Reality (VR) based innovative model of evaluation of the performance and potentiality of young mentally/psychically disabled subjects with learning difficulties. Using an immersive PC-based VR system, the study investigated the characteristics of 150 disabled subjects in the EU funded project "Horizon O.D.A. - Catania-1998-2000". The result is the definition of an individual neuropsychological "Integrated Profile", based on VR performance, that allows an objective functional benchmark between different subjects. This model can be used to investigate the possibility of job integration for mentally/psychically disabled subjects.

1. Introduction

The primary goal of the Virtual Reality (VR) activity, inserted in the EU funded project "Horizon O.D.A. Catania 1998 - 2000" , is the definition of an innovative model of evaluation of an individual's potentiality in a real working context, which can also be used to evaluate the ability / performance of young disabled subjects with learning difficulties [1].

1.1 Background

The computer system used in the study consists of 2 HP Kayak redundant and connected workstations, fitted with a Sony Glasstron peripheral viewer, integral helmet-Glove 5DT (sx and dx), Fast Track / position tracking system, Inter Trax / integrated aim on viewer system, 21 in. monitor (effect Desktop), using Superscape VRT software version 4.56. The lay-out of the VR postings, VR activity spaces and CSVR Operators were suited for the conditions and characteristics of the disabled subjects [2].

To achieve the important aim of integration, an innovative system is proposed, with the acquisition of Psychosocial Clinical date from one Handy.Net for 800 people, addressing the intervention towards personalized consultation for 150 subjects.

2. Objectives, Method and Tools

The characteristic content of VR activity was: the experimentation and verification of the VR innovative model, integrated with other standard models of psychosocial clinical and of orientation / formation; for the global investigation of the disabled persons inserted in the project, with the model of integration developed according to the standard scheme: Objective VR Activities - Contents VR Tool - *Verification Virtual Reality* - Objective Orientation - Contents Disabilities; the formulation and presentation of the tool *Integrated Profile VR.*

2.1 The basic Indicators

The basic indicators of the method are:

- 150 disabled subjects followed by VR application - aged 14 - 46 years.
- Formulation and control of actions with the disabled subject for standard methods and procedures.
- The entire VR activity as a Psychosocial Clinical Setting was programmed with the creation of a standard protocol and application of 4 tests / virtual worlds in sequence and a standard protocol of diagnostic evaluation (the type and degree of disabilities are suitable for Public Health Committee).
- The indicators of evaluation and results derive from factors external to the subjects pre-during-post VR application and from factors internal to the VR activity during VR applications.
- The times-phases of VR activity were assigned to the elaboration / evaluation component.

2.2 Standard Procedures

The standard procedures of CSVR activity were conducted as follows:

1. Accompaniment of disabled subject by support operator throughout CSVR.
2. Heading VR and Form 1 compilation.
3. Activity in posting VR – observation – survey – recording – support, with 4 VR tests in sequence.
4. Compilation of Technical Survey Cards in VR test (virtual world) applications.
5. Technical evaluation of single VR test
6. Evaluation of single Psychological VR test sector and general VR sector
7. Compilation and evaluation of SelfEvaluation Questionnaire.
8. Verification and description of insertion data in Integrated Diagnostic VR Model.
9. Verification and description of data processing in Diagnostic VR Model for the innovative orientation.
10. Compilation and evaluation of the Functional VR Diagnosis integrated in the Integrated VR Profile

2.3 Tools for the innovative intervention with Virtual Reality activity in CSVR

The specialized model was initially designed and structured for the global insertion of VR activity data in terms of the activity / type, functionality, method and times of evaluation / compilation / control and integration of the results [3].

This model, denominated VR Activity Data Insertion Form, contains all the sectors, tools and procedures to achieve the project aim and consists of a basic integrated diagnostic in Neuro-Psychosocial Investigation with pre-evaluation, of 3 VR sectors in VR tests (education-learning-orientation/training), an Integrated VR Diagnostic Model in 7 areas of Psychological evaluation, and the final and complete Integrated VR Profile Model.

In particular, the tools developed for use with the disabled subjects, were:

- *Form 1*, for the acceptance of in CSVR by disabled subjects, with case indications.
- *Card of Technical Survey of VR test*, to note the effects-results of each VR test performed (educational / learning / orientation) with the single disabled subject.
- *VR SelfEvaluation Questionnaire*, for the immediate comparison with the disabled subject post-VR application [4].
- *Forms of VR activity Investigation*, in Integrated Diagnostic VR Model, for the database to elaborate and to complete the Integrated VR Profile

2.4 The Integrated Diagnostic VR Model

This is the complex system of assignment, elaboration, correlation of all data (observations, degrees of effect) and results obtained from the activity of a single subject.

It was purpose - built with the following factors and scheme.

- 1) Recording in the model of all the scores marked in 4 VR tests and in the SelfEvaluation Questionnaire, with scale: *2 (none) 4 (insufficient) 6 (fair) 8 (good) 10 (excellent)* for 150 specialized items of evaluation in 7 psychological areas assigned to the single test and divided into *Personality/Emotional/Affective Sector - Interactional/Relational/Behavioral Sector - Cognitive/ Intellectual Sector - Sensorial Sector - Psychomotor/Perceptive Sector - Expressive/Communicational Sector – Neuropsychological Sector*; for all adaptations by the subject to the VR instrumentation, initial and final, to single VR test, for the different degree s of support (guidance) given in single VR tests.
- 2) Analysis and verification of the correlation found in the recording of the model computer form data, with the quantitative description of the score obtained in the 7 areas of psychological evaluation marked in each VR test performed and in the overall VR activity developed by the subject; with further assignment of the scores (again with the scale 2 - 4 - 6 - 8 - 10, for connection and statistic function) referring to:

a)   degree of necessity - *Autonomy* – recorded in each VR test;
b)   level reached in each VR test and for each psychological sector in the evaluation parameters: *Recovery - Consolidation - Expansion;*
c)   level reached in the correlation between a) and b) for each psychological sector with 3 evaluative parameters of *Ability Competence - Potential Evolution - Self Efficacy.*

3. The "Integrated VR Profile" Model

This is the definitive tool obtained from the entire VR activity and represents the result of all the data for each disabled subject in CSVR and from personalized consultation. It contains the following indicators of evaluation: personal / individual and general reference data of the VR activity, correspondence data with the Handy.Net (7 descriptions), VR profile evaluation with the important indicators of:

◆   Recording in the model of the subject's personal data derived from the Handy.Net and Form 1, for the elaboration of assignments and the correlation in the Integrated Diagnostic VR Model. The principle references and diagnostic indicators were: *Age - Sex -Typology of Disabilities – Degree of Disabilities - Left / Right Gradient – Pharmacological Treatment – Sight Handicap – Motor Handicap – Post VR Support – Experience in Education, Rehabilitation, Formation, Work.*

◆   Recording in the model of the subject's personal data for *Ability Competence – Potential Evolution – Self Efficacy,* with the score value min = 1, max = 10.

◆   Recording in the model for 5 sectors: *Personality / Motivational Sector, Interactional Sector, Cognitive / Neuropsychological Sector, Sensorial Sector, Innovative / Orientation Sector,* with the score value min = 1, max = 10.

◆   Compilation of *Integrated Functional VR Diagnosis,* with analytical description of the fitness found in the innovative orientation and of the proposals / individual necessity for occupational integration.

3.1 The Evaluation of Integrated tool VR Profile and VR activity for Disabled People

The *Evaluation* is important to highlight the main, and most difficult, methodological content on which the present formulation and activities are based. While providing important and reliable results; evaluation has been, and will be even more so in the near future, a decisive factor in documenting the effectiveness of innovative tools and their results and benefits for people with difficulties [5].

This is the most complex methodological question raised by the VR activity applied in the UE project "Horizon O.D.A. Catania 1998 - 2000", contemporarily deepening, for every disabled subject, in every result / effect / area of survey, the dubiousness and the typicality in the areas: personality - cognitive - neuropsychological - formative of the single subject, application - potentiality of the innovative Virtual Reality tool, significance - validation of the VR method for the innovative orientation [6].

There was also an overall investigative method assessment (evaluation *in itinere* and post) of functions in terms of: *effectiveness* of the methodology suited for the content and objectives, *validity* of the VR results with the single subject in the Integrated VR Profile, *signification* of the VR test / applications with the subjects / disability range [7] [8].

4. Results of VR activity for Disabled People

We describe some of the principle results of the activity developed by the Centro Sistemi Virtual Reality, following the methodological characteristics to achieve the objective of the project.

The objective was reached with the standardization of the principal tool *Integrated VR Profile.* This model, in addition to being the concrete synthesis of the whole activity and VR method performed with CSVR, represents a unique tool of its kind to identify, describe, integrate and confirm the important and individual / personal / characteristics with some basic typical functions related to the specific orientation for young disabled subjects.

The primary characteristic was the identification of a meaningful *fitness* for integration in the workforce for the disabled, analyzed-structured-obtained by application of the innovative Virtual Reality method.

The principle parameters finalized to VR activity were:

- Typology of Disability for each subject, described as Mental Disabilities - Psychic Disabilities - Difficulty of Learning Disabilities;
- Degree of the Disabilities associated to the Typology for each subject with Medium-Serious, Medium, Medium-Light and Light;
- Age divided into 3 Areas of survey - 14/18 - 19/26 - 27/46;
- Gender (Table 1).

Table 1. Basic parameters for Disabled People in VR activity

Parameters	Numerical Values	Percentage Values
Number Examined Subjects	150	-
Male	110	73%
Female	40	27%
Psychic Disabilities	14	9%
Mental Disabilities	112	75%
Difficulty of Learning Disabilities	24	16%
Degree Medium - Serious	5	3%
Degree Medium	57	38%
Degree Medium - Light	50	33%
Degree Light	38	25%
Age 14/18	59	39%
Age 19/26	52	35%
Age 27/46	39	26%

4.1 Principal results and functions (indicators and variables)

The specific results of the Virtual Reality activity, are directly correlated to the individual characteristics of each subject and were correlated *in itinere* to a specialist evaluation conducted on the overall VR activity developed by all 150 subjects. The principal results - indicators used were:

- Subjects with Right Gradient: 85%, Left Gradient: 15%, Pharmacological Treatment: 29%, Sight Handicap: 33%, Motor Handicap: 7%, Post VR Support: 9%, other Guidance in post VR: 3%.
- Recognition of the Emotional and Motivational Status of each subject [9]. Emotional Status is intended as the mean function that the subject self-evaluates in the degree of emotion / worry pre-during-post VR activity. Motivational Status is intended as the mean function that the subject self-evaluates for the degree of satisfaction / interest post VR tests. The positive score recorded shows the high motivational / emotional value of the Virtual Reality activity, and analysis of these data is currently in progress.
- Time recording of the VR test - application, with the results: Time <30' = 59%, Time >30' / <40' = 38%, Time >40' = 3%, Average Total Time of VR tests: = 30 minutes. The particular indicators of Variations and Adaptations in the sequence of the VR tests were also appraised [10]. Variations and adaptations to VR instrumentation and to space post VR is intended as the increase, during the execution of all VR tests, on the factors of viewer/desktop/helmet functionality, movement in space, functionality of the glove in the 4th VR test.

As parameters internal to the tests and meaningful parameters for diagnostic evaluation, the indicators of *Recovery – Consolidation – Expansion* were used. The positive score recorded show the high dynamic value of the Virtual Reality activity. Analysis of these data is currently in progress.

- Recognition of experience type, pre - VR activity for typology disabilities / age [11]. The results: in video games = 57%, in educational = 74%, in formation / orientation = 67%, in rehabilitation = 83%, in work experience = 7%.

4.2 Results of Psychological Evaluation and Support Sectors in VR activity.

In Table 2, percentages are described on a scale from least to sufficient for every positive value of all psychological sectors and for each degree of necessity / support found in all subjects. In particular, there is *a meaningful score in the Interactional and Personality Sector* , considering that this is a completely new approach for the subject; *a meaningful score for the Sensorial Sector* considering that this is a dimension/activity with a notable index of inexperience and novelty of the sensorial situation; *only one under average score in the Cognitive Sector*, demonstrating that the subjects indeed manifest in this sector the principal aspects of the disabilities ascertained; *a notable score for necessity of guidance / support to perform VR tests,* demonstrating that the Virtual Reality activity requires appropriate support during execution and that the majority of subjects needed constant guidance.

Table 2. Psychological and Support Sectors in VR activity for Disabled People

Parameters	Percentage Values
Personality Sector	67%
Interactional Sector	74%
Cognitive Sector	44%
Sensorial Sector	60%
Psychomotor Sector	53%
Expressive Sector	53%
Neuropsychological Sector	56%
Support	69%

4.3 Results of Indicators for Ability Competence - Potential Evolution - Self Efficacy

In Table 3, it can be seen that in *Abilities* and *Self Efficacy* (*Effectiveness*) the most indicative area is recorded on the score >5 = 6, while in *Potentialities* the most indicative area is recorded on the score >6 = 7.

This confirms the validity and importance of the VR activity in the specific observation – survey – coherence of the *potential increases in every disabled subject's possession* [12] [13].

Table 3. The final values of Ability Competence, Potential Evolution, Self Efficacy

Parameters	Percentage Values
Ability Competence < 4 = 5	9%
Ability Competence > 5 = 6	*43%*
Ability Competence > 6 = 7	38%
Ability Competence > 7 = 8	9%
Ability Competence > 8 = 9	1%
Potential Evolution < 4 = 5	6%
Potential Evolution > 5 = 6	27%
Potential Evolution > 6 = 7	*37%*
Potential Evolution > 7 = 8	26%
Potential Evolution > 8 = 9	4%
Self Efficacy < 4 = 5	21%
Self Efficacy > 5 = 6	*39%*
Self Efficacy > 6 = 7	24%
Self Efficacy > 7 = 8	16%
Self Efficacy > 8 = 9	1%

4.4 Results of Fitness of the "Integrated VR Profile" tool

This data describes the general value of *Fitness* to integration in the workforce integration, determined by the complex innovative orientation activity performed. In the Integrated VR Profile, the principal characteristics of evaluation of each subject were have suited to the 5 sectors: *Personality - Motivational - Interactional - Cognitive/Neuropsychological - Sensorial* and quantify the indicators of *Ability Competence – Potential Evolution – Self Efficacy.*

The resultant of these sectors and indicators determines the conclusive evaluation for the sector *innovative orientation.* In the *Integrated Functional VR Diagnosis* of every subject profile, the values of the indicators and sectors are analytically described, proposing *Fit* those subjects who show sufficient or more than sufficient values in all three indicators, and *Partially Fit* or *Unfit* those subjects who show one or more insufficiencies in the three indicators (Table 4).

Table 4. Fitness values for Disability Typology – Age

Parameters	Percentage Values
Psychic 14-18 Fit	67%
Psychic 19-26 Fit	75%
Psychic 27-46 Fit	57%
Mental 14-18 Fit	58%
Mental 19-26 Fit	48%
Mental 27-46 Fit	41%
Difficulty of Learning 14-18 Fit	88%
Difficulty of Learning 19-26 Fit	75%

5. Final note

The study would seem to show that great abilities and potentialities still emerge in subjects during the phase of important development / evolution, and above all that of a meaningful and important correspondence which is strongly highlighted in an innovative activity such as that of *Virtual Reality* and also the innovative response shown by subjects performing VR tests to the difficulties they encountered [14].

In particular, despite the evident needs and consistent cognitive difficulties, the disabled subjects performing VR activity showed concrete, positive, important and coherent results in the sectors evaluated (Table 3). There is also a valid evolution of the subjects in *Neuropsychological / Expressive and Psychomotor Sectors* (Table 2).

It should be noted that for the mental and difficulty of learning disabilities there is a decrease in the characteristic of fitness with the age of the subject, while for the *Psychic Disabilities* (also with a less significant number of subjects) a different distribution is found (Table 4).

The most evident result is that the *"Integrated VR Profile"* is confirmed as a valid, significant and effective tool which can help develop adequate perspectives towards education, rehabilitation, orientation and work integration required by every disabled subject, on the basis of individual and diverse characteristics.

A first important conclusion seems to emerge: if the orientation to disabled people with the Virtual Reality method is understood and verified as a process of evaluation and development of abilities and consequent potentialities of the single subject with handicap - difficulty, then the Virtual Reality innovation is potentially presented as an extremely suitable and effective tool.

The study will proceed by considering the following aspects: to program a more profitable formative - training program, select the most suitable areas of areas education and learning and underline further important rehabilitation necessities, so as to address and program the most suitable orientation to the goals of integration in the workforce.

References

[1]   C. Guaita Diani, P. A. Piccini, M.C. Boudart Filippi, M. J. Santoveña, ACCES - Integration and Disabilities. FrancoAngeli (ed), Milano, 2000.

[2]   P.A. Piccini,and M. Turrisi, Summary of Virtual Reality Activity in CSVR for Project U.E. Horizon – Opera Diocesana Assistenza - O.D.A. Catania. In: web site centrosistemivr.org

[3]   C. Youngblut, Educational uses of Virtual Reality technology. IDA Document D - 2128. Log: H 98000105. January 1998.

[4]   B.G. Witmer, M.J. Singer, Measuring Presence in Virtual Environments: A Presence Questionnaire. In: Presence, Vol 7, No 3, June 1998, 225-240.

[5]   A. Rizzo, and J.G. Buckwalter, Virtual Reality and Cognitive Assessment and Rehabilitation: The State of Art. IOS Press, Amsterdam, 1998.

[6]   C.H. Lewis, and M.J. Griffin, Human Factors Consideration in Clinical Application of Virtual Reality. IOS Press, Amsterdam, 1998.

[7]   J. Moline, Virtual Reality for Health Care: a survey. IOS Press, Amsterdam, 1998.

[8]   M. M. North, S. M. North, and J. R. Coble, Virtual Reality Therapy: An Effective Treatment   for Psychological Disorders. IOS Press, Amsterdam, 1998.

[9]   G. Riva, Virtual Reality as Assessment Tool in Psychology. IOS Press, Amsterdam, 1998.

[10] F.D. Rose, E.A. Attree and B.M. Brooks, Virtual Environments in Neuropsychological Assessment and Rehabilitation. IOS Press, Amsterdam, 1998.

[11] K.M. Stanney, R.R. Mourant, R. Kennedy, Human Factors Issues in Virtual Environments: A Review of the Literature. In: Presence, Vol 7, No 4, August 1998, 327-351.

[12] D. Strickland, Virtual Reality for the Treatment of Autism. IOS Press, Amsterdam, 1988.

[13] J.P. Wann, S.K. Rushton, M. Smith and D. Jones, Virtual Environments for the Rehabilitation of Disorders of Attention and Movement. IOS Press, Amsterdam, 1998.

[14] G.C. Vanderheiden, J. Mendenhall, T. Andersen, Access Issues related to Virtual Reality for People with Disabilities. IOS Press, Amsterdam, 1999.

Virtual Environment System for Motor Tele-Rehabilitation

Lamberto PIRON*, Paolo TONIN§, Andrea Massimiliano ATZORI§, Elena ZANOTTI§, Cristiano MASSARO§, Elena TRIVELLO* and Mauro DAM*

Department of Neurology and Psychiatry University of Padova, via Giustiniani 5, 35100 Padova, § Department of Neurorehabilitation San Camillo Hospital, via Alberoni 70, 30011 Lido di Venezia, Italy.

Abstract

The present cutting-edge communication technology applied to the rehabilitation may change the real possibility of providing therapeutic treatments to the patients at their home. In order to confirm this assertion a current study on motor telerehabilitation was undertaken. Through a virtual reality based system, and a complementary video conference apparatus, we supplied five post stroke patients with a motor rehabilitation therapy. The rehabilitation technique was based on the augmented feedback. Subjects underwent the telerehabilitation program for six weeks. Before and after the therapy, arm motor performance and the activities of daily living were evaluated by the means of clinical scales and measuring the affected arm velocity (end-effector). This pilot study suggested that telerehabilitation could promote the learning of arm motor abilities at distance from the health facilities. From an economic point of view, it could be proposed also as an opportune strategy for saving resources.

1. Introduction

In the field of rehabilitation the possibility of providing treatments at distance has been identified as Telerehabilitation. Although the first pioneering telerehabilitation systems date back to the late seventies, with simple device for the augmentative communication, only recent developments in Telemedicine and Information Technology have allowed the possibility of a real remote support for disabled people [1-3]. In this context, the opportunity of developing innovative systems for motor telerehabilitation is strongly supported by the increasing number of people surviving from severe neurological lesions and due to the lack of available rehabilitative resources. In the United States, for example, there are more than three million stroke survivors, with different degrees of neurological disability, requiring various levels of assistance and rehabilitation therapy [4]. For the majority of these patients, the possibility of a prolonged rehabilitative motor training from their home would be very desirable.

In Italy, as in many others industrialized countries, the National Health System (NHS) is under a consistent organizing and economic adjustment in order to improve the quality of the health service with a real economic saving. The NHS guidelines indeed recommend to optimize the resources with the shortening of the impatient hospitalization, in both the acute and the long-term facilities. This recommendation is paradoxical for stroke survivors, clearly it is not in agreement with the idea of improving their motor recovery, their quality of life and hence their autonomy.

In the attempt to go beyond the above impasse, the present investigation was undertaken for experimenting a motor telerehabilitation system in patients with arm motor deficits long lasting from the stroke.

The purpose of this study was hence to evaluate the success of the rehabilitative therapy from patient's homes and its efficiency from an economic point of view. To carry out these aims we have used a Virtual Reality (VR) based system connected to a 3D motion tracking device [5-7].

2. Methods

Five patients with mild/intermediate arm motor impairment due to a stroke, occurring several months before (average 17 ± 15.8 months), were recruited for the study. All patients were affected by an ischemic cerebrovascular lesion in the territory of the middle cerebral artery (three in the left side, two in the right one). All subjects did not have clinical evidence of severe cognitive impairment or language disturbances interfering with verbal comprehension at the start of the study.

The rehabilitation program consisted of one hour of VR tele-therapy daily, five days per week, for six weeks. Before the telerehabilitation program, subjects were exposed to a training period (two weeks) with the VR therapy in the Hospital.

The VR telerehabilitation system consisted of two PC workstations: Patient and Therapist computer. The two workstations (Pentium III 1000 MHz processor, with 256 MB of RAM, a 64MB video card and graphics accelerator) were linked with a point-to-point ISDN phone connection (128 Kbps), communicating through a TCP/IP protocol. A 3D motion tracking system (Polhemus 3Space Fastrack, Vermont, U.S.A.) was connected to the patient's PC to capture the patients arm movements by a magnetic receiver. The receiver was usually attached to an object, grasped by the patient, or directly to a glove, worn by the subject. The static accuracy of the position signal was 0.76 mm RMS and 0.15 degrees RMS for orientation. Resolution was 0.0005 cms/cm. The receiver latency was 4 msec and the sampling rate was 120 Hz.

A specific software VRRSnet (Virtual Reality Rehabilitation System for the net, VRmotion Ltd., Padova , ITALY) was built on the Windows 2000^{TM} platform for processing motion data deriving from the tracking device and to represent the patient arm movement in the virtual environment (VE). Also the software ensured that the physical therapist (PT) was able to manage remotely the patient's PC console via the TCP/IP protocol.

During each therapy session, the PT managed remotely the sequence of virtual tasks that the patient had to perform. Virtual tasks were mainly motor skills which resembled activities of daily living, i.e. pouring water from a glass, using the hammer, posting an envelope into a mailbox slot, etc. [7]. The software represented the patient's arm movement simultaneously to the correct trajectory prerecorded by the PT.

A dedicated video conference apparatus (VCA) was set up for telemonitoring the patient during the therapeutic session and for assuring the safety in every phase. The VCA provided high-quality video conference using up to 384Kbs on six ISDN channels. It allowed a remote control of the video-camera mobility and the zoom.

While the patient executed the tasks in the VE, the PT could continuously monitor him with the VCA and control his movement represented on the PT computer screen.

The subscore of the Fugl-Meyer scale for the upper extremity (Fugl-Meyer UE) and the FIM scale were used for clinically assessing respectively the motor deficit and the quality of daily living activities before and after the study.

Before and after the telerehabilitation program, the end-effector (magnetic receiver) mean velocity of 10 consecutive reaching movements was calculated for each patient (speed-test). The T test was used to determine the statistical significance of the differences in the mean velocity of reaching movements, before and after the therapy.

Statistical significance was considered at $p \leq 0.05$.

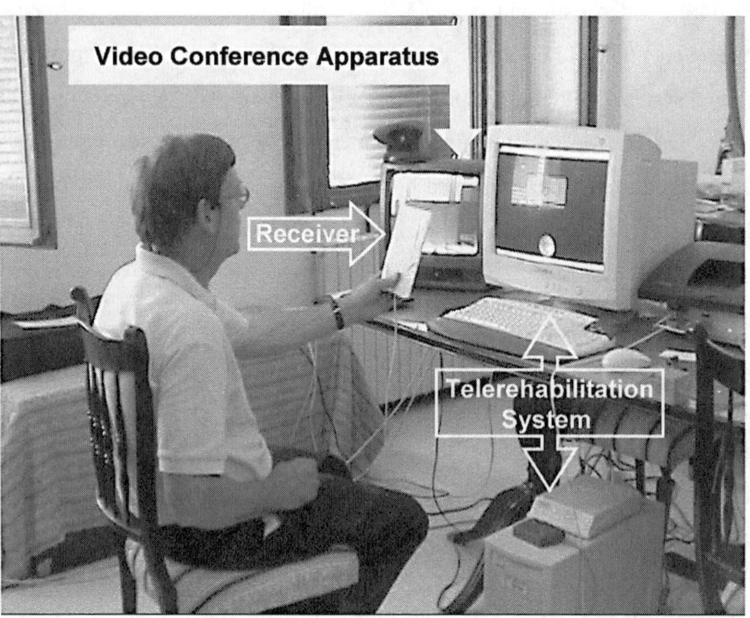

Fig. 1: The telerehabilitation setup: the patient console.

3. Results

The mean velocity of the speed-test performed with the affected arm significantly changed after the program. The mean of all patients' means velocity in the speed-test improved from 10.9 ± 1.1 to 14.5 ± 0.9 cm/sec (35.9 % faster).

No patients reported side effects due to the interaction with the VE. Patients did not report any real complexity in managing the PC workstation or the VCA. Sometimes the ISDN phone lines generated some complications in the transferring of data with several system breakdowns.

The mean of patients Fugl-Meyer UE scores before treatment was $56.8 + 8$ becoming

62.0 ± 4.2 after the telerehabilitation program. The means of FIM scores was 121 ± 4,7 before and 124,3 ± 2,1 after therapy.

Representative patients' arm trajectories before and after telerehabilitation program are shown in figure 2.

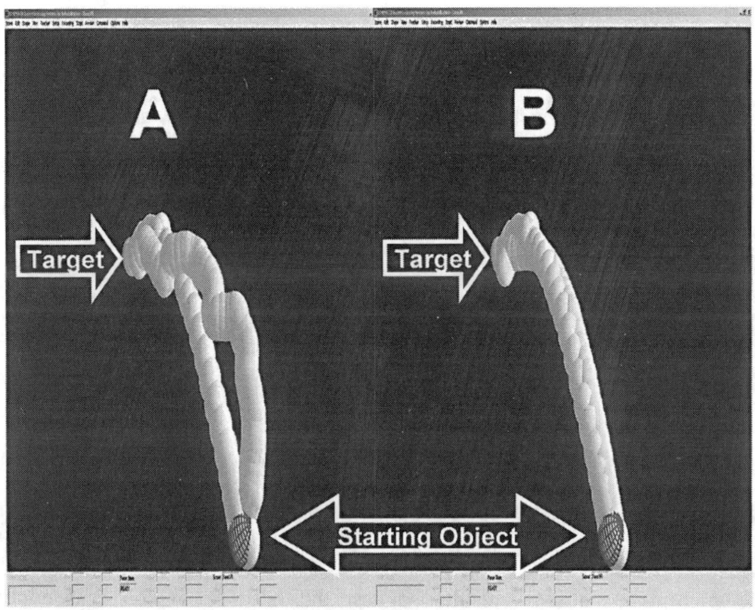

Fig. 2: A virtual reaching task: correct prerecorded trajectory is the wither trace, patient is the darker trace. **A** trajectory before therapy, **B** trajectory after therapy

4. Discussion

In this study, we evaluated the efficacy of our telerehabilitation system in providing arm rehabilitation treatment to patients at their domicile. Specifically, we studied the possibility of delivering a motor training focused on the impaired movements while the PT could visually monitor the patient.

All the subjects were soon familiarized with the experimental procedure without complaining of any discomfort related to the interaction with the VE or to the complexity of the system. The VCA was appreciated by the patients, who felt much more safe and positive in undergoing the therapy sessions.

We observed that the arm mean velocity during the speed-test significantly improved in response to the therapy program and the arm trajectories became straighter and linear. Moreover, all the clinical scale scores improved after the treatment.

These results were consistent with previous observations, obtained in the Hospital facilities with the same VR system, showing the validity of the VR approach with the augmented feedback in post stoke patients [8].

The data confirmed the crucial role in promoting motor learning played by the augmented feedback, which is the neurophysiological mechanism underlying in our VR rehabilitation system. In these settings, indeed, the augmented feedback consisted of showing the correct trajectory of the motor tasks, prerecorded by the PT, and pointing out differences with the patients' movement. Subjects, hence, could improve their arm motion by comparing continuously their own arm trajectory with the correct one already displayed on the screen.

PTs could modify the complexity of the existing virtual tasks and setup a variety of new reproducible skills remotely from the hospital console.

In conclusion, the present investigation was a pilot study for testing the success of a rehabilitation program for the treatment of patients at home, managed remotely by the PTs. The clinical scores confirmed the effectiveness of this rehabilitation strategy.

The preliminary clinical results suggest the need to exploit and continue the telerehabilitation program. Firstly, due to patient satisfaction and lack of drawbacks in administering and monitoring the program. Secondly, from an economic and geographic perspective the program is ideal for people who do not live near to the rehabilitation facilities and would therefore have difficulties commuting in a daily basis. Using the telerehabilitation program would offer such patients the means and the opportunity for rehabilitation.

5. **References**

1.   RB Burns, D Crislip, P Daviou, A Temkin *et al*. Using telerehabilitation to support assistive technology. Assistive Technology 1998;10(2):126-133

2.   GH Sell, GL Stratford, ME Zimmerman, M Youdin, D Milner. Enviromental and typewriter control system for high-level quadriplegic patients: evaluation and

prescription. Arch Phys Med Rehabil 1979;60:246-252

3. SA Holme, EM Kanny, MR Guthrie, KL Johnson. The use of environmental control units by occupational therapists in spinal cord injury and disease services. American Journal of Occupational Therapy 1997;51:42-48

4. Prescott. Survey shows stroke to be one of the most expensive medical illness in the United States. Int Med World Rept 1994;9(12):1-5

5. FD Rose, EA Attree, DA Johnson. Virtual reality: an assistive technology in neurological rehabilitation. Curr Opin Neurol 1996:9:461-467

6. PN Wilson, N Foreman, D Stanton. Virtual reality, disability and rehabilitation. Disability and Rehabilitation 1997;19:213-220

7. L. Piron, F. Cenni, P. Tonin and M. Dam. Virtual reality as an assessment tool for arm motor deficits after brain lesions. In J.D. Westwood, HF Hoffman, RA Robb, GT Mogel, D Stredney (ed.), Medicine Meets Virtual Reality 2001. IOS Press, Amsterdam 2001, pp 386-392

8. L. Piron, M. Dam, E. Trivello et al. Virtual Environment Training Ameliorates Motor Deficits in Post-Stroke Patients. Neurology 1999;52(2):A138

Medicine Meets Virtual Reality 02/10
J.D. Westwood et al. (Eds.)
IOS Press, 2002

Shared Virtual Environments for Telerehabilitation

George V. Popescu[1], Grigore Burdea and Rares Boian

Center for Advanced Information Processing,
Rutgers University, Piscataway, N.J. 08854, USA.
http://www.caip.rutgers.edu/vrlab

Abstract.
Current VR telerehabilitation systems use offline remote monitoring from the clinic and patient-therapist videoconferencing. Such "store and forward" and video-based systems cannot implement medical services involving patient therapist direct interaction. Real-time telerehabilitation applications (including remote therapy) can be developed using a shared Virtual Environment (VE) architecture. We developed a two-user shared VE for hand telerehabilitation. Each site has a telerehabilitation workstation with a videocamera and a Rutgers Master II (RMII) force feedback glove. Each user can control a virtual hand and interact haptically with virtual objects. Simulated physical interactions between therapist and patient are implemented using hand force feedback. The therapist's graphic interface contains several virtual panels, which allow control over the rehabilitation process. These controls start a videoconferencing session, collect patient data, or apply therapy. Several experimental telerehabilitation scenarios were successfully tested on a LAN. A Web-based approach to "real-time" patient telemonitoring - the monitoring portal for hand telerehabilitation – was also developed. The therapist interface is implemented as a Java3D applet that monitors patient hand movement. The monitoring portal gives real-time performance on off-the-shelf desktop workstations.

1. Introduction

Recent research investigates Virtual Environments use for home-based orthopedic rehabilitation [2,3,4,7]. Haptics increase patient immersion and participation and could potentially lead to faster recovery. Several networking solutions were proposed for home-based telerehabilitation [6,7,9]. These systems use a "store and forward" architecture for data collection and videoconferencing for patient-therapist interaction.

The VR-based telerehabilitation architecture presented in [7] is the reference point for our current work. The architecture supports offline interaction between therapist and a VR-enabled patient site. The telerehabilitation system contains a PC workstation, a novel Multipurpose Haptic Control Interface, the Rutgers Master II (RMII) force feedback glove, and videoconferencing hardware. The Client/Server software architecture implements a "store and forward" type of system. The Client (patient home) runs VR simulations and

---

[1] Currently with IBM T.J. Watson Research Center

collects real-time patient data. The Server (clinic site) stores patient medical records and runs data analysis and visualization software. Pilot clinical trials were performed in 1999 at Stanford Medical School (client site), with rehabilitation progress being monitored remotely from Rutgers University (Server site) [2].

The "store and forward" system described above is insufficient for implementing telerehabilitation services involving patient-therapist direct interaction. Shared Virtual Environments technology can be used to implement real-time interactions between physician and patient. This technology would require high-speed, low-latency communication networks in addition to advance human-machine interfaces. Currently such network infrastructure (e.g. Internet 2 [5]) is only available for research prototyping. In the future, these networks along with broadband consumer access (DSL, cable modem) will have the potential of supporting real-time telemedicine services.

This paper proposes a shared Virtual Environment telerehabilitation architecture. Simulated physical interactions between therapist and patient are implemented using force feedback. Data transmitted between the two sites includes audio, video, images, scene graph information, force, and control commands. The shared VE telerehabilitation system is presented in Section 2. Section 3 describes several "real-time" hand telerehabilitation experiments implemented on the shared VE platform. A Web-based approach to "real-time" patient telemonitoring - the monitoring portal - is presented in Section 4. Section 5 concludes this paper.

2. The Shared VE Telerehabilitation System

The shared VE telerehabilitation system is a software platform for real-time patient-therapist interactions. Its two sites are each equipped with a workstation, a video camera and an RMII force feedback glove [1]. The VE allow user control of virtual hands and haptic interaction with virtual objects. The shared VE uses a replicated database of virtual objects. All static content (3D objects, textures, sounds, etc.) is stored locally at each site. Therefore only dynamic updates (3D positions and rotation angles) are transmitted during the simulation. Additional data transmitted between the two sites include audio, video, forces, images, graphs and control commands.

Hand positions and finger joint angles are continuously sent over the network from each site, in order to animate the corresponding remote hand. Additionally, the forces displayed to the patient's hand are sent over the network to the clinic site. This information is used to display at both sites force and effort - calculated as an integral of forces displayed at patient's hand - visual feedback. Simulated physical interactions between therapist and patient are implemented using hand force feedback. This is achieved by replicating on the remote user the forces felt by the local user. Force data read from a local haptic glove is sent over the network and displayed on the remote glove.

Another component of the shared VE telerehabilitation system is the videoconferencing window. CuSeeMe videoconferencing software [12] is installed at the clinic and patient sites and runs as a separate program. The VE contains graphic elements (push buttons) which allow either the therapist or the patient to open a video consultation channel.

The architecture of the shared VE telerehabilitation system is presented in Fig. 1 [8]. The application was developed using WorldToolKit [10] graphics library. In addition to the graphics loop, separate threads run the database update, force feedback loop and the network communication loop. Both sites include an application controller, which implements the control logic of the simulation. Patient force and motion data are continuously available at the therapist site and can be stored on demand in the clinical database. The haptic thread displays the interaction forces on the RMII glove. The network protocol threads are responsible for formatting/parsing the messages and sending them to the remote site at specified update rates. The position and patient force data are sent at the graphics frame rate speed. The forces can be sent at either graphics or haptics thread update rates, depending on the application control mode.

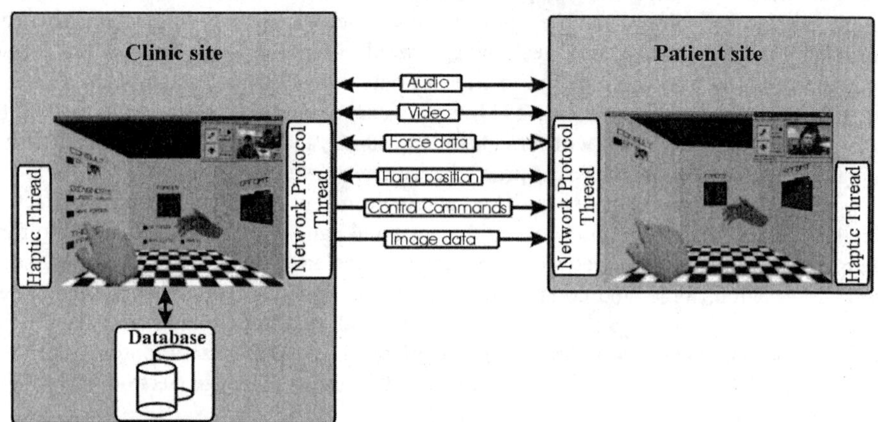

Figure 1: The Shared Virtual Environment Telerehabilitation System [8]. © 2001 Rutgers University.

2.1 The Shared Virtual Rehabilitation Room

The *Shared Virtual Rehabilitation Room* (SVRR) is a VE application implementing the above telerehabilitation architecture (Fig. 2). The environment contains virtual displays, user hands (local and remote) and control panels. The virtual displays are used to visualize the force and effort exerted by the patient's hand. Each VE shows two virtual hands, one controlled by the local user and the other one controlled by the remote user. At each site, the remote hand is displayed in transparent blue (50% transparency), so that it doesn't obstruct the local user view of the 3D buttons. The transparency is also an intuitive way to identify the remote objects.

In addition to the shared objects, the *SVRR* contains customized control elements: master control panels at the therapist site and a slave panel at the patient site. The master system virtual panels allow the therapist to control the rehabilitation process. The therapist can start a videoconferencing session ("consult" panel), collect patient data ("diagnosis" panel) or apply therapy ("therapy" panel). The "consult" panel allows the therapist or the patient to start the videoconferencing window by pushing the on/off button on the wall. The "diagnosis" panel has two buttons: one for measuring finger joint angles and the other for measuring the maximum forces exerted by the patient's hand. The "therapy" panel has a single entry. When this is activated, the therapist can send a control command at the patient site to indicate the force level. Possible options are: "no forces"; "constant" - set constant level forces; "spring" - set forces proportional with finger displacement; "replicated" – send the target forces applied to therapist hand to be replicated at the patient site.

In addition to these panels, a "graphic board" switch is used to display a virtual whiteboard. The whiteboard can display a sequence of images, similar to a slide projector. The images - representing X-ray, patient reports, graphs, drawings, etc. - are displayed as textures mapped on the whiteboard.

The slave panel at the patient site has limited interaction modalities, its primary task being to feedback force and visual information. The forces rendered here are either the result of patient's hand interaction or commanded by the therapist from the remote site. The only control items in the Virtual Environment are the "consult" and whiteboard switches. These allow the patient to start a videoconsultation session and to select the desired image to be displayed on the whiteboard.

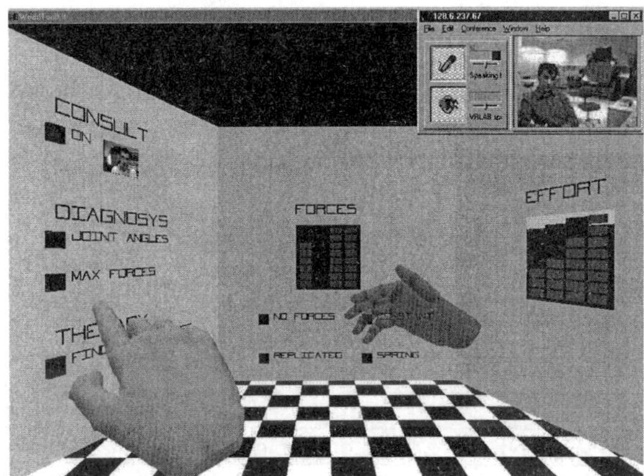

Figure 2: The Shared Virtual Rehabilitation Room (clinic site) [8]. © 2001 Rutgers University.

2.2 Application Control Logic

The session control diagram of the clinic site applications is shown in Fig. 3. A similar state machine is used to control the client application [8]. Synchronization of the two sites is based on a command protocol, which sets the application state in one of several modes: *diagnosis*, *therapy*, *graphic board* and *neutral*.

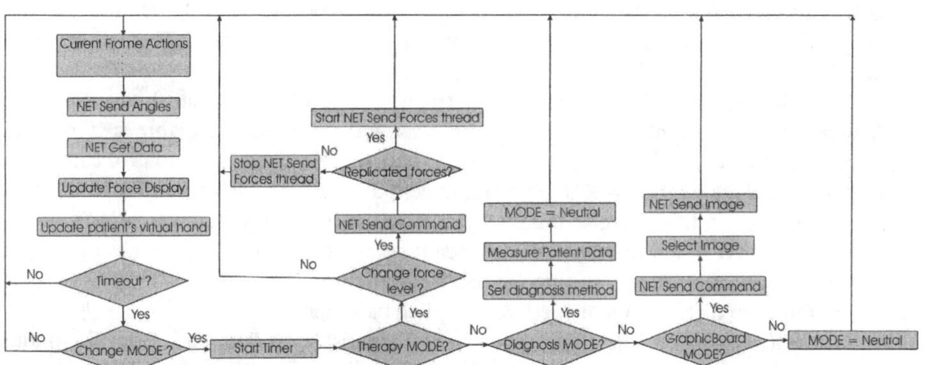

Figure 3: *SVRR* Session Management and Communication Diagram - Clinic site.[8]

The *diagnosis* mode allows patient force and range measurements. The *therapy* mode sends finger forces from the therapist site to the patient site similarly to a robotics telemanipulation application. Since these forces are used as targets for force feedback control the transmission rate should match the force feedback loop update rate (about 200 updates per second for the RMII glove [1]). Therefore when this mode is selected, the applications start an additional network thread, which runs at the above-mentioned speed.

In *graphic board* mode images are sent remotely from clinic site for display on the patient's whiteboard.

The shared VE application described above uses a custom communication protocol. There are five types of message: angles, positions, forces, images and commands. The packet format of the network protocol is <*tag, data, length*>. The tag is used to identify the message type. Each type of message is parsed and processed differently by the network protocol thread (e.g. when *tag*=NET_ANGLES the *data* package contains 20 hand joint angles). The command messages used for session management synchronize the application modes between the two shared-VE sites. Thus when the therapist site changes to replicated force mode, the patient site is switched to the same mode. Table 1 shows the message formats used by the protocol.

Table 1: SVRR message formats

Tag	Message type	Bytes
NET_ANGLES	Hand Joint Angles	80
NET_POSITION	Hand Position	24
NET_FORCES	Finger Forces	16
NET_IMAGE	Image	Variable
NET_COMMAND	Command	1

3. Shared Virtual Rehabilitation Room Experiments

The *SVRR* application was tested on a LAN at the Center for Advanced Information Processing, Rutgers University. Two PCs with high performance graphics cards, videoconferencing capabilities and RMII haptic interfaces were used in the experiment. The shared VE contains about 8000 Gouraud shaded polygons. The two systems had different processing power, and therefore ran the graphic and network loops at different speeds. In order to prevent the overflow of the slower computer, the graphic and network update rate was limited to 20 fps at both sites. Patient force data were logged in the clinical database during the tests. Force data were sampled one time per graphic frame. This experimental setup was used for several telerehabilitation experiments:

a) Teletherapy: The teletherapy experiment allows the therapist to control the patient's hand movements. The force control method using replicated forces from clinic site was used to control the forces applied to the patient's hand (position control can also be implemented). This method was used to implement a standard hand rehabilitation exercise: *finger stretching.* In this exercise the therapist is virtually molding the patient's hand. The current RMII glove could only be used to open up patient's hand, as it provides one degree of force feedback per finger (opening the hand). In addition to *replicated* forces, *spring* and *constant* forces of different intensities were applied to patient's hand.

b) Telediagnosis: The *SVRR* allows the therapist to collect data from the patient during a real-time session. The videoconference application allows the therapist to give instructions to the patient ("open hand", "close hand", "grasp", etc.) and asks the patient to execute standard tests for evaluation purposes. The therapist measures joint angles, finger mobility, maximum force, and hand range of motion, which are automatically entered in the clinical database.

c) Telemonitoring: The therapist monitors patient hand movement, forces and mechanical effort applied by the patient's hand. Since both virtual hands (local and remote) are displayed in the shared virtual environment, the therapist can observe unusual hand movements and incorrect routine execution. The graphic panels mounted on the walls of SVRR provide force and effort information feedback.

To characterize *SVRR* traffic requirements, several network traffic sessions were recorded. As expected, the network traffic (in a LAN) produced during therapy and diagnosis modes is almost constant. The application uses only 45 Kbps on average in these modes. Switching to *graphic board* mode creates bursty traffic. An average bandwidth of 1.2 Mbps was needed in order to transmit high quality images during a graphic frame (the image transmission interval can be set higher in order to accommodate lower bandwidth). Videoconferencing creates network traffic of about 300 Kbps, depending on the quality (size, compression) of the transmitted video. The critical parameter for force replication is the network round trip time (RTT). Haptic data requires a maximum time delay of less than 100 ms for stable control. This requirement is easily met in a LAN setup (RTT in the order of couple of milliseconds), but can also be satisfied by Internet2 connections (measured RTT for Rutgers-Stanford connection is about 80 ms).

4. Web-based telemonitoring portal

A web-based telemonitoring portal was implemented as an extension of the shared VE telerehabilitation platform. The portal running at the clinic site allows telemonitoring of hand motion and patient data collection. The patient site runs several VR rehabilitation exercises [7]. The data flow in this case is unidirectional (from patient to clinic). The server application at the clinic receives sets of sensor data and exercise monitoring parameters. Similarly to the architecture presented in Fig. 1 the server continuously samples and stores patient data in the clinical database.

The web-portal is implemented as a Java3D [11] applet that displays a virtual hand model controlled by the data read from the monitoring server (Fig. 4). A simplified virtual hand model was chosen over a more realistic one to make the finger angles more obvious. Also, the simplified model contains fewer polygons, which is important for the performance of Java3D applets running in a browser. The monitored patient could be easily chosen from a select list in the applet window.

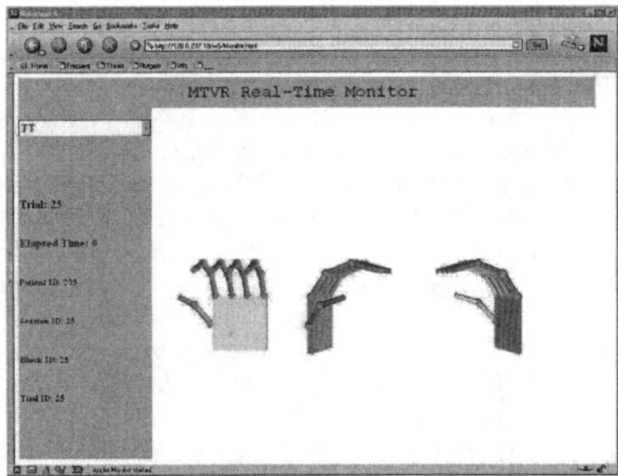

Figure 4: Web monitoring applet. © 2001 Rutgers University.

The main advantage brought by the web-based monitoring portal is the flexibility offered to the therapist. Any computer with Internet access can serve as monitoring station. The therapist can also monitor multiple patients simultaneously by either switching between them in one applet window or by opening a separate window for each.

To test the performance of the web monitor we used three computers with T1 Internet connection. The location of the monitoring server was in New Brunswick, New

Jersey. The client workstations were located in Newark New Jersey. The results obtained are presented in Table 2.

Table 2 - Monitoring applet performance

Computer	Frame Rate
PentiumII 400MHz, 256MB RAM	6 fps
PentiumII 700MHz, 256 MB RAM	13 fps
Dual PentiumIII 833MHz, 256 MB RAM	27 fps

5. Conclusions

A shared VE telerehabilitation system was designed to support real-time communication and remote interaction between patient and therapist. Each site has a telerehabilitation workstation with a videocamera and an RMII force feedback glove. Both users can control a virtual hand and interact hapticly with virtual objects. The shared sense of space and presence allow patient-therapist interactions mediated by haptic devices. The system allows the therapist to apply remote physical therapy and collect patient data. Several experimental telerehabilitation scenarios were successfully tested in a LAN.

A Web-based approach to "real-time" patient telemonitoring - the monitoring portal for hand telerehabilitation – was also developed. The therapist interface is implemented as a Java3D applet that monitors patient hand movement. The web-based portal has less functionality than *SVRR* but offers portability and flexibility advantages. The therapist can monitor multiple patients simultaneously.

Acknowledgments

Research reported here was supported by grants from the National Science Foundation and from the New Jersey Commission on Science and Technology.

References

[1] Bouzit M., G. Burdea, G. V. Popescu, and R. Boian. 2000. "The Rutgers Master II-ND Force Feedback Glove", submitted to *IEEE Transactions on Mechatronics*, July.

[2] Burdea, G., Popescu, V., Hentz, V., Colbert, K. 2000. "Virtual Reality-Based Orthopedic Telerehabilitation", *IEEE Transactions on Rehabilitation Engineering*, Vol. 8, No. 3, pp. 430-432.

[3] Deutsch, J., J. Latonio, G. Burdea and R. Boian. 2001. "Post-Stroke Rehabilitation with the Rutgers Ankle System - A case study," *Presence*, MIT Press, Vol. 10(4), pp. 416-430, August 2001.

[4] Girone, M. J., G. C. Burdea, M. Bouzit, V. Popescu, and J. E. Deutsch. 2000. "Othopedic Rehabilitation Using the 'Rutgers Ankle' Interface," In *The Proc. of Medicine Meets Virtual Reality 2000*.

[5] Internet2. 2000. [Online]. Available: http://www.internet2.edu. [2001, October 15].

[6] Peifer, J., A. Hooper and B. Sudduth. 1998. "A Patient-Centric Approach to Telemedicine Database Development," *Proceedings of Medicine Meets Virtual Reality 6*, IOS Press, Amsterdam, pp. 67-73, 1998.

[7] Popescu, V., G. Burdea, M. Bouzit and V. Hentz MD. 2000. "A Virtual Reality-based Telerehabilitation system with Force Feedback," *IEEE Transactions on Information Technology in Biomedicine*, vol. 4, No. 1, pp. 45-51.

[8] Popescu G. V. 2001. *Design and Performance Analysis of a Virtual Reality-based Telerehabilitation System*, Ph.D. Thesis, Rutgers University, January.

[9] Trepagnier, C., M. Rosen, C. Lathan. 1999. "Telerehabilitation and Virtual Reality Technology for Rehabilitation: Preliminary Results." *CSUN's Conference Proceedings*. [Online]. Available: http://www.dinf.org/csun_99/session0241.html [2001, October 15].

[10] Sense8 Co., WorldToolKit User's Manual, Sausalito, CA, 1994.

[11] Sowizral, H., K. Rushforth, M. Deering. 1997. *The Java 3D API Specification*. Addison Wesley.

[12] WhitePine, CuSeeMe User manual, 1998.

Medicine Meets Virtual Reality 02/10
J.D. Westwood et al. (Eds.)
IOS Press, 2002

A New Approach for the Synthesis of Glistening Effect in Deformable Anatomical Objects Displayed with Haptic Feedback

C. E. Prakash[1], Jung Kim[2], Manivannan M.[2], M. A. Srinivasan[2]

[1]*Division of Software Systems, Nanyang Technology University,*
Singapore 639798

[2]*Laboratory for Human and Machine Haptics,*
Massachusetts Institute of Technology, Cambridge, MA 02139

Abstract. An environment mapping approach for texture mapping of anatomical objects with glistening was studied and implemented in surgical simulation. A classifier based on the generalized goal of achieving glistening effect, which depends on the underlying physics and the mapped data, was used as a visual metric and shown to be realistic in the presence of achieving the desired quality in real time in the presence of haptic feedback. The proposed approach was compared with the standard texture mapping approaches used in existing surgical simulation methods that generally suffer from texture stretching and with little or no glistening effect. In our work, we have successfully applied environment mapping techniques for realistic real-time rendering of anatomical objects. We also show several examples of anatomical objects with glistening effects that mimic real anatomical objects.

1. Introduction

The problem of texture mapping [1], where texture parameters are not explicitly given or when the underlying geometry is non-planar and non-rectilinear, but rather available as complex shapes that occur in anatomical objects, is of considerable importance in virtual surgery simulation [2,3] and in a variety of 3D graphics applications [4,5,6,7]. Unfortunately, all the previous work on texture mapping approaches for 3D complex surfaces focus on solving the texture stretching problem place very little emphasis on photorealism with glistening effects. The only exceptions are images produced for visual effects in movies that are not done in real time. The need for perceptually based rendering procedures that produce synthetic images that are visually indistinguishable from real-world environments has been emphasized in recent years. Realistic rendering has been a challenge when it comes to representation of non-geometric structures. Visual realism is essential to make the simulation life-like and that is the goal of our work described here.

The problem we addresses is the following: given one or more arbitrary meshed and their associated RGB texture to render them in real time, with glistening effects similar to that obtained using expensive ray casting. The grid can deform at the same time as well. Some of the issues are listed below.

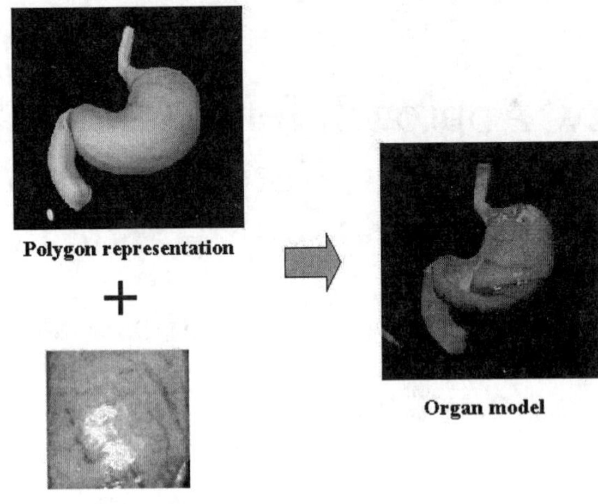

Figure 1 The process of texture mapping on a polygonal organ model

Multiple objects: The problem we model here is for surgery simulation with multiple anatomical organs. Each object has a large number of polygons and in most cases is a topologically closed object. The performance issue here arises especially when the rendering context switches between the different objects in the scene. Our goal is to have smooth models and more than one of such objects in the scene.

Multiple textures: Each organ model can have one or more textures associated with it. Multiple textures are required especially when constructing a two-sided surface where the textures on both sides of the mesh may be different. In the case of environment mapping we present, multiple textures may be needed for one object. The goal here is to ensure that multiple textures should be supported.

Deformable objects: One good example of a deformation is palpation where a surgeon needs to examine the organs by poking via probes. The deformation of the organ models leads to the update of vertex positions and polygon orientations that need to be computed for rendering. Since real time display of deformations is essential in surgical simulation, the texture mapping technique should be capable of displaying the deformation of the underlying surfaces.

Force feedback: Force feedback or haptic feedback is necessary in surgical simulation to improve realism of the simulator. When the force feedback is involved in the system in addition to visual display of deformation, high update rate (at least a few hundreds of Hz) is required to provide realistic feeling to the users in real time. It imposes an additional constraint to generate a response/feedback to the users.

Glistening effect: The smooth glistening appearance of the internal organs is partly due to the lining by the serous membrane (serosa). The complexity associated with modeling multi-layered thin films and the physical behavior of light by explicitly tracing the light rays throughout a scene has led to the exploration of alternative techniques to simulate realistic reflections. Since the simulation of glistening effects by conventional ray casting requires considerable computational effort, it is difficult to simulate such effects at interactive rates.

2. Texture Map for Anatomy

2.1 Texture Mapping for Range Images

One possible approach for texture mapping is to extend the techniques used for 3D digitization. In the approach proposed by Lee [4], the texture construction for facial texture mapping, two images are accomplished by assembly from the front and side views. A cylindrical projection of each image is obtained. The projected images are cropped at the eye extremes vertically. A multi-resolution assembling is performed to ensure smooth boundaries. The problem of texture fitting is to identify texture points for all points on the anatomical object. Texture coordinates of feature points are obtained from position data and a function applied for texture image generation. A cylindrical projection is applied to every point on the head surface. Extra points are added to obtain a convex hull containing all the points, so that coordinate of every point is located on an image. Then a Voronoi triangulation on control points and extra points are processed and the local Barycentric coordinates of every point with a surrounding Voronoi triangles are calculated [8]. The texture coordinates of each point on a 2D texture image are obtained using the texture coordinates of control points, extra points and the corresponding Barycentric coordinate [9]. This method has been successfully applied for facial models and the results are impressive, except that it takes few minutes to texture map each frame and hence not suitable for our work [10].

2.2 Tiled Texture Mapping

Another possible approach for texture mapping of anatomical objects is the so-called Tiled texture maps. Texture mapping of general non-rectilinear surfaces synthesize textures on the surface itself. There are several research efforts that map textures on manifolds (polyhedron) from tiled texture images. Delinguette [11] uses a tiled texture mapping technique to display a liver model. The our lab has presented results that use a simple texture mapping supported by Open Inventor from TGS for the bile duct exploration simulation [12]. Although they show a certain degree of realistic appearance of anatomy models, they suffer from the texture-stretching problem, which is an undesirable feature, and in addition have no glistening effect.

2.3 Other Possible Approaches

A simpler approach would be to have an oriented projective texture map where we project the surface texture onto scaled projection coordinates of the texture map available on orthogonal planes. The projected location and its texture or function of the texture is used to obtain the pixel texture. An alternate but fast solution is to use environment maps used in our research. The properties of environment maps and the algorithms are described in the next section.

3. Environment Mapping

Environment mapping technique is an efficient technique to compute the reflection vectors without adding real time computations. Although this technique was developed around the 1970s [13], this became available in PC level workstations recently due to the advance of computer graphics hardware.

In general, human beings perceive the properties of surfaces by the degree to which light is absorbed and reflected. To simulate this fully, the complicated modeling of light is required to specify the direction of secondary rays from the surfaces. In real time applications, it imposes extra computational burden on system, which have limited computing capacity. Therefore, some realistic effects requiring this computation, for example a glistening effect, are difficult to be simulated in real time surgical simulation due computational burden on the system. The environment mapping approach uses a simple form of reflection-vector dependent texturing and pseudo ray tracing computations. In other words, by projecting 3D environments surrounding the object onto a 2D environment map, reflections can be approximated with some degree of accuracy and significantly reduced real time computations.

3.1 Environment Map Design Issues for Anatomical Objects

For practical environment mapping the following processes are involved:

- Texture comes from encoded images of the environment in all directions and its converted images depend on mapping methods. In case of cube mapping, the images are mapped onto cubes, while the images are mapped onto spheres in sphere mapping
- Reflection vectors are precomputed and mapped to texture coordinates to reduce real time computations in the simulation

Environment mapping technique has several advantages over traditional texture mapping techniques for surgical simulation. First, the connectivity on a projected texture is maintained, because normal vectors change smoothly from one texture to another. Second, it is not necessary to flatten the entire surface of the anatomical object. Just one triangle is flattened at a time. So we don't need to worry about flattening neighborhoods. Finally, topology of the model is maintained, because a triangle can be projected always to one of the cube faces. The local texture orientation is implicitly maintained, so that no uneven scaling or stretching occurs as in traditional texture mapping techniques.

However, in spite of the computational speed and quality of the mapping, there are several limitations to environment mapping, such as no self-reflection properties. Therefore, careful consideration for obtaining and implementing are required to apply it in surgical simulation.

3.2 Anatomical Environment Map Algorithm

This section describes the procedure used for the construction and rendering of the anatomical objects. We used OpenGL v1.2 to implement this technique in a WinNT based computer.

Anatomical Environment Map Algorithm
OpenGL Environment Map Setup Usage

Step 1. Binding to a environment map texture
    Step 2. Loading environment map textures
 	
OpenGL Environment Map Rendering Usage
    Step 1. Enabling an environment map texture

```
                    glEnable(GL_TEXTURE_ENV_MAP);
Step. 2. Generated environment map coordinates (explicit or implicit)
        glTexCoord3f(vx, vy, vz); // (vx,vy,vz) is unnormalized direction
        vector
Step. 3. Generate anatomical object with textures
```

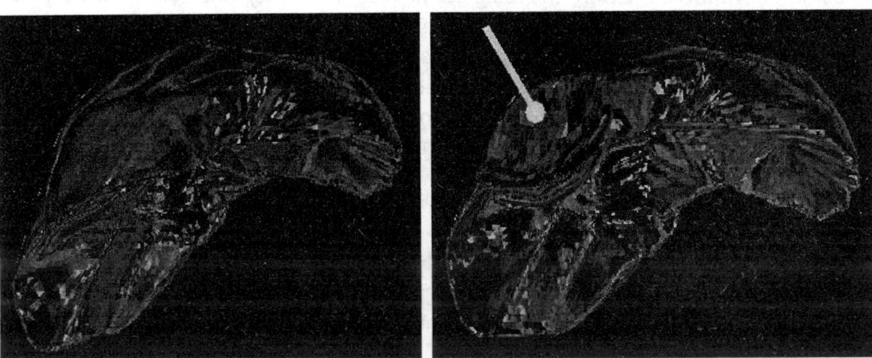

Figure 2. Glistening liver rendered using a Cube map (left panel) and Glistening liver deformed and rendered using a Sphere map (right panel)

4. Discussion

Experiments were performed to test the environment map for anatomical objects with glistening effects. In our experiments, we assumed that the textures are loaded during the initialization of the program. The texture images are captured from the laparoscopic video images of a real medical procedure.   In the current graphics hardware, two kinds of environment mapping techniques are available depending on the shape of a map: sphere mapping and cube mapping. The sphere mapping is less computationally expensive, but has view point dependency such as warping or distortion.

4.1 Experiment One-Cube map

This experiment was designed to test cube maps for different anatomical objects. The emphasis here was to generate a glistening effect. Fig. 2 left panel shows the rendering with glistening effects for a deformed model. The rendered image has the following properties. First, the rendered image shows the glistening effect that was the original goal. Second, the rendering can be done in real time. Third, the results produced are far superior to the results reported in the literature.

4.2 Experiment Two – Sphere Map

This experiment was designed to test the glistening effects obtained from sphere maps instead of cube maps. The sphere map instead of a cube map uses the reflection over the sphere and uses a single texture. Although it requires less memory and computation, the image is a little bit distorted. Fig. 2 right panel. shows the rendering of the deformed liver, which is another major goal of this research. The anatomical models have to be deformed as well. In the ideal situation the deformation has to be done in real-time.

4.3 Experiment Three – Performance Evaluation for Environment map

This section describes the performance evaluation obtained through analyses, simulation and some timing measurements. Table 1 summarizes these results. We used GEForce 2 from NVIDIA, which provides hardware-supported environment mapping features and E&S Tornado 3000 from E&S, which has only software emulated environment mapping techniques. From table 1, we observe that the cube mapping and sphere mapping using GEForce 2 shows better performance in rendering organ models with glistening effects. If we simulated the same effect by using conventional texture mapping techniques, it is very difficult to achieve real time performance due to the huge amount of computations required for ray tracing. We also observe that the software emulated environment mapping technique is not recommendable for rendering of complicated anatomy objects due to its poor performance as shown in Table 1. The graphics cards with hardware support of environment mapping are three times faster than graphics cards which do not support an environmental mapping technique in the simulation of complicated effects.

Table 1 Rendering Performance of Environmental Mapping

Object	Grid Size	Rendering capacity per second		
		Cube Map (GeForce2) MTriangles/sec	Sphere Map (GeForce2) MTriangles/sec	Sphere Map (E&S Tornado 3000) MTriangles/sec
Liver	17536	1.714	1.121	0.387
Stomach	51264	1.645	1.477	0.377
Lung	27648	1.714	1.593	0.388
Kidney	16512	1.710	1.408	0.371
Intestine	68456	1.581	1.656	0.412

5. Conclusion

We have analyzed and described the results of the use of environment mapping for deformable organ models. The novel aspect of the results presented here is that glistening effects of organ models can be achieved in real time. The quality of the effect is comparable to ray tracing. Such a technique has not been reported before in literature. The significance of the results is that deformation with glistening effect can be displayed in real time together with force feedback. Such an effect has a significant impact on the realism that can be achieved in interacting with virtual environments for surgical simulation.

6. Acknowledgments

Our thanks to Dr. Suvranu De, Hyun Kim, Blasander Raju, Dr. David Rattner, and Boon Tay, for sharing their technical expertise for this project. This work was supported by a grant from the Harvard Center for Minimally Invasive Surgery.

References

[1] Fabrice Neyret and Marie-Paule Cani, Pattern-Based Texturing Revisited, SIGGRAPH 99 Conference Proceedings, 1999, ACM SIGGRAPH, Addison Wesley, Aug, pp. 235 - 242.

[2] M. Bro-Nielsen, D. Helfrick and *et al.*, VR simulation of abdominal trauma surgery, Medicine Meets Virtual Reality 6 (MMVR-6), San Diego, California, 1998

[3] S. Cotin, H. Delingette and N. Ayache, Real-time Elastic Deformations of Soft Tissues for Surgery Simulation., IEEE Transactions On Visualization and Computer Graphics, 5(1) , 62-73, January-March 1999.

[4] Won-Sook Lee, Elwin Lee, and et al., Real Face Communication in a Virtual World.

[5] P. V. Sander, J. Snyder, and *et al.*, Texture Mapping Progressive Meshes, Computer Graphics, Proceedings of SIGGRAPH 2001.

[6] Paul Heckbert and Michael Herf, Fast Soft Shadows., SIGGRAPH '96 Visual Proceedings, pp. 145. Aug. 1996.

[7] William Reeves, David Salesin and Robert Cook, Rendering Antialiased Shadows with Depth Maps. Computer Graphics, Volume 21, Number 4, July 1987.

[8] Mark Segal, Carl Korobkin and *et al.*, Fast shadows and lighting effects using texture mapping, Proceedings of the 19th annual conference on Computer graphics July 27 - 31, 1992, Chicago, IL USA, pp. 249-252

[9] J. I. Toriwaki, S. Yokoi, Voronoi Related Neighbors on Digitized Two-Dimensional Space with Applications to Texture Analysis, Computational Morphology, pp. 207-228, North-Holland, 1988.

[10]John F. S. Yau and Neil D. Duffy, A Texture Mapping Approach to 3-D Facial Image Synthesis, *Computer Graphics Forum*, 7(2), pp. 129-134, June 1988.

[11]H. Delingette. Towards realistic soft tissue modeling in medical simulation. *Proceedings of the IEEE : Special Issue on Surgery Simulation*, pages 512-523, April 1998.

[12]Basdogan C, Ho C. and Srinivasan MA, Virtual Environments in Medical Training: Graphical and Haptic Simulation of Laparoscopic Common Bile Duct Exploration, IEEE/ASME Transactions on Mechatronics, 2001.

[13] J.F. Blinn and M.E. Newell, Texture and Reflection in Computer Generated Images, CACM, 19(10), October 1979, pp. 542-547

Medicine Meets Virtual Reality 02/10
J.D. Westwood et al. (Eds.)
IOS Press, 2002

Qualitative and Quantitative Analysis of Pressure Sensor Data Acquired by the E-Pelvis Simulator During Simulated Pelvic Examinations

Carla M. Pugh, MD, PhD.* and Jacob Rosen, PhD**
Stanford University Medical Media and Information Technologies Group, Stanford University and Department of Electrical Engineering, University of Washington***

1. Introduction

Incorporation of pressure sensors into simulation devices enables capture and analysis of various types of Human performance data (1-2). Analysis of such data is imperative in objectively evaluating user performance and simulator validity (2-4).

2. Materials and Methods

In a study involving 87 medical students enrolled in an Introduction to Pre-Clinical Medicine course, performance data were collected using the E-Pelvis simulator. The E-Pelvis is a newly designed device that consists of a partial mannequin– umbilicus to mid thigh – constructed in the likeness of an adult human female. The mannequin is instrumented internally with several electronic sensors that communicate indirectly with a computer-generated interface for providing immediate visual feedback. While students performed simulated clinical female pelvic examinations on the mannequin, electronic data were collected at a sampling frequency of 30hz and stored in individual data files for off-line analysis. Evaluation of these data involved the use of both quantitative and qualitative methods to determine if the sensors functioned properly throughout the study, and to validate the simulator as a reliable measurement tool.

Quantitative analysis of sensor function was performed in two parts. The first part involved the creation of baseline pressure variables for each sensor. Using the assumption that the calculated modes for each sensor were equal to the baseline pressure, SPSS (Statistical Package for the Social Sciences) descriptive statistics functions were used to extract baseline pressure data from the sensor readings. Secondly, scatter plots were used to determine which pressure variables failed to meet the initial assumption. Figure 1 shows scatter plots for the right posterior cervix sensor (c_rp_base) and the fundus sensor (c_f_base) on Simulator C (Ortho-McNeil Gynny® Model with an anteverted uterus). Those values that are encircled represent values that were targeted for further investigation. Qualitative analyses were used for investigating those values that failed to meet the initial assumption.

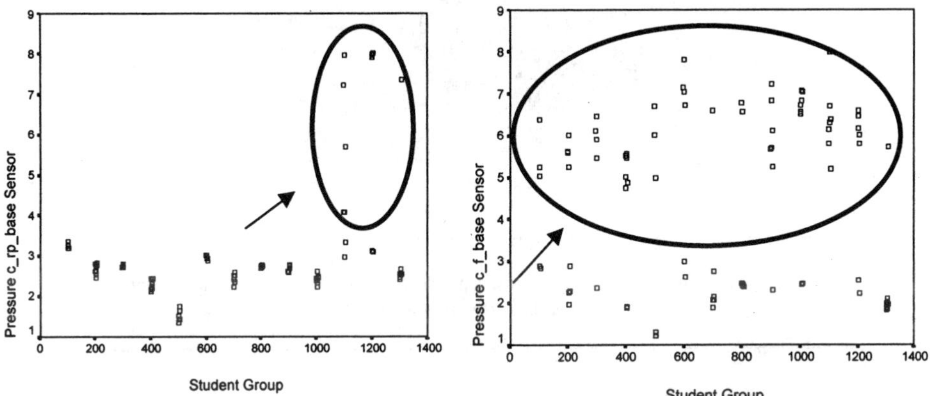

Figure 1. Scatter plots showing sensor readings marked for further investigation

During the qualitative investigation, graphs generated from the raw sensor data for each student were individually analyzed using visual analyses of the graphs and histograms of the sensors' readings. This process confirmed the true baseline readings for those pressure sensor values that were targeted for further evaluation after failing to meet the initial assumption. Figure 2, a histogram for the fundus sensor readings on Simulator C shows the bimodal distribution of the data. Those values near 2.0 pressure units represent

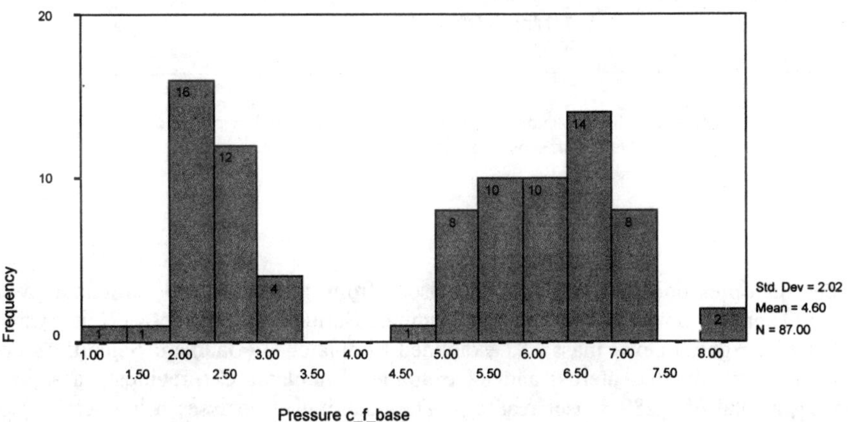

Figure 2. Histogram of the baseline readings for the Fundus sensor on Simulator C

the true baseline, whereas those values near 6.5 represent the pressure that was used when examining the fundus. Figures 3 and 4 depict sample graphs showing the sensor readings that were designated as the modal values and the sensor readings that represent the true baseline.

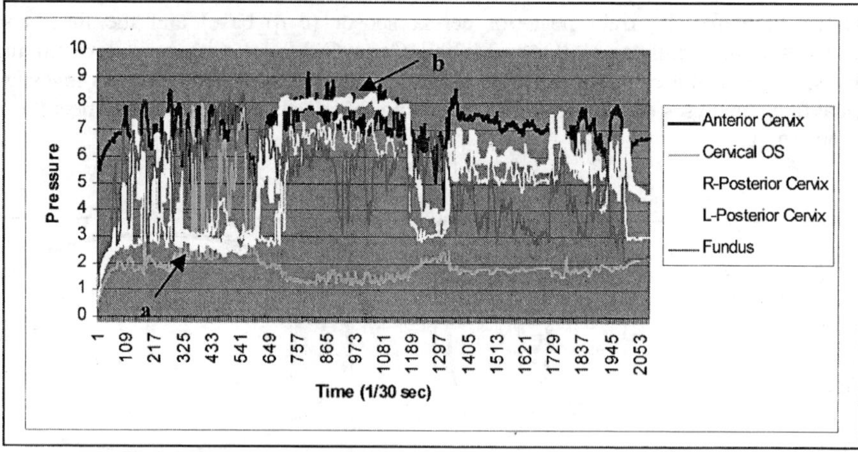

Figure 3. Graphic depiction of raw sensor data: a- the baseline pressure for the right posterior cervix sensor, b - the detected modal values.

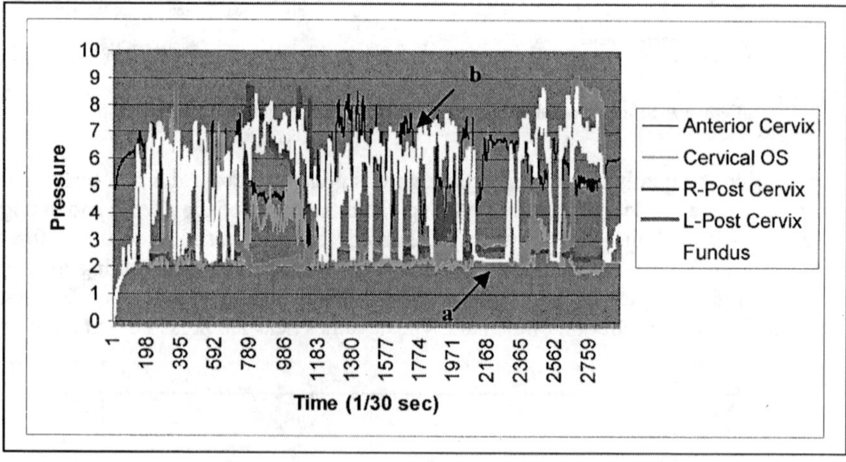

Figure 4. Graphic depiction of raw sensor data: a- the baseline pressure for the Fundus sensor, b – the detected modal values.

3. Results

The baseline pressure readings for 16 sensors from three different simulators were analyzed (Table 1). Seventy-four students examined Simulator A (Ortho-McNeil Gynny® Model with a right adnexal mass), 82 examined Simulator B (Gaumard Scientific Zoe® Model with a retroverted uterus) and 87 examined Simulator C (previously described) generating a total of 1,289 sensor readings. The quantitative analyses using scatter plots and histograms revealed that 94.18% of the baseline pressures captured for all of the sensors met the initial assumption that the sensors' modal values equaled the baseline pressures. The remaining pressure readings, 75 in total, which failed the initial assumption, were evaluated using qualitative methods and the true baseline pressures were determined. During the qualitative analyses, all of the graphs analyzed using visual analyses had one quality in common; a sensor that the user held constant digital pressure on for a time period that exceeded the amount of time in which the true baseline reading was recorded. This quality enabled the higher, constant pressure sensor readings to be recorded as the modal value. Overall, the findings from the quantitative and quantitative analyses confirm that 100% of the sensors functioned properly throughout the ten-week study period.

Sensor	Simulator A (n=74)	Simulator B (n=82)	Simulator C (n=87)
Anterior Cervix	.21	.47	6.0
Cervical OS	.01	.01	2.22
R-Posterior Cervix	.58	.84	2.5
L-Posterior Cervix	.01	.55	2.75
Fundus	.00	.01	2.0
Adnexa	4.0	-	-
Number of Sensors Targeted (number analyzed)	1 (444)	4 (410)	70 (435)

Table 1. Baseline pressure readings and number of sensors targeted for qualitative investigation for Simulators A-C.

4. Conclusion

This is the first report detailing analysis of sensor function for the E-Pelvis simulator. The findings reported here validate the simulator as a reliable measurement tool.

References

1) Rosen J, Solazzo M, Hannaford B, Sinanan M. Objective laparoscopic skills assessments of surgical residents using Hidden Markov Models based on haptic information and tool/tissue interactions. Stud Health Technol Inform. 2001;81:417-23.

2) Pugh CM. Evaluating Simulators for Medical Training: The case of the pelvic exam model. Bell & Howell - UMI Dissertations Publishing, Ann Arbor, MI. 2001.

3) Pugh CM, Srivastava S, Shavelson R, et. al. The effect of simulator use on learning and self-assessment: The Case of Stanford University's E-Pelvis simulator. Stud Health Technol Inform. 2001;81:396-400

4) Pugh, CM, Heinrichs, WL, Dev, P, et al – Objective Assessment of Clinical Skills with a Simulator. JAMA. 2001 Sep 5;286(9):1021-3

Medicine Meets Virtual Reality 02/10
J.D. Westwood et al. (Eds.)
IOS Press, 2002

Visual Representations of Physical Abilities: Reverse Haptic Technology?

Carla M. Pugh, MD, PhD., Sakti Srivastava, MD. and Wm. LeRoy Heinrichs, MD, PhD.
Stanford University Medical Media and Information Technologies
Stanford University School of Medicine

1. Introduction

Haptic technology allows users to 'touch', navigate and experience images, and virtual environments, usually with the aid of a graphics interface [1-2]. In contrast, the technique we have developed uses a graphical interface to depict the consequences and measurements of touch and physical interactions occurring in the real world.

2. Methods & Tools

We developed a graphical interface to depict the quality and location of individual users' hand movements while examining or touching critical areas within the E-Pelvis simulator. The E-Pelvis is a newly-designed teaching and assessment tool consisting of a partial mannequin– umbilicus to mid thigh – constructed in the likeness of an adult human female. The mannequin is instrumented internally with several electronic sensors that communicate indirectly with a graphical interface, providing immediate visual feedback. Students performing clinical pelvic exams on the simulator are able to receive immediate visual feedback regarding the location and intensity of their touch.

Eighty-seven medical students were randomly assigned to three different teaching groups: the mannequin group with visual feedback, the mannequin group without visual feedback and a control group. After completion of the teaching sessions, the students participated in a simulator assessment and an assessment by skilled patient educators. Both quantitative and qualitative data were collected during the study.

3. Results

Quantitative analysis of the simulator assessment variables revealed that both mannequin groups had similar technical skills performance. However, those students trained using the visual feedback method had significantly shorter exam completion times when compared to their colleagues trained without visual feedback, $p < 0.05$. Results from the patient educator assessments indicate that there were no significant differences in technical skills when comparing the overall examination techniques of the three groups. However, the patient educators rated those in the visual feedback group as having significantly better rapport compared to their colleagues trained without visual feedback, $p < 0.05$.

Combining the quantitative findings with qualitative findings, the results also indicate that students readily process the additional information provided by the visual feedback interface and use it to better understand specific content and skills that need to be improved. Our analyses also indicate that students prefer immediate visual feedback compared to verbal feedback from experienced clinicians and appear to be more confident in their clinical examination skills than those trained without this visual feedback method.

4. Conclusion

The search for understanding the full potential of the human mind is, in some ways, a quest for new ways of processing information. The visual feedback interface provides access to information that has never been available while students prepare for their first real-life clinical experience. This study indicates that students readily process visual representations of human performance and use this additional information for their personal educational benefit. Visual representations of human performance offers an innovative method of   accurate, immediate feedback with the potential to produce trainees with higher and more uniform levels of experience. We present this novel method as an adjunct to haptic technology.

References

1) Burdea, GC, Force and Touch Feedback for Virtual Reality, July 1996, John Wiley & Sons, New York, NY, USA

2) Salisbury, K, Haptics: The Technology of Touch HPCwire Special to HPCwire Nov. 10, 1995 www.sensable.com/community/haptwhpp.htm

Medicine Meets Virtual Reality 02/10
J.D. Westwood et al. (Eds.)
IOS Press, 2002

Simulation of bleeding during laparoscopic herniorrhaphy

Lakshminarasimhan Raghupathi M.S.[1]
Venkat Devarajan Ph.D.[1]
Robert Eberhart Ph.D.[2, 3]
Daniel B. Jones. M.D.[2]

[1] *Virtual Environment Lab*
Department of Electrical Engineering
The University of Texas at Arlington
P.O. Box 19016
Arlington TX 76019 USA

[2] *Southwestern Center for Minimally Invasive Surgery*
The University of Texas Southwestern Medical Center at Dallas

[3] *Bio-Medical Engineering Program*
The University of Texas at Arlington and
The University of Texas Southwestern Medical Center at Dallas

Abstract: Simulation of intragastric bleeding due to an accidental cut by the surgeon is an important component of a virtual laparoscopic herniorrhaphy trainer. We present a method for simulating bleeding during laparoscopic herniorrhaphy here. The various approaches used in previous research work are reviewed and our present approach is justified. Physically based fluid models used in computer graphics are used to simulate bleeding.

1. Introduction

Hernia is diagnosed by careful inspection and palpation of the inguinal region. Surgeons are mindful of the area between the spermatic vessels and the vas deferens in proximal to iliac vessels called the *"triangle of doom"* [1]. Complications like damage to the spermatic cord, nerves and blood vessels may occur within the triangle. Since laparoscopic herniorrhaphy requires a longer learning curve for the surgeon than for more conventional repairs [2], our objective is: 1) to provide realistic bleeding simulation during virtual laparoscopic herniorrhaphy, 2) to train residents to avoid entering the triangle. To this end, we have developed a physics-based approach to bleeding simulation. During training, any attempt by the surgeon to enter the forbidden region is instantly detected and bleeding simulation is initiated.

2. Previous work

One of the most accurate methods for describing fluid behavior is the Navier-Stokes (NS) equation. However, computational fluid dynamics (CFD) methods based on NS equation provide accurate but time-consuming models for fluid flow that are unsuited for real-time applications. Kass and Miller [6] using a simplified form of NS equations developed a realistic model. Although, later, many researchers such as Chen et al [9] and Foster et al [10] in the computer graphics community have developed sophisticated fluid models to account for more complex behavior, they are difficult to implement in real-time applications such as surgical simulation. Hence many researchers have used the earlier Kass model for bleeding simulation. A surface-bleeding scheme based on simple texture animation technique was developed in [4]. An interesting technique was suggested by Oppenheimer et al [5], where video captures of blood flow are rendered. But this method may not be suitable when the underlying tissue geometry changes or when the flow otherwise needs more realism.

Since in the Kass model fluid is represented as a single-valued height field, it alone cannot exhibit phenomenon such as breaking waves and splashing. Hence O'Brien and Hodgins [8] further extended the Kass approach to account for phenomenon such as splashing. Based on this approach, our method simulates a variety of in-plane and out-of-plane bleeding situations.

3. Method

To simulate bleeding occurring during surgery, we used different models for various blood flow situations. The volume model accounts for basic movement of fluid columns, whose neighbors are connected by virtual pipes. The disconnected particle system illustrates the free-flow of blood particles. Finally, the surface flow model renders the visible part of the blood over the tissue surface.

3.1 The volume model

The main volume of blood is modeled by a rectilinear grid of connected columns as suggested in [8]. We assume that all fluid properties within a column remain a constant. Further, we define a set of virtual pipes that connect neighboring columns. The equations of flow between the pipes derived from hydrostatic laws is given as:

$$P_{ij} = h_{ij}\rho g + p_0 + E_{ij}$$

where ρ is the density of fluid, p_0 is the atmospheric pressure in the system, and h_{ij} is the height of the column at the position (i,j) and E_{ij} is the external pressure due to the impact of particles as described in the next section.

The height of the column is related to the volume of that column, V_{ij}, by

$$h_{ij} = \frac{V_{ij}}{d_x d_y}$$

where d_x and d_y are the distance between the mesh points in the x and y directions respectively.

The difference in the pressure between neighboring columns results in the flow of fluid between these columns. For a fluid column at (i, j), the neighboring columns are defined by η_{ij}. The flow of fluid between the pipe at (i, j) and one of its neighbors at $(k,l) \in \eta_{ij}$ is defined by $Q_{ij \to kl}$. The net volume of change of a column during a time interval is given as:

$$\Delta V_{ij} = \Delta t \sum_{kl \in \eta_{ij}} \left[\frac{Q_{ij \to kl}^{t+\Delta t} + Q_{ij \to kl}^{t}}{2} \right]$$

Volume conservation was applied by making the flow at one end of the pipe equal in magnitude, but in opposite direction to the flow at the other end. Further if a column has a negative volume of fluid, then all the pipes drawing fluid from the column are reversed.

3.2 Particle system model

We have to model the blood spurting out over free space, when the practicing surgeon accidentally cuts/maneuvers near a vessel. During the practice surgery, the haptic device constantly monitors the position of the virtual instrument. Any maneuver near the area of surgical danger is detected and blood flow simulation routine is initiated. To this extent we have developed a particle-based system based on the classical paper by Reeves [7]. Each blood particle created in the system has the properties such as position, velocity and lifetime. The initial position of flow was obtained from the surface contact point of the haptic device and the initial flow parameters were determined based on best visual appearance. The position and velocity values of each particle are updated in each direction over each time step as given by:

$$p_{x,y,z}^{t+\Delta t} = p_{x,y,z}^{t} + v_{x,y,z} . \Delta t$$

Further, to model the effect of gravity we update the velocity in the y direction by:

$$v_y^{t+\Delta t} = v_y^{t} + g . \Delta t$$

The blood particles were appropriately texture mapped to give a realistic appearance.

3.3 Surface flow algorithm

This section describes the flow of blood over a tissue surface. In an actual surgery, blood emanating from the vessel flows in free space until it collides with an obstacle such as tissue surface. We implemented a collision detection routine based on a simple nearest neighbor method, i.e., the particle collides to the column, which is the closest among the set of neighboring columns. The particle impact causes an increase in the external pressure in the fluid equation, which causes it to flow over to adjacent columns through the virtual pipes. The particle is appropriately removed from the system immediately after collision. The fluid now represented as a height field is rendered by the auxiliary surface method suggested by Basdogan et al [3]. Accordingly, the initial fluid volume is placed just below the tissue surface. After the particles collide on the inguinal floor, the height field values are updated by the fluid dynamics routines. From the resulting new height values, only the portion of fluid above the tissue surface is rendered.

4. Results

The snapshots in Figure 1 were rendered from the data generated using the methods described above. For added realism we included models of a sample tissue surface and a blood vessel in the graphical scene. The simulation runs at interactive speeds (around 32 frames per second (fps) for 11x11 fluid grid). The bleeding simulation presented here will be a part of the overall laparoscopic herniorrhaphy trainer. In the simulation, one will be able to see the flow of blood particles over free-space till it collides with tissue surface and flows over it.

A dynamic real-time demonstration of our results is available as a companion to this paper at http://omega.uta.edu/~laks/demos/demo.html

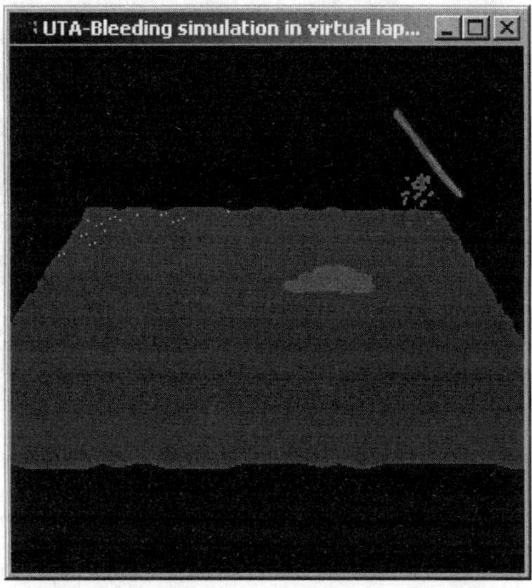

Figure 1a Initial blood particles from the blood vessel collides with the surface and forms a blood patch

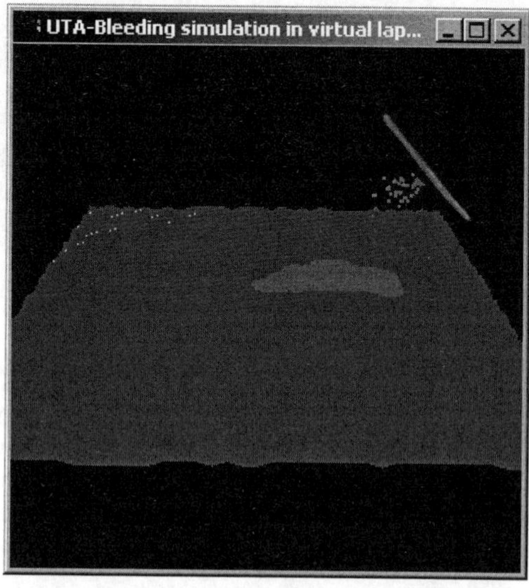

Figure 1b More blood particles fill the blood surface as blood spreads over the surface

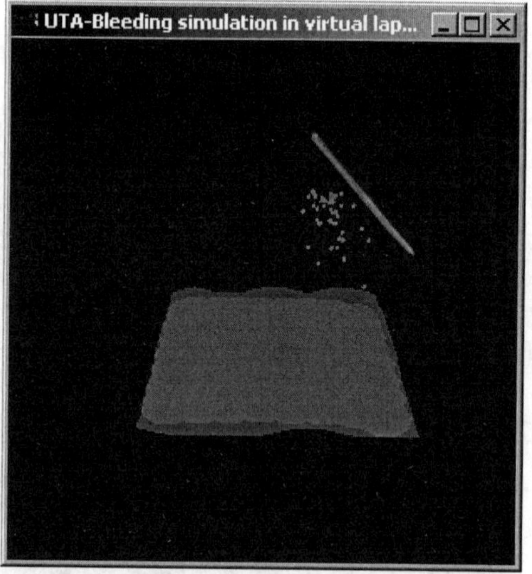

Figure 1c Illustration of a condition where the entire tissue surface is covered with blood

Figures 1a, 1b and 1c Snap shots of the bleeding simulation runs for an 11x11 fluid grid at 32 frames/sec

5. Conclusion

We have presented a method for bleeding simulation as a part of our virtual laparoscopic herniorrhaphy trainer. Laparoscopic herniorrhaphy requires more pre-surgical training than other minimally invasive procedures to avoid operative complications. Simulations of bleeding such as implemented here will add more visual realism to the surgeon during the virtual practice phase of training.

6. Acknowledgements

This work is funded in part by the Advanced Research Project Grant No. 003656-0079-1999 from the Texas Higher Education Coordinating Board and by grants from US Surgical/Tyco.

References

[1] Jones D.B. et al., *"Laparoscopic Surgery: Principles and Procedures"*, Quality Medical Publishing Inc., 1997, pp. 233-246.

[2] Avital S. et al., *"Conventional versus Laparoscopic Surgery for Inguinal-Hernia Repair"*, The New England Journal of Medicine, No. 337, Oct. 1997, pp. 1089-1090.

[3] Basdogan C. et al., *"Simulation of Tissue Cutting and Bleeding for Laparoscopic Surgery Using Auxiliary Surfaces"*, Proceedings of Medicine Meets Virtual Reality, 1999, pp. 38-44.

[4] Cakmak H.K., Kuhnapfel U., *"Animation and simulation techniques for VR-training systems in endoscopic surgery"*, Computer Animation and Simulation 2000, Proceedings of the Eleventh Eurographics Workshop, Springer-Verlag, Wien, Austria, 2000, pp.173-185.

[5] Oppenheimer P., Gupta A., Weghorst S., Sweet R. and Porter J., *"The representation of blood flow in endourologic surgical simulations"*, Proceedings of Medicine Meets Virtual Reality, 2001, pp. 365-371.

[6] Kass M. and Miller G., *"Rapid, stable fluid dynamics for computer graphics"*, Computer Graphics, Vol. 24, No. 4, Aug. 1990, pp. 49-57.

[7] Reeves W.T., *"Particle Systems - A Technique for Modeling a Class of Fuzzy Objects"*, Computer Graphics, Vol. 17, No. 3, Jul. 1983, pp. 359-376.

[8] O'Brien J. F. and Hodgins J. K., *"Dynamic Simulation of Splashing Fluids"*, Proceedings of Computer Animation `95, Geneva Switzerland, April 19-21 1995, pp. 198-205.

[9] Chen J.X. and Lobo N.V., *"Toward interactive-rate simulation of fluids with moving obstacles using Navier-Stokes equations"*, Graphical Models & Image Processing, Vol. 57, No. 2, March 1995, pp.107-16

[10] Foster N. and Metaxas D., *"Realistic animation of liquids"*, Proceedings. Graphics Interface '95. Canadian Inf. Process Soc. Toronto, Ont., Canada, 1996, pp. 204-12.

Medicine Meets Virtual Reality 02/10
J.D. Westwood et al. (Eds.)
IOS Press, 2002

A New Haptic Interface for VR Medical Training

Robert Riener[1] and Rainer Burgkart[2]
[1]*Institute of Automatic Control Engineering and*
[2]*Clinic for Orthopedics and Sport-Orthopedics, Klinikum Rechts der Isar,*
Technische Universität München (TUM), 80290 Munich, Germany

Abstract. Successful applications of haptic displays are limited to tool-based interfaces that simulate haptic effects on surgical and other medical instruments. However, no satisfactory haptic display exist so far, that enable the simulation of high fidelity palpation of human tissue or body segments. Existing approaches developed for medical training fail due to unrealistic haptic effects, time-consuming donning and doffing, and inconvenient use (e.g., mechatronic tactile and kinesthetic displays) or due to restricted function and adjustability (e.g., passive mannequins). The key idea of the new haptic interface is to attach artificial organs or segments (e.g. a plastic leg) to a force actuating mechatronic unit (e.g. robot). A set of different materials combined in certain layers yield components that look and feel like real objects. When the user touches the artificial object the contact forces and position changes are measured and fed into a model-based controller. Thus, the actuator moves the object so that the user gets the impression that he had induced the movement. The new haptic display has been verified with a setup developed for the training of functional joint evaluation after knee injuries. Compared to classical approaches, this display is convenient to use, provides realistic tactile properties and can be partly adjusted to different system properties (e.g. pathological joint properties). This kind of new interface can be applied to many different medical applications, where the clinician directly touches human limbs or tissue, such as in obstetrics, reanimation, organ palpation, etc.

1. Introduction

Due to limited simultaneous access to a greater pool of patients an effective training of medical students or young physicians is difficult [1]. Simulation environments based on VR technologies can support medical education and training. Certain VR applications profit considerably from haptic feedback, that not only improve user immersion but also increase the functional spectrum. However, successful applications of haptic displays are limited to tool-based interfaces, where the contact forces are transmitted to the user via a medical or surgical instrument that is handheld by the physician. Numerous approaches were developed to simulate haptic effects in laparoscopic [2], arthroscopic [3], and other medical interventions [4].

Unfortunately, no satisfactory haptic display exist so far, that enable the simulation of high fidelity palpation of human tissue or body segments and, additionally, is easy to don and doff and convenient to use. Thus, previous approaches were not well accepted by the users. The realization of such "palpative" displays is challenging, because not only kinesthetic but also tactile feedback into the fingers must be provided to simulate realistic contact phenomena that occur during palpation.

Two converse strategies exist so far. On the one hand mechatronic devices such as the PHANToM™ [5], the CyberGrasp™, or other force displays [6] are used to apply kinesthetic feedback to the fingers and pin arrays are used to provide tactile feedback to the finger tips [7], [8]. Although these devices can be adjusted to varying situations, pathologies, and individual subject properties the quality of the haptic effect is often unsatisfactory and donning and doffing is cumbersome and time-consuming.

The second approach are passive mannequins [9] and body segments/components. They are used for medical training to provide insight into anatomy and biomechanics. Some of them are fabricated by different layers of plastic and rubber materials, so that they feel like real human tissue or skin. Several systems were developed for training of breast cancer detection [10], [11], palpation of organs [12], [13], practicing external cardiac massage [14], etc. These approaches provide realistic tactile properties and are convenient to use but they cannot be adjusted to different situations or subjects.

In this paper a novel mechatronic system is presented that allows a realistic display of haptic contact information typically generated, when touching, palpating, and moving human anatomy (organs, segments, etc.). It arises from a combination of the two existing palpative approaches and comprises the advantages of both.

2. Method: Principle of the new haptic display

The key idea of the new haptic interface is to attach artificial organs or segments (e.g. a plastic leg) to a force actuating mechatronic unit (e.g. robot arm), see Fig. 1. A set of different materials combined in certain layers yield components that look and feel like real objects (Fig. 2). When the user touches such an artificial object the contact forces and position changes are measured by sensors and fed into a model-based controller. The controller output drives the actuator, which then moves the object so that the user gets the impression that he had induced the movement.

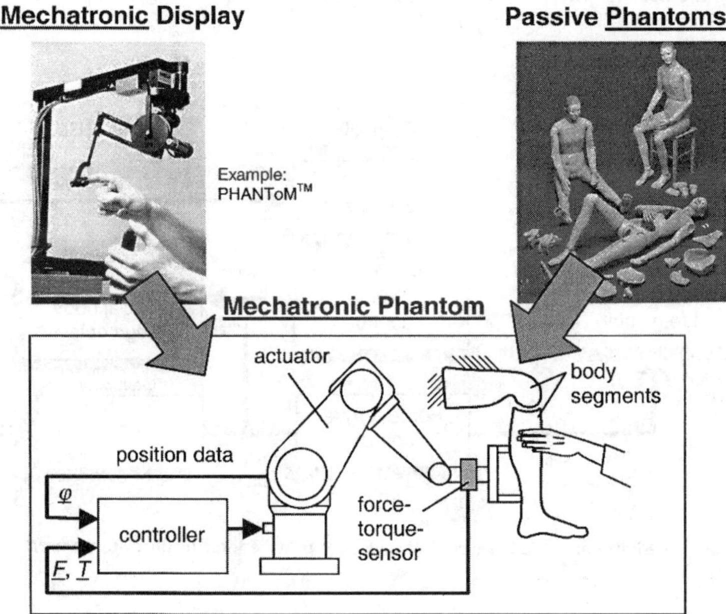

Figure 1: The new haptic interface as it arises from classical approaches

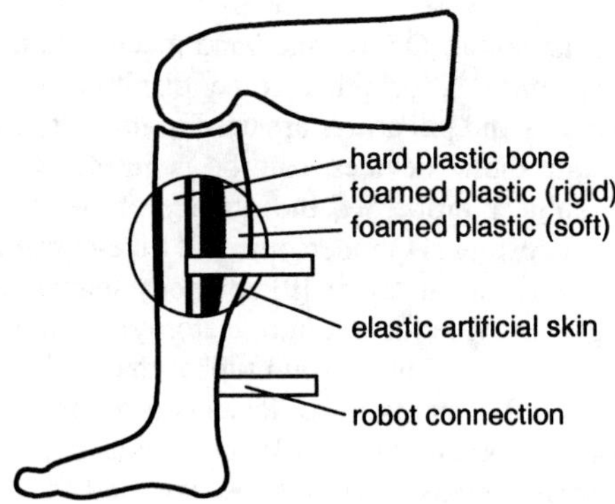

Figure 2: Artificial body segment of a shank. Layers of different
viscoelastic materials provide natural anatomical properties

Different control strategies can be applied to provide mechanical interactivity between
the actuated body segments and the user. One of those is known as admittance control (Fig.
3). When the user touches such an artificial object the contact forces are measured by a
force-moment-sensor mounted between artificial object and actuator (Figs. 1, 3). A
biomechanical model computes the motion of the object that results from the contact forces
applied. By controlling the position or velocity of the actuator, the object is moved in a
way so that the user gets the impression he had induced the motion. An alternative force
control method is impedance control, where the motion commanded by the user is detected
and the respective force is applied by the actuator.

System properties can be changed by modifying biomechanical model parameters, thus
enabling the user to simulate different physiological and pathological situations.

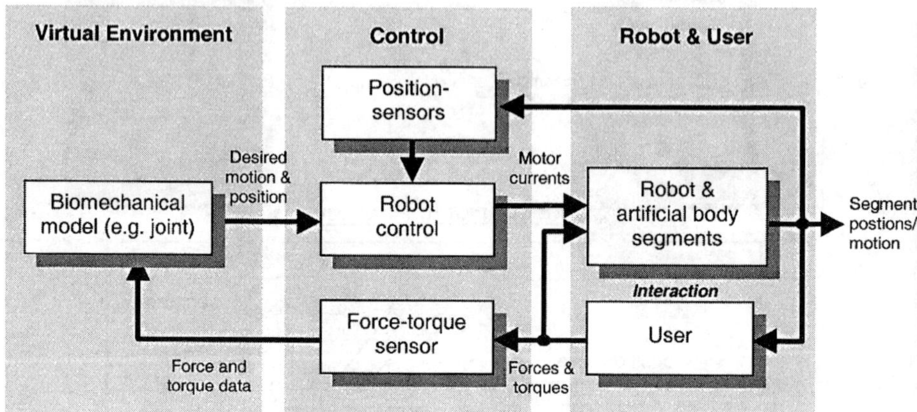

Figure 3: Admittance control scheme to provide force feedback to the user.

In a second mode, the actuated segments can be moved actively in order to teach the user how to perform certain tests on the human body. In this case the actuator is simple driven by a position control strategy, which is well known from classical robot applications. The user can observe the presented movements visually or touch the artificial segments during the movement in order to memorise how the test is performed correctly. Similar ideas have been presented by others, for example to teach the user how to play tennis or golf [15].

The haptic display can be enhanced by adding also a visual display (monitor, head-mounted display) that provides an insight into the internal of the body. Anatomical data can be obtained from CT and MRI data that is segmented and reconstructed in order to depict 3D shapes of bones, muscles, joint tissue, etc. The anatomical components on the visual display moves synchronously with the haptic display. The challenge for future investigations will be the animation of soft tissue motion.

Immersion within the virtual environment can be further improved by adding acoustic feedback, which provides realistic sounds, when touching and moving the human body. A suggested approach is to call a specific sound sample from a set of different pre-recorded sounds and sent to a pair of speakers, whenever a certain command is received from the modelling process. This can include also a sound uttered by the patient due to pain.

3. First Results

The new haptic display has been verified with a setup developed for the training of functional joint evaluation after knee injuries (Fig. 4). An artificial plastic leg with realistic anatomical structure and landmarks (e.g., femur condyles, fibula head, tuberositas tibiae, achilles tendon, see Figs. 2, 4) represents the leg of a patient. The shank is attached to a 6 DOF Stäubli RX 90 robot so that it can be translated and rotated in three dimensions. The thigh was rigidly connected in space. In the area of the knee joint, thigh and shank are contactless. A 6 DOF force-torque sensor (JR3) records the forces and moments that act between user and the actuated shank. The admittance control loop allows the user to touch and move the shank like a real shank and feel and assess the biomechanical knee joint properties. In the current version this movement is limited to movements in anterior-posterior directions. When moving the artificial shank, it feels as if it is connected to the thigh by natural joint tissue, although thigh and shank are not in contact. For training purposes different pathologies and injuries can be easily adjusted by changing the model parameters of the simulated knee joint [16].

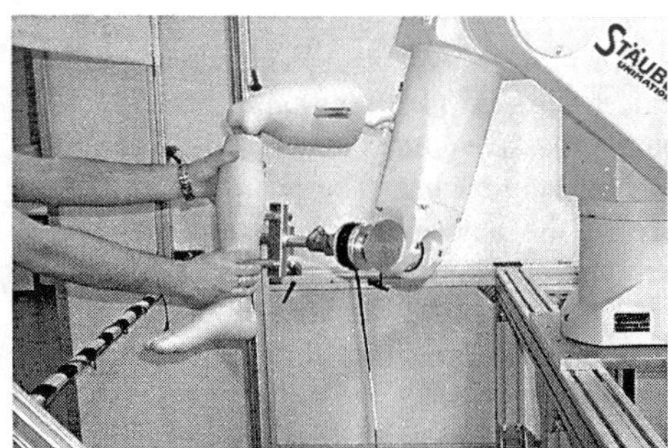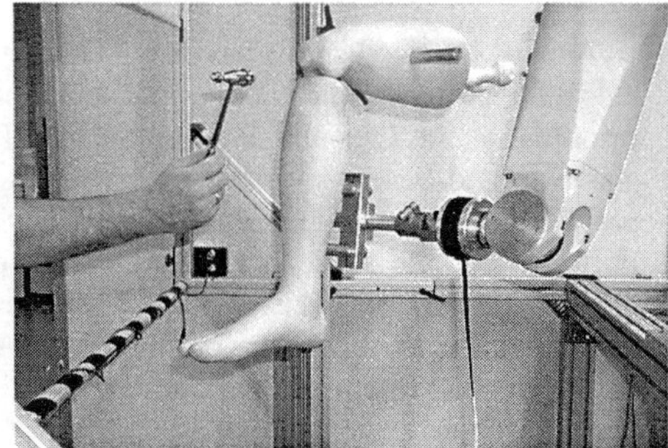

Figure 4: New haptic display for training of knee evaluation tests (left photograph) and the patella tendon test (right photograph).

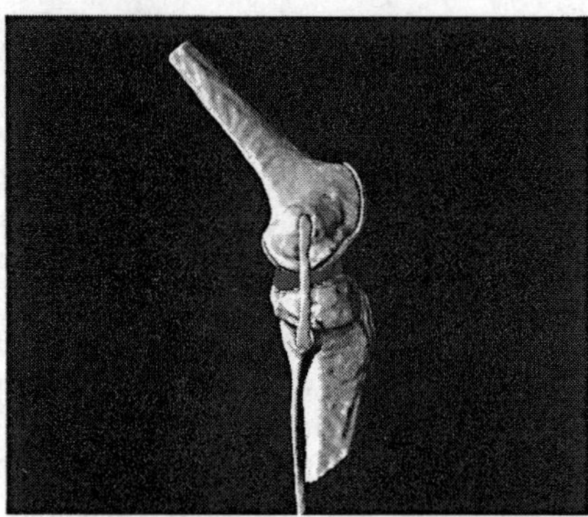

Figure 5: Graphical representation of the knee anatomy
as displayed on the monitor.

With the knee simulator further knee functions can be evaluated. For example, for neurological tests the patella tendon reflex can be activated. To induce a reflex response, the shank has to be beaten with a reflex hammer (Fig. 4, right photograph) in a certain region of the distal patella tendon and the contact force and force gradient have to be above certain threshold values. Both location and force are computed from the signals registered by the force-torque sensor.

Also the "teaching mode" has been implemented. In this mode the user is guided by the actuated shank so that he or she can learn different clinical test movements. More than 60 tests exist for the assessment of knee joint stability. They are essential for the correct diagnosis and therapy planning such as arthroscopy or open surgery. Prior to the use of the teaching mode the desired movement trajectories were recorded by the contactless motion acquisition system Ascension^{TM} and then fed into the knee joint simulator software.

In both modes anatomical components were segmented and reconstructed from MRI data and depicted on a monitor (Fig. 5). The knee animation comprises bones (femur, tibia, fibula, patella), ligaments (medial and lateral collateral ligament, anterior and posterior cruciate ligament), menisci, and joint cartilage. However, for motion simulation only the flexion-extension movement of the bones and collateral ligaments has been considered so far.

4. Conclusion and Outlook

A new haptic display has been developed that is easy to use and enables realistic palpation and movement of virtual anatomical structures. The new haptic interface is a combination of two classical approaches (purely passive components and mechatronic displays) and benefits from the advantages of both approaches. The passive components provide realistic tactile properties and the use of the device is simple and convenient. Furthermore, the force actuated mechatronic unit allows to be used for a variety of different situations. The concept has been verified for the simulation of knee joint movements. First results are promising and show that the knee joint simulator can be used for the training of clinical knee joint evaluation.

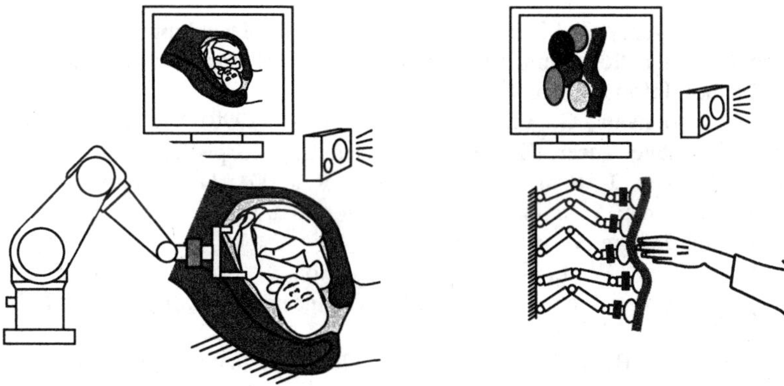

Figure 6: Further applications of the new haptic display.
Left: birth simulator; right: simulation of soft tissue palpation

This kind of new haptic display can be applied to many different medical applications, where the physician or other clinical staff touches human body segments or organs. There is a high potential that this will support training of joint evaluation, obstetrics, reanimation, organ palpation, examination of maxilla, pharyngeal, or throat, etc. (Fig. 6). A very promising application field is gynecology: by exchanging the shank and thigh by a plastic model of a baby and a mothers pelvis, respectively, a birth simulator is obtained, which can be used to train birth complications or difficult prenatal manual therapies. The acoustic display can then be used to depict the labor pains of the mother as well as the heart sound of the baby.

5. Acknowledgements

We thank Thomas Pröll, Martin Frey, Felix Regenfelder, Jens Hoogen, Jure Rejc, Rudolf Merzendorfer, Günther Schmidt, and Reiner Gradinger for their support in this study. Furthermore, we are indebted to Thomas Link and Karl-Hans Englmeier for their assistance in image data acquisition and processing. This work was supported in part by the German Ministry for Education and Reseach (BMBF) within the project network on "Virtual Orthopaedic Reality" (VOR).

References

[1] Riener, R., Burgkart, R. (2001) A survey for the development of VR technologies in orthopedics, Stud. Health Technol. Inform. 81, p. 407-409.

[2] Kühnapfel, U., Kuhn, C., Hübner, M., Krumm, H. G., Maaß, H., Neisius, B. (1997) The Karlsruhe endoscopic surgery trainer as an example for virtual reality in medical education. Minimally Invasive Therapy and Allied Technologies 6, p. 122-125.

[3] Ward, J. W., Wills, D. P., Sherman, K. P., Mohson, A. M. (1998) The development of an arthroscopic surgical simulator with haptic feedback. Future Generation Computer Systems Journal 14, p. 243-251.

[4] Dang, T., Annaswamy, T. M., Srinivasan, M. A. (2001) Development and evaluation of an epidural injection simulator with force feedback for medical training. Stud. Health Technol. Inform. 81, p. 97-102.

[5] Burdea, G., Patounakis, G., Popescu, V., Weiss, R. (1999) VR-based training for diagnosis of prostate cancer. IEEE Trans. Biomed. Eng. 46, p. 1253-1260.

[6] Riener, R., Hoogen, J., Schmidt, G., Burgkart, R. (2001) Development of a multi-modal virtual human knee joint for education and training in orthopaedics. Stud. Health Technol. Inform. 81, p. 410-416.

[7] Howe, R. D., Peine, W. J., Kontarinis, D. A., Son, J. S. (1995) Remote palpation technology for surgical applications. IEEE Engineering in Medicine and Biology Magazine 14, p. 318-323.

[8] Kammermeier, P., Buss, M., Schmidt, G. (2000) Actuator array for display of distributed tactile information - design and preliminary experiments. Proc. of the 9th Symposium on Haptic Interfaces for Virtual Environment and Teleoperator Systems, ASME IMECE 2000, Orlando, Florida, November 5-10, p. 1315-1321,

[9] Baldwin, J. F. (1988) Training mannequin. US Patent Nr. 4 773 865.

[10] Fasse, W. G. (1975) Breast cancer detection training device. US Patent Nr. 4 001 951.

[11] Goldstein, M. K. (1989) Breast cancer detection model and method for using same. US Patent Nr. 4 867 686.

[12] Greenfield, C. L., Johnson, A. L. (1993) Anatomically correct artificial organ replicas for use as teaching aids. US Patent Nr. 5 518 407.

[13] Voights, D. L. (1982) Palpation and ascultation teaching method and apparatus. US Patent Nr. 4 411 629.

[14] Kohnke, O., B. (1992) Training manikin for practising external cardiac massage. European Patent Nr. 560 440.

[15] Yokokohji, Y., Hollis, R. L., Kanade, T., (1996) Toward machine mediated training of motor skills. IEEE Int. Workshop on Robot and Human Communication, p. 32-37.

[16] Peters, J., Riener, R. (2000) A real-time model of the human knee for a virtual orthopaedic trainer. Proceedings of the International Conference on Biomedical Engineering, Singapore, December, 6-9, p. 110-111.

The VEPSY UPDATED Project:
Technical and Clinical Rationale

G. Riva, Ph.D. [1-2], M. Alcañiz [3], L. Anolli, Ph.D. [2], M. Bacchetta, Psy.D. [1],
R. Baños, Ph.D. [9], F. Beltrame, Ph.D. [4], C. Botella, Ph.D. [5], C. Galimberti, Ph.D. [2], L.
Gamberini, M.S. [11], A. Gaggioli, M.S. [1], E. Molinari, Ph.D. [2-6],
G. Mantovani, Ph.D. [11], E. Klinger, Ph.D. [7], G. Optale, M.D. [8], G. Orsi, M.S. [12],
C. Perpiñá, Ph.D. [9], R. Troiani, M.S. [10]

[1] *Applied Technology for Neuro-Psychology Lab., Istituto Auxologico Italiano, Verbania, Italy*
[2] *Department of Psychology, Catholic University, Milan, Italy*
[3] *MedIClab- Universidad Politécnica de Valencia, Valencia, Spain*
[4] *DIST, University of Genoa , Genoa, Italy*
[5] *Universitat Jaume I, Castellon de la Plana, Spain*
[6] *Laboratorio Sperimentale di Psicologia, Istituto Auxologico Italiano, Verbania, Italy*
[7] *GREYC, Université de Caen, Caen, France*
[8] *Associazione Medici Psicoterapeuti, Venice, Italy*
[9] *Universidad de Valencia, Valencia, Spain*
[10] *VRHealth Multimedia Consulting, Milan, Italy*
[11] *Department of General Psychology, University of Padua, Padua, Italy*
[12] *TSD Projects, Milan, Italy*

Abstract: The emergence of new shared media, such as the Internet and virtual reality are
changing the ways in which people relate, communicate, and live. Health care, and in particular
clinical psychology, is one of the areas that could be most dramatically reshaped by these new
technologies. To exploit and understand this potential is the overall goal of the " Telemedicine and
Portable Virtual Environment in Clinical Psychology" -VEPSY UPDATED – an European
Community funded research project (IST-2000-25323, http://www.vepsy.com) whose specific
goal is the development of different PC based virtual reality modules to be used in clinical
assessment and treatment. In particular the developed modules have been using to address the
following pathologies: anxiety disorders; male impotence and premature ejaculation; obesity,
bulimia and binge-eating disorders. The chapter details the general technical and clinical
characteristics of the developed modules.

Introduction

As recently noted by Jerome and Zailor [1], "emerging technology will perpetually alter the
ealth care environment, continuously changing the tools and options that are available to
erapists. It is thus important to study the impact of these changes as they occur, and it is
nperative that new technological competencies be developed as clinicians integrate these
chnologies into their research and practice" (p. 478).

In fact, even if many clinicians have the naive assumption that couches and conversation are the
est used therapeutic tools in mental health care, the tools for supporting psychotherapy are
volving in a much more complex environment than a designer's made chaise-longue. In particular,
e use of Virtual Reality (VR) offers many new possibilities to therapists.

Previous work has shown that even relatively unsophisticated Virtual Reality tools can prove a
aluable tool in psycho-neurological assessment and rehabilitation [2-5] .To date however the use
f VR-technologies *has been limited to single locations* – typically hospital or rehabilitation centers.

In theory new multi-user VR technologies combined with rapid increases in Internet bandwidth a performance and steep reductions in the cost of hardware and software, make it possible to bri distributed VR environments directly to clients' homes – thereby offering improved access for use who are inadequately served by current services. *In order to achieve this goal it will first necessary to overcome a number of clinical, ergonomic, technological and organization challenges.* Main contribution of the European Community funded "Telemedicine and Portat Virtual Environment for Clinical Psychology" – VEPSY UPDATED – research project innovation in this area is to design, test and validate solutions to these challenges [6].

In fact, the main objective of the project is to prove the technical and clinical viability of usi Virtual Reality Therapy (VRT) in clinical psychology. In particular, the project designed a developed 4 clinical modules and their associated clinical protocols, to be used for the assessme and treatment of the following disorders:

- panic disorder and agoraphobia;
- male impotence and premature ejaculation;
- obesity, bulimia and binge-eating disorders;
- social phobia.

2. VEPSY UPDATED: The technical platform

2.1 The emergence of PC based virtual reality

Even if the history of VR is based on expensive graphic workstations, the significant advances PC hardware that have been made over the last three years, are allowing the appearance of low c VR systems. While the cost of a basic desktop VR system has not changed much, the functional has improved dramatically, both in terms of graphics processing power and VR hardware such head-mounted displays (HMDs). The availability of powerful PC engines based on Intel's Pentiu III/IV, AMD's Athlon and Motorola's Power PC G4, and the emergence of reasonably priced accelerator cards allow high-end PCs to process and display 3D simulations in real time.

A standard Celeron/Duron 1 Ghz system with as little as 128 Mb of RAM can offer sufficie processing power for a bare-bone VR simulation, a 1.8 Ghz Pentium III//Athlon with 256 Mb RAM, can provide a convincing virtual environment, while a dual 1.8 Ghz Pentium IV XEC configuration with OpenGL acceleration, 512 Mb of RAM and 64/128 Mb of VRAM running Windows 2000, can match the horsepower of a graphics workstation.

Immersion is also becoming more affordable. For example, Virtual I-O (USA) and now have HMD that costs less than $1000 and has built in head tracking. Sony distributes its basic Glasstr headset for about $600 without headtracking. Two years ago HMDs of the same quality were abc 10 times more costly. A HMD with VGA quality produced by Sony is now about $2,000. Howevv this price will probably decrease during the next five years.

Presently, input devices for desktop VR are largely mouse- and joystick-based. Although the devices are not suitable for all applications, they can keep costs down and avoid the ergonom issues of some of the up-to-date I/O devices such as 3D mouses and gloves. Also, software has be greatly improved over the last three years. It now allows users to create or import 3D objects, apply behavioral attributes such as weight and gravity to the objects, and to program the objects respond to the user via visual and/or audio events. Ranging in price from free (ALICE 99 http://www.alice.org; BLENDER - http://www.blender.nl; CYBERWORLD Personal Edition http://ww3.cyberworldcorp.com/corpsite/products/products_personal.html) to $6,000, the toolk are the most functional among the available VR software choices. While some toolkits re exclusively on C or C++ programming to build a virtual world, others offer simpler point-and-cli operations for simulation.

A further attempt to spread the diffusion of low-cost VR comes from the development and
creasing diffusion of the *Virtual Reality Modeling Language* (VRML). The VRML is a file format
d run-time description of 3D graphics for use on the World Wide Web. It includes interaction and
imation elements as well as interfaces to scripting languages, thereby providing more general
nulation behaviors and interfaces in network services [7]. Today VRML worlds can be scripted
th Java and JavaScript, both of which are familiar to most web programmers.

The first version of VRML (1.0) allowed the creation of virtual worlds with limited interactive
havior. These worlds can contain objects that have hyper links to other worlds, HTML
cuments, or other valid Multimedia Internet Mail Extensions (MIME). The second version of
RML (2.0), available now, allows the user for richer behaviors, including animations, motion
ysics, and real-time multi-user interaction.

The general experience of VRML worlds on the Internet will be vastly improved over the next
w years as basic technologies such as 2nd generation graphics accelerators and network
chnologies such as Asymmetric Digital Subscriber Line (ADSL) become available. Up to now,
plications of VRML for telemedicine VR are available in visualization and training [8].

To ensure the broadest user base, the developed modules have been developed as shared
lemedicine tools available through Internet by using a plug-in for the most common browsers
xplorer and Navigator) and as portable tools based on Speed-Step notebook PCs (PentiumIII/IV,
8/256 Mb Ram) This choice ensures wide availability, an open architecture and the possibility of
nefiting from the improvements planned for these machine by INTEL, mainly faster processors
d enhanced multimedia support. Both solutions allow the support of end-users in their living
vironment.

2 VEPSY UPDATED: The Hardware

All the VR-based clinical modules were developed to be used on the following PC platforms:

Pentium IV/Athlon XP desktop VR system:
- o   1500 mhz or better,
- o   256 mega RAM or better,
- o   minimum specification for the graphic engine: Matrox MGA 550 32Mb WRam or
     Nvidia GeForce 2 MX 32Mb VRam

Pentium IV/Athlon based portable VR system:
- o   1000 mhz or better,
- o   128 mega RAM or better,
- o   minimum specification for the graphic engine: ATI Radeon 16Mb VRam or Nvidia
     GeForce 2 MX 16Mb VRam

The hardware also includes:

- *a head mounted display (HMD) subsystem.* The HMDs used are:
  - o   Glasstron PLM-A35/PLM-S700 from Sony Inc (http://www.sel.sony.com/SEL/). The
       Glasstron uses LCD technology (two 0.7" active matrix color LCD's) displaying 180000
       pixels (PLM-A35: 800H x 225V) or 520000 pixels (PLM-S700: 832H x 624V) to each
       eye. Sony has designed its Glasstron so that no optical adjustment at all is needed, aside
       from tightening a two ratchet knobs to adjust for the size of the wearer's head. There's
       enough "eye relief" (distance from the eye to the nearest lens) that it's possible to wear
       glasses under the HMD. The motion tracking is provided by Intersense through its
       InterTrax 30 serial gyroscopic tracker (Azimuth: ±180 degrees; Elevation: ±80 degrees,
       Refresh rate: 256Hz, Latency time: 38ms ± 2).

o   VFX-3D from Interactive Imaging Systems Inc (http://www.iisvr.com). The VFX-3D uses LCD technology (two 0.7" active matrix color LCD's) displaying 360000 pixel (800H x 400V) to each eye. The HMD doesn't require any optical adjustment. It can be easily worn using the patented flip-up visor. Included is also an accelerometer based serial tracker (Pitch & Roll Sensitivity +/- 70 degrees +/- ~0.1 degrees; Yaw Sensitivity 360 degrees +/-0.1 degrees)

-   *a two-button joystick-type input device* to provide an easy way of motion: pressing the upper button the operator moves forward, pressing the lower button the operator moves backwards. The direction of the movement is given by the rotation of operator's head.

2.3 VEPSY UPDATED: The Software

Each module was created by using the software Virtools Dev. 2.0 (http://www.virtools.com). Based on a building-block, object-oriented paradigm, Virtools makes interactive environments and characters by importing geometry and animation from several animation packages, including Discreet 3D Studio MAX (http://www.discreet.com), Alias Wavefront Maya (http://www.aliaswavefront.com), Softimage (http://www.softimage.com), and Nichimen Nendo and Mirai (http://www.nichimen.com), and combining them with an array of more than 200 basic behaviors. By dragging and dropping the behavior blocks together the user can combine them to create complex interactive behaviors.

The Virtools toolset consists of Virtools Creation, the production package that constructs interactive content using behavior blocks; Virtools Player, the freely distributable viewer that allows anyone to see the 3D content; Virtools Web Player, a plug-in version of the regular player for Netscape Navigator and Microsoft Internet Explorer; and the Virtools Dev for developers who create custom behaviors or combine Virtools with outside technology. Virtools Dev includes a full blown software development kit (Virtools SDK) for the C++ developer that comes with code samples and an ActiveX player which can be used to play Virtools content in applications developed with tools such as Frontpage, Visual Basic or Visual C++.

Content created with Virtools can be targeted at the stand-alone Virtools Player, at web pages through the Virtools Web Player, at Macromedia Director, or at any product that supports ActiveX. Alternatively, the Virtools SDK allows the user to turn content into stand-alone executable files. Virtools's rendering engine supports DirectX, OpenGL, Glide and software rendering, although hardware acceleration is recommended.

3. VEPSY UPDATED: The clinical rationale

Virtual reality offers a blend of attractive attributes for the psychologists. The most basic of these is its ability to create a 3D simulation of reality that can be explored by patients. In this sense VR can be considered a special, sheltered setting where patients can start to explore and act without feeling threatened. In this sense the virtual experience is an "empowering environment" that therapy provides for patients. As noted by Botella and colleagues [9] nothing the patient fear can "really" happen to them in VR. With such assurance, they can freely explore, experiment, feel, live experience feelings and/or thoughts. VR thus becomes a very useful intermediate step between the therapist and the real world.

Besides, it is unnecessary to wait for situations to happen in the real world because any situation can be modeled in a virtual environment, thus greatly increasing self-training possibilities. In addition, VR allows the situation to be graded so the patient can start at the easiest level and progress to the most difficult. Gradually, because of the knowledge and control afforded by interaction in the virtual world, the patient will be able to face the real world.

Given to its flexibility, VR is an excellent source of information on self-efficacy. In fact, as
derlined by Botella and colleagues [9] "different environments can be designed to practically
sure success in all of the patient's virtual adventures; and occasional difficulties, challenges, and
ilures can be posed for the patient to overcome. This means that patients are able to discover that
fficulties can be defeated. They also have the experience of a competent, effective, empowered
lf, and can attribute all this personal competence to internal factors: perseverance and effort." (p.
').

These general features of a VR experience are used in the specific clinical protocols used by the
fferent modules. The use of VR can improve the treatment of phobias. The typical clinical
proach to the treatment of phobias is the graded exposure of the patient to anxiety-producing
muli (Systematic Desensitization) generated either through the patient's imagination or in vivo.
s mentioned, social phobias offer a particular challenge, which virtual reality is particularly suited
solve.

VR tools, like current imaginal and in vivo modalities, are able to generate stimuli that could be
ed in desensitization therapy with patients who have difficulty in imagining scenes and/or are too
iobic to experience real situations. Moreover, these tools have some unique advantages. The use
computer graphics techniques allows the creation of stimuli of much greater magnitude than
indard in vivo techniques. Since the virtual environment may be under patient control, it appears
fer than in vivo desensitization and at the same time more realistic than imaginal desensitization
0]. Finally, the low cost of actual PC based VR platforms, adds the advantage of greater
ficiency and economy in delivering the equivalent of in vivo systematic desensitization within the
erapist's office.

Moreover, VR may enhance cognitive therapy in the treatment of obesity, bulimia and binge-
ting disorders by addressing two key topics that are somewhat neglected by current clinical
iidelines: body experience disturbances and motivation for change [11, 12]. The advantages of a
R-based treatment are clear. It minimizes distortion in self-report, since there is no script for
nforming clients to parrot or oppositional clients to reject; a typical behavior of anorexic
dividuals. VR-based therapy is also able to circumvent power struggles because the therapist can
invisible to the patient and presents no direct arguments to oppose. Finally, evidence is more
nvincing and conclusions better remembered because they are one's own. As noted by many
erapists, people are "more persuaded by what they hear themselves say than by what other people
ll them" [13].

In the treatment of male impotence and premature ejaculation, the use of VR enables the patient
quickly develop memories and emotions that are worked through with the psychotherapist at the
d of the session. In particular, the patient follows pathways in the virtual experience that
celerate a psycho-dynamic process which eludes cognitive defenses and directly stimulates the
bconscious, hence also everything related to his experience in the sexual sphere. The obstacles
at lead to sexual dysfunction are thus brought to light and the patient becomes aware that the
uses of his sexual dysfunction can be modified.

Finally, the ability to control virtual environments (VEs) and then to introduce a predetermined
t of stimuli can also enhance the standard approach used in psychological assessment. Moreover,
e additional capabilities that are inherent in VEs can lead to greater flexibility in the adaptation to
e patient's individual problems, improving the efficacy of the rehabilitation process. VEs are
ghly flexible and programmable. They enable the therapist to present a wide variety of controlled
muli and to measure and monitor a wide variety of responses made by the user. Both the synthetic
ivironment itself and the manner in which this environment is modified by the user's responses
n be tailored to the needs of each client and/or therapeutic application. It is also possible for the
erapist to follow the user into the synthesized world [14].

4. Conclusions

The VEPSY UPDATED VR modules addresses the following pathologies that have a stron
impact on the actual health care policies:

- The *Anxiety Disorders* modules are aimed at the assessment and treatment of specific phobia
  and social phobias . In Europe, twenty-one million subjects will suffer from an anxiety disorde
  at some time in their life, with anxiety disorders being the fifth most common diagnosis i
  primary care and the most common psychiatric diagnosis made by primary care physicians.
    - o *Specific Phobias*, which are one type of anxiety disorder, are the most prevalent ment;
      health disorder, more common than alcohol abuse, alcohol dependence, or majc
      depression. Moreover, thirty-three percent of patients presenting with chest pair
      abdominal pain, or insomnia actually have an anxiety disorder, as do 25% of those wit
      fatigue, headache, or joint pain. The average person with an anxiety disorder has te
      encounters with the health-care system before being correctly diagnosed, increasin
      health-care costs, and causing frustration on the part of both the patient and physician.
    - o *Social phobia*, is thought to be one of the largest mental health care problems, wit
      about 7% of the population experiencing significant social anxiety, and about 2% soci;
      phobia. The Royal College of Psychiatrists estimates that about 1-2% of men and 2-3%
      of women develop full social phobia, with the danger of subsequent development of
      depressive illness. Nevertheless social phobia is one of the least researched an
      neglected of all mental health problems, and yet has extremely debilitating effects fc
      sufferers. It significantly limits people from from forming relationships by generatin
      severe phobic responses at the prospect of human social contact, causing suffer
      significant impairment of their professional and private lives.
- *The Impotence module* is aimed at supporting the treatment of or erectile dysfunction, th
  inability to reach or maintain an erection sufficient for sexual performance. Erectile dysfunctio
  is undoubtedly a more wide-spread phenomenon than had been estimated up to today. Sinc
  approximately one hundred million men in the world suffer just from erectile dysfunction (i
  Italy 3 million, 3 to 5 million in Germany, 14-18 million in Europe, 18 million in U.S.), and w
  know that a psychogenous component is always present even when the primary cause i
  organic, contributing to maintain a vicious circle. The natural sense of shame, which afflict
  individuals affected by this pathology, is probably the reason that only a fraction of the cases i
  brought under medical observation. Impotence causes a loss of self-esteem, and may lead th
  patient, beyond a depressed condition, to be so skeptical about the chances of treatmer
  (preferably simple, and above all, immediate) so as to keep him from willingly asking
  therapist for help, making him ready to stop treatment not giving quick results.
- The *Eating Disorders* module is aimed at the assessment and treatment of obesity and eatin
  disorders, pathologies with an increasing diffusion in Europe. Obesity, in addition of having
  high priority in nutritional health policies of several industrialized countries it has bee
  recognized as a growing problem that must be corrected and prevented, not only as a nutrition;
  disease, but also as a risk factor for diet-related chronic diseases, such as coronary heart diseas
  hypertension and type II diabetes. The latter includes overweight (BMI>25) and not only sever
  obesity with BMI>35. *Body image disturbances and eating disorders* are increasing in femal
  adolescents making these the most prevalent psychological disorders in this community with
  penetration ranging from 5 to 15% according to the EU country.

The number of potential users for the tools developed by the project is very high: as a roug
estimate figures, within Europe there are more than 10000 hospitals and health-care centers wit
concrete needs for using the developed tools. However, we feel that there are now serious barrier
to the possibility for health care centers to gain advantages from the use of virtual reality. Due to th

iiqueness of the solution (the system will use standard components) and its relative low cost when •mpared with usual investments in this area, the final VR system will be available to a wide •ectrum of potential users - hospitals, universities and research centers - who will benefit to a large :tent from the advantages of this new technology: a penetration of 3% within 2 years from product /ailability (Spring 2005) seems quite realistic.

cknowledgment

The present work was supported by the Commission of the European Communities (CEC),)ecifically by the IST programme through the VEPSY UPDATED (IST-2000-25323) research ·oject (http://www.vepsy.com).

eferences

]   L. W. Jerome and C. Zaylor, Cyberspace: Creating a therapeutic environment for telehealth applications, *Professional Psychology: Research and Practice* **31** (2000) 478-483.

]   G. Riva, M. Bolzoni, F. Carella, C. Galimberti, M. J. Griffin, C. H. Lewis, R. Luongo, P. Mardegan, L. Melis, L. Molinari-Tosatti, C. Poerschmann, A. Rovetta, S. Rushton, C. Selis, and J. Wann, Virtual reality environments for psycho-neuro-physiological assessment and rehabilitation, in *Medicine Meets Virtual Reality: Global Healthcare Grid*, K. S. Morgan, S. J. Weghorst, H. M. Hoffman, and D. Stredney, Eds. Amsterdam: IOS Press, 1997, pp. 34-45.

]   G. Riva, B. Wiederhold, and E. Molinari, Virtual environments in clinical psychology and neuroscience: Methods and techniques in advanced patient-therapist interaction. Amsterdam: IOS Press, 1998, pp. 249.

·]   G. Riva and C. Galimberti, Towards CyberPsychology: Mind, Cognition and Society in the Internet Age, in *Emerging Communication: Studies on New Technologies and Practices in Communication*, G. Riva and F. Davide, Eds. Amsterdam: Ios Press. Online: http://www.emergingcommunication.com/volume2.html, 2001.

]   G. Riva and F. Davide, Communications through Virtual Technologies: Identity, Community and Technology in the Communication Age, in *Emerging Communication: Studies on New Technologies and Practices in Communication*, G. Riva and F. Davide, Eds. Amsterdam: Ios Press. Online: http://www.emergingcommunication.com/volume1.html, 2001.

·]   G. Riva, M. Alcañiz, L. Anolli, M. Bacchetta, R. M. Baños, F. Beltrame, C. Botella, C. Galimberti, L. Gamberini, A. Gaggioli, E. Molinari, G. Mantovani, P. Nugues, G. Optale, G. Orsi, C. Perpiña, and R. Troiani, The VEPSY Updated project: Virtual reality in clinical psychology, *CyberPsychology and Behavior* **4** (2001) 449-455.

·]   M. Pesce, *VRML: Browsing and building cyberspace.* Indianapolis, IN: New Riders, 1995.

·]   G. Riva and L. Gamberini, Virtual Reality in Telemedicine, *Telemedicine Journal* **6** (2000) 325-338.

·]   C. Botella, C. Perpiña, R. M. Baños, and A. Garcia-Palacios, Virtual reality: a new clinical setting lab, *Studies in Health Technology and Informatics* **58** (1998) 73-81.

0]   F. Vincelli, From imagination to virtual reality: the future of clinical psychology, *CyberPsychology & Behavior* **2** (1999) 241-248.

1]   M. Alcañiz, C. Perpiña, R. Baños, J. A. Lozano, J. Montesa, C. Botella, and A. Garcia, A new realistic 3D body representation in virtual environments for the treatment of disturbed body image in eating disorders, *CyberPsychology and Behavior* **3** (2000) 421-432.

2]   G. Riva, M. Bacchetta, M. Baruffi, G. Cirillo, and E. Molinari, Virtual reality environment for body image modification: A multidimensional therapy for the treatment of body image in obesity and related pathologies, *CyberPsychology & Behavior* **3** (2000) 421-431.

3]   G. Riva, M. Bacchetta, M. Baruffi, C. Defrance, F. Gatti, C. Galimberti, P. Nugues, G. Samuelli Ferretti, and A. Tonci, VREPAR 2: VR in Eating Disorders, *CyberPsychology & Behavior* **2** (1999) 77-79.

4]   G. Riva, Design of clinically oriented virtual environments: A communicative approach, *CyberPsychology & Behavior* **3** (2000) 351-358.

Medicine Meets Virtual Reality 02/10
J.D. Westwood et al. (Eds.)
IOS Press, 2002

e-Health in Eating Disorders: Virtual Reality and Telemedicine in Assessment and Treatment

Giuseppe Riva, Ph.D. [1-3]; Monica Bacchetta, Psy.D. [2], Gianluca Cesa, M.S. [2],
Sara Conti, M.S. [2], Enrico Molinari, Psy.D. [2-3]

[1] *Applied Technology for Neuro-Psychology Lab., Istituto Auxologico Italiano, Verbania, Italy*
[2] *Laboratorio Sperimentale di Ricerche Psicologiche, Istituto Auxologico Italiano, Milan, Italy*
[3] *Department of Psychology, Università Cattolica del Sacro Cuore, Milan, Italy*

Abstract: e-health, the integration of telehealth technologies with the Internet and shared virtual reality could become a significant enabler of consumer health initiatives. In fact, they provide an increasingly accessible communication channel for a growing part of the population. In the past decade medical applications of virtual reality (VR) and telemedicine have been rapidly developing, and the technology has changed from a research curiosity to a commercially and clinically important area of medical informatics technology.
The chapter details the characteristics of the Experiential Cognitive Therapy (ECT), an integrated inpatient/outpatient (4 weeks) and telemedicine approach (24 weeks) that tries to enhance the classical cognitive-behavioral method used in the treatment of eating disorders, through VR sessions and telemedicine support in the follow-up stage. Particularly, using VR and telemedicine, ECT is able to address body experience disturbances, interpersonal relationships, self efficacy and motivation to change, key issues for the development and maintenance of eating disorders that are somehow neglected by actual clinical guidelines.

1.   Introduction

For many years, research and practice in eating disorders and weight management have been based largely on a one-dimensional, simplistic, weight-loss/weight-gain paradigm because of the common assumption that the major cause of obesity is overeating. Despite this widespread assumption, however, a review of the literature does not support the notion that fat individuals consume more calories than their lean counterparts.

A review of 20 studies by Wooley and colleagues [1] and the findings of two more reviews [2, 3] suggest that, generally, fat people probably do not consume more calories than people who are not overweight. Thus, if fat people do not necessarily eat any more than thinner people, the prescription of a diet may not be warranted or reasonable. This is probably why the long-term success rate for persons using this paradigm has been low. Moreover, more recent follow-up studies after a weight loss intervention have shown how frequent dieters usually have significantly more weight regain than less frequent dieters [4].

To overcome this unsuccessful approach, our work follows some new thinking in this area of weight and eating disorders treatment that recognizes the dangers of chronic dieting and proposes a focus on body image, motivation for change, self-efficacy, self-acceptance and better nutrition.

Specifically our program stresses the following: (a) understanding the origins and reinforcement of negative attitudes toward body image; (b) redefining beauty with regard to fatness and thinness; (c) examining, treating, and decreasing the restriction in activities and negative feelings many eating disordered patients experience; (d) teaching clients empowerment techniques to support motivation to change and self-efficacy, and (e) developing individualized treatment plans regarding eating behaviors and exercise. We hypothesize that the proposed approach would be effective increasing the number and variety of clients' daily activities, decreasing their fat phobic attitude and depression, and increasing their self-esteem.

Experiential-Cognitive Therapy: the clinical rationale

Experiential-Cognitive Therapy for eating disorders is a relatively short-term, integrated, patient
iented approach that focuses on individual discovery [5]. The treatment lasts about 28 weeks - 4-
:ek inpatient/outpatient treatment and 24-week telemedicine (Internet based) treatment - and it is
ministered by therapists having a cognitive-behavioral orientation who work in conjunction with
)sychiatrist as far as the pharmacological component is concerned.

When a multidisciplinary treatment is mandatory (e.g., a suicidal patient), Experiential CT is
nducted on an inpatient basis. However, Experiential CT can be profitably applied also to non
·spitalized patients. Here, the treatment has to include nutritional counseling and physical activity
 help patients learn to regulate their eating and cope with specific high-risk situations (i.e.,
creased availability of food or limited control) that cannot be adequately addressed during
.tpatient therapy.

During the first phase, the different therapists carry out one *step* of the psychological process,
·th with individual and group sessions. The individual work regards assessment through
ychometric tests, weekly supportive psychological talks, sessions for assessment and therapy
rried out using Virtual Reality (VR), and psycho-pharmacological assessment and control. The
ychological group therapy is based on weekly group meetings ("closed" group of 5/6 persons) of
·o hours each. The work group aims both at training for development and acquisition of assertive
ills, and at training for assessment and consolidation of motivation.

Moreover, during the first phase of the treatment the subjects participate to both bi-weekly
ycho-nutritional groups held by nutritionists and to daily group sessions of physical activity. The
ovided physical activities are:

- Postural gymnastics (in the gymnasium);
- Abdominal exercises, floor exercises, stretching, etc. (60 minutes);
- Aerobic activity by cycloergometers (30 minutes);
- Walks in the open with different levels of difficulty (30 minutes).

During the telemedicine phase the patient has periodical individual contacts - through text, audio
 video chat depending on the technologies at patient's disposal - with the therapist who followed
 m/her during the inpatient/outpatient stage. These contacts will be fortnightly during the first two
onths and monthly during the third and fourth months. Six months after dismission, there will be a
al individual face-to-face session held in our day-hospital. Each patients is also given the
ssibly of contacting the therapist by e-mail in case of urgencies or emergencies for a maximum of
·o added contacts each month. Here the therapist decides, according to the characteristics of the
quest, the most suitable modality of response among e-mail, chat or telephone. The family of the
tient, too, can have a monthly contact by e-mail with the therapist.

During the telemedicine phase are also scheduled six monthly group meetings based on 1-hour
kt based chat sessions. The groups are composed by the same patients who took part in the group
ssions of the inpatient/outpatient phase. In this way the patients already know each other and can
scuss with the therapist both on pre-defined subjects concerning assertiveness, self-esteem,
otivation to change, prevention of relapses, and on other specific individual problems faced
.ring this phase. The patients are also allowed to keep in touch after the group sessions. This
ciprocal support (self-help group) can be very useful especially in the early phases of the
.tpatient stage: they can feel stronger and less alone in facing the difficulties and the problems of
ily life.

Finally, during the telemedicine phase, the patients have to download from Internet at monthly
tervals specific text based (booklets) or video based (educational videos) material to be used both
·r exercises and for the preparation of the individual and group sessions. The topics discussed

include assertiveness, self-esteem, body image disturbances, motivation to change and preventio of relapses.

Recently, some researchers have tried to use telehealth in the treatment of eating disorder Particularly, an American group examined *Student Bodies*, an Internet-delivered computer-assiste health education program designed to improve body satisfaction and reduce weight/shape concerr [6-8]. In a controlled study they evaluated whether an 8-week program offered over the Intern was able to target body image dissatisfaction, disordered eating patterns, and preoccupation wit shape/weight among women at high risk for developing an eating disorder. The results suggest th; technological interventions may help for reducing disordered eating patterns and cognitions amon high-risk women [8].

Moreover, the findings of the next research coming from the same group showed that an Intern intervention with limited face-to-face contact was more effective in improving body image an reducing disordered attitudes and behaviors than a purely face-to-face psycho education; intervention [6].

3. VREDIM: Virtual Reality for Eating DIsorders Modification

Starting from the above rationale the VEPSY UPDATED – Telemedicine and Portable Virtu; Environments for Clinical Psychology - European Community funded project (IST-2000-2532; has developed the Virtual Reality for Eating DIsorders Modification - VREDIM – VR system to t used in the Experiential Cognitive Therapy. VREDIM is an enhanced version of the original Virtu; Reality for Body Image Modification (VEBIM) immersive virtual environment, previously used i different preliminary studies on non-clinical subjects [9, 10]

3.1 VREDIM: Hardware

VREDIM is implemented on a Thunder 1800/C virtual reality system by VRHealth, Milan, Ital (http://www.vrhealth.com). The Thunder 1800/C is a Pentium IV based immersive VR syste (1800 mhz, 512 mega RAM, graphic engine: Matrox MGA 550, 32Mb WRam) including a hea mounted display (HMD) subsystem. The HMD used is the Glasstron from Sony Inc. The Glasstrc uses LCD technology (two active matrix color LCD's) displaying 180000 pixels each. Sony ha designed its Glasstron so that no optical adjustment at all is needed, aside from tightening a tw ratchet knobs to adjust for the size of the wearer's head. There's enough "eye relief" (distance fro the eye to the nearest lens) that it's possible to wear glasses under the HMD. The motion tracking provided by Intersense through its InterTrax 30 gyroscopic tracker (Azimuth: ±180 degree Elevation: ±80 degrees, Refresh rate: 256Hz, Latency time: 38ms ± 2).

We used a two-button joystick-type input device to provide an easy way of motion: pressing tf upper button the operator moves forward, pressing the lower button the operator moves backward The direction of the movement is given by the rotation of operator's head.

3.2 VREDIM: the 3D Healing Experiences™

VREDIM is composed by 14 3D Healing Experiences™ (see Table 1), different immersiv virtual environments, each one individually used by the therapist during ten 45-minute sessior with the patient.

Each 3D Healing Experience™ was created by using the software Virtools Dev. 2 (http://www.virtools.com). Based on a building-block, object-oriented paradigm, Virtools mak interactive environments and characters by importing geometry and animation from sever animation packages, including Discreet 3D Studio MAX (www.discreet.com), Alias|Wavefro Maya (www.aliaswavefront.com), Softimage (www.softimage.com), and Nichimen Nendo ai Mirai (www.nichimen.com), and combining them with an array of more than 200 basic behaviors.

By dragging and dropping the behavior blocks together the user can combine them to create complex interactive behaviors.

Table 1*: 3D Healing Experiences™ used in VREDIM*

1st 3D Healing Experience	Virtual balance
2nd 3D Healing Experience	Sitting room
3rd 3D Healing Experience	Kitchen
4th 3D Healing Experience	Bedroom
5th 3D Healing Experience	Bathroom
6th 3D Healing Experience	BIVRS
7th 3D Healing Experience	9 doors room
8th 3D Healing Experience	Shopping centre
9th 3D Healing Experience	Supermarket
10th 3D Healing Experience	Gymnasium
11th 3D Healing Experience	Pub
12th 3D Healing Experience	Clothes shop
13th 3D Healing Experience	Restaurant
14th 3D Healing Experience	Swimming pool + beach

Each session is divided in three phases:

- 15 minutes of psychological individual interview;
- 15 minutes of immersion into the 3D Healing Experience™;
- 15 minutes of psychological interview.

During the first interview the therapist investigates the feelings of the subject, describes the course of the therapy and introduces the virtual reality session. In the second interview, the therapist discusses what emerged from the immersion in the 3D Healing Experience™ and analyses emotions, behaviors and cognitions of the patient.

The main goal of the first session is to introduce the patient to the procedure and to the instruments needed for exploring the virtual environments (HMD and joystick), The first session is also used to assess any body-related stimula that could elicit abnormal eating behavior. Specifically the attention is focused on the patient's concerns about body image, eating, shape and weight. This assessment is normally part of the Temptation Exposure with Response Prevention protocol.

At the end of the first 3D Healing Experience™ the therapist uses the *miracle question*, a typical approach used by the solution-focused brief therapy [11]. According to this approach, the therapist asks the patient to imagine what life would be like without her/his complaint. Answering to this question in writing the patient constructs her/his own solution, which then guides the therapeutical process. According to deShazer [11] this approach is useful for helping patients establish goals that can be used to verify the results of the therapy.

The next eight sessions are used to assess and modify:

- *the symptoms of anxiety related to food exposure.* This is done by integrating different cognitive-behavioral methods: Countering, Alternative Interpretation, Label Shifting, Deactivating the Illness Belief and Temptation Exposure with Response Prevention.
- *the body experience of the subject.* Particularly in VREDIM we used the virtual environment in the same way as guided imagery [12] is used in the cognitive and visual/motorial approach.
- *the approach to critical interpersonal settings*: using the virtual environments the patient can experience or re-experience critical interpersonal situations and *reframe* them, using different cognitive-behavioral methods: Countering, Alternative Interpretation and Label

Shifting. Moreover, the therapist presents the patients applicable ways of honestly *communicating their feelings* during the interaction (assertiveness training).

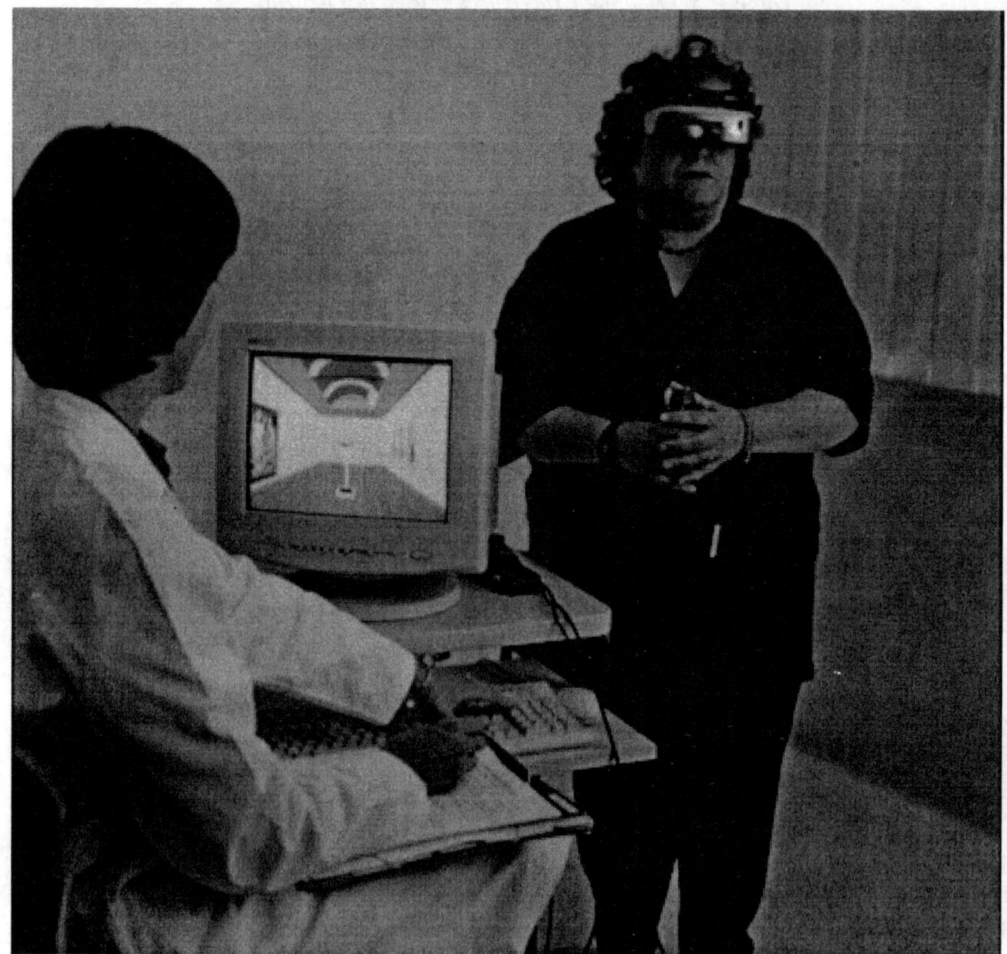

Figure 1: *A session of the Virtual Reality for Eating DIsorders Modification - VREDIM*

The conclusive session is used for a final analysis of the inpatient/outpatient phase with particular attention to the reached goals, prevention of relapses and maintenance of the therapeutic compliance in the forthcoming outpatient phase.

In all the sessions, the therapists followed the Socratic style: they used a series of questions, related to the contents of the virtual environment, to help clients synthesize information and reach conclusions on their own.

4. Results and Discussion

The preliminary version of this approach, not including the telemedicine treatment, was tested in different studies on clinical and non clinical samples [13-16]. The results show that ECT can be successful in improving the clinical practice in this area. Its multidisciplinary approach, ranging from cognitive-behavioral therapy to motivational group sessions seems to be suitable to the peculiar characteristics of eating disorders. Particularly the use of VR was effective in dealing with two key features of these disturbances not always adequately addressed by CBT therapy: body experience disturbances and motivation for change.

The first obtained result is the significant change induced by the treatment on the body image of the patients. In a sample of non-clinical subjects two single cases with anorectic and bulimic patients, and in three preliminary clinical trials with 18 obese, 25 binge-eating and EDNOS patients, ECT produced a significant change in the body image, usually associated to a reduction in problematic eating and social behaviors [13-16]. Actual body-image treatment involves a cognitive/behavioral or a visuomotor therapy that needs many sessions. The possibility of inducing a significant change in body image and its associated behaviors using a short-term therapy can be useful to improve the efficacy of the existing approaches. As such, the procedure can be considered as a comprehensive treatment package to break through the "resistance" to treatment in clinical subjects.

VR also immerses the patient in a real-like situation that she/he is forced to face. It can minimize distortion in self-report, since there is no script for conforming clients to parrot or oppositional clients to reject. Moreover, it circumvents power struggles because the therapist can be invisible to the patient and presents no direct arguments to oppose. Finally, evidence is more convincing and conclusions better remembered because they are one's own.

Change often requires the recognition of the distinction between an assumption and a perception. Until revealed to be fallacious, assumptions constitute the world; they seem like perceptions, and as long as they do, they are resistant to change. By using VR, the therapist can actually prove that what looks like a perception doesn't really exist. Once this has been understood, individual maladaptive assumptions can then be challenged more easily. As underlined by social cognitive theory, performance-based methods are the most effective in producing therapeutic change across behavioral, cognitive, and affective modalities [17]. In fact, the proposed experiential approach could help patients to discover that difficulties can be defeated, so improving their cognitive and behavioral skills for coping with stressful situations.

The final interesting result is the lack of side effects and simulation sickness after the experience in the virtual environment, confirming the possibility of using VREDIM in Experiential CT. This result, confirmed in both studies, is even more interesting given the sample used. In fact, females tend to be more susceptible to motion sickness than males [18].

Acknowledgments

The present work was supported by the Commission of the European Communities (CEC), in particular by the TELEMATICS programme (Project VEPSY UPDATED – IST- 2000-25323, http//www.psicologia.net; http://www.vepsy.com).

Moreover, the authors have benefited from support and contributions coming from many other colleagues. These people include Eugenia Borgomainerio, Margherita Baruffi, Gianluca Castelnuovo, Andrea Gaggioli, Fabrizia Mantovani, Letizia Petroni, Silvia Rinaldi and Francesco Vincelli.

References

[1]   O. W. Wooley, S. C. Wooley, and S. R. Dyrenforth, Obesity and women—II. A neglected feminist topic., *Woman's Studies International Quarterly* **2** (1979) 81-92.
[2]   K. D. Miller, Body-image therapy, *Nursing Clinics of North America* **26** (1991) 727-736.
[3]   E. D. Rothblum, Women and weight: fad and fiction, *Journal of Psychology* **124** (1990) 5-24.

[4]   W. J. Pasman, W. H. Saris, and M. S. Westerterp-Plantenga, Predictors of weight maintenance, *Obesity Research* **7** (1999) 43-50.

[5]   G. Riva, M. Bacchetta, M. Baruffi, S. Rinaldi, F. Vincelli, and E. Molinari, Virtual reality based Experiential Cognitive Treatment of obesity and binge-eating disorders, *Clinical Psychology and Psychotherapy* **7** (2000) 209-219.

[6]   A. A. Celio, A. J. Winzelberg, D. E. Wilfley, D. Eppstein-Herald, E. A. Springer, P. Dev, and C. B. Taylor, Reducing risk factors for eating disorders: comparison of an Internet- and a classroom-delivered psychoeducational program, *Journal of Consulting & Clinical Psychology* **68** (2000) 650-7.

[7]   M. F. Zabinski, M. A. Pung, D. E. Wilfley, D. L. Eppstein, A. J. Winzelberg, A. Celio, and C. B. Taylor, Reducing risk factors for eating disorders: Targeting at-risk women with a computerized psychoeducational program, *International Journal of Eating Disorders* **29** (2001) 401-8.

[8]   A. J. Winzelberg, D. Eppstein, K. L. Eldredge, D. Wilfley, R. Dasmahapatra, P. Dev, and C. B. Taylor, Effectiveness of an Internet-based program for reducing risk factors for eating disorders, *Journal of Consulting & Clinical Psychology* **68** (2000) 346-50.

[9]   G. Riva, L. Melis, and M. Bolzoni, Treating body image disturbances, *Communications of the ACM* **40** (1997) 69-71.

[10]   G. Riva, Modifications of body image induced by virtual reality, *Perceptual and Motor Skills* **86** (1998) 163-170.

[11]   S. deShazer, *Keys to solutions in brief therapy*. New York: W.W. Norton, 1985.

[12]   H. Leuner, Guided affective imagery: a method of intensive psychotherapy, *American Journal of Psychotherapy* **23** (1969) 4-21.

[13]   G. Riva and L. Melis, Virtual reality for the treatment of body image disturbances, in *Virtual reality in neuro-psycho-physiology: Cognitive, clinical and methodological issues in assessment and rehabilitation*, G. Riva, Ed. Amsterdam: IOS Press, 1997, pp. 95-111.

[14]   G. Riva, M. Bacchetta, M. Baruffi, S. Rinaldi, and E. Molinari, Virtual reality based experiential cognitive treatment of anorexia nervosa, *Journal of Behavioral Therapy and Experimental Psychiatry* **30** (1999) 221-230.

[15]   G. Riva, M. Bacchetta, M. Baruffi, S. Rinaldi, F. Vincelli, and E. Molinari, Virtual reality-based experiential cognitive treatment of obesity and binge-eating disorders, *Clinical Psychology and Psychotherapy* **7** (2000) 209-219.

[16]   G. Riva, M. Bacchetta, M. Baruffi, G. Cirillo, and E. Molinari, Virtual reality environment for body image modification: A multidimensional therapy for the treatment of body image in obesity and related pathologies, *CyberPsychology & Behavior* **3** (2000) 421-431.

[17]   A. Bandura, *Social foundation of thought and action: A social cognitive theory*. Englewood Cliffs, NJ: Prentice Hall, 1985.

[18]   M. J. Griffin, *Handbook of Human Vibration*. London: Academic Press, 1990.

Medicine Meets Virtual Reality 02/10
J.D. Westwood et al. (Eds.)
IOS Press, 2002

Training and Assessment of Laparoscopic Skills using a Haptic Simulator

Göran Rolfsson, Anna Nordgren, Stefan Bindzau, J-P Hagström,
John McLaughlin, Lennart Thurfjell
Reachin Technologies AB, Stockholm, Sweden

Abstract: Surgical simulation is a promising technique for training of laparoscopic surgery. Computer based simulation provides not only a cost effective alternative to traditional training but also a way to assess the surgeons performance. In this paper, we present a haptic simulator that allows for training and assessment of basic laparoscopic skills. The skills trained are modeled around a cholecystectomy procedure and include bi-manual dissection, clips setting, catheter insertion and cutting. The system uses accurate anatomic models of the organs involved in the procedure. This combined with effective methods for soft tissue deformation and haptic feedback, giving the surgeon a precise feeling of the interaction between organs and surgical instruments, provides a realistic training environment. The system has been designed with procedural training in mind and by putting together the individual tasks it will be possible to train on performing a complete cholecystectomy procedure.

1. Introduction

The working conditions in laparoscopic surgery are very different from those during open surgery with a major difficulty lying in the hand-eye coordination. Therefore extensive training is needed. The most common training method is apprenticeship, where an experienced surgeon guides the student. This may be combined with training using closed box trainers. However, there are several limitations with these techniques including cost, risk for the patient and lack of feedback to the student. To overcome some of these limitations, training using virtual reality (VR) based simulators has been proposed [1]. In this paper, we present a haptic simulator that allows for training of basic laparoscopic skills. The system has been designed with a focus on skills assessment.

2. Methods

2.1 Simulator design

The skills trained in the Reachin Laparoscopic Trainer are modeled around a cholecystectomy procedure. Therefore, laparoscopic cholecystectomy was studied in depth and the clinical procedure was modeled using UML's activity diagrams combined with activity specifications. The modeling resulted in an algorithmic description of the procedure that was the basis for the development of the system. With this description as input, we identified a number of basic skills involved and went on with the design of the different

lessons in the system. For the first version of the Laparoscopic Trainer we have decided to include the following lessons:
- Dissection of connective tissue using diathermy (liberating gall bladder from liver).
- Dissection of covering tissue using diathermy (fat around cystic duct).
- Setting clips around tubular structures and cutting them.
- Cutting a hole in a tubular structure and inserting a catheter (cholangiography).

In addition to the simulator there is a Lesson Management System (LMS), which is an administrative system for setting up users and assigning lessons to them. The lessons are run from the LMS environment, and in each lesson a number of parameters are recorded and subsequently used for assessment.

2.2   Geometric models

The anatomic models are based on the male Visible Human data set. These have been textured and reshaped so that the organs' positions reflect the changes that occur when the abdomen is inflated. In addition, we have built realistic models of all tools used (scissors, pliers, diathermy hook etc.)

2.3   Development platform and hardware

The development of the simulator is based on the Reachin API extended with the Reachin Medical Toolkit. The Reachin API was developed as the first scene-graph API that fully integrates graphics with haptics, and is designed as a general API for development of haptics applications. All functionality specific to medical applications is collected in the Reachin Medical Toolkit, which extends the functionality of the API [2]. As input devices we are currently using two Impulse Engines (Immersion Corp.) that have been mounted together. The system runs on a dual Pentium, Windows NT/2000 platform.

3.   Results

This paper describes work in progress. The first versions of the dissection and setting clips lessons have been implemented. The student can use a bi-manual technique where tissue is grabbed and pulled using one instrument while the other hand holds a diathermy hook or diathermy pliers, which is used to remove tissue (figure 1 and 2).

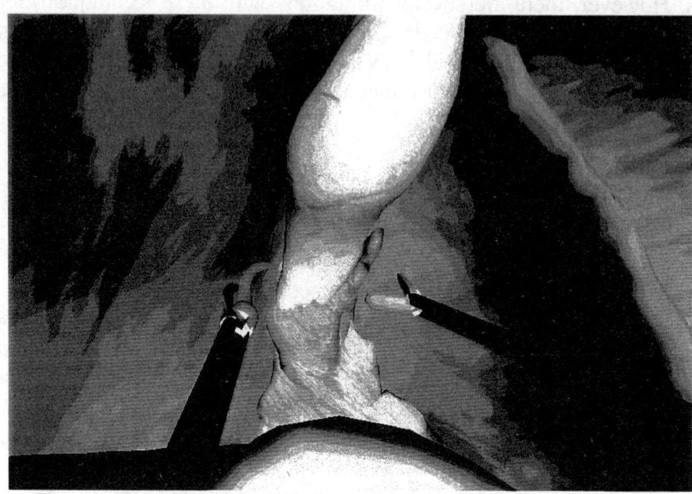

Figure 1. The gallbladder, cystic duct and surrounding fat before dissection.

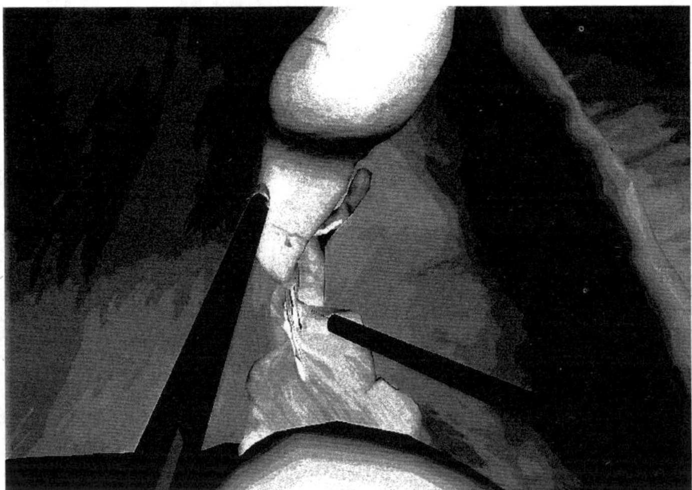

Figure 2. The gallbladder, cystic duct and surrounding fat after dissection.

Using this technique, the student can free the cystic duct from surrounding fat. In the next lesson the student can train setting clips around the cystic duct and cystic artery and cut them.

A large number of parameters are collected during the lessons. These include time spent, path for instruments, tool collisions, failure of using bi-manual and bi-lateral techniques, diathermy applied to the wrong tissue as well as a number of other parameters.

Although we have not addressed validation in this paper, it is important to emphasize that a surgical simulator is not useful until it has been validated. It is also important that a complex simulator such as our cholecystectomy application is validated first module-by-module and then as a whole. This work is currently underway and will be carried out in multi-center studies in collaboration with our clinical partners.

4. Discussion

We believe that realism is important for achieving an efficient training environment and we have paid great attention to develop a system with realistic haptic and visual impression. The first version of the simulator includes lessons for training of basic skills but by tying these together it will be possible to train a complete cholecystectomy procedure. Future versions will include anatomic variation and training of complication management.

5. Acknowledgments

Gold Standard Multimedia, Tampa, Florida, has developed all anatomic models used in the project.

References

[1] Kühnapfel U, Çakmak H. K, Maass H. Endoscopic Surgery Training using Virtual Reality and deformable Tissue Simulation. In *Computer & Graphics*, volume 24 (2000), pp. 671-682, Elsevier, 2000.
[2] Thurfjell L, Lundin A, McLaughlin J, A Medical Platform for Simulation of Surgical Procedures, In Westwood et al. (Eds), Medicine Meets Virtual Reality, IOS Press, 2001; pp. 509-514.

Medicine Meets Virtual Reality 02/10
J.D. Westwood et al. (Eds.)
IOS Press, 2002

The Blue DRAGON - A System for Monitoring the Kinematics and the Dynamics of Endoscopic Tools in Minimally Invasive Surgery for Objective Laparoscopic Skill Assessment

Jacob Rosen, Ph.D. (1), Jeffrey D. Brown BSE. (2), Marco Barreca, M.D. (3), Lily Chang, M.D. (3)
Blake Hannaford, Ph.D. (1), Mika Sinanan, M.D., Ph.D. (3)

(1) Department of Electrical Engineering, Box 352500, University of Washington, Seattle, WA
(2) Department of Bioengineering, Box 352500, University of Washington, Seattle, WA
(3) Department of Surgery, Box 356410, University of Washington, Seattle, WA

`<rosen, jdbrown, mbarreca, lchang, mssurg, blake>` `@u.washington.edu`
Biorobotics Lab: http://brl.ee.washington.edu
Center of Videoendoscopic Surgery: http://depts.washington.edu/cves/

ABSTRACT

Minimally invasive surgery (MIS) involves a multi-dimensional series of tasks requiring a synthesis between visual information and the kinematics and dynamics of the surgical tools. Analysis of these sources of information is a key step in mastering MIS surgery but may also be used to define objective criteria for characterizing surgical performance. The BlueDRAGON is a new system for acquiring the kinematics and the dynamics of two endoscopic tools along with the visual view of the surgical scene. It includes two four-bar mechanisms equipped with position and force torque sensors for measuring the positions and the orientations (P/O) of two endoscopic tools along with the forces and torques applied by the surgeon's hands. The methodology of decomposing the surgical task is based on a fully connected, finite-states (28 states) Markov model where each states corresponded to a fundamental tool/tissue interaction based on the tool kinematics and associated with unique F/T signatures. The experimental protocol included seven MIS tasks performed on an animal model (pig) by 30 surgeons at different levels of their residency training. Preliminary analysis of these data showed that major differences between residents at different skill levels were: (*i*) the types of tool/tissue interactions being used, (*ii*) the transitions between tool/tissue interactions being applied by each hand, (*iii*) time spent while performing each tool/tissue interaction, (*iv*) the overall completion time, and (*v*) the variable F/T magnitudes being applied by the subjects through the endoscopic tools. Systems like surgical robots or virtual reality simulators that inherently measure the kinematics and the dynamics of the surgical tool may benefit from inclusion of the proposed methodology for analysis of efficacy and objective evaluation of surgical skills during training

1. INTRODUCTION

Alternatives to the traditional apprenticeship model of surgical training are necessary in today's age of cost containment and increasing oversight of professional competency. There is an impetus not only for the demonstration of continuing competency among surgeons, but also for the instillation of basic competency early on, even before a resident reaches the operating room. Elements of this surgical skill include 1) expert knowledge of anatomy and the pathophysiology of the disease process, 2) visuospatial and eye-hand coordination, 3) team leadership and 4) critical decision making - in the prosecution of specific goals and often under conditions of incomplete information where error may have devastating consequences. Tests of technical competency currently available, beyond crude patient outcomes data such as survival, length of stay, or complication rates, have been directed at measurement of one or two specific elements of this expertise such as visuospatial ability. No currently validated systems exist for integrating or measuring surgical skill across all elements.

Performing minimally invasive surgery (MIS) involves a multi-dimensional series of tasks requiring a synthesis between visual information and the kinematics and dynamics of the surgical tools. One of the more difficult tasks in surgical education is to teach and objectively assess the optimal application of instrument forces and torques and the associated tools' kinematics necessary to conduct an operation. This is especially problematic in the field of MIS where the teacher is one step removed from the actual conduct of the operation. Along with the progress in developing MIS techniques, two additional modalities emerged in the last decade including teleoperated surgical robots and virtual reality simulators incorporating haptic technology as preoperative training tool. All these three modalities associated with MIS shared the same user interface in which both visual and kinesthetic information is flowing at the interface between the surgeon and the tools.

The proposed methodology for objective assessment of technical skill in MIS is based on the kinematics and the dynamics of the surgical tools measured at the tool/hand interface. The power of this methodology arises from decomposing the surgical task into its fundamental elements, and therefore it is independent from the modality being used (in-vivo surgery, robotic surgery or virtual reality simulators). Pervious research focused on measurement and analysis of the forces and torques being applied by the surgeons on a single endoscopic tool during two common laparoscopic procedures: cholecystectomy and Nissen fundoplication [1, 2].. In addition, Markov models were used to analyze and predict the skill level of the surgeon, based solely on the forces and torques they apply. The aim of the study was to develop a system of acquiring data in a real MIS setup and a methodology for decomposing two handed surgical task using Markov models (MM). These models enable objective assessing surgical skills.

2. TOOLS AND METHODS

2.1 The BlueDRAGON System

The BlueDRAGON is a system for acquiring the kinematics and the dynamics of two endoscopic tools along with the visual view of the surgical scene (Fig. 1). The system includes two four-bar passive mechanisms attached to endoscopic tools [4]. The four bar mechanisms translate the tool's rotation around the pivot point located in the port into the mechanism's joints incorpotaying position sensors. These translation is enabled when the base axes and the tool's shaft axis intersect the port's pivot point (Fig. 2). Moreover, the mechanism's axes alignment prevented any additional moments applied on the skin and internal tissues except the ones that are generated intentionally by using the tools. The gravitational forces applied on the surgeon's hand when the mechanism is away from its neutral position are compensated by an optimized spring connecting the bases and the first two coupled links.

The two mechanisms are equipped with three classes of sensors: (i) position sensors (multi turn potentiometers - Midori America Corp.) are incorporated into four of the mechanisms' joints for measuring the positions, the orientations and the translation of the two instrumented endoscopic tools attached to them. In addition, two linear potentiometer (Penny & Giles Controls Ltd.) that are attached to the tools' handle are used for measuring the endoscopic handle and tool tip angles; (ii) three-axis force/torque (F/T) sensors (ATI-Mini sensor) are located at the proximal end of the endoscopic tools' shaft, as well as force sensors inserted into the tools' handles for measuring the grasping forces at the hand/tool interface and (iii) contact sensors providing binary indication of any tool/tissue contact. Data measured by the BlueDRAGONs' sensors are acquired using two 12-bit National Instruments USB A/D cards sampling the 26 channels (3 rotations, 2 translations, 1 tissue contact, and 7 channels of forces and torques from each instrumented grasper) at 30 Hz. In addition to the data acquisition, the synchronized view of the surgical scene is incorporated into a graphical user interface displaying the data in real-time.

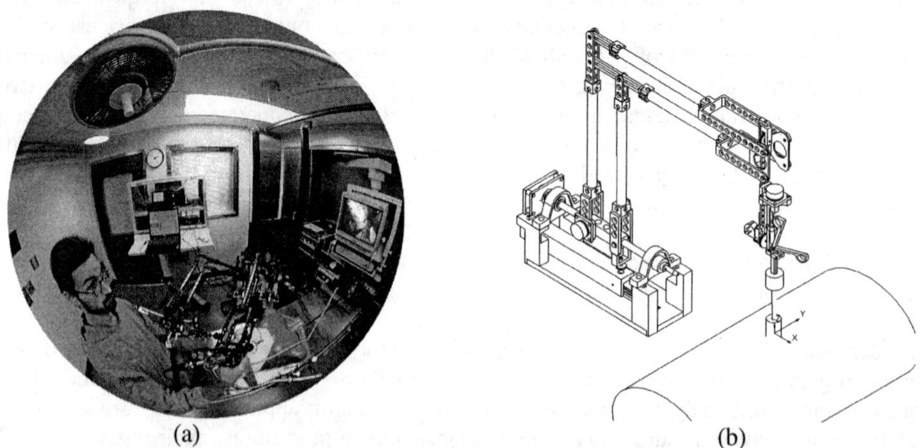

(a)   (b)

Figure 1: The BlueDRAGON system: (a) The system integration into a minimally invasive surgery setup (b) CAD drawing of the mechanism and its coordinate system.

2.2 MIS Task Decomposition

The methodology of decomposing surgical task is based a fully connected, symmetric finite-states (28 states) MM where the left and the right hands are represented by 14 states each (Fig. 2). Each one of the 14 states corresponded to a fundamental tool/tissue interaction based on the tool kinematics and associated with unique F/T signatures defined as observations and measured at the hand/tool interface (Table 1). In view of this model, any MIS task can be describe as a series of finite state. In each state the surgeon is applying a specific F/T signature, out of several F/T signatures which are typical to that state, on the tissue by using the tool. The surgeon may stay at that state for specific time duration applying different F/T signatures associated with that state and then perform a transition to another state. The surgeon may utilize any of the 14 states by the using the left and the right tools independently. However, the states representing the tool/tissue interactions of the left and the right tools are mathematically and functionally linked.

The 14 tool/tissue interactions can be further divided into three types based on the number of movements performed simultaneously (Table 1). The fundamental maneuvers are defined as Type I. The 'idle' state was defined as moving the tool in space (abdominal cavity) without touching any internal organ. The forces and torques developed in this state represented mainly the interaction with the trocar and the abdominal wall, in addition to the gravitational and inertial forces. In the 'grasping' and 'spreading' states, compression and tension were applied to the tissue by closing and opening the grasper handle, respectively. In the 'pushing' state, the tissue was compressed by moving the tool along the Z axis. 'Sweeping' consisted of placing the tool in one position while rotating it around the X and/or Y axes (trocar frame). The rest of the tool/tissue interactions in Types II and III were combinations of the fundamental ones defined as Type I.

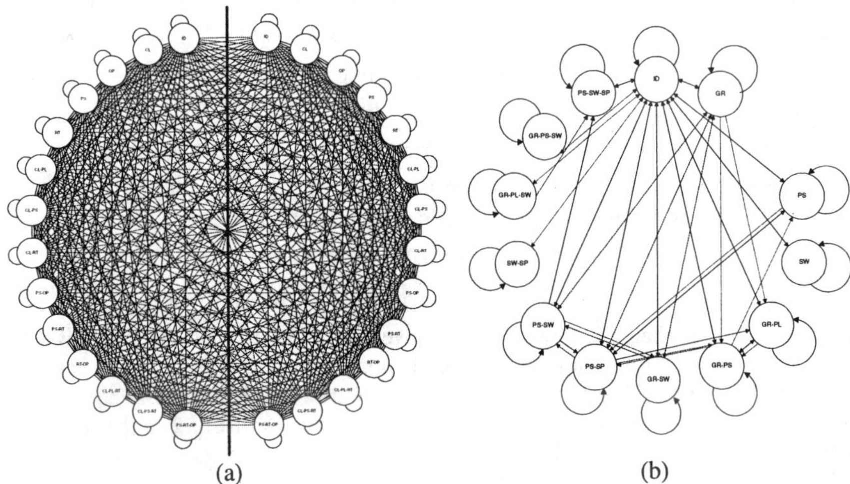

(a)   (b)

Figure 2: *Finite State Diagrams (FSD) - (a) Fully connected FSD for decomposing MIS. The tool/tissue interactions of the left and the right endoscopic tools are represented by the 14 fully connected sub models. Circles represent states whereas lines represent transitions between states. Lines that cross the center line represent different combination of states preformed by the left and the right tool. Force/torque signature associated with each state were omitted for simplifying the diagram; (b) Finite state diagram of MIS tissue dissection preformed by using endoscopic tool held by the right hand (Dashed line - transitions preformed by an expert surgeons - ES, Dotted line - transitions preformed by novice surgeons - first year residences R1, Solid line - transitions preformed both by R1 and ES)*

Type	No.	State Name	State Acronym	Tissue Contact	$\theta_x,\dot\theta_x$	$\theta_y,\dot\theta_y$	$\theta_z,\dot\theta_z$	$L_z,\dot L_z$	$\theta_g,\dot\theta_g$	F_x	F_y	F_z	T_x	T_y	T_z	F_g
I	1	Idle	ID	-	$\pm\varepsilon_{\theta_x}$	$\pm\varepsilon_{\theta_y}$	$\pm\varepsilon_{\theta_z}$	$\pm\varepsilon_{L_z}$	$\pm\varepsilon_{\theta_g}$	$\pm\varepsilon_{F_x}$	$\pm\varepsilon_{F_y}$	$\pm\varepsilon_{F_z}$	$\pm\varepsilon_{T_x}$	$\pm\varepsilon_{T_y}$	$\pm\varepsilon_{T_z}$	$\pm\varepsilon_{F_g}$
	2	Closing Handle (Grasping / Cutting)	CL	•	$\pm\varepsilon_{\theta_x}$	$\pm\varepsilon_{\theta_y}$	$\pm\varepsilon_{\theta_z}$	$\pm\varepsilon_{L_z}$	$\dot\theta_g > \varepsilon_{\theta_g}$	$\pm\varepsilon_{F_x}$	$\pm\varepsilon_{F_y}$	$\pm\varepsilon_{F_z}$	$\pm\varepsilon_{T_x}$	$\pm\varepsilon_{T_y}$	$\pm\varepsilon_{T_z}$	$F_g > \varepsilon_{F_g}$
	3	Opening Handle (Spreading)	OP	•	$\pm\varepsilon_{\theta_x}$	$\pm\varepsilon_{\theta_y}$	$\pm\varepsilon_{\theta_z}$	$\pm\varepsilon_{L_z}$	$\dot\theta_g < -\varepsilon_{\theta_g}$	$\pm\varepsilon_{F_x}$	$\pm\varepsilon_{F_y}$	$\pm\varepsilon_{F_z}$	$\pm\varepsilon_{T_x}$	$\pm\varepsilon_{T_y}$	$\pm\varepsilon_{T_z}$	$F_g < -\varepsilon_{F_g}$
	4	Pushing	PS	•	$\pm\varepsilon_{\theta_x}$	$\pm\varepsilon_{\theta_y}$	$\pm\varepsilon_{\theta_z}$	$\dot L_z < -\varepsilon_{L_z}$	$\pm\varepsilon_{\theta_g}$	$\pm\varepsilon_{F_x}$	$\pm\varepsilon_{F_y}$	$F_z < -\varepsilon_{F_z}$	$\pm\varepsilon_{T_x}$	$\pm\varepsilon_{T_y}$	$\pm\varepsilon_{T_z}$	$\pm\varepsilon_{F_g}$
	5	Rotating (Sweeping)	RT	•	$\dot\theta_x > \|\varepsilon_{\theta_x}\|$	$\dot\theta_y > \|\varepsilon_{\theta_y}\|$	$\pm\varepsilon_{\theta_z}$	$\pm\varepsilon_{L_z}$	$\pm\varepsilon_{\theta_g}$	$F_x > \|\varepsilon_{F_x}\|$	$F_y > \|\varepsilon_{F_y}\|$	$\pm\varepsilon_{F_z}$	$T_x > \|\varepsilon_{T_x}\|$	$T_y > \|\varepsilon_{T_y}\|$	$\pm\varepsilon_{T_z}$	$\pm\varepsilon_{F_g}$
II	6	Closing - Pulling	CL-PL	•	$\pm\varepsilon_{\theta_x}$	$\pm\varepsilon_{\theta_y}$	$\pm\varepsilon_{\theta_z}$	$\dot L_z > \varepsilon_{L_z}$	$\dot\theta_g > \varepsilon_{\theta_g}$	$\pm\varepsilon_{F_x}$	$\pm\varepsilon_{F_y}$	$F_z > \varepsilon_{F_z}$	$\pm\varepsilon_{T_x}$	$\pm\varepsilon_{T_y}$	$\pm\varepsilon_{T_z}$	$F_g > \varepsilon_{F_g}$
	7	Closing - Pushing	CL-PS	•	$\pm\varepsilon_{\theta_x}$	$\pm\varepsilon_{\theta_y}$	$\pm\varepsilon_{\theta_z}$	$\dot L_z < -\varepsilon_{L_z}$	$\dot\theta_g > \varepsilon_{\theta_g}$	$\pm\varepsilon_{F_x}$	$\pm\varepsilon_{F_y}$	$F_z < -\varepsilon_{F_z}$	$\pm\varepsilon_{T_x}$	$\pm\varepsilon_{T_y}$	$\pm\varepsilon_{T_z}$	$F_g > \varepsilon_{F_g}$
	8	Closing - Rotating	CL-RT	•	$\dot\theta_x > \|\varepsilon_{\theta_x}\|$	$\dot\theta_y > \|\varepsilon_{\theta_y}\|$	$\pm\varepsilon_{\theta_z}$	$\pm\varepsilon_{L_z}$	$\dot\theta_g > \varepsilon_{\theta_g}$	$F_x > \|\varepsilon_{F_x}\|$	$F_y > \|\varepsilon_{F_y}\|$	$\pm\varepsilon_{F_z}$	$\pm\varepsilon_{T_x}$	$\pm\varepsilon_{T_y}$	$\pm\varepsilon_{T_z}$	$F_g > \varepsilon_{F_g}$
	9	Pushing - Opening	PS-OP	•	$\pm\varepsilon_{\theta_x}$	$\pm\varepsilon_{\theta_y}$	$\pm\varepsilon_{\theta_z}$	$\dot L_z < -\varepsilon_{L_z}$	$\dot\theta_g < -\varepsilon_{\theta_g}$	$\pm\varepsilon_{F_x}$	$\pm\varepsilon_{F_y}$	$F_z < -\varepsilon_{F_z}$	$\pm\varepsilon_{T_x}$	$\pm\varepsilon_{T_y}$	$\pm\varepsilon_{T_z}$	$F_g < -\varepsilon_{F_g}$
	10	Pushing - Rotating	PS-RT	•	$\dot\theta_x > \|\varepsilon_{\theta_x}\|$	$\dot\theta_y > \|\varepsilon_{\theta_y}\|$	$\pm\varepsilon_{\theta_z}$	$\dot L_z < -\varepsilon_{L_z}$	$\pm\varepsilon_{\theta_g}$	$F_x > \|\varepsilon_{F_x}\|$	$F_y > \|\varepsilon_{F_y}\|$	$F_z < -\varepsilon_{F_z}$	$\pm\varepsilon_{T_x}$	$\pm\varepsilon_{T_y}$	$\pm\varepsilon_{T_z}$	$\pm\varepsilon_{F_g}$
	11	Rotating - Opening	RT-OP	•	$\dot\theta_x > \|\varepsilon_{\theta_x}\|$	$\dot\theta_y > \|\varepsilon_{\theta_y}\|$	$\pm\varepsilon_{\theta_z}$	$\pm\varepsilon_{L_z}$	$\dot\theta_g < -\varepsilon_{\theta_g}$	$F_x > \|\varepsilon_{F_x}\|$	$F_y > \|\varepsilon_{F_y}\|$	$\pm\varepsilon_{F_z}$	$T_x > \|\varepsilon_{T_x}\|$	$T_y > \|\varepsilon_{T_y}\|$	$\pm\varepsilon_{T_z}$	$F_g < -\varepsilon_{F_g}$
III	12	Closing - Pulling - Rotating	CL-PL-RT	•	$\dot\theta_x > \|\varepsilon_{\theta_x}\|$	$\dot\theta_y > \|\varepsilon_{\theta_y}\|$	$\pm\varepsilon_{\theta_z}$	$\dot L_z > \varepsilon_{L_z}$	$\dot\theta_g > \varepsilon_{\theta_g}$	$F_x > \|\varepsilon_{F_x}\|$	$F_y > \|\varepsilon_{F_y}\|$	$F_z > \varepsilon_{F_z}$			$\pm\varepsilon_{T_z}$	$F_g > \varepsilon_{F_g}$
	13	Closing - Pushing - Rotating	CL-PS-RT	•	$\dot\theta_x > \|\varepsilon_{\theta_x}\|$	$\dot\theta_y > \|\varepsilon_{\theta_y}\|$	$\pm\varepsilon_{\theta_z}$	$\dot L_z < -\varepsilon_{L_z}$	$\dot\theta_g > \varepsilon_{\theta_g}$	$F_x > \|\varepsilon_{F_x}\|$	$F_y > \|\varepsilon_{F_y}\|$	$F_z < -\varepsilon_{F_z}$	$T_x > \|\varepsilon_{T_x}\|$	$T_y > \|\varepsilon_{T_y}\|$	$\pm\varepsilon_{T_z}$	$F_g > \varepsilon_{F_g}$
	14	Pushing - Rotating - Opening	PS-RT-OP	•	$\dot\theta_x > \|\varepsilon_{\theta_x}\|$	$\dot\theta_y > \|\varepsilon_{\theta_y}\|$	$\pm\varepsilon_{\theta_z}$	$\dot L_z < -\varepsilon_{L_z}$	$\dot\theta_g < -\varepsilon_{\theta_g}$	$F_x > \|\varepsilon_{F_x}\|$	$F_y > \|\varepsilon_{F_y}\|$	$F_z < -\varepsilon_{F_z}$	$\pm\varepsilon_{T_x}$	$\pm\varepsilon_{T_y}$	$\pm\varepsilon_{T_z}$	$F_g < -\varepsilon_{F_g}$

Table 1: *Definitions of the 14 states based on spherical coordinate system with an origin at the port (trocar). Each state is characterized by a unique set of angular velocities forces and torques. A non zero threshold value is defined for each parameter by ε. The states' definitions are independent from the tool tip being used e.g. the state defined as Closing Handle might be associated with grasping or cutting if a grasper or scissors are being used respectively.*

The MM is defined by the compact notation (7). Each Markov sub model representing the left and the right tool is defined by λ_L and λ_R (Eq. 1). The sub model is defined by: (*i*) The number of states - N whereas individual states are denoted as $S = \{s_1, s_1, \ldots s_N\}$, and the state at time as q_t.; (*ii*) The number of distinct observation symbol -

M whereas individual symbols are denoted as $V = \{v_1, v_1, ... v_M\}$; (*iii*) The state transition probability distribution matrix $- A = \{a_{ij}\}$, where $a_{ij} = P[q_{t+1} = s_j | q_t = s_i]$ $1 \leq i, j \leq N$; (*iv*) The observation symbol probability distribution matrix $- B = \{b_j(k)\}$, where for state j $b_j(k) = P[v_k \text{ at } t | q_t = s_j]$ $1 \leq j \leq N, 1 \leq k \leq M$; (*v*) The initial state distribution vector$- \pi$ where $\pi_i = P[q_1 = s_i]$ $1 \leq i \leq N$. The two sub models are linked to each other by the left-right interstate transition probability distribution matrix $- C = \{c_{lr}\}$, where $c_{lr} = P[q_{tL} = s_l \cup q_{tR} = s_r]$ $1 \leq l, r \leq N$

The probability observing the state transition $Q = \{q_1, q_2, ... q_T\}$ and the associated observation sequence $O = \{o_1, o_2, ... o_T\}$ given the two MM sub models (Eq. 1) and interstate transition probability distribution matrix is defined by Eq. 2a

$$\lambda_L = (A_L, B_L, \pi_L) \qquad \lambda_R = (A_R, B_R, \pi_R) \tag{1}$$

$$P(Q, O | \lambda_L, \lambda_R, C) = \pi_{q_L} \pi_{q_R} \prod_{t=0}^{T} a_{q_t q_{t+1} L} b_{q_t L}(o_t) a_{q_t q_{t+1} R} b_{q_t R}(o_t) c_{q_{tL} q_{tR}} \tag{2}$$

Due to the fact that probabilities by definition have numerical value in the range of 0 to 1. For relatively short time duration the probability calculated by Eq. 2 converge exponentially to zero and therefore exceed the precision range of essentially any machine. Hence by using logarithmic transformation the resulting values of Eq. 2 in the range of [0 1] are mapped by eq. 3 into [$-\infty$ 1].

$$Log(P(Q, O | \lambda_L, \lambda_R, C)) = Log(\pi_{q_L}) + Log(\pi_{q_R}) + \sum_{t=1}^{T} Log(a_{q_t q_{t+1} L}) + Log(b_{q_t L}(o_t)) + Log(a_{q_t q_{t+1} R}) + Log(b_{q_t R}(o_t)) + Log(c_{q_{tL} q_{tR}}) \tag{3}$$

Once the MMs were defined for specific subjects with specific skill levels, it is then possible to calculate the statistical distance between them. This statistical distance is considered to be an objective criterion for evaluation skills level if for example the statistical distance between a subject under study and an expert is being calculated. Given two MMs λ_1 and λ_2 the statistical distances between them $D(\lambda_1, \lambda_2)$ and $D(\lambda_2, \lambda_1)$ are defined by Eq. 4

$$D(\lambda_1, \lambda_2) = \frac{1}{T_{O_2}}[logP(O_2, Q_2 | \lambda_1) - logP(O_2, Q_2 | \lambda_2)] \tag{4}$$

$$D(\lambda_2, \lambda_1) = \frac{1}{T_{O_1}}[logP(O_1, Q_1 | \lambda_1) - logP(O_1, Q_2 | \lambda_2)]$$

$D(\lambda_1, \lambda_2)$ is a measure of how well model λ_1 matches observations and the state sequence generated by model λ_2 relative to how well model λ_2 matches observations and the state sequence generated by itself whereas T_{O_1}, and T_{O_2} stand for the time duration of the observation vectors O_1 and O_2 respectively. Since $D(\lambda_1, \lambda_2)$ and $D(\lambda_2, \lambda_1)$ are nonsymmetrical, The natural expression of the symmetrical statistical distance version is defined by Eq 5.

$$D_S(\lambda_1, \lambda_2) = \frac{D(\lambda_1, \lambda_2) + D(\lambda_2, \lambda_1)}{2} \tag{5}$$

2.3 Experimental Protocol

The experimental protocol included seven standard MIS tasks performed in-vivo on an animal model (pig) by 30 surgeons at different levels of their residency training (5xR1,R2,R3,R4,R5 where the numeral denotes year of training and Expert Videoendoscopic surgeons). These tasks were 1) Running the bowel right to left; 2) Running the bowel left to right 3) Dissecting Mesenteric Arteries;
4) Passing a Suture; 5) Tying a Knot; 6) Suturing the Colon; 7) Passing Stomach behind the Esophagus. All animal procedures were performed in an AALAC-accredited surgical research facility under an approved protocol from the institutional animal care committee of the University of Washington.

3. RESULTS

Typical raw data of forces torques and tool tip position were plotted in a 3D space showing the kinematics and the dynamics of the left and the right endoscopic tools measured by the BlueDRAGON while examining 0.762m of the bowel (Fig. 2b). The forces and torques can be described as vectors with an origin at the center of the sensor and the coordinate system aligned with the tool coordinate system. These vectors are constantly changing both their magnitudes and orientations as a result of the F/T applied by the surgeon's hand on the tool while interaction with the tissues. The F/T as vectors can be depicted as arrows attached to the origin and changing their lengths and orientations as a function of time. Fig.3 a,b describes the traces of the tips of these vectors as they were changing during the surgical procedure. In a similar fashion the traces of the tool tips position were plotted in Fig 3c. The forces along the Z axis (in/out of the trocar) were higher compared to the forces in the XY plane. On the other hand, torques developed by rotating the tool around the Z axis were extremely low compared to the torques generated while rotating the tool along the X and Y axis while sweeping the tissue or performing lateral retraction. Similar trends in terms of the F/T magnitude ratios between the X, Y, and Z axes were found in the data measured in other MIS tasks. These raw data demonstrated the complexity of the surgical task. Deeper understanding of the MIS task is gained by decomposing it to its prime elements.

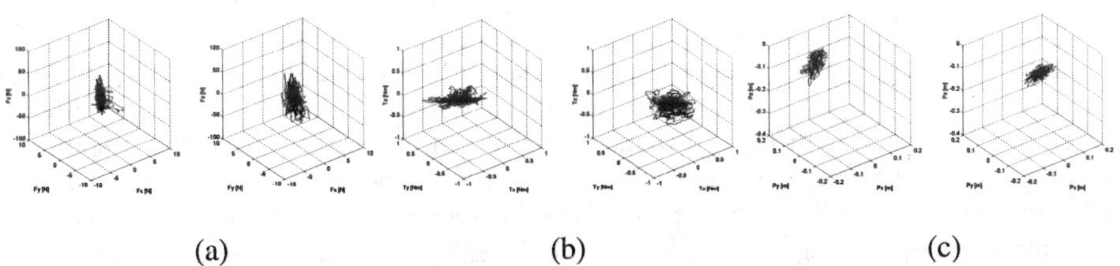

(a)   (b)   (c)

Figure 3: The kinematics and dynamics data of the left and the right endoscopic tools measured by the Blue DRAGON while sequentially examining sections of the bowel (For coordinate system definition see Fig. 1b) - (a) Forces; (b) Torques (c) Tool tip position.

A cluster analysis using the K-means algorithm was preformed for defining typical F/T signatures in the database [3]. This decoding process allowed to decompose the surgical task and depict it as a finite state diagram (Fig 2b). The Idle state is the only state connected to all the other states in the diagram. This state, in which no tool/tissue interaction was performed, was mainly used by both expert and novice surgeons to move from one operative state to the other. However, the expert surgeons used the idle state only as a transition state while the novices spent a significant amount of time in this state planning the next tool/tissue interaction. Another major difference between surgeons from different skill groups was related to the tool/tissue interaction and tool/tissue transitions used by these two groups. Surgeons took different paths to reach the same goal. Each group utilized states and transitions not used by the other group.

Further analysis of the F/T associated with each state showed that the F/T magnitudes were found to be task dependent. High F/T magnitudes were applied by novices compared to experts during tissue manipulation, and vice versa during tissue dissection. High efficiency of surgical performance was demonstrated by the expert surgeons and expressed by shorter tool tip displacements, shorter periods of time spent in the 'idle' state, and sufficient application of F/T on the tissue to safely accomplish the task.

4. DISCUSSION

Minimally invasive surgery is a complex task that requires a synthesis between visual and kinesthetic information. Analyzing MIS in terms of these two sources of information is a key step towards developing objective criteria for training surgeons and evaluating the performance in different modalities: real surgery, master/slave robotic systems or virtual reality simulators incorporating haptic technology.

In developing the BlueDRAGON system several alternatives were examined as a 3D position tracking system including systems that are based on optical, acoustic, electromagnetic, and mechanical sensors. Considering the surgical scene with multiple instruments that might block the line of sight required by optical and acoustic systems, and the massive amount of metallic devises that might generate magnetic interference to the electromagnetic systems, a mechanical system utilizing a passive mechanism incorporating linear and rotary potentiometers and attached to the surgical tool provides a simple and robust solution for tracking the position and the orientations of the surgical tool.

The Markov model proved to be a very powerful method encompassing multi modal sources of information into compact mathematical representation of a complex task such as surgery. Moreover, once the model's architecture is determined and the model's parameters are calculated it provides quantitative and objective measure of surgical performance. A feasible analogy to the proposed methodology for decomposing the surgical task is the human language. Based on this analogy the basic states - tool/tissue interactions are equivalent to 'words' of the MIS 'language' and the 14 states are forming the MIS 'dictionary'. In the same way as a single word is pronounced differently by different people, the same tool/tissue interaction is performed differently by different surgeons while applying different F/T magnitudes, yet they all share the same meaning, or outcome, as in the realm of surgery. The cluster analysis was used to identify the typical F/T associated with each one of the tool/tissue interactions in the surgery 'dictionary', or using the language analogy, it characterized different pronunciations of a word. Utilizing the 'dictionary' of surgery, the MM was then used to define the process of each task or step of the surgical procedure, or in other words, 'dictating chapters' of the surgical 'story'. The proposed methodology regains its power by decomposing the surgical task to its prime elements - tool/tissue interactions. These elements are inherent in MIS no matter which modality is being used.

ACKNOWLEDGMENTS - This research was funded by a major grant from US Surgical, a division of Tyco, Inc. to the University of Washington, Center for Videoendoscopic Surgery.and a gift from Washington Research Foundation Capital.

REFERENCES

[1] Richards, C., Rosen, J., Hannaford, B., MacFarlane, M., Pellegrini, C., Sinanan, M., Skills Evaluation in Minimally Invasive Surgery Using Force/Torque Signatures, Surgical. Endoscopy., 14(9):791-8.

[2] Rosen J., Solazzo, M., Hannaford, B., Sinanan, M., Objective Laparoscopic Skills Assessments of Surgical Residents Using Hidden Markov Models Based on Haptic Information and Tool/Tissue Interactions, Stud. Health Tech. Inform. 81:417-23, 2001.

[3] Rosen J., B. Hannaford, Richards C., M. Sinanan, Markov Modeling of Minimally Invasive Surgery Based on Tool/Tissue interaction and Force/Torque Signatures for Evaluating Surgical Skills, IEEE Transactions on Biomedical Engineering Vol. 48. No. 5, pp. 579-591 May 2001.

[4] Madhani, A.J., Niemeyer, G., Salisbury, J.K., Jr., 1998, "Black Falcon: A Teleoperated Surgical Instrument For Minimally Invasive Surgery," Proceedings, 1998 IEEE/RSJ International Conference on Intelligent Robots and System

Medicine Meets Virtual Reality 02/10
J.D. Westwood et al. (Eds.)
IOS Press, 2002

A tutorial platform suitable for surgical simulator training (SimMentor™)

Jan Sigurd Røtnes, MD,PhD[1,2], Johannes Kaasa, MSc[1],
Geir Westgaard, PhD[1], Eivind Myrold Eriksen, BSc[1],
Per Øyvind Hvidsten, MSc[1], Kyrre Strøm, PhD[1],
Vidar Sørhus, PhD[1], Yvon Halbwachs, MSc[1], Einar Haug, PhD[1],
Morten Grimnes, PhD[1], Hugues Fontenelle. BSc[1],
Tom Ekeberg, MSc[3], Jan B. Thomassen, PhD[4],
Ole Jakob Elle, MSc[2], Erik Fosse, MD, PhD[2]

1) *SimSurgery AS, email: j.s.rotnes@simsurgery.no*
      URL: www.simsurgery.no
2) *Interventional Centre, National Hospital, Rikshospitalet,*
      N-0027 Oslo, Norway, email: j.s.rotnes@klinmed.uio.no
         URL: www.interventionalcentre.com
3) *Mobile Media, N-0027 Oslo, Norway,*
         URL: www.MobileMedia.com
4) *Sintef, N-0027 Oslo, Norway,*
         URL: www.sintef.no

Abstract: Background: The introduction of simulators in surgical training entails
the need to develop pedagogic platforms adapted to the potentials and limitations
provided by the information technology. As a solution to the technical challenges in
treating all possible interaction events and to obtain a suitable pedagogic approach,
we have developed a pedagogic platform for surgical training, SimMentor™.
Methods: In SimMentor™ the procedure to be practiced is divided into a number
of natural phases. The trainee will practice on one phase at a time, however he can
select the sequence of phases arbitrarily. A phase is taught by letting the trainee
alternate freely between 2 modes:
1: A 3-dimensional animated guidance designed for learning the objectives and
challenges in a procedure.
2: An interactive training session through the instrument manipulator device
designed for training motoric responses based on visual and tactile responses
produced by the simulator.
The two modes are interfaced with the same virtual reality platform, thus
SimMentor™ allows a seamless transition between the modes.
Results: We have developed a prototype simulator for robotic assisted endoscopic
CABG (Coronary Artery Bypass Grafting) procedure by first focusing on the
anastomosis part of the operation. Tissue, suture and instrument models have been
developed and integrated with a simulated model of a beating heart comprises the
elements in the simulator engine that is used in construction a training platform for
learning different methods for performing a coronary anastomosis procedure.
Conclusion: The platform is designed for integrating the following features: 1)
practical approach to handle interactivity events with flexible-objects 3D simulators,
2) methods for quantitative evaluations of performance, 3) didactic presentations, 4)
effective ways of producing diversity of clinical and pathological training scenarios.

1. Introduction

A challenging task in developing simulator technology for surgical training is to establish algorithms that can handle all possible events that can follow the interaction between simulated objects. There are methods for detecting collisions between rigid and soft tissue objects, but a sequence of collisions between objects with the subsequent effect on the complete three-dimensional (3D) model may very well produce an unpredicted scene that does not contain sufficient information to further simulate realistic responses.

A pedagogic method in learning new skills is first to copy techniques provided by experts before trainees are allowed to improvise on their own. Expert experience is often provided by both animated sequences and videos from real operations. Such illustrations provide the objectives for training with the simulator. The learning sequence is first to see and understand the objectives, then to perform tasks. However, often there are substantial differences in the displayed images from real operations compared to images produced by the simulator, especially in regard to the realization of how the interactivity with soft tissue is simulated. Lack of realism in image display and elestodynamical behavior of soft tissue has consequences for training on image-guided decision making and how to optimally maneuver instruments with important anatomical structures in the 3D surroundings.

In our development of a coronary anastomosis simulator (SimCor^{TM}) we have designed a platform, SimMentor^{TM} that exploits a common 3D model both for simulating interactivity during performance and for the animated 3D visualization used during learning of the objectives in training sessions. Thus, SimMentor^{TM} is a platform where a common 3D model ("simulation engine") is used in different modes for construction, visualization, performance and evaluation of tasks. By exactly defining the tasks to be performed with the simulator we achieve a pedagogic approach where the objectives are very precise, and at the same time we avoid the challenge where a sequence of collisions brings the simulator into an undetermined state from where the model is not able to calculate further realistic responses. This platform (SimMentor^{TM}) where the common 3D "simulator engine" is applied in tasks design, guidance and performance, render an optimal situation for evaluating performance since the objectives of the training are defined by a 3D animated visualization identical to the simulated environment, and from where the performance is conducted.

The visual appearance during task guidance and task performance should be very similar. For the SimCor^{TM} simulator we have obtained realism with deformable soft tissue objects by applying a new 3D modeling technique ideal for anatomical structures undergoing reconstructive topological changes (Sim3DM^{TM}) [1,2].

2. Material & Tools

In SimMentor™ the procedure to be practiced is divided into a number of natural **phases**. The trainee will practice one phase at a time, however he can select the sequence of phases arbitrarily. A phase is taught by letting the trainee alternate freely between 2 modes (figure 1):

1: A 3-dimensional animated guidance designed for learning the objectives and challenges in a procedure.

2: An interactive training session through the instrument manipulator device designed for training motoric responses based on visual and tactile responses produced by the simulator.

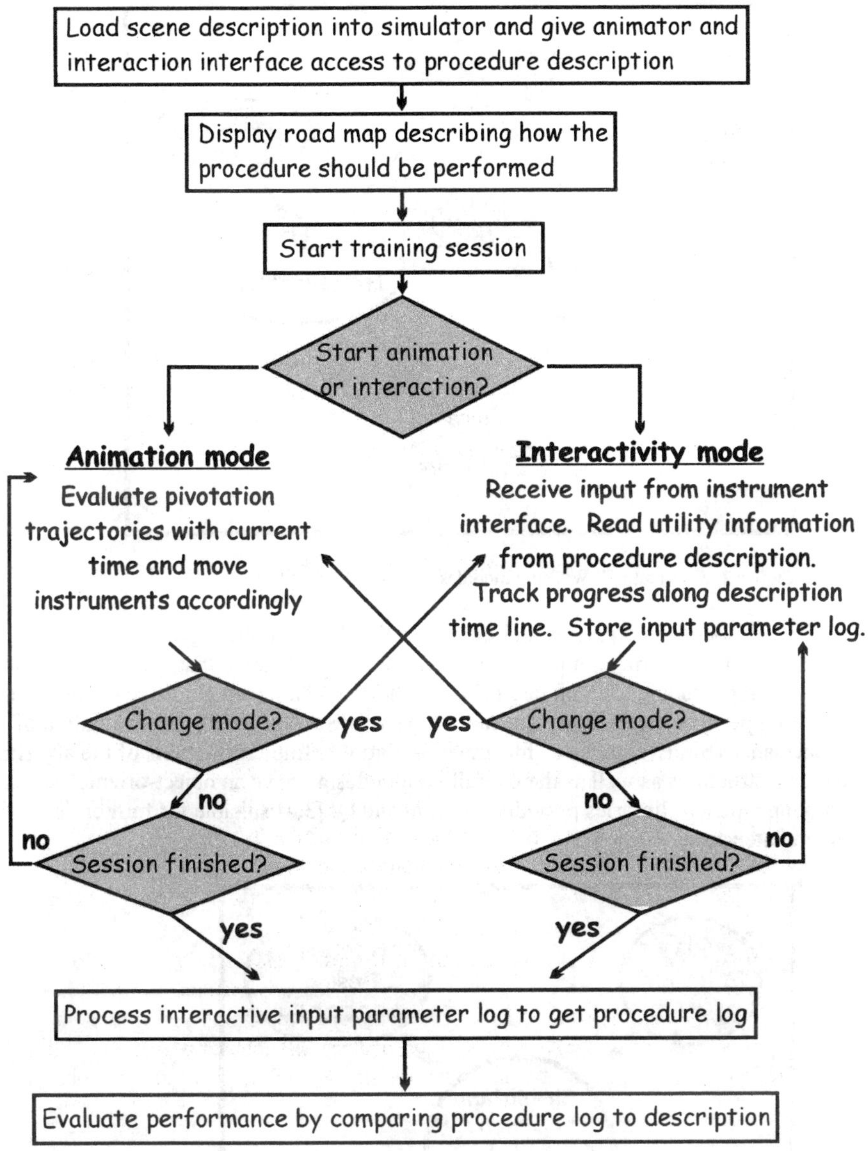

Figure 1 SimMentor™ Task Chart

The two modes are using the same virtual reality platform, thus SimMentor™ allows a seamless transition between the modes. The mode switch can be performed at any time during the training phase. For training longer procedural sequences several phases can be assembled into a long super-phase. The seamless transition between 3D animation and interactivity is also an important feature in designing and modifying tasks as illustrated in figure 2. Since the objectives of the tasks are precisely defined, quantitative analysis of the results are easily derived from the difference between the performance obtained from the trainee log file and the parameters guiding the animator.

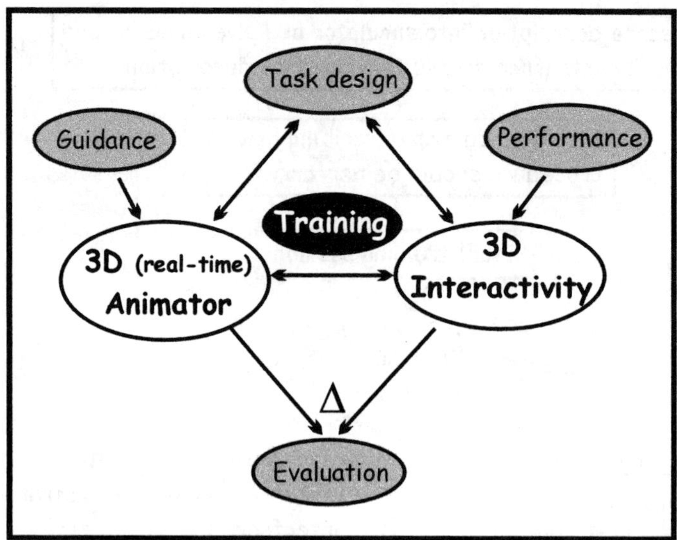

Figure 2 SimMentor™ Working modules

The tissue models, instruments and the interaction between the objects are all integrated in a common 3D platform simulation, animation and visualization that is used by all the modules in producing training tasks (SimDesign), 3D animated guidance (SimPlayer), recording performance and use during task design (SimRecorder), and evaluation of performance (SimEvaluator) as illustrated in figure 3. Implementations of the algorithms and data structures as well as the overall system design have an object-oriented structure applying OpenGL libraries provided by Coin and Qt [3,4] suitable for further development and maintenance.

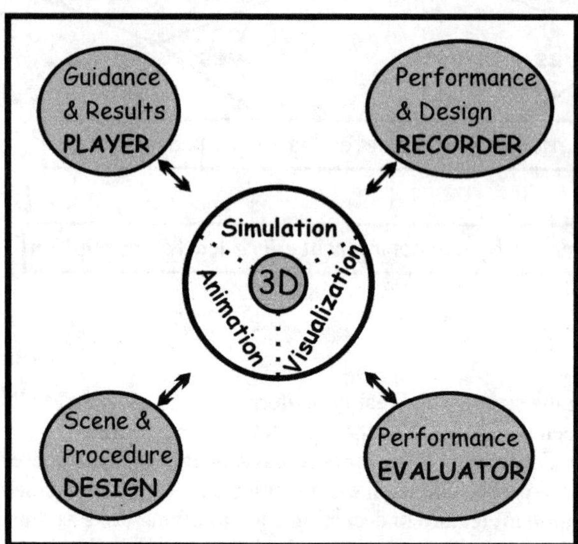

Figure 3 SimMentor™ Software Modules

3. Results

Virtual reality surgical training is an educational method ideal for telemanipulating [5,6] systems. We have developed a prototype simulator (SimCor^{TM}) for robotic assisted endoscopic Coronary Artery Bypass Grafting (CABG) procedure by first focusing on the anastomosis part of the operation, and surgical planning regarding the robotic system setup as indicated in figure 4 and 5. Tissue, suture and instrument models have been developed and integrated with a simulated model of a beating heart. These comprise the elements in the simulator engine that is used for constructing a training platform for learning different methods for performing a coronary anastomosis procedure [1,2,7]. The experience obtained from simulating a conventional anastomosis procedure will be exploited to extend the repertoire of training sessions, and in the future other training methods applicable to conventional techniques.

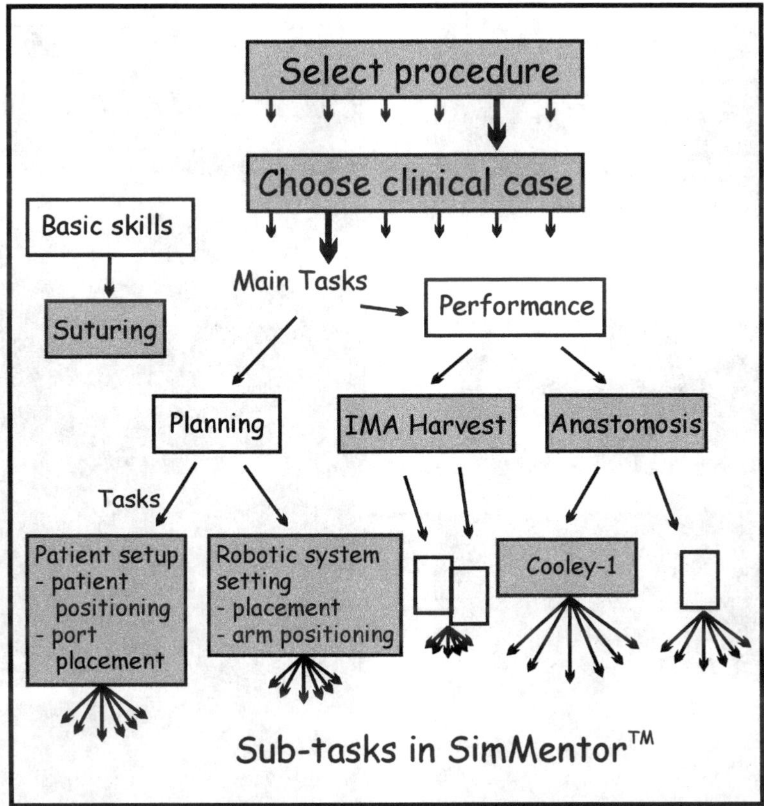

Figure 4 SimCor^{TM} Flow Chart

Figure 5 (next page) A-J Snapshots obtained from training on anastomosis procedure with the robotic system Zeus [5] and planning robotic system setup.
Simulation training in the operation room with the robotic system Zeus, but where the robotic arms are interacting with a virtual reality beating heart. B) Simulation training where the Zeus master consol controls a virtual reality robot interacting with a virtual reality patient. C) As B) but now the surface is made transparent and instruments are viewed from inside. D) Simulating the robotic system setting where two arms collide. E) Simulating robotic system setting where one instrument falls out. F-I) Stapshots obtained during training. J) Modelling with SimDesign

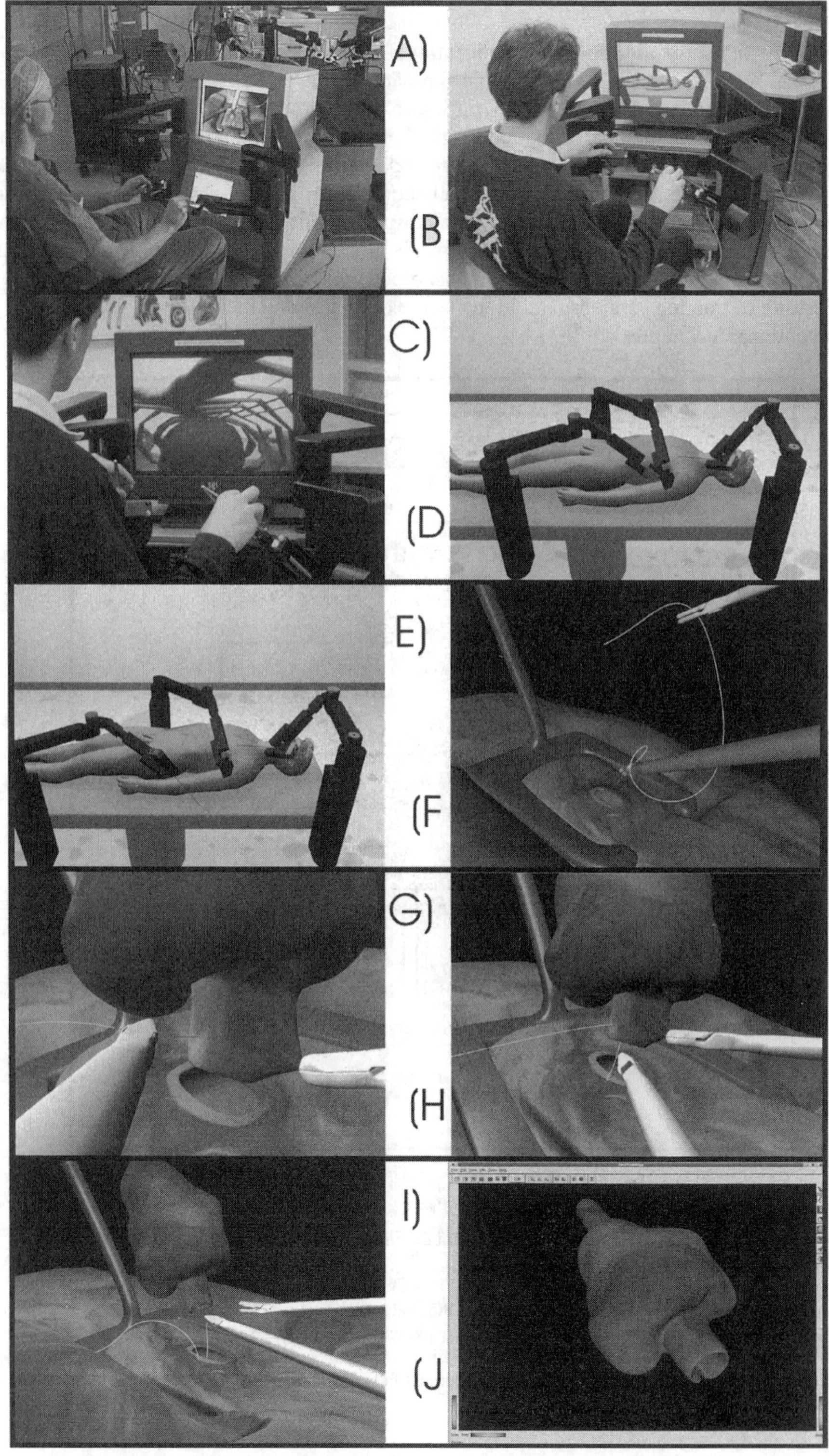
A)
(B
C)
(D
E)
(F
G)
(H
I)
(J

Based on our Sim3DM^{TM} technology, an application development tool has been developed so that anatomical and physical properties together with object textures can be included, according to the needs defined during application development as illustrated in figure 6.

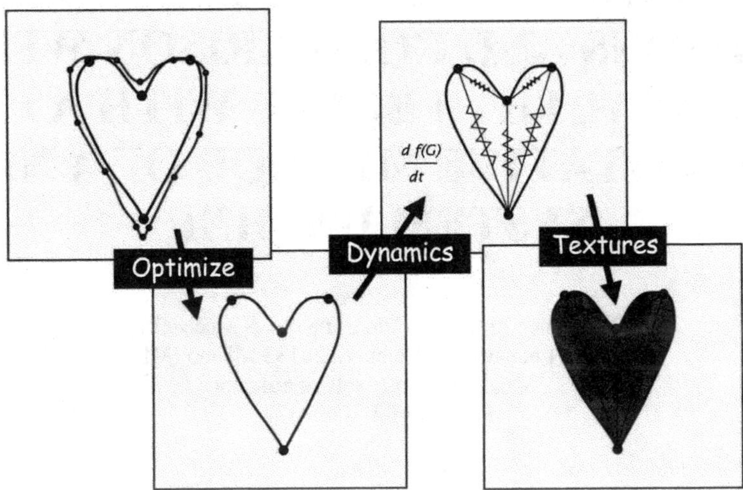

Figure 6 Sim3DM^{TM} application designer and developer tool

4. Discussion

The SimMentor™ platform is based on a pedagogic and effective method for implementing simulator technology in surgical training.

The platform is designed for integrating the following features: 1) practical approach to handle interactivity events with deformable-objects 3D simulators, 2) methods for quantitative evaluations of performance, 3) didactic presentations, 4) effective ways of producing diversity of clinical and pathological training scenarios.

5. References

[1] Røtnes J.S., et al., Digital trainer developed for robotic assisted cardiac surgery
     Medicine Meets Virtual Reality 2001, Technology and Informatics 81
     ISBN 1 58603 143 0 (IOS Press), 424-430, 2001
[2] Røtnes J.S., et al., Realism in surgical simulators with free-form geometric modelling
     Computer Assisted Radiology and Surgery, CARS/SMIT 2001, ISBN 0-444-50866-X , 997-1002, 2001
[3] Systems In Motion, www.sim.no
[4] Trolltech, www.trolltech.com
[5] Computer Motion, www.computermotion.com
[6] Intuitive Surgical, www.intusurg.com
[7] Austad, A., Elle, O.J., Røtnes, J.S., Computer aided planning of trocar placement and robot settings in
     robot assisted surgery, Computer Assisted Radiology and Surgery, CARS/SMIT 2001,
     ISBN 0-444-50866-X, 981-986, 2001

Medicine Meets Virtual Reality 02/10
J.D. Westwood et al. (Eds.)
IOS Press, 2002

PROTOCOLS FOR CLINICAL TESTS ON PARKINSON DISEASE AFFECTED PERSONS AND COMPARISON WITH HEALTHY PEOPLE WITH A QUANTITATIVE METHOD OF A NEW SYSTEM DAPHNE

A. Rovetta
Politecnico di Milano, Dipartimento di Meccanica
Piazza Leonardo da Vinci, 32 20133 Milano (MI)
E-Mail: alberto.rovetta@polimi.it
Fax: +39-02-70638377

Keywords: clinical protocols, biorobotics, Parkinson disease, new equipment

Abstract

This paper deals with Daphne, a portable equipment for the evaluation of the state of health in Parkinson disease. The protocols have been developed, according to the design, to the characteristics, to the performances of the system. Tests on patients and healthy persons are presented, as application of protocols.

1. Introduction

In the Laboratory of Robotics is on development the final prototype of the portable system Daphne for the measure of the neuromotor conditions and of the attention of a person. The

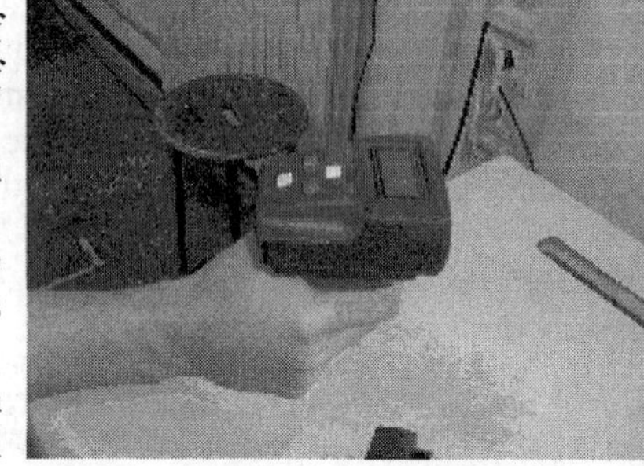

research has been dedicated to a new system for the immediate diagnosis of the neuromotor state of health. Methodologies of design and development of new engineering for the medicine have been adopted. The clinical tests want to validate the prototype with test protocols which have demanded a deep attention. Also for the applications in sport and for the domestic application lighter and flexible protocols have been proposed.

The measurement on the health of a person with reference to neuromotor and psychological conditions requires a quantitative data. At present time some parameters are easily measured, as the response time in front of active audio and visual signals. Also the measurement of force parameters under stress are measured. No integrated quantitative measure in the same time actually exists. Daphne system, here presented, offers the possibility of measurement with active protocol (Ref. [1] to [4]).

The research has been born from a biorobotic analysis and the developed system has been patented from ST Microelectronics.

2. Problem

The measurement in unhealthy conditions, and also in sport and in home care, must be referred to numerical quantitative data, and not only to the impression of the medical doctor or of the trainer. A protocol which reports some regularities in test must be performed and adopted in health, sport and home care analysis of the neuromotor condition (Ref. [5] to [10]).

3. Methods and Tools used

The DAPHNE system has been applied with a protocol applied to the measurement of a soft touch of a finger of the right and / or left hand. The finger touches softly a button; the measurement occurs for the time response, for the velocity of the finger, for the applied force, for the tremor, for the voice response.

As a result of such formulation, the protocols and the design of the system, the clinical tests and the analysis of the results have been developed in a parallel way. The system Daphne has been presented in previous works, which described the scientific phases for the construction of a table system and of a portable system.

4. Design of the system Daphne and protocols.

Instantaneous engineering, concurrent engineering in the project Daphne are adopted in the construction of the mechanical system in order to press the push-button adapted to persons of various age and force. Moreover the screen must be wide and readable, without stressing the action of the person. Daphne may transmit the data in network via infrared rays.

A microprocessor receives and processes the signals and gives as output a complete analysis of the results for the person and the specialist of support by Internet or network to a Center of health. New engineering in

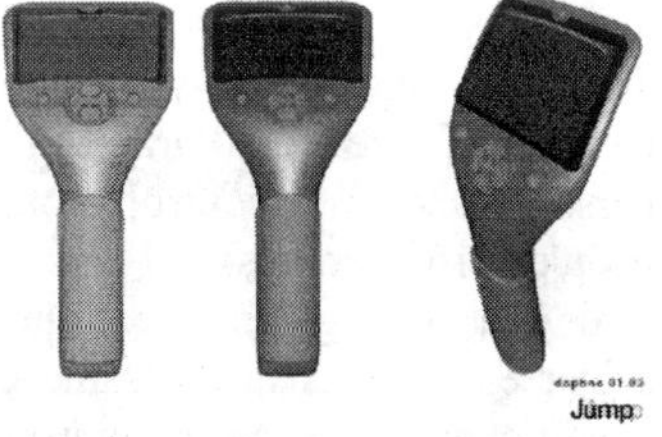

medicine transforms also the relationship with the medicine. Objective of Daphne is to realize an International network, collecting the experiences of telehealth at world-wide level.

The design and the materials of the system Daphne influence the protocols. The shape of the push-button and the feeling of the person who executes the test must be of extreme simplicity and comfort. The stress, even if minimum, which could change the psychological condition in the test, must be avoided. Also the materials influence the test, and consequently the protocol. The person does not have to try physical hard work in supporting the device, neither must receive disturbing feelings, also at unconscious level.

5. Performing the tests.

The movement of the hand and of the fingers in particular indicates very well the psychomotor state of health of a person. The person seizes the grip of the system Daphne without any difficulty. It is light, easy to hold, both with the right hand and with the left hand,

and the reading on the small screen is easy. The grasping is sure, the hand is not tired, no effect of stress disturbs the person. A sound signal orders the start of the touch, that must be soft and fast. The person presses the push-button, reaches the maximum of the flexion and of the force.

The sensors measure the time of reaction, the speed of the finger, the final force exercised on the push-button, the tremor. The project is sophisticated because these measurements happen in various moments, and the measure is not carried out on the same phenomenon but it is executed on various phenomena. In fact Daphne measures the time of reaction at the beginning of the movement, the speed of the finger during the movement, the force at the end of the movement and the tremor, without that operator knows it, for some seconds before the test begins. Design influences deeply the realization of the protocols, because, according to the screen and the type of push-button, the person must execute various tests. The recent Daphne uses a display wide 12 cm for 10 cm, and a not linear restoring force with a stroke of 25 millimeter (1 inch).

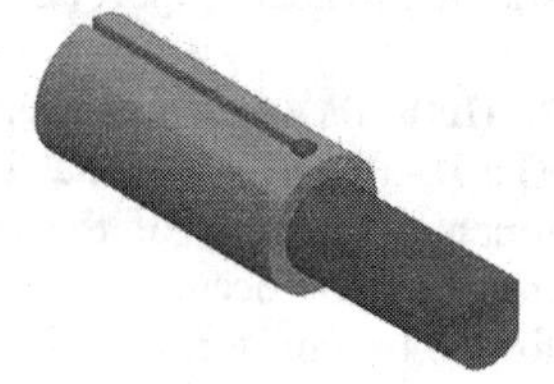

Moreover the display offers also the option of virtual simulation. On the display an element shaped as a finger appears: it simulates the movement that the human hand must execute. The person must follow with his finger the movement of the virtual finger; the images must overlap.

6. Tests and results

The tests have been performed on adult patients affected by Parkinson disease (18 persons) and on a control group of healthy people (16 persons) . The samples are analogous for age and sex. They have been subjected to tests in the same experimental conditions, inn the same environment and in the same hour time (10 a.m. – 1 p.m.).

The figures report the Reaction Time RT, the tremor T for Parkinsonian people (P) and Non Parkinsonian people (NP). The segment reports the variance of the value.

Data on the finger velocity, on the force and on the tremor are significant. On the contrary, the differences on the reaction time are not so large for the two groups. The execution time for the Parkinsonian is longer than for healthy people.

The force is lower for the Parkinsonian people. The tremor is higher, as foreseen.

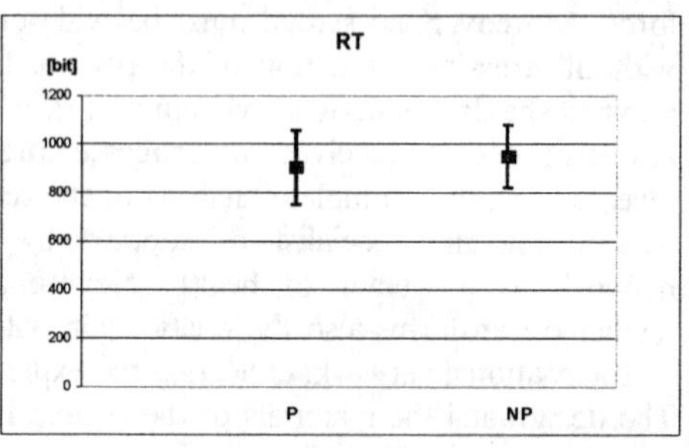

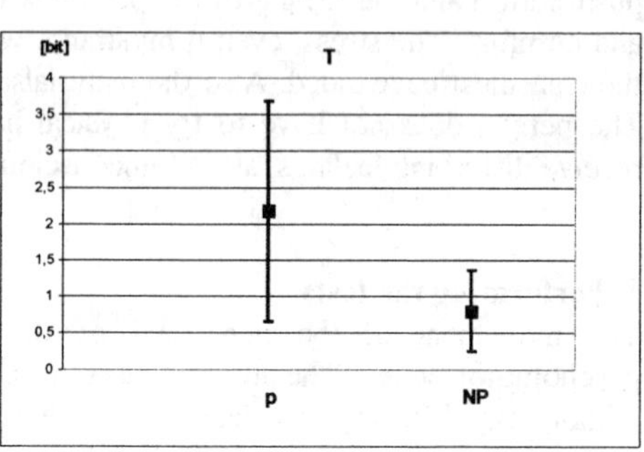

The variability of the data in the confidence interval is higher for unhealthy people in comparison with unhealthy people, with a same amplitude for the right and left hand. The variability is higher for Parkinsonian people, with the same character for both the hands. The variability is connected with the level of the illness. For the force, on the contrary, the confidence interval is more narrow. The patients present more variability between right and left hand.

7. Considerations

Daphne represents a project for the health and a product which is proposed for the diagnosis of the Parkinson disease. The developed protocols, in use and on process, can enrich the fields of application of Daphne also in the sport field, in the domestic care and in special fields, like the automotive field. The measured and expressed quantitative values of Daphne represent a new element in the field of the diagnostic care to detect the disturbs which cause stress and neuromotor affections.

Tests offer a large variability of results and they strictly correspond to the level of sickness of the persons affected by the Parkinson disease. The comparison with healthy people systematically demonstrates the efficiency of the Daphne device.

8. Novelty

The system has measured and tested person healthy (16 persons) and unhealthy, affected by Parkinson disease (18 persons) and has demonstrated that a multiparametric measurement in the same time and in the same conditions offer a diagnostic analysis useful for medical doctors and for rehabilitation purposes.

The novelty is that:
- the system may foresee the birth and the beginning of disease in neuromotor control and in psychology action with quantitative measurement;
- the virtual reality screen presents image of the finger and the time reaction of Parkinsonian persons is very similar to the time reaction of healthy people, as demonstration that the brain and mind activity of Parkinsonian in a first phase of the sickness are very active;
- the system is portable and may be used in every part of the world, in every moment and the protocol of test is clearly presented for tests, which transmit the data to a medical / training centre;
- the disease may be interpreted in its first phase also as difference of behaviour of right / left hand.

This portable device can potentially revolutionise the relationship between a person and his/her own body and give him/her a better knowledge of own health state.

9. Project data.

The participants to the DAPHNE project, which is an European Union Project, consist of two complementary groups. Industry (3 participants) and academia (2 representatives) encompassing people with technical and clinical background. This gives the necessary multidisciplinary to the consortium which is essential for successfully carrying out the work in this project. The participants are: Prof. Rita Pegoraro, Politecnico di Milano, Dr. Tonino Cucé, STMicroelectronics Srl, Italy; Prof. Fausto Baldissera, Physiology Institute of the

University of Milano, Italy; Dott.ssa Elena Della Torre, Agilent Technologies Europe, The Netherlands; Arch. Antonio Gardoni, Jump Studios, United Kingdom
For more information on the project you can refer to the DAPHNE WWW site: http://www.crema.unimi.mi/presenze/st/daphne/
The tests have been performed by Prof. Antonini, Institute for the Parkinson Disease, Milano, whom we thank.

References

[1]   A. Rovetta, F. Lorini, M. Canina, Virtual Reality in the Assessment of Neuromotor Diseases: Measurement of Time Response in Real and Virtual Environments, in "Virtual Reality in Neuro-Psycho-Physiology", IOS Press, 1997

[2]   G. Riva, A. Rovetta et al., Virtual Reality Environments for Psycho-Neuro-Physological Assessment and Rehabilitation, MMVR, IOS Press, 1997

[3]   A. Rovetta, A. Cucè , M. Bisogni, R. Pegoraro, Innovative biorobotic system DDX for the analysis of neuro-motor conditions: methodology and results, ICAR 2001, International Conference on Advanced Robotics, Budapest, 22-26 August

[4]   Antonini, A. Rovetta, R. Fariello, et al, A novel device in the evaluation of motor impairment in Parkinson Disease, Fifth International congress of Parkinson's Disease and Movement Disorders, New York, October 10-14, 1998

[5]   G. Miscio, P. Pinelli, Prefrontal Cortex, Working Memory and Delayed Reactions, Collane Maugeri, Pavia, 1998

[6]   European Union, Biomedical and Health Research, IOS Press, 1995

[7]   J. Rothwell, Control of Human Voluntary Movement, Crook Helm, 1987

[8]   P. Pinelli, Brain Control of Behaviour, Karger, 1997

[9]   A. Dal Monte, La valutazione funzionale dell'atleta, Ed. Sansoni, 1983

[10]   J. V. Basmajian, Muscles alive, Their functions revealed by Electromyography, Baltimore, 1971

Medicine Meets Virtual Reality 02/10
J.D. Westwood et al. (Eds.)
IOS Press, 2002

FIRST CLINICAL TRIALS FOR NEUROMOTOR ANALYSIS

A. Rovetta (*), A. Antonini (**), F. Pignatelli (*), V. A. Ragone (*)
(*) Politecnico di Milano, Dipartimento di Meccanica
Piazza Leonardo da Vinci, 32 20133 Milano (Itala)
E-Mail: alberto.rovetta@polimi.it
(**) ICP, Dept. of Neurosciences,
Via Bignami 3, 20100 Milano (Italy)

Keyword: Parkinson disease, Pathological analysis, Diagnostic tools

Abstract
This paper deals with a first test model of DAPHNE system, called DDX, which may measure the reaction time, the velocity of a finger, the force exerted on a button, the tremor of the person, and also the time delay on pronouncing a word which appears in the screen of the display. The system is made by a button and a spring, with sensors which detect all the parameters. Tests on healthy and unhealthy people have been performed to check the validity of the instrument and the possibility to use the results in diagnosis and in therapy.

1. Introduction
The clear measure and the easy monitoring of the state of health on the psychophysical activity is a requirement for the therapies of many diseases. Also for sport and for home care a portable system is required, with the use of network and of recording of data, to continuously monitor patients' state of health. The system DAPHNE must measure simple conditions of motion and must be capable to give a large series of data to the medical doctor, to recognise the conditions of health of a person, also during a day, a week, for a diagnosis and a possible therapy, also by means of centres connected in Internet.

2. Tests
The tests have shown that the measurements are constant for the same person with a small range of variations. This is done in an automatic way through a multi-parametric analysis and according to statistic observation supported by clinical validation The differences are detected on the course of the day, and in front of stress (travels, exams, particular conditions of working, etc). The age represents an important factor. Particular typical conditions are detected by the instrument. Some tests have shown that the reaction time in quick response test is comparable for healthy and unhealthy persons. The force, on the contrary, is less than 40% in Parkinson disease affected people. The tremor occurs in unhealthy people, but the device has shown that many healthy persons are disturbed by tremor, even if not in critical conditions. The index of efficiency shows a strong relation between the neuromotor condition and the psychophysical condition. In virtual reality tests, the response time is low also for unhealthy people, while dynamic action is slower and less strong.

3. Results

Patients affected by neuro-motor diseases will be able to use the system at home and send the results to own Clinicians by means of a data telecommunication system integrated in the device. In the same time the device will be a prevention system able to warn about an incoming illness and furthermore the patient will have the possibility to actively participate to his/her on-going care. Here are reported the results of the processing by mathematics-statistics of the data.

Descriptive statistics

	PARKINSON				NOT PARKINSON			
	RT	V	T	F	RT	V	T	F
Average	900,8359	498,9869	2,172162	71,55077	945,4102	362,8016	0,801382	91,26275
Standard Error	45,45405	31,30424	0,455533	2,907427	45,4944	15,90411	0,192414	3,503337
Median	841,5787	432,0745	1,183333	71,97222	904,6667	296	0,4	94,29167
Shunting line standard	301,5081	207,6488	3,021667	19,28569	257,3552	89,96724	1,088455	19,81787
Variance collection of samples	90907,12	43118,03	9,130472	371,9378	66231,69	8094,105	1,184735	392,748
Curtosi	-0,6963	2,001168	9,681466	-0,45999	-0,52063	0,73706	0,880685	-0,40468
Asymmetry	0,674496	1,499998	2,712906	-0,12583	0,50088	1,2207	1,41499	-0,45153
Interval	1051,333	839,8	16	77,56667	921,8	315,4	3,54881	77,2
Minimal	470,3333	295,8	0	33,6	547,8	295,6	0	46,6
Maximum	1521,667	1135,6	16	111,1667	1469,6	611	3,54881	123,8

Averages and Shunting lines standard

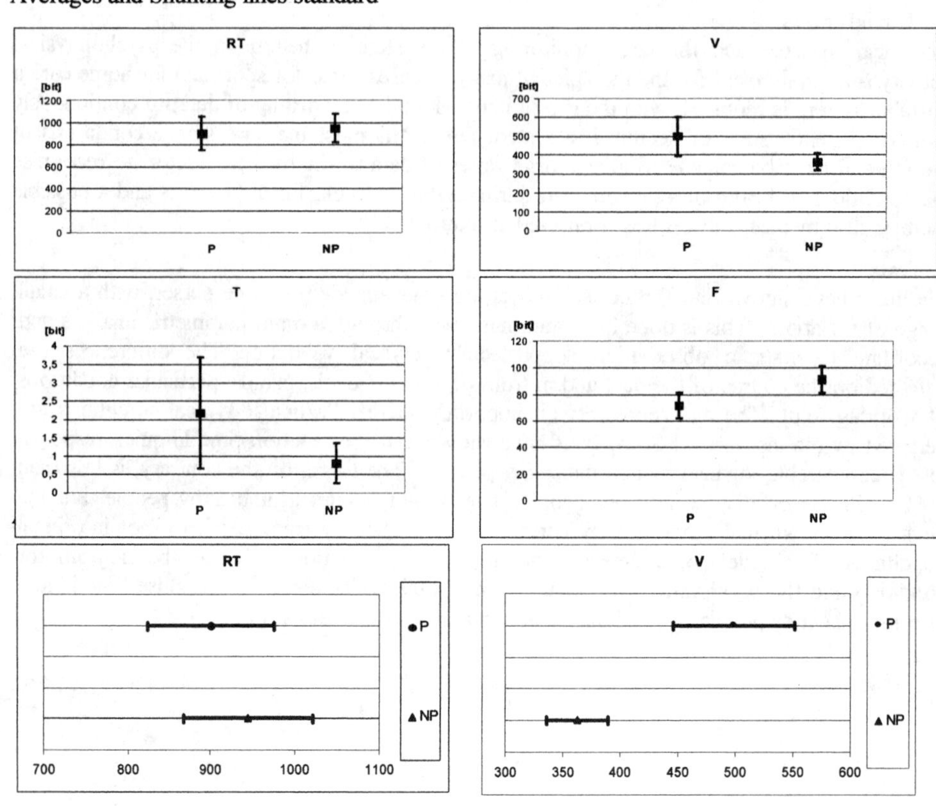

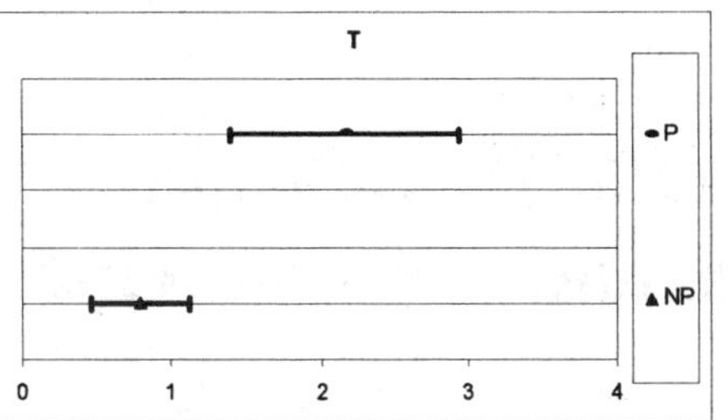
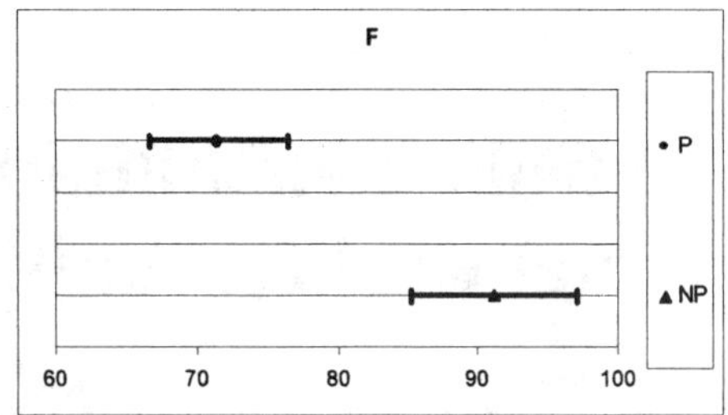

The data inserted have been calculated applying a medium operator on a cycle of "n" consecutive test executed in short time interval (some minutes), with a protocol DDX- fast Parkison (p), DDX- fast Not Parkison (NP). RT is Reaction Time in ms; V is Velocity time in ms; T is tremor in cycles for second; F is force in grams. The variables studied in the DDX follow asymptotically the Gaussian distribution.

4. Conclusions

Thanks to the integration of suitable sensors, the new device will be able to measure all the parameters that in the previous versions were separately recorded: reaction time, hand tremor, speed and strength of button pressing and vocal parameters for a verbometric analysis. The result is also the calculation of an index for the neuromotor efficiency. This device can potentially revolutionise the relationship between a person and his/her own body and give him/her a better knowledge of own health state.

The participants to the DAPHNE project, which is an European Union Project, are: Dept. Mechanics, Lab. Robotics, Politecnico di Milano; STMicroelectronics Srl, Italy; Physiology Institute of the University of Milano, Italy; Philips, The Netherlands; Jump Studios, United Kingdom

References

[1] A. Rovetta et al., Teleoperator Response in a Touch Task with Different Display Conditions, IEEE Transactions on System, Man, and Cybernetics, Vol. 25, No.5, pp.878-881, May, 1995.
[2] A. Antonini, A. Rovetta, R. Fariello, et al, A novel device in the evaluation of motor impairment in Parkinson Disease, Fifth International congress of Parkinson's Disease and Movement Disorders, New York, October 10-14, 1998.

Medicine Meets Virtual Reality 02/10
J.D. Westwood et al. (Eds.)
IOS Press, 2002

Stroke Rehabilitation at Home using Virtual Reality, Haptics and Telemedicine

Martin Rydmark, MD, Ph.D.[1], Jörgen Broeren, OTR, B.Sc.[1,2],
Ragnar Pascher, M.Sc.[1]

[1] *Mednet , The Sahlgrenska Academy at Göteborg University*
[2] *Department of Rehabilitation Medicine, Sahlgrenska University Hospital.*

Mednet (The Computer Laboratory of the Sahlgrenska Academy)
Box 417, SE 405 30 GÖTEBORG (SWEDEN)
E: martin.rydmark@mednet.gu.se, URL: http://www.mednet.gu.se

Abstract: The objective of this pilot study is to identify the level of difficulty in which subjects with left hemisphere damage in the acute phase after stroke can start practicing in a virtual environment. Second, to test an application of Virtual Reality technology to existing occupational treatment methods in stroke rehabilitation and develop a platform for home rehabilitation controlled telemedically. The findings indicate that the system shows potential as an assessment and training device. The feasibility study setup is working well likewise the assessment method. Developing and increasing the complexity of the tasks must be based on the patient individual neurology, and that the cinematic motion patterns of the patient's are the basis for exercise design.

1. Introduction

In Sweden stroke is one of the most common diseases and a major cause of disablement. The incidence rate is about 30,000 individuals a year (population: 9,000,000). Approximately 80% of stroke patients survive the acute phase [1]. Individuals who survive a severe stroke face long-term problems with impairments, which create deficits in motor control and cognitive function [2]. About 85% show an initial deficit in the hemiplegic arm, they are unable to produce well coordinated, smooth, efficient movements and have difficulties in producing enough force to manage every day activities. This problem remains in 55% to 75% of all patients, three to six months later [3]. Arm/hand function recovery is poor and loss of arm/hand function is perceived as a major problem by stroke survivors [4]. There is a need to develop active treatment methods for upper extremity function [5]. The results of the Feys *et al.* study suggest that motor recovery after stroke improves due to a specific intervention of the upper limb [3]. The use of an impaired limb can promote functional recovery [7]. The recovery is dependent on regularity, compliance and intensity in training. Motor learning is built on theories of the brain's own ability to relearn and re-adjust, and that functional training (i.e. training of motor tasks) may in itself be remedial [2]. Thus subjects receiving more intensive therapy should make more rapid progress and this should result in an earlier discharge from hospital.

Several reports show that VR rehabilitation can improve motor recovery [7, 8, 9]. Benefits are: increased duration, frequency and intensity in therapy. Furthermore, the exercises can be made engaging which is important in terms of the patient's motivation [10]. However, none of these studies have reported on the setting of training level for patients in the acute phase after stroke. We asked whether a rehabilitation program with the use of virtual reality and haptics could be implemented within 6 weeks after stroke.

The primary objective of this pilot study is to identify the level of difficulty in which subjects with left hemisphere damage in the acute phase after stroke can start practicing in a virtual environment. The second stage is to test an application of Virtual Reality technology to existing occupational treatment methods in stroke rehabilitation and develop a platform for home rehabilitation controlled telemedically.

2. Materials and Methods

2.1 Subjects

Three subjects (Table I) were included in this study, they all underwent inpatient rehabilitation in the Dept. of Rehabilitation Medicine at Sahlgrenska University Hospital. The criteria for inclusion in this study were (1) patients who have had a stroke, i.e.cerebrovascular accident (CVA), which has caused a partial paresis in the right arm; (2) have their first stroke; (3) have an obvious deficit of the upper limb (Box and Blocks score lower then 45) [11] (4) have normal spatial competence and body awareness and also the ability to understand information; (5) minimum age of 18.

Table 1. Patient Characteristics

Subjects	Age	Gender	Dominate hand	Type of stroke	Post stroke	Box and Blocks score
Subject 1	58 y	Male	Right	Thromboses	12 weeks	6 blocks
Subject 2	29 y	Male	Right	Hemorrhage	6 weeks	31 blocks
Subject 3	48 y	Male	Right	Thromboses	9 weeks	43 blocks

2.2 VR System

The VR system (Figure 1) consists of a PHANToM haptic device (SensAble Technologies Inc.), which is connected to an Intergraph Zx10 ViZual Workstation (2 x 750 MHz Pentium III with 512 Mb RAM and a WildCat 4110 graphics card, Windows NT 4.0) [12]. Haptic properties are added using Magma 2.5 from ReachIn Technologies AB [13]. Magma® is a programming API/environment allowing interactive manipulation of a 3D model using a haptic interface. Haptic force feedback is provided using the PHANToM haptic device. Visualization can be accomplished using a standard stereoscopic CrystalEyes CE-2 setup [14].

2.3 VR Exercise

A coordination task was developed. The subjects have to reach for, grasp and move the PHANToM haptic device to different targets (generated positions) on the screen (task analysis see table II).

Table 2. Task analysis for pointing at a prefixed spot on the screen.

Exercise	Function deficit
• Reach for, grasp and move the PHANToM haptic device to different targets (randomized positions) on the screen	• Difficulty in reaching. • Difficulty in grasping. • Difficulty in moving • Difficulty in locating the target. • Difficulty in lifting. • Difficulty in holding while striking the spot. • Difficulty in coordinating.

At the start of the exercise a handle becomes visible on the screen. The position of the handle appears randomly, depending on how the subject lifts the PHANToM haptic device. The subjects now have to point at different targets, which appear on the screen randomly, except the first target which always appears in the lower part of the right hand side of the computer screen. As soon as the subject touches the target it changes color, disappears and a new target becomes visible. There were three different exercise programmed (Figure 1). There was no time limit to complete the exercise.

Figure 1. Illustration of three exercises.

Exercise 1	*Exercise 2*	*Exercise 3*

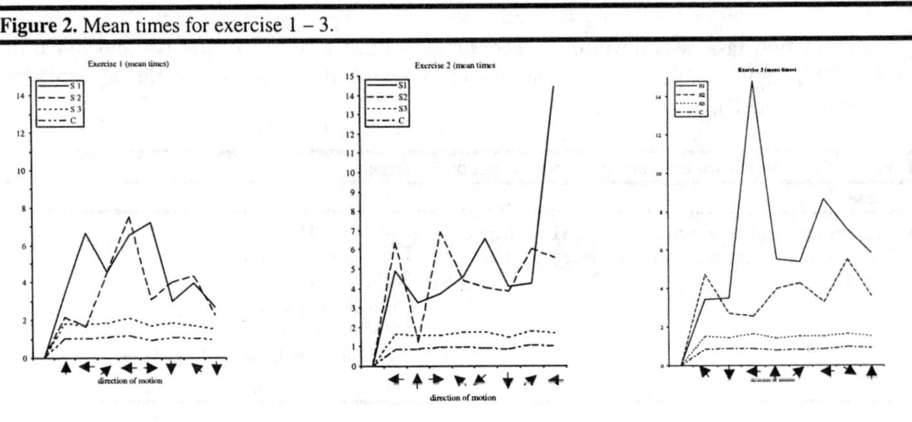

2.4 Data analysis

For the purpose of comparison a control group of 7 subjects (C) was added to the study. The subjects in the control group were healthy employees at the Dept. of Rehabilitation Medicine, Sahlgrenska University Hospital who were asked to carry out the same exercises. To analyze the data retrieved, the motions of the upper limb were divided in different directions, i.e. sideways (left – right and right – left), up and down, diagonal (left – right) up and down. The time taken to complete the exercise was also a criterion by which the performance was evaluated.

3. Results

The PC based setup of the home rehabilitation system is working well with visualization and haptics. The preliminary results (Figure 2) show that subject 1 (S1) and subject 2 (S2) had difficulties with motions in all directions. Subject 3 (S3) had a uniform quality of motion, but was generally slower in performing the exercises than the control group (C). The grand mean of the control group was 0,9 sec. (median 0,95 sec.), standard deviation 0,1 and the 95 % tolerance limits 0,7 – 1,2 sec.

Figure 2. Mean times for exercise 1 – 3.

4. Discussion

Initial work with the VR/haptic system is encouraging. The findings indicate that the system shows potential as an assessment and training device. Rehabilitation of the upper limb in patients with CVA in the left side of the brain appears to be successful. S1 and S2 are clearly patients who would benefit training in a virtual environment. S3 box and blocks test score (43) was too high to participate in the study although his score was far below the average score for his age group.

Unilateral neglect (UN) is a relatively common functional disorder caused by stroke in the right side of the brain which causes a partial paresis in the left arm. As a result of this phenomenon patients with UN have difficulty seeing objects and people to their left, and/or have a lack of awareness of their own left side. To increase awareness of body movements in the neglected field it would be challenging to develop procedures with the VR/haptic system which reduce neglect following stroke. We believe that developing and increasing the complexity of the tasks must be based on the patient's individual neurology, and that the cinematic motion patterns of the patient are the basis for exercise design.

The telemedical connection is for patient to health care consultation and for continuous assessment of training results and setting of new rehabilitation goals.

5. Conclusions

The feasibility study setup is working well, likewise the assessment method. The unique aspects of this system are not the individual components, but the assembly to a low cost VR system for rehabilitation placed in the patient's home and telematically connected to the rehabilitation center for assessment and setting of training levels. The next step is to extend the clinical use and to produce more templates for exercises.

6. References

[1]   National Board of Health and Welfare. State of the Art - Stroke. 1997. [Cited 2000 March 3]. Available from: URL: http://www.sos.se/mars/sta029/sta029.htm.

[2]   Carr JH, Shepherd RB. A motor relearning program for stroke. Oxford: Butterworth – Heineman; 1996.

[3]   Feys HM, De Weerdt WJ, Selz BE, Cox Steck GA, Spichiger R, Vereeck LE, Putman KD, Van Hoydonck GA. Effect of a therapeutic intervention for the hemiplegic upper limb in the acute phase after stroke: a single blind, randomized, controlled multicenter trial. Stroke. 1998; 29(4): 785-92.

[4]   Kwakkel G, Wagenaar RC, Twisk JW, Lankhorst GJ, Koetsier JC. Intensity of leg and arm training after primary middle-cerebral-artery stroke: a randomized trial. Lancet. 1999. 354, (9174), 191-6.

[5]   Broeks JG, Lankhorst GJ, Rumping K, Prevo AJH. The long-term outcome of arm function after stroke: results of a follow–up study. Disability and Rehabilitation. 1999. 21 (8): 357-364.

[6]   Nudo RJ, Friel KM. Cortical plasticity after stroke: implications for rehabilitation. Rev Neurol. 1999; 155(9): 713-7.

[7]   Jack D, Boin R, Merians A, Adamovich SV, Tremaine M, Recce M, Burdea GC, Poizner H. A Virtual Reality-Based Exercise program for Stroke Rehabilitation. Proceedings of ASSETS; 2000 November 13-15; Arlington Virginia, USA.

[8]   Holden M, Todorov E, Callahan J, Bizzi E. Virtual Environement training improves motor performance in two patients with stroke: case report. 1999. NEUROL–REP. 23 (2): 57–67.

[9]   Holden M, Dettwiler A, Dyar T, Niemann G, Bizzi E. Retraining Movement in Patients with Acquired Brain Injury using Virtual Environment. Proceedings of Medicine Meets Virtual Reality; 2001 January 24-28; Newport Beach USA. California; 2001.

[10] Broeren J. The potential of Virtual Reality-technology in occupational therapy treatment for motor impaired persons. 2000. [Cited March 2001]. Available from: URL: http://www.mednet.gu.se.

[11] Mathiowetz V, Volland G, Kashman N, Weber K. Adult norms for the Box and Block Test of manual dexterity. Am J Occup Ther. 1985; 39(6):386-91

[12] SensAble Technologies Inc. 2000. [Cited 2000 Mai 17]. Available from: URL: http://www.sensable.com.

[13] ReachIn Technology AB. 2001. [Cited 2001 March 5]. Available from: URL: http://www.reachin.se.

[14] Stereographics®. 2001. [Cited 2001 March 7]. Available from: URL http://www.stereographics.com.

Medicine Meets Virtual Reality 02/10
J.D. Westwood et al. (Eds.)
IOS Press, 2002

Feature Preserving Refinement of Surfaces for Web-based Surgical Simulation

Mitsuaki Saito* Takamichi Hayashi* Yoshifumi Takebe**
Akira Wakita**   Masahiro Kobayashi***   Hiroaki Chiyokura*
*Faculty of Environmental Information, Keio University, Japan
**Graduated School of Media and Governance, Keio University, Japan
***Faculty of Nursing And Medical Care, Keio University, Japan

Abstract. In plastic surgery, 3D models of the affected part are often used for the purpose of visualizations and surgical simulations. The optimal models for web-based surgical simulations keep high accuracy in affected parts and keep low accuracy in other parts. Consequently, the data size becomes small. In this research, we propose a method to generate free-form surfaces based on Lattice Structure from polygonal meshes. The polygonal meshes are generated automatically from CT and MRI data using Marching Cubes. By changing the resolution of input images, the accuracy of output meshes is controlled. Free-form surfaces based on Lattice Structure are fitted to polygonal meshes. Lattice Structure is a method to manage a free-form surface with a simple base polygonal mesh. The data size is quite small because surface shape is converted and saved as a simple polygon. A free-form surface is quickly generated and high accuracy is maintained. Moreover, users can input character lines and they are reflected as boundaries of patches. The models generated with this method are partly accurate and compact. These data make it possible to simulate surgery on the WWW , because they can be quickly transferred

1. Optimum Models for Web-based Surgical Simulations

The objective of our method is to generate meshes for medical education and surgical simulations. The data size of the output models should be small because real time calculation and fast transmission are necessary in web-based surgical simulations. Accuracy of the models is also important. However high quality meshes consist of quite large numbers of polygons. We reduce data size by providing both high quality models of the affected part and low quality models of the other parts. By combining the above two models, a compact but high quality model can be generated without decreasing the accuracy of the organ models of interest. The input of character lines is also important for preserving the information that is critical for clinical use. Preservation of character lines makes possible to visualize incision lines and boundaries between organs obviously.

2. System

The system consists of two modules called ARS(Automatic Reconstructive System) and Haniwa Modeler. ARS generate polygonal meshes from CT and MRI data. The system outputs two kinds of meshes, that are high quality meshes of the affected part and low quality meshes of the entire model. Haniwa Modeler fits surfaces to the above two kinds of meshes. Character lines are also input at this step.

3. Generation of Polygonal Meshes

A volume model from CT and MRI is converted into polygonal meshes by using Marching Cubes[1]. By changing the resolution of the input image, the accuracy of output meshes is controlled. Because the accuracy of affected parts is critical, high-resolution image are applied and consequently high quality meshes are generated. High quality meshes of the affected part are shown in Fig. 1.

Where the accuracy is not important, coarse and low quality meshes are generated by applying large cubes. The data size of these meshes is quite small, however the appearance is enough because of smoothing operations. Fig. 2 shows the low quality meshes of the skull after smoothing operations are applied.

By combining the high quality meshes of affected parts on the low quality meshes of the whole model, the integrated meshes are generated (Fig. 3). The data size is quite small, however the accuracy of the important area is maintained

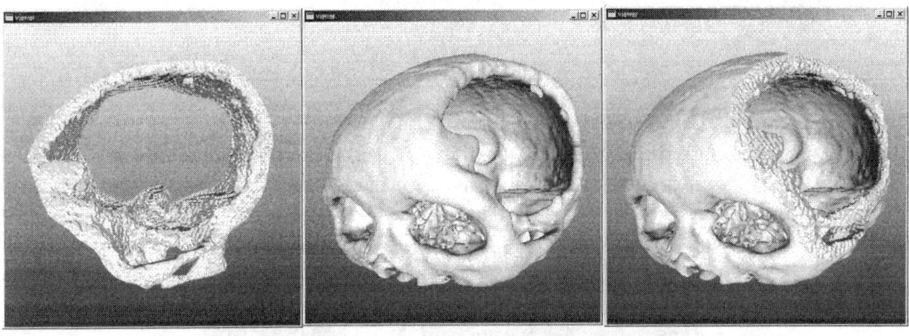

Fig 1　　　　　　　　　　Fig 2　　　　　　　　　　Fig 3

Fig. 1: The high quality meshes of the affected part (the cave-in part of a skull).

Fig. 2: Low quality skull meshes after smoothing operations.

Fig. 3: The final output mesh.

4. Fitting Surfaces Reflecting Character Lines

Our method is an extend version of Tanaka's technique [3], a technique fitting free-form surfaces to dense polygonal meshes. We have extended their technique to reflect character lines intentionally as boundaries between patches. First, we specify character lines on the input meshes. Lines are drawn on the screen with tablet interface. By projecting the meshes on the screen plane, the character lines are projected on the meshes. Second, we fit free-form surfaces by utilizing QEM-based mesh simplifications[2]. At each simplification steps, edges which have high QEM value are not deleted. By making use of this feature of QEM, we set high values to character edges and execute reductions. Consequently, character edges are reflected as boundaries of patches. Fig. 4 (left) is the head model generated by ARS, and Fig. 4 (right) is the model reduced and fitted free-form surfaces by Haniwa Modeler without decreasing the accuracy.

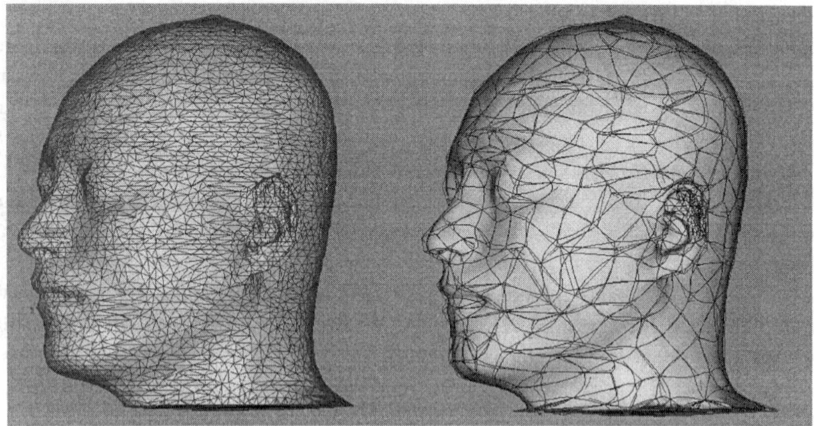

Fig. 4

5. Web-based Surgical Simulators

We have developed a web-based surgical simulator of hemi facial microsomia. Hemi facial microsomia is a case of disease that one side of ramus of mandibular is longer than the other side.

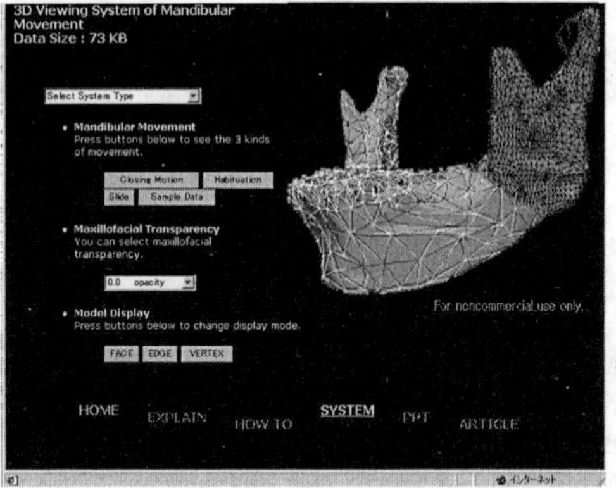

6. Conclusion

We have presented a method to generate medical surface models in which character lines input and adaptive accuracy control can be realized. Because the models generated by our method have realized coexistence of small data size and high data accuracy, the models can be used in variety of web-based surgical simulators. It is also possible to generate more advanced simulators because incision lines and boundaries between organs can be explicitly represented.

References

[1] W. Lorensen, and H. Cline, Marching Cubes: A High Resolution 3D Surface Construction Algorithm, SIGGRAPH 87, 1987.

[2] S. Takeuchi, T. Kanai, H.. Suzuki, K. Shimada and F. Kimura, Subdivision Surface Fitting with QEM-based Mesh Simplification and Reconstruction of Approximated B-spline Surfaces, *Pacific Graphics 2000*, pp202-212, 2000.

[3] Daigo Tanaka, M. Kobayashi, H. Chiyokura, T. Nakajima and T. Fujino: Web-based Educational Tool for Cleft Lip Repair using XVL, Medicine Meets Virtual Reality 2001

Medicine Meets Virtual Reality 02/10
J.D. Westwood et al. (Eds.)
IOS Press, 2002

Risk Reduction in Craniofacial Surgery using Computer-based Modeling and Intraoperative Immersion

Tobias Salb[+], Oliver Burgert[+], Tilo Gockel[+], Jakob Brief[*], Stefan Hassfeld[*],
Joachim Muehling[*], Ruediger Dillmann[+]

[+] *Industrial Applications of Informatics and Microsystems (IAIM)*
Chair Prof. Dr.-Ing. R. Dillmann
Building 07.21, Department for Computer Science
Universität Karlsruhe (TH), 76128 Karlsruhe, Germany
Tel.: ++49 721 608 7126, Fax: ++49 721 608 8270
Email: salb@ira.uka.de, WWW: http://wwwiaim.ira.uka.de/

[*] *Department of Oral and Maxillofacial Surgery*
University of Heidelberg, 69120 Heidelberg, Germany
Email: jbrief@med.uni-heidelberg.de

Abstract. We present a two-stage concept for risk reduction in craniofacial surgery, consisting of preoperative risk modeling and intraoperative risk reduction. Preoperatively it is important to find and to visualize risk sources in order to minimize them. Our risk model is composed by superimposition of an isotropic risk potential and an anisotropic tissue field constituent. It is being applied to preoperative planning and simulation of craniofacial surgeries, for example to determine an access path with least overall risk value.
In the operation room risks arise mainly from the absence of preoperative planning and simulation data in the operation field. We use a see-through head-mounted display to optimize this situation in order to allow the surgeon to maintain accuracy in the whole process of computer aided surgery. Main steps of the intraoperative immersion are optical tracking of the surgeon wearing the head-mounted display and of the patient, registration of preoperatively calculated planning data with the patient and visualization of the data within the glasses.

1 Introduction

Every surgery holds different kinds of risks to the patients affected by it. Risks may arise from complexity of surgical interventions, occlusion of target areas by surrounding anatomical structures, anatomical anomalies or absence of knowledge in clinical treatment for a certain defect. For safety of the patient it is necessary to localize and to minimize these risks in surgery.

Our approach to solve this problem concentrates on two parts of computer aided surgery. For enhancement of preoperative computer-based modeling and simulation of surgeries, we decided to describe existing risks using a widely applicable, patient specific and variously configurable mathematical risk model. Based on this model, risks can be visualized or palpated and it is possible to achieve a risk reduction in planning and simulation of interventions. The second part of our work concentrates on the transfer from preoperatively achieved planning and simulation results into the operation field. In order to maintain accuracy and to reduce risks in the operation room, augmented reality is used to visualize preoperatively calculated data and to superimpose this information with the operation field.

Nowadays, clinical risk treatment is restricted to postoperative risk scores and preoperative risk estimations, both of which are statistical analysis without usage of any model. Computer-based modeling of critical areas has been performed for access planning in neurosurgery [1] and for detection of nerves in the lower human jaw [2], similar approaches are known for modeling and simulation of permitted and tabooed areas in mobile robotics [3]. All these models are restricted to and adapted to special surgical applications, most of them are not arbitrarily configurable and can therefore not be used for risk estimation and reduction in general.

Intraoperative support for surgeons with augmented reality is being realized using standard computer monitors [4], half-silvered mirrors [5], superimposition within a surgical endoscope or microscope [6], video projection [7] or digital holography [8]. Intraoperative immersion is also realized by using see-through head-mounted displays in different technical solutions and for various clinical fields [9,10,11,12]. Many groups are working in the field of augmented reality for clinical applications but almost all systems are still prototypes with different problems and restricted usability.

2   Methods

2.1   Risk Modeling

The idea of our risk model is to assign a unique scalar risk value to each voxel of a patient data set, taking into account the patient specific anatomy and the surgical action to be performed. For the first implementation of the model called *RISKMIN – RISK MINimization* the Visible Human data set is used and a simple planar cut is assumed as surgical action. Arbitrary CT or MRI data can be used as basic input data, but the tissue classes to be included in the risk model have to be segmented first.

The model is realized as the superimposition of an isotropic part called risk potential and an anisotropic part, the tissue field [13]. The weighted sum of these components forms the risk distribution:

$$Risk(X) = \lambda_1 P(X) + \lambda_2 F(X)$$

For each tissue type the risk potential determines the harm a surgeon does by cutting, drilling or in any other way affecting this kind of tissue. The risk potential of a tissue type G_i is calculated by the application of a tissue specific risk function ρ on an Euclidian distance transformation *dist* for this tissue class:

$$P_{G_i}(\vec{x}) = \rho(dist(\vec{x}, G_i))$$

ρ has been chosen as a decreasing exponential function in our experiments. The overall risk potential for all tissue classes has been determined by superimposing the single potentials using a maximum norm:

$$P(X) = \int_X (\sum_i P_{G_i}(\vec{x}))\, do$$

Figure 1 shows risk potentials for the head of the Visible Human data set, where the tissue types bone, eye and optic nerve and all cerebral tissue classes have been included. The lighter a point appears in the image, the higher is the risk value for this voxel.

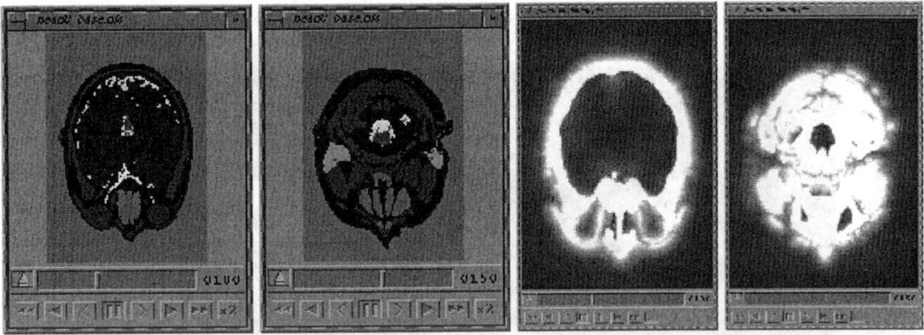

Figure 1: Anatomical Basis Data (leftmost and Center left) and corresponding Risk Potentials (Center right and rightmost) for Head of Visible Human Data Set

The second part of the risk model, the tissue field, takes into account the direction of the surgical action relative to the fiber orientation of the tissue. It has been realized as a vector field, where the direction of the field corresponds to the direction of the tissue fiber orientation and the vector norm defines the relevance of this direction for a certain voxel:

$$\vec{v}: \Re^3 \rightarrow \Re^3, \vec{n} \perp X$$

Basis data for fibre orientation can be taken from anatomical atlases and has also been provided by the Institute of Biomedical Engineering at Universität Karlsruhe (TH) [14]. The overall tissue field is calculated by superimposition using the maximum norm:

$$F(X) = \int_X (\vec{v} \cdot \vec{n})^2\, dc$$

Basis data and results of tissue field calculation are shown in the following figure.

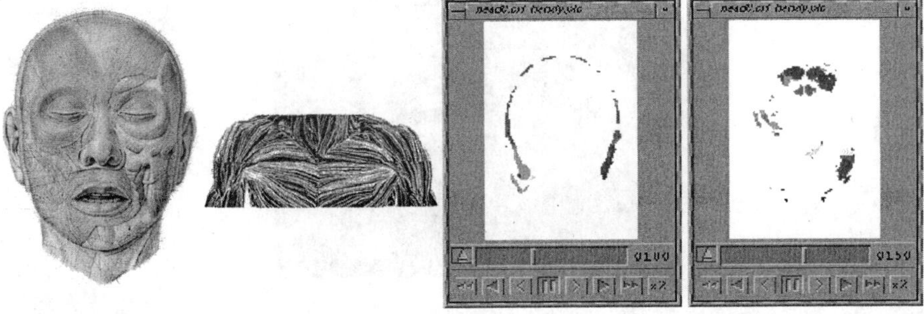

Figure 2: Fiber Orientation Data in Anatomical Atlas (leftmost) or calculated by IBT [14] (Center left) and Tissue Fields (Center right and rightmost) for Head of Visible Human

The resulting risk model can be haptically mediated using a SensAble PHANTOM™ device or can be displayed graphically as 2D or 3D image. First application of the model has been automatic cut trajectory optimization. In order to reduce risks, one had to find a global minimum of the following function, where $\vec{t}$ is the target area of X:

$$Opt(X) = \lambda_1 P(X) + \lambda_2 F(X) + \lambda_3 tdist(X,\vec{t})$$

The search for the best cut trajectory has been realized using a simplex descent algorithm within a seven dimensional search space. In figure 3 (left), one can see the seven different solutions in a screenshot where the darkest solution is the best one found so far.

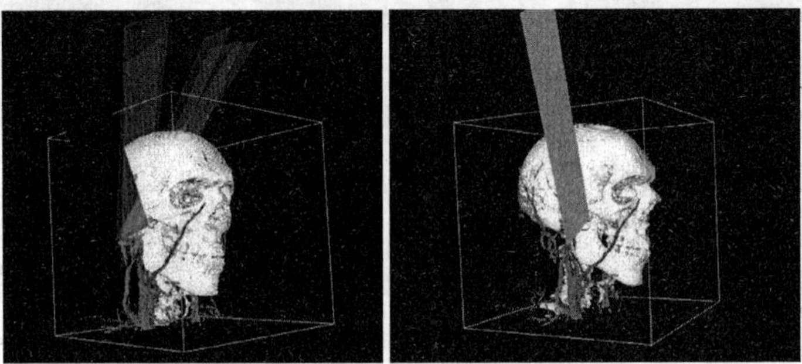

Figure 3: Automatic Cut Trajectory Optimization with Risk Minimization: In Progress (left) and finished with Solution found (right)

Currently we are working on the integration of the risk estimation in existing planning and simulation software tools [15] and on extensive clinical tests of the system.

2.2   Intraoperative Presentation

Intraoperative support of surgeons for minimization of risks concentrates on technical help for the transfer of preoperatively calculated planning and simulation results into the operation field. In our system, called *INPRES – INtraoperative PRESentation*, a see-through head-mounted display is used for overlay of the virtually generated data with the patient in the operation room [16]. The display device is shown in figure 4.

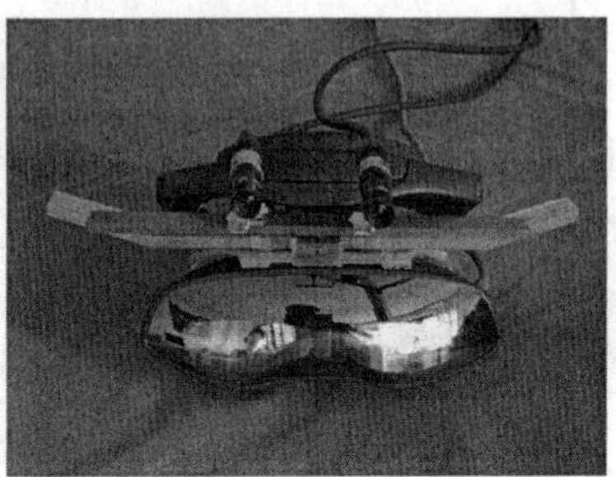

Figure 4: Sony Glasstron LDI-D100BE with Teli CS-6100P Miniature Cameras and Passive Tracking Target for NDI Polaris P4 Tracking System

Most challenging tasks of this work are tracking of the display device and the patient, registration of preoperatively calculated data with the patient and finally data display and overlay [17]. For tracking of the display device and the patient three approaches have been realized: Our first approach, a stereo camera system with active infrared tracking targets, didn't meet the specifications for clinical usage [18]. A NDI Polaris device is now being used instead as standard tracking system providing a translational accuracy in the submillimeter range. Special passive tracking targets for our Sony Glasstron device can be seen in figure 5. For the third tracking approach we use a 360° panorama camera to be mounted on the head of a surgeon and artificial landmarks for localization [19]. The panorama image is first transformed into the *HSV* format (Hue, Saturation, Value) and bounding boxes corresponding to the circles of the landmarks are being searched. If dedicated landmark criteria are fulfilled, an ellipse is placed in the blobs of the circles, and the center of gravity of the ellipse is used for position and orientation reconstruction. In figure 5 one can see a camera image of our experimental setup und the belonging calculated centers of gravity of the landmarks found in the image.

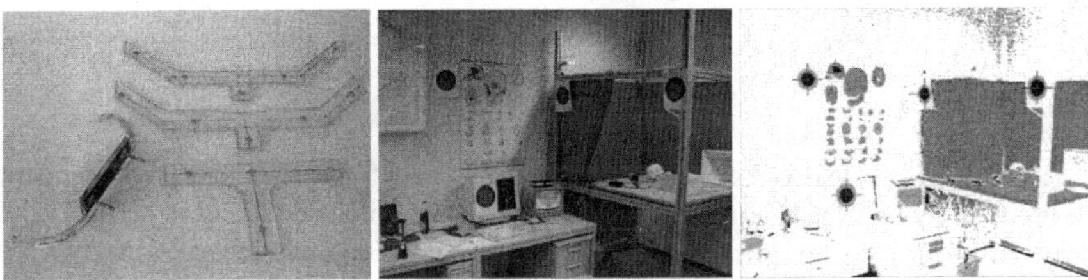

Figure 5: Handmade passive Tracking Bodies for Sony Glasstron Device to be tracked by NDI Polaris System (left), Raw Image of Panorama Camera Remote Reality S360C (Center) and Processed Camera Image (right)

Visualization of data within the see-through head-mounted display is done using Open Inventor as graphics library on a standard PC. In addition to planning and simulation data, it is also possible to visualize risk estimations or any other kind of radiological or medical data in the glasses. Data to be displayed in the glasses is calculated from CT or MRI images. Registration is done using titanium mini screws which can be segmented preoperatively in the data sets and touched intraoperatively with a pointer.

One problem of the system is the occurrence of occlusions when visualizing data in the glasses. The two miniature cameras mounted on the display device have been used for creation of a depth map in order to detect occlusions, one result is shown in figure 6. However, the algorithm is not fast enough so far. Clinical tests have been done with the Sony Glasstron device in order to check its functionality and the display parameters to be used for visualization [20]. The overall INPRES system still has to be clinically evaluated.

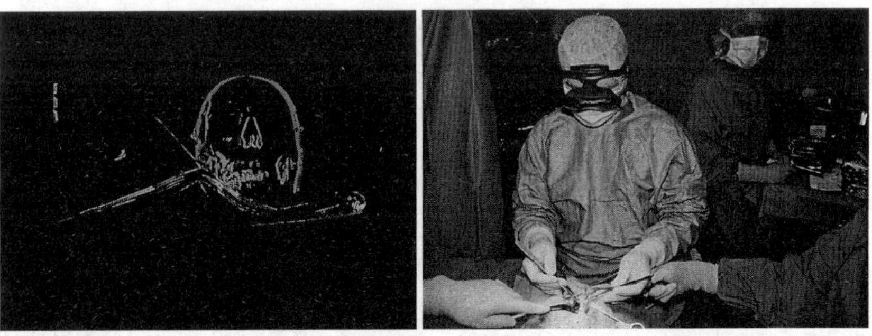

Figure 6: Depth Map created with Miniature Cameras (left), first Clinical Tests with the Sony Display (right)

3   Results

The risk model as described above has been implemented and applied to Visible Human data sets of thigh and head. We also have applied the model to selective craniofacial patient data sets. The model itself works well, it can be parameterized in various ways as clinically indicated. First application of the model for an automatic cut trajectory optimization also works well. Currently we are working on the integration of the risk estimation in existing planning and simulation software tools [15] and on extensive clinical tests of the system.

The prototype for Intraoperative Presentation has also been established and is currently being evaluated in the laboratory. It shows real-time behavior unless used with huge data sets. Overall accuracy has not been determined in detail but should be in the range 1 to 5 millimeters as estimated so far. At the moment we are preparing a clinical field study which is scheduled for the beginning of 2002.

4   Conclusion

For reduction of surgical risks we presented a risk model and a system for intraoperative support of surgeons. The risk model has already been implemented and is being evaluated currently, a prototype for Intraoperative Presentation is also available. Future work will concentrate on the intraoperative support of surgeons, especially on the investigation of the influence of eye movements on data display, on the development of an intuitive user interface to be displayed directly in the glasses, on the detection of occlusions and on markerless registration.

Acknowledgement

This research was performed at the Universität Karlsruhe (TH), Department of Computer Science, Group for Industrial Applications of Informatics and Microsystems, Chair Prof. Dr.-Ing. R. Dillmann. The work is being funded by the Special Research Area 414 „Information Technology in Medicine – Computer and Sensor Supported Surgery" of the National German Science Foundation (Deutsche Forschungsgemeinschaft).

References

[1]   Jendrysiak, U., Gregg, S. and Weinert, J.: Virtual Access Planning for Neurosurgery with NeurOPS. Proceedings of Conference: Computer Assisted Radiology (CAR), Tokyo, Japan, June 1997.

[2]   Stein, W.: Computertomogrammbasierte 3D-Planung für die dentale Implantologie. Ph. D. Thesis, Universität Karlsruhe (TH), Germany, 1999.

[3]   Brock, O. and Kathib, O.: Real-Time Replanning in High-Dimensional Configuration Spaces Using Sets of Homotopic Paths. Proceedings of Conference: IEEE International Conference on Robotics and Automation (ICRA), San Francisco, CA, April 2000.

[4]   Grimson, E., Leventon, M., Ettinger, G., Chabrerie, A., Ozlen, F., Nakajima, S., Atsume, H., Kikinis, R. and Black, P.: Clinical Experience with a high Precision Image-Guided Neurosurgery System. Proceedings of Conference: Medical Image Computing and Computer-Assisted Intervention (MICCAI), Boston, MA, 1998.

[5]   Liao, H., Nakajima, S., Iwahara, M., Kobayashi, E., Sakuma, I., Yahagi, N. and Dohi, T.: Intra-operative Real-Time 3-D Information Display System Based on Integral Videography. Proceedings of Conference: Medical Image Computing and Computer-Assisted Intervention (MICCAI), Utrecht, The Netherlands, 2001.

[6] Edwards, P., King, A., Hawkes, D., Fleig, O., Maurer, C., Hill, D., Fenlon, M., de Cunha, D., Gaston, R., Chandra, S., Mannss, J., Strong, A., Gleeson, M. and Cox, T.: Stereo Augmented Reality in the Surgical Microscope. Proceedings of Conference: Medicine Meets Virtual Reality (MMVR), Newport Beach, CA, 1999.

[7] Hoppe, H., Däuber, S., Raczkowsky, J., Wörn, H. and Moctezuma, J.: Intraoperative Visualization of Surgical Planning Data using Video Projectors. Proceedings of Conference: Proceedings of Conference: Medicine Meets Virtual Reality (MMVR), Newport Beach, CA, 2001.

[8] Bergman, W., Tse, V., Schulz, R., Geil, G., Shatsky, S. and Bao, L.: An Improved Stereotactic Technique for Cyst Cannulation. Proceedings of Conference: Medicine Meets Virtual Reality (MMVR), Newport Beach, CA, 1999.

[9] Birkfellner, W., Figl, M., Huber, K., Watzinger, F., Wanschitz, F., Hanel, R., Hummel, J., Ewers, R. and Bergmann, H.: Calibration of a Head-Mounted Operating Microscope for Augmented Reality Visualization in CAS. Proceedings of Conference: Computer Assisted Radiology and Surgery (CARS), Berlin, Germany, June 2001.

[10] Rosenthal, M., State, A., Lee, J., Hirota, G., Ackerman, J., Keller, K., Pisano, E., Jiroutek, M., Muller, K. and Fuchs, H.: Augmented Reality Guidance for Needle Biopsies: A Randomized, Controlled Trial in Phantoms. Proceedings of Conference: Medical Image Computing and Computer-Assisted Intervention (MICCAI), Utrecht, The Netherlands, 2001.

[11] Dubois, E., Nigay, L., Troccaz, J., Carrat, L. and Chavanon, O.: A Methodological Tool for Computer-Assisted Surgery Interface Design: Its Application to Computer-Assisted Pericardial Puncture. Proceedings of Conference: Proceedings of Conference: Medicine Meets Virtual Reality (MMVR), Newport Beach, CA, 2001.

[12] Wildermuth, S., Thonier, G. and Montgomery, K.: An Augmented Reality System for Endoluminal Aortic Stent Placement. To appear in Proceedings of Conference: Proceedings of Conference: Medicine Meets Virtual Reality (MMVR), Newport Beach, CA, 2002.

[13] Salb, T., Brief, J., Burgert, O., Hassfeld, S. and Dillmann, R.: Haptic based risk potential mediation for surgery simulation. Proceedings of 1. International Workshop on Haptic Devices in Medical Applications (HDMA), within the scope of CARS 1999, Paris, June 1999.

[14] Sachse, F., Wolf, P., Werner, D. and Dössel, O.: Extension of Anatomical Models of the Human Body: Three-Dimensional Interpolation of Muscle Fiber Orientation based on Restrictions, Journal of Computing and Information Technology, 6(1), 1998

[15] Burgert, O., Salb, T., Gockel, T., Dillmann, R., Hassfeld, S., Brief, J., Krempien, R., Walz, S. and Muehling, J.: A System for Facial Reconstruction using Distraction and Symmetry Considerations . Proceedings of Conference: Computer Assisted Radiology and Surgery (CARS), Berlin, Germany, June 2001.

[16] Salb, T., Brief, J., Burgert, O., Hassfeld, S., Muehling, J. and Dillmann, R.: An Augmented Reality System for Intraoperative Presentation of Planning and Simulation Results. Proceedings of 2nd Workshop: European Advanced Robotic Systems Development - Medical Robotics, Pisa, Italy, September 1999.

[17] Salb, T., Brief, J., Burgert, O., Hassfeld, S. and Dillmann, R.: Intraoperative Presentation of Surgical Planning and Simulation Results using a Stereoscopic See-Through Head-Mounted Display. Proceedings of Conference: Stereoscopic Displays and Applications, Part of Electronic Imaging / Photonics West (SPIE), San Jose, CA, January 2000.

[18] Salb, T., Burgert, O., Gockel, T., Giesler, B. and Dillmann, R.: Comparison of Tracking Techniques for Intraoperative Presentation of Medical Data using a See-Through Head-Mounted Display. Proceedings of Conference: Medicine Meets Virtual Reality (MMVR), Newport Beach, CA, January 2001.

[19] Weyrich, T.: Entwicklung eines Kopfverfolgungssystems auf der Basis einer Panoramakamera und künstlicher Landmarken. Diploma Thesis, Universität Karlsruhe (TH), Germany, 2001.

[20] Brief, J., Hassfeld, S., Salb, T., Burgert, O., Muenchenberg, J., Pernozzoli, A., Grabowski, H., Redlich, T., Raczkowsky, J., Krempien, R., Kotrikova, B., Woern, H., Dillmann, R., Muehling, J. and Ziegler, C.: Clinical Evaluation of a See-Through Display for Intraoperative Presentation of Planning Data. Proceedings of Conference: Israeli Symposium on Computer-Integrated Surgery, Medical Robotics and Medical Imaging (ISRACAS), Haifa, May 2000.

Medicine Meets Virtual Reality 02/10
J.D. Westwood et al. (Eds.)
IOS Press, 2002

ADAPTIVE HYBRID INTERPOLATION TECHNIQUES FOR DIRECT HAPTIC RENDERING OF ISOSURFACES

Ganesh Sankaranarayanan[1]
Venkat Devarajan Ph.D[1]
Robert Eberhart Ph.D[2,3]
Daniel. B. Jones M.D[2].

[1]*Virtual Environment Lab*
Department of Electrical Engineering
The University of Texas at Arlington
P.O. Box 19016
Arlington TX 76019 USA

[2] *Southwestern Center for Minimally Invasive Surgery*
The University of Texas Southwestern Medical Center at Dallas

[3]*Bio-medical Engineering Program*
The University of Texas at Arlington and
The University of Texas Southwestern Medical Center at Dallas

Abstract: Direct Haptic rendering of voxels from an anatomical dataset provides patient specific haptic feedback vital for diagnosis and surgical planning. Our algorithm uses zero sets of scalar trivariate function for polynomial interpolation with sixty-four neighborhood points to generate isosurfaces on the fly for haptic rendering. This approach gives continuity in surfaces as well as better capture of isosurface features of the medical dataset. The detailed algorithm is presented along with the description of results from haptically rendering medical datasets.

1.Introduction

Virtual environments provide an efficient way for training, surgical planning and diagnosis. Such environments coupled with tactile feedback greatly increase the realism of the simulation. Fa update rate in the order of 1KHz is required for stable haptic rendering which severely limits the u of conventional graphical primitives for simulation. Haptic algorithms, which can render surfaces of the fly, can use the readily available and rich anatomical datasets for simulation.

.Background

Several algorithms exist to simulate palpation in hard isosurfaces [1, 2]. These algorithms use spring damper model for rendering haptic walls by generating restoring forces, which resist enetration [3]. For accurate restoring force calculation, a good tracking and tracing algorithm is eeded since the magnitude and direction of the force depend on the accuracy of the contact point losest to the surface and its normal. This need to calculate the contact point in real time has limited hese models to planes and polygons [2, 4]. However, volumetric datasets produce large numbers of olygons making haptic rendering difficult with these models.

The other method [5] use volumetric datasets for haptic interaction without generating any urfaces making it unsuitable for rendering hard isosurfaces. Haptic texture [7] and force shading [8] nethods do not provide patient specific haptic clues.

Haptic rendering of implicit surfaces [6] enables rendering of complex graphical objects epresented by implicit functions. Anatomical datasets were haptically rendered on the fly [9] with ri-linear interpolation providing a real feel of the complex anatomical surface. However, tri-linear nterpolation provides the continuity of the visualized scalar function but not continuity of the first nd higher derivatives. This makes the rendered surfaces discontinuous over adjacent voxel oundaries. A higher order polynomial interpolation could provide smooth and continuous surface ;enerating a real feel of the anatomical surfaces.

Implicit functions for representing surfaces of higher order are difficult to compute in real – ime as the voxel dataset is probed. Various implicit surface representations have been proposed in he area of solid modeling [10,11,12] which can be used for higher order surfaces but cannot be lirectly implemented in a haptic application requiring a fast update rate. Freeform sculpting using he extraction of a constant isosurfaces from the scalar trivariate functions [13] provides a means of urface testing thereby making it suitable for haptic rendering.

.Methods

We propose an algorithm for haptic rendering of a constant isosurface from a uniform calar B-spline trivariate function, which we believe, will provide higher order interpolation and ontinuity of the haptic surface.

To render the isosurface, a surface contact point (SCP) is established and slid along to the osition that minimizes the distance from the probe point inside the volumetric object. The hysical restriction of the SCP on the surface generates a restoring force proportional to the lepth of the probe point from the SCP. This approach effectively generates a hard surface to feel.

The scalar trivariate B - spline function can be represented as

$$\sum_{i=0}^{l-1} \sum_{j=0}^{m-1} \sum_{k=0}^{n-1} PijkBi(u)Bj(v)Bk(w) \tag{1}$$

vhere $Bi(u)$, $Bj(v)$, $Bk(w)$ are the uniform basis functions and $Pijk$ are the scalar coefficients of he volumetric datasets of the size l x m x n.

The zero set of the function can be represented as F (u, v, w) = T for a given threshold value which represents the isosurface. This model is C^k continuous with B-spline functions of order (k+2). The representation of these surfaces is in parametric form, which can be easily ranslated to the Euclidian space by using the structured grid property of the anatomical datasets.

The anatomical dataset lies on a regular grid. Therefore, the B-spline is represented in 3D as a tensor product of 1D splines eliminating the parametric representation [14]. This is generally true for the surfaces generated from CT data. The 3D formulation can be developed from the analogous 2D case. Consider a B-spline patch on regular uniform 2D grid of unit length (fig1) with $P_{x,y}$ representing the scalar function in 2D .

$$F(x,y) = SMPM^{T}T^{T} \quad 0 \leq x, y \leq 1 \tag{3}$$

where the well-known B-spline basis matrix [15].

$$M \;=\; 1/6 \begin{vmatrix} -1 & 3 & -3 & 1 \\ 3 & -6 & 3 & 0 \\ -3 & 0 & 3 & 0 \\ 1 & 4 & 1 & 0 \end{vmatrix}$$

$$S=[y^{3}, y^{2}, y, 1] \text{ and } T=[x^{3}, x^{2}, x, 1]$$

$$P = \begin{vmatrix} p_{i-1,\,j-1} & p_{i,\,j-1} & p_{i+1,\,j-1} & p_{i+2,\,j-1} \\ p_{i-1,\,j} & p_{i,\,j} & p_{i+1,\,j} & p_{i+2,\,j} \\ p_{i-1,\,j+1} & p_{i,\,j+1} & p_{i+1,\,j+1} & p_{i+2,\,j+1} \\ p_{i-1,\,j+2} & p_{i,\,j+2} & p_{i+1,\,j+2} & p_{i+2,\,j+2} \end{vmatrix}$$

The matrix P consists of the control point in 4X4 neighborhood centered on the patch $P_{i,j}$, $P_{i,j+}$ $P_{i+1,j}$, $P_{i+1,j+1}$ and the scalar value is constrained to lie within the convex hull of the 16 control points.

Extending the same to the 3D we can represent the trivariate B-spline function in 3D uniform grid coordinate as

$$F(x, y, z) = RM \begin{vmatrix} SM & P_{k-1} & M^{T}T^{T} \\ SM & P_{k} & M^{T}T^{T} \\ SM & P_{k+1} & M^{T}T^{T} \\ SM & P_{k+2} & M^{T}T^{T} \end{vmatrix}$$

$$R=[z^{3}, z^{2}, z, 1]$$

Where P_{k-1}, P_{k}, P_{k+1}, P_{k+2} represent the 4 X 4 X 4 neighborhood (figure 2) sixty four control points and F (x,y,z) represents the scalar distribution of the volume bounded by the central nodes

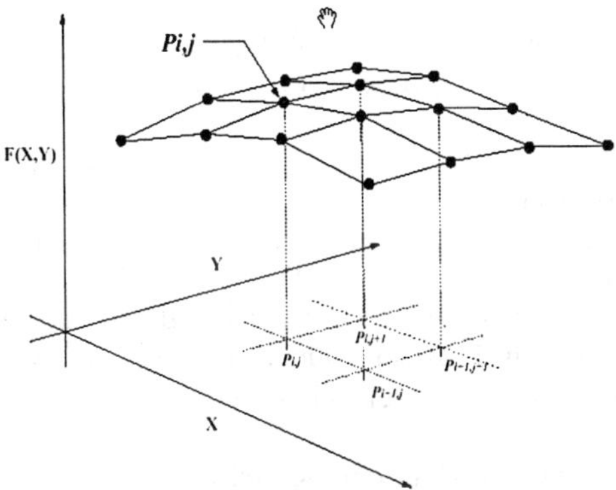

Figure 1. 2D B –Spline Cubic patch with 16 control points forming the convex hull

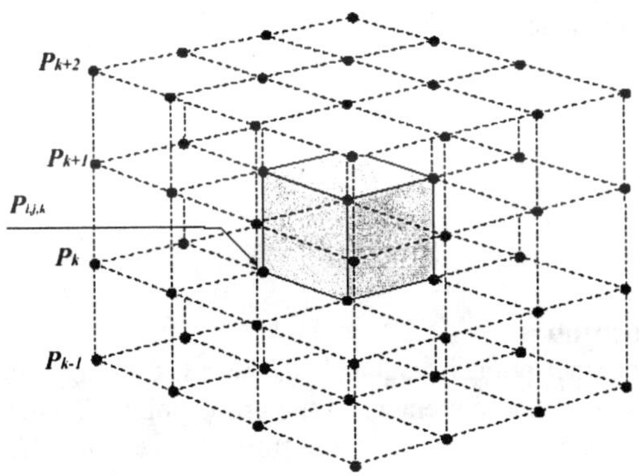

Figure 2. 3D Cubic B-Spline with 64 control points

3.1 Haptic Rendering Algorithm.

For generating isosurface for haptic rendering the implicit form of the surface is taken as

$$F(x,y,z)-T=0 \qquad (4)$$

which is an isosurface representing the threshold value T. It is now easy to test whether the probe has intersected the volume by examining the value of the function F(x,y,z). The normal is calculated for any point on the surface directly from the trivariate function as shown in equation 5.

$$N = (\ \partial F(x,y,z)/\partial x,\ \partial F(x,y,z)/\partial y,\ \partial F(x,y,z)/\partial z) \qquad (5)$$

The haptic rendering consists of two parts. The first part is to find the intersection point where the probe enters the surface for the first time. The second part does the tracking once the SCP is established on the surface.

3.2 Part 1 intersection algorithm

As the probe enters the volume for the first time the intersection to the surface is found using the binary search method. From the previous probe position P and the present position P^l a parametric line equation is formed and the intersection point t will be between $[0-1]$. The resolution of the parameter t as well as the number of steps are taken as the stopping criteria because of the requirement for fast haptic refresh rate.

Algorithm for finding the surface contact point

If probe is inside the surface for the first time **then**
While (numsteps !=max **and** t>=resolution)
        t=(begin+end)/2.0
        $X^l = P_x + t*(P^l_x - P_x)$
        $Y^l = P_y + t*(P^l_y - P_y)$
        $Z^l = P_z + t*(P^l_x - P_z)$
        If $F(X^l, Y^l, Z^l) < 0$ then
        end=t
        else
        begin=T
end while
SCP=(X^l, Y^l, Z^l)

3.3 Surface tracking algorithm

Once the surface contact point is established, the tracking algorithm moves the SCP on the volumetric surface based on the movement of the probe point. The new SCP^l is found as the projection of the probe point on to the tangent plane from the previous SCP as shown in equation 6.

$$SCP^l = SCP + dP \qquad (6)$$
$$dP = (D.N)N/|N|^2 \qquad (7)$$

Where D= P^l-SCP and N is the surface normal at the SCP.

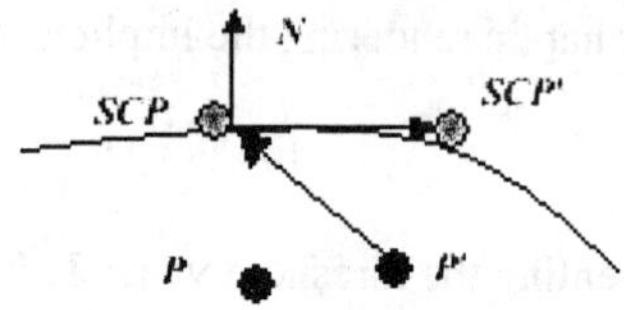

Figure 3. The movement of SCP to a new position SCP^l

Algorithm for surface tracking

If probe is inside the surface **then**
N=surface normal at SCPD= P^l-SCP
dP=(D.N)N/$|N|^2$
SCP^l=SCP+dP
Return F=k(SCP^l - P^l)
Else
Return F= K(0,0,0)

The algorithm was implemented using the PHANToM haptic feedback device and tested with various datasets. During testing it is found that at times the algorithm fails to maintain the surface thereby rendering zero force vector. To overcome this problem the implicit condition was modified with a small tolerance value ϕ as shown in equation 8.

$$F(x,y,z)\text{-}T\text{-}\phi=0 \tag{8}$$

This improved the surface capture and made the simulation much more realistic.

4.Results

The algorithm was first tested on a volumetric cube (figure 4) of constant scalar value of 600 assigned to each voxels. The scalar value calculated at SCP was used for the restoring force for haptic rendering. The surface was found to be smooth as expected of the B-spline interpolation. The scalar value was then varied thereby changing the restoring force and the feel of the surface.

The algorithm was tested with a CT data (figure 5,6) of a patient first thresholded to bone (threshold=1150) and then to skin (threshold =600) and haptically rendered. With ϕ =0, the haptic surface rendered was smooth but somewhat discontinues whenever there was a large change in the surface. These occur when the change in the value is small relative to the size of the B-spline support. By varying the value of ϕ better surface feature was observed. For the threshold value of 600 ϕ was varied from 0 to 100 and the surface variation felt was a close approximation to the actual surface.

The algorithm was also tested with a simulated MRI dataset with varying density value. The algorithm was able to render the surface with detail as long as the changes in the density were within the B-spline support. The B-spline tends to smooth small features making the haptic rendering even smoother.

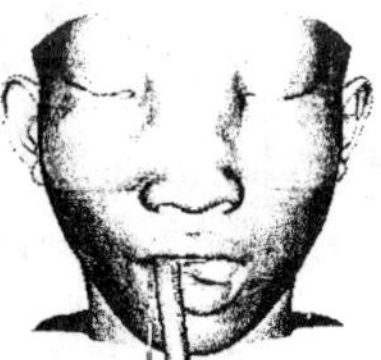

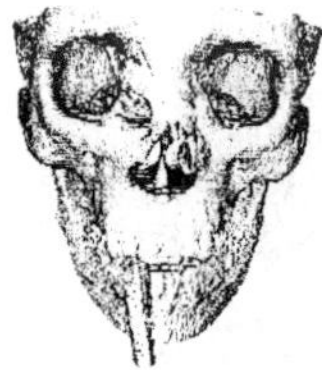

Figure 4: A Volumetric Cube   Figure 5:skin isosurfaces extracted   Figure 6:Bone isosurfaces
from a CT Dataset   from a CT Dataset

5.Conclusions and Future Work

Haptic rendering of isosurfaces using polynomial interpolation with sixty-four neighborhood points provided a smooth and realistic palpation sensation. The isosurfaces extracted was within the limit of the B-spline support. We intend to investigate the use of local interpolation algorithm such as proximity and density mean with the proposed algorithm to capture smaller variations in the anatomy.

6. References

1. R.B. Gillespie and M.R. Cutkoksy, *"Stable user-specific haptic rendering of the virtual wall"*, Proceedings of the 1996 international mechanical engineering congress and exhibition, ASME, 1996, DSC 58,pp. 397-406
2. C.B. Zilles and J.K. Salisbury, *"A constraint-based God-object method for haptic display"*, ASME haptic interfaces for virtual environment and teleoperator systems, 1994, Vol. 1,pp. 146-150
3. J.E. Colgate and G. Schenkel, *"Passivity of a class of sampled-data systems: Application to Haptic interfaces"*, In Proceedings of the American Control Conference, AIAA, 1994, pp. 3236-3240
4. W. R. Mark, S. C. Randolph, M. Finch and J. M. Van Verth, *"UNC-CH Force-Feedback Library, Revision C"*, University of North Carolina at Chapel Hill, Department of Computer Science, Jan. 1996
5. R. S. Avila and L. M. Sobierajski, *"A haptic interaction method for volume visualization"*, IEEE proceedings on visulaization'96, Oct. 1996, pp. 197-203
6. J.K. Salisbury and C. Tarr, *"Haptic rendering of surfaces defined by implicit functions"*, ASME Haptic interfaces and teleoperator system, Nov. 1997, pp. 61-67
7. J. P. Fritz and K. E. Barner, *"Stochastic models for haptic texture"*, Proceedings of the SPIE international symposium of intelligent systems and Advanced manufacturing-telemanipulator and telepresence technologies III, Nov. 1996
8. H.B. Morgenbesser, *"Force shading for shape perception in haptic virtual environments"*, Masters dissertation, Massachusetts Institute of Technology, Department of Electrical Engineering and Computer Science, 1995
9. D. J. Blezek and R. A. Robb, *"Haptic rendering of isosurfaces directly from medical images"*, Proceedings oif the Medicine Meets Virtual Reality Conference, IOS Press, 1999, pp. 67-73
10. H. Nishimura, M. Hirai, T. Kawai, T. Kawata, I. Shirkawa and K. Omura, *"Object modeling by distribution and a method of image generation"*, Transactions of the Institute of Electronics and Communication Engineers of Japan, J68-D(4),1985, pp. 718-725
11. G. Taubin, *"An improved algorithm for algebraic curve and surface fitting"*, Proceedings of the fourth international conference on computer vision, 1993, pp. 658-665
12. G. Wyvill, C. McPheeters and B. Wyvill, *"Data structures for soft objects"*, The visual computer, 2(4), 1986, pp. 227-234
13. A. Raviv and G. Elber, *"Three Dimensional Freeform Sculpting via Zero Sets of Scalar Trivariate Functions"*, ACM Fifth symposium on solid modeling, 1-58, 1999, pp. 246-257
14. J. Carr, *"Surface reconstruction in 3-D medical imaging"*, Ph.D dissertation, University of Canterbury, New Zealand, Feb. 1996
15. J. D. Foley, A. van Dam, S. K.Feiner, J. F. Hughes and R. L.Phillips, *"Introduction to computer graphics"*, Addison-wesley Publishing company, Reading Massachusetts, 1990

An Augmented Reality System for Ultrasound Guided Needle Biopsies

Frank Sauer, Ali Khamene, Benedicte Bascle, and Sebastian Vogt

Siemens Corporate Research
755 College Road East
Princeton, NJ, 08540

Abstract

We have developed an augmented reality visualization system that helps the physician perform ultrasound guided needle biopsies. For a needle biopsy, the needle has to be inserted into an anatomical target to remove a tissue sample. Ultrasound guidance is routinely used e.g. for breast needle biopsies. The real-time ultrasound images allow the physician to locate the target and to monitor the needle position.
Our system uses a combination of an optical laser guide and a virtual guide in the augmented image to provide intuitive guidance for the needle placement. There is no need to track the needle, i.e. there is no need to instrument the needle for tracking.
In phantom tests, users have performed well with the system without prior training. This paper describes special features of our system and the workflow for the needle placement procedure.

Introduction

For a needle biopsy, the needle has to be inserted into an anatomical target to remove a tissue sample. Ultrasound guidance is routinely used e.g. for breast needle biopsies. The real-time ultrasound images allow the physician to locate the target and to monitor the needle position.
The procedure is usually performed "in-plane". With the ultrasound transducer being in a position where the target is visible in the image, the needle is placed in the ultrasound plane, oriented so that it points to the target. When the needle is now inserted, it will appear in the ultrasound image, and the progress along its path towards the target can be monitored.
Performing such an ultrasound guided needle biopsy requires considerable skill and training. It is not easy to estimate the correct orientation of the needle based on the ultrasound image displayed on the scanner's monitor, nor is it easy to place the needle in the ultrasound plane to begin with.
Augmented Reality (AR) visualization has the potential to make the needle placement more intuitive and precise. In fact, Augmented Reality visualization of ultrasound images was the first AR application suggested and pioneered in the medical field [1]. The group from UNC at Chapel Hill has further developed their initial system and reported on it in [2, 3, 4].
We developed a system similar to the UNC system, in that it is also based on a stereoscopic video-see-through head-mounted display. We use a head-mounted tracker camera in combination with a set of optical markers attached to the transducer and another set of optical markers fixed to the workspace, giving us the pose of the transducer with respect to the observer's viewpoint and with respect to a stationary world coordinate system. The user can see the ultrasound image overlaid onto the view of the actual patient, registered to the position of the transducer. A structure seen in the ultrasound image appears at the location of the actual anatomical structure.
In this paper, we describe our AR system for ultrasound guided needle biopsy. It provides intuitive guidance without the need for needle tracking. Special features include a laser guide for in-plane alignment of the needle. Furthermore, we implemented a user interface that allows one to mark the target and the desired needle path in the 3D world coordinate system, creating a virtual needle guide.

System Description

For the demonstration experiments, the user sits at a table, which is mounted on a tripod for portability. A set of markers is attached to the ultrasound transducer; a set of stationary markers can be positioned above the workspace (Fig. 1). The user wears a custom video-see-through head-mounted display (HMD) (Fig. 2). Two color video cameras attached to the HMD provide a stereo view of the scene; a third head-mounted video camera is added for tracking. The video images are augmented with the live images from the ultrasound scanner. The ultrasound images are registered to the pose of the ultrasound transducer. Hence, structures in the ultrasound images are perceived at the locations of the actual physical structures. Figure 3 is an example of such an augmented view, with the ultrasound image overlaid on the video image of the breast biopsy phantom in a registered way.

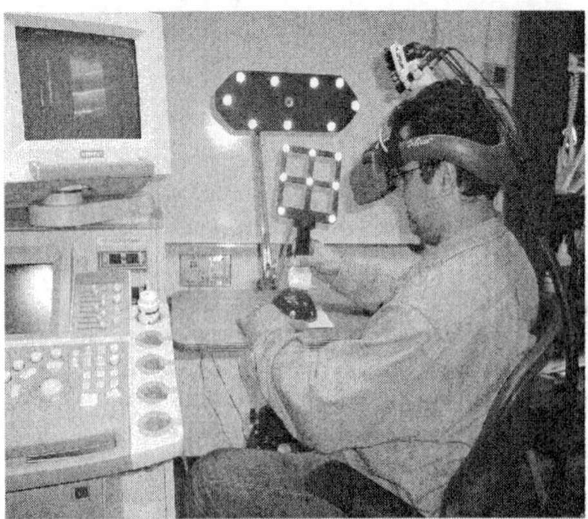

Figure 1. Demonstration of the ultrasound workspace.

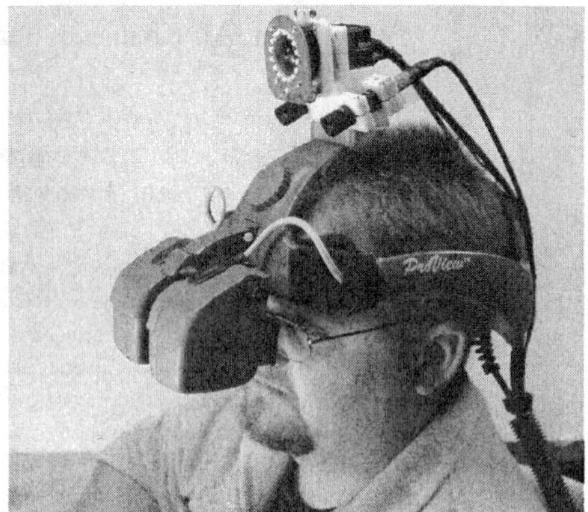

Figure 2. Video-see-through head-mounted display.

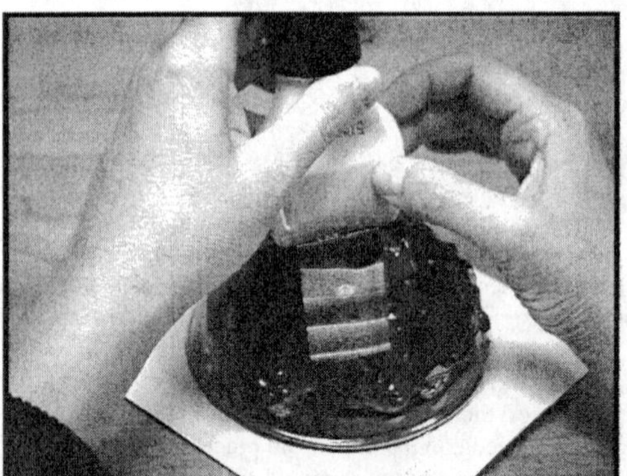

Figure 3. Augmented view of biopsy phantom.

Our system runs on three SGI PCs and achieves real-time performance with 30 frames per second with a latency of about 0.1 sec, generating a stable augmentation with no apparent jitter visible in the composite images. The registration accuracy of the augmentation measured in object space is around 1 mm. More system details are described in [4,5].

System Calibration

Two stages of calibration have to be performed. We need to determine the internal and relative external camera parameters for our camera triplet [5]. And we need to register the ultrasound image correctly to the transducer. We designed a special object for this latter calibration task [6]. With this method, we achieved a calibration accuracy of 1.05 mm RMS and 1.6 mm max deviation. The literature describes a number of other calibration approaches for 3D free-hand ultrasound [7-11].

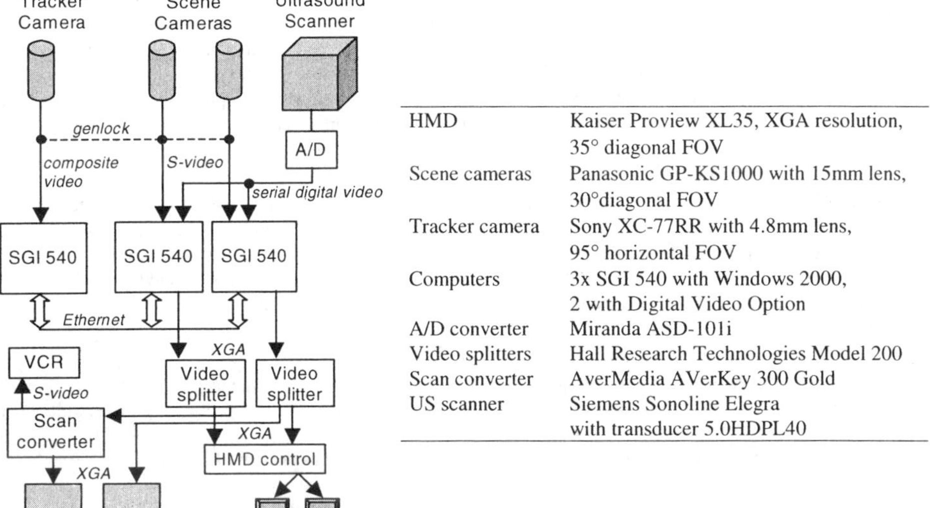

HMD	Kaiser Proview XL35, XGA resolution, 35° diagonal FOV
Scene cameras	Panasonic GP-KS1000 with 15mm lens, 30°diagonal FOV
Tracker camera	Sony XC-77RR with 4.8mm lens, 95° horizontal FOV
Computers	3x SGI 540 with Windows 2000, 2 with Digital Video Option
A/D converter	Miranda ASD-101i
Video splitters	Hall Research Technologies Model 200
Scan converter	AverMedia AVerKey 300 Gold
US scanner	Siemens Sonoline Elegra with transducer 5.0HDPL40

Figure 4. System block diagram.

Table 1. Hardware Components.

To demonstrate the accuracy of the AR overlay, we fabricated a small phantom with visible rubber structures. When one observes this phantom from approximately the normal direction, refraction does not displace the internal structures in the optical image, and one can appreciate the accuracy of the ultrasound overlay (Fig. 5).

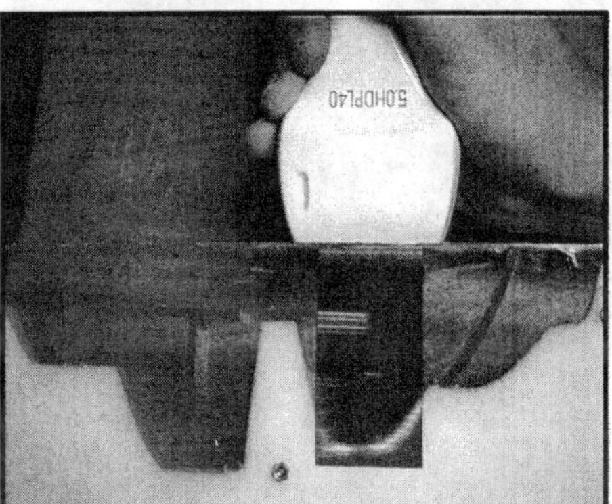

Figure 5. Test phantom for visualizing the ultrasound overlay accuracy.

Procedure for needle placement

1. Positioning of transducer

A usual, the user positions the ultrasound transducer so that the target structure appears in the ultrasound image.

2. Marking of target in 3D

The user can mark the target in 3D by simply aiming his/her gaze toward it. The position, where the optical axis of the user's artificial "left eye" (left scene camera) intersects with the ultrasound image, is visualized as a yellow circle (Fig. 6). The user aims this yellow circle at the target structure by moving his/her head accordingly, and then presses a foot switch. The target is then marked with a graphics object such as a sphere, which appears fixed in space (i.e. fixed relative to the stationary workspace coordinate system) (Fig. 7).

3. Positioning of needle in ultrasound plane

The in-plane needle positioning is facilitated with an optical guide. Figure 8 shows how a laser attached to the transducer projects a line of light that marks the intersection between the plane of the ultrasound image and the surface of the patient. Hence, the laser line marks all the possible in-plane entry points for the needle.
After the needle tip is placed on a suitable point of the laser line, the needle can be rotated around its tip until it lights up along its length. The needle is now positioned in the ultrasound plane.

4. Adjusting in-plane needle angle

Next the user tilts the needle in the ultrasound plane so that it points towards the target. We introduce a virtual guide that facilitates this alignment procedure. To mark the virtual needle guide, the user now points his/her gaze towards the needle entry point and again presses the foot switch. That prompts the system to visualize guidelines connecting the in-plane entry point with the target, which has been marked before (Fig. 9).

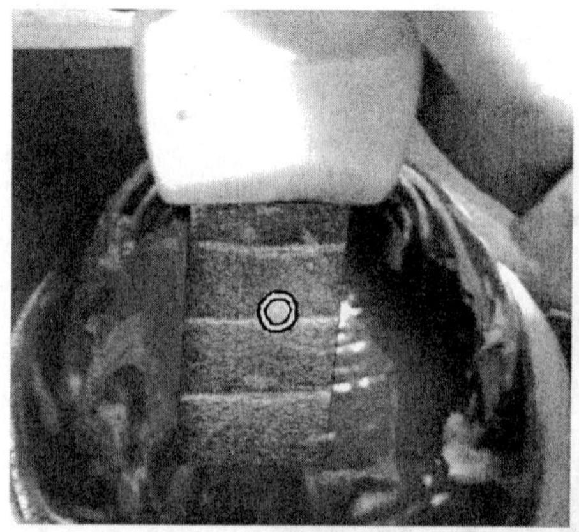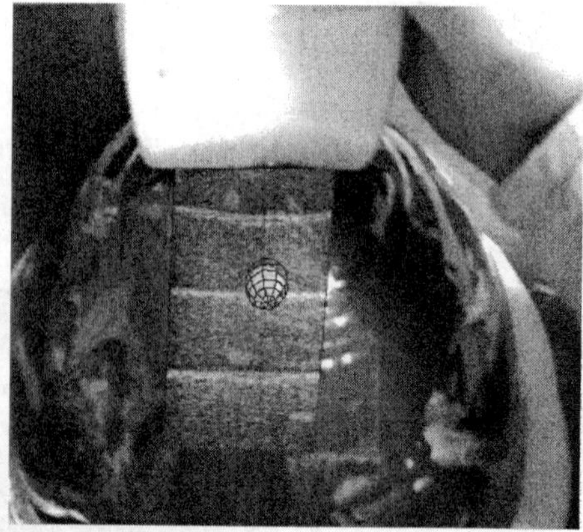

Figure 6. The use aims his/her gaze, visualized as a circle at the intersection with the ultrasound plane, at the target.

Figure 7. After pressing the foot switch, the target is marked by a red sphere, fixed in 3D.

5. Inserting needle

The aligned needle can now be inserted and will appear in the ultrasound image on its way towards the target.

Results

Several test users successfully inserted needles into targets of the breast biopsy phantom, guided by the augmented reality system. The process is intuitive and does not require specialized training.

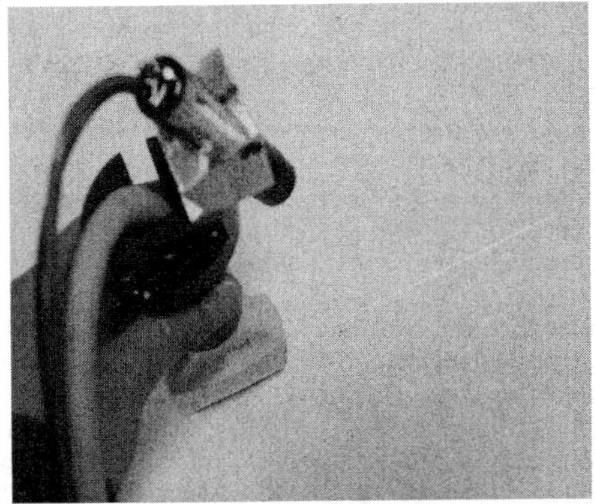

Figure 8. Laser guide marks ultrasound plane.

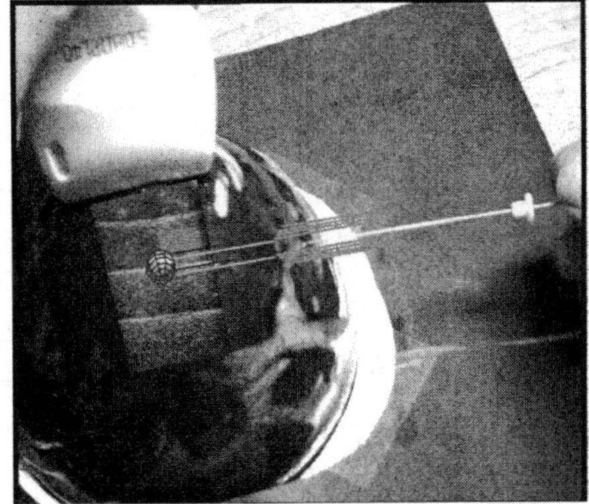

Figure 9. Virtual guidelines help to align the needle towards the target.

Conclusion

We developed an augmented reality ultrasound workspace where the user wears a video-see-through head-mounted display and observes the ultrasound slices *in-situ*, i.e. in their actual location. The ultrasound-to-video and ultrasound-to-workspace registration is performed with a head-mounted tracker camera that tracks markers attached to transducer and workspace.

The system provides intuitive guidance for needle placement without the need to instrument the needle for tracking. An optical laser guide facilitates the placement of the needle in the ultrasound plane, and the augmented view facilitates the aiming of the needle towards the target within the ultrasound plane. A virtual guide that connects the target with the needle entry point supports the aiming process. To mark target and entry point, the user simply directs his/her gaze towards them and presses a foot switch.

Non-medical users have performed well using the system for phantom tests. We are planning to evaluate the system in a clinical setting.

References

[1] M. Bajura, H. Fuchs, and R. Ohbuchi. "Merging Virtual Objects with the Real World: Seeing Ultrasound Imagery within the Patient." Proceedings of SIGGRAPH 92 (Chicago, IL, July 26-31, 1992). In Computer Graphics 26, #2 (July 1992): 203-210.

[2] State, Andrei, Mark A. Livingston, Gentaro Hirota, William F. Garrett, Mary C. Whitton, Henry Fuchs, and Etta D. Pisano (MD). "Technologies for Augmented-Reality Systems: realizing Ultrasound-Guided Needle Biopsies." Proceedings of SIGGRAPH 96 (New Orleans, LA, August 4-9, 1996). In Computer Graphics Proceedings, Annual Conference Series 1996, ACM SIGGRAPH, pgs. 439-446.

[3] Fuchs, Henry, Andrei State, Etta D. Pisano, William F. Garrett, Gentaro Hirota, Mark A. Livingston, Mary C. Whitton, and Stephen M. Pizer. "(Towards) Performing Ultrasound-Guided Needle Biopsies from within a Head-Mounted Display." Proceedings of Visualization in Biomedical Computing 1996, (Hamburg, Germany, September 22-25, 1996), pgs. 591-600.

[4] Rosenthal M et al., Augmented Reality Guidance for Needle Biopsies: A Randomized, Controlled Trial in Phantoms, In Forth Int. Conf. on Medical Image Computing and Computer-Assisted Intervention (MICCAI '01), pages 240-248, Utrecht, Netherlands, October 2001.

[5] F. Sauer, F. Wenzel, S. Vogt, Y.Tao, Y. Genc, and A. Bani-Hashemi, "Augmented Workspace: Designing an AR Testbed," IEEE and ACM Int. Symp. On Augmented Reality – ISAR 2000 (Munich, Germany, October 5-6, 2000), pages 47-53.

[6] F. Sauer, A. Khamene, B. Bascle, S. Vogt, "Augmented Reality Visualization of Ultrasound Images: System Description, Calibration, and Features," IEEE and ACM Int. Symp. On Augmented Reality – ISAR 2001 (NYC, New York, October 28-29, 2001)

[7] R.W. Prager, R.N. Rohling, A.H. Gee and L. Berman. Rapid calibration for 3-D freehand ultrasound. Ultrasound in Medicine and Biology, 24(6): 855-869, July 1998.

[8] R.W. Prager, A.H. Gee and L. Berman. Stradx: real-time acquisition and visualization of freehand three-dimensional ultrasound. Medical Image Analysis, 3(2):129-140, 1999.

[9] R.W. Prager, R.N. Rohling, A.H. Gee et al: Rapid calibration for 3-D freehand ultrasound. Ultrasound Med Biol 24:855--869, 1998

[10] A. Hartov, S. D. Eisner, D. W. Roberts, K. D. Paulsen, L. A. Platenik, and M. I. Miga. Error analysis for a free-hand three-dimensional ultrasound system for neuronavigation. Neurosurg Focus 6 (3):Article 5, 1999

[11] J. M. Blackall, D. Rueckert, C. R. Maurer Jr., G. P. Penney, D. L. G. Hill, and D. J. Hawkes. An image registration approach to automated calibration for freehand 3D ultrasound. In Third Int. Conf. on Medical Image Computing and Computer-Assisted Intervention (MICCAI '00), pages 462-471, Pittsburgh, PN, 2000.

Medicine Meets Virtual Reality 02/10
J.D. Westwood et al. (Eds.)
IOS Press, 2002

Automatic patient registration in computer assisted maxillofacial surgery

O. Schermeier [a], T. Lueth [a], J. Glagau [a], D. Szymanski [a], R. Tita [a],
D. Hildebrand [b], M. Klein [b], K. Nelson [b], J. Bier [b]

[a] *Berlin Center for Mechatronic Medical Devices*
Fraunhofer IPK – Charité • Campus Virchow, [b] *Clinic for Maxillofacial Surgery*
Augustenburger Platz 1, 13353 Berlin / Germany
olaf.schermeier@charite.de

Abstract. In this paper, a new approach for patient registration in computer assisted maxillofacial surgery is presented. The method uses a unique structure of markers embedded in a reference frame for the automatic detection of the coordinate system of the medical imaging data during the surgical intervention. With the new method, the inaccurate and time consuming process of manually identifying markers in the data volume and manually teaching them to a navigation system can be replaced. The method and algorithms for the automatic marker detection are described in this paper. Experiments with 45 data sets of patients proove the robustness, usability and safety of the new method. The method has been integrated into the navigation system RoboDent for dental implant surgery.

1. Introduction

Several applications for navigation and robotic systems in maxillofacial surgery have been presented so far [3][4]. The navigated insertion of dental implants is a new promising field for computer aided surgery [1][2][9]. These systems use optical localizers to calculate the locations of instruments and patients. The deviation between preplanned geometries and the current instrument location is displayed on monitors or on displays that allow the surgeon to view the information without moving the eyes from the operation scenario [1][10].

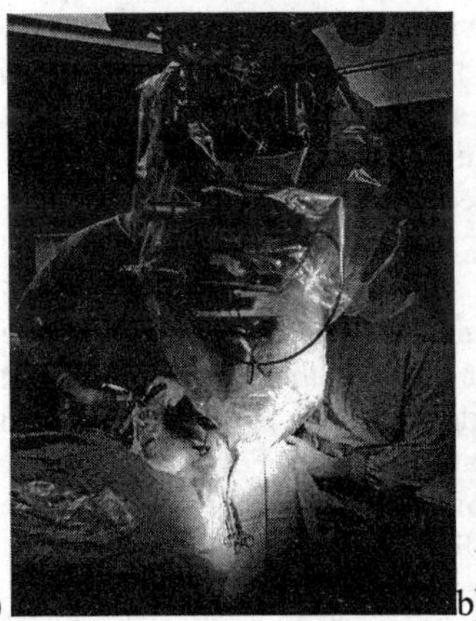
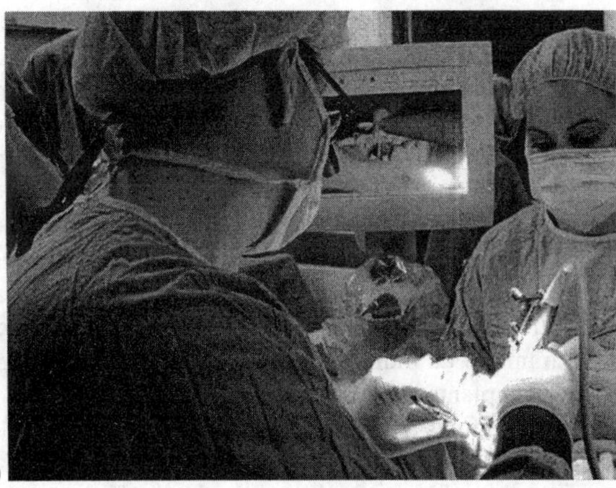

Fig. 1   a) Robot assisted operation in maxillofacial surgery and b) navigated insertion of dental implants in the clinic for maxillofacial surgery, Charité, Berlin.

Due to the fact that for most dental implantations the patients are not under anaesthetic, the patients head cannot be fixed to the chair. Thus, the location of the patient's head has to be measured during the intervention. This can be realized by using an individual impression of the remaining teeth or of temporary implants. This non-invasive impression is capable of securing a tracking device to the patients jaw. Since the location of this device in relation to the jaw bone is reproducable, it can also be used for the registration of the patient. The problem remains, that the registration process for high precision navigation systems is still done manually. The locations of fiducial markers in the medical imaging data are identified manually. These markers again have to be measured by a pointer device during the navigated intervention. Both processes are time consuming and a potential source of error caused by inaccuracies of the human.

This paper presents a method for the registration of a patient's head or jaw without any interaction with the user of the system. The preoperative detection of fiducial markers is done automatically by a fast, robust and secure algorithm that can handle even sets of data distorted by metallic artefacts from teeth, crowns or fillings. The intraoperative registration of these positions to the operation scene is calculated by CAD-Data of precision manufactured reference bodies. The principles of the new approach and experiments with 45 data sets of patients are presented in this paper.

2. Problem description

Patient registration can be carried out on the basis of points, polygons, surfaces or volumes [5], but is usually based on the manual definition of the user in the patient data and/or manual measurements during the intervention. Using point to point registration, fiducial markers are fixed to the area that is to be navigated to build the transition coordinate system between image data and navigation system.

The fiducials are mostly small bone screws that are fixed to the bone or to dental impressions. The locations of the projections of the screws in the medical imaging data is determined by identifying regions of the same density in the volume by selecting them with an input device on two dimensional views of the data volume. The inaccuracies in the perception of markers in the volume make the exact identification of certain positions, like the head of the screw or the center, impossible by manual processing. Reasons are artifacts or the limited resolution of the image data.

During the intervention, the reference between patient data and patient location in space can be registered by defining the marker positions with a navigated pointer device. The error of this procedure is dominated by the jitter and inaccuracies of the human hand and eye. Another source of error is the measurement error of the navigation system [6][7].

To overcome these limitations, a method for the automatic identification of the fiducials and the automatic intraoperative registration has been developed.

3. Automatic patient registration

The method relies on the assumption that a reference frame with known geometry is fixed to the patient's jaw during the medical image aquisition and during the surgical intervention. The location of the frame in relation to the bone is reproducible. This is reached by connecting the frame to an individual dental impression of the patient's teeth. For endentulous jaws, temporary implants can be used to secure the proper seat of the impression.

The frame defines a coordinate system that can be identified in the medical imaging data and during the surgical intervention. The identification in the data is done by an algorithm that recognizes the reference body automatically. This is achieved by the identification of known geometry structures that are integrated in the body.

For the intraoperative registration, the body has a connector to a precise manufactured tracking device. Since the geometries of reference body and tracking device are known, the transformation between the coordinate system of the reference body and the coordinate system, that is measured by the localizer, is known. With the transformation of the automatic marker detection, the patient registration is performed without any user interaction.

Since the tracking device is fixed rigidly to the frame in a given configuration, the design of the devices has to be adapted to the application. The transformations between the sensor and the reference frame and between the reference frame connector and the geometric structures in the reference frame can be calculated by a CAD-Software.

The algorithm for the automatic detection of the reference frame is described in the following.

4. An algorithm for automatic marker detection

The structure, that is integrated in the reference frame is defined by the geometry of a number v_{max} of fiducial markers with $v_{max} \geq 4$. Three markers are used for defining the transition coordinate system, the remaining markers are used to validate the geometry of the structure. The volume of these markers has a projection of voxels with gray values in a known range in the voxel volume of the medical imaging system. The gray values of the markers differ from grayvalues of tissue. Using CT-data small titanium spheres or cylinders can be integrated in the reference frame.

Each voxel in the data volume is defined by the vector $\mathbf{n}$ of its three index coordinates. The range of gray values for the chosen imaging device is H_M. For each voxel, the gray value h is determined by the projection function Λ_{idx}. The function Ω_{idx} is the projection of index coordinates in metric coordinates $^{dat}\mathbf{p}$ of each voxel $\mathbf{n}$:

$$\Lambda_{idx} : \mathbf{n} \longrightarrow h \mid h \in H_M, \mathbf{n} \in \aleph^3 \tag{1}$$

$$\Omega_{idx} : \mathbf{n} \longrightarrow {}^{dat}\mathbf{p}^{vox} \mid {}^{dat}\mathbf{p}^{vox} \in \Re^3 \tag{2}$$

The function Ω_{idx} also supports data volumes with non parallel slices and non constant slice distances [11] as they are produced by high precision imaging systems as described in [8].

To calculate the transformation between the metric coordinate system of the data volume *dat* and the coordinate system defined by the markers, the centers of gravity of the voxel groups, that are the projections of the fiducials in the data volume have to be identified and their order has to be classified.

The range of gray values of the chosen material of the markers is H_M^m. The markers are defined in the volume as connected areas of voxels with a projection

$$\Lambda_{idx}(\mathbf{n}_{k,i}^m) \in H_M^m . \tag{3}$$

The k_{max} groups of voxels $\mathbf{n}_{k,i}^m$ with $i_{max}(k)$ voxels each can be separated by region growing or neighborhood operations.

As mentioned before, many other areas in a human mouth have a grayvalue similar to the choosen material. If titanium is used, areas of all metallic and ceramic material in the mouth have a similar range, dental implants have the same range. The number of voxel groups with a gray value in the range of titanium is approx. four times as large as the number of markers in the reference frame. To get a robust and secure result, several criteria are inspected for each group to identify the groups that are projections of markers.

The exact dimensions of the markers in the frame are known. This information is used to perform a consistency check with the identified groups. The size of the bounding box of a group of voxels, that is a projection of a marker, must not be much lower than the minimum diameter d_m^{min} or much higher than the maximum diameter d_m^{max} of the marker. Having a cylindrical marker with the diameter d_{cld} and the length l_{cld}, the function $G(k)$ determines if a group has the right size to be the projection of one of these cylinders:

$$G(k) = \begin{cases} 1, & \text{if } d_m^{\min} \leq d(k) \leq d_m^{\max} & \to \text{possible marker} \\ 0, & \text{else} & \to \text{no marker} \end{cases} \tag{4}$$

$$d_m^{\min} = l_{cld}, d_m^{\max} = \sqrt{2} \cdot l_{cld} \text{ for } l_{cld} >> d_{cld} \tag{5}$$

$$d(k) = \left\| \Omega_{idx}\left(\mathbf{n}_{max}^{j}\right) - \Omega_{idx}\left(\mathbf{n}_{min}^{j}\right) \right\| \tag{6}$$

where $\mathbf{n}_{\min}^{k}$ and $\mathbf{n}_{\max}^{k}$ are the minimum and maximum coordinates of the bounding box of the group k. Additionally, the volume of the group can be compared to the volume of the original marker.

After the diameter inspection, the geometry between the remaining q_{max} groups q is compared to the geometry of the real markers. Therefore, a vector to the center of gravity $^{dat}\mathbf{p}^{cog}(q)$ of all voxels of each group is calculated in metric coordinates in the medical imaging volume that is defined by the coordinate system *dat*.

$$^{dat}\mathbf{p}^{cog}(q) = \frac{1}{i_{max}(k^*)} \sum_{i=1}^{i_{max}(k^*)} \left(\Omega(\mathbf{n}_{k^*,i}^{m}) \right) \Big| \; \forall k^* \Big| G(k^*) = 1 \tag{7}$$

This calculation assumes, that all voxels have the same size. For different voxel dimensions, the metric vectors of equation (7) should be multiplied by the voxel volume as a weighting function.

The centers of the original markers, which are inserted in the reference frame by a computer driven machine, are defined by the CAD-Software as vectors $^{pin}\mathbf{p}^{cnc}(v)$, $v = [1, v_{max}]$ in any coordinate system *pin*. The correlation between the geometry defined by $^{pin}\mathbf{p}^{cnc}(v)$ and the geometry defined by $^{dat}\mathbf{p}^{cog}(q)$ is done in a three dimensional geometry verification. The goal of this investigation is the assignment of each vector $^{pin}\mathbf{p}^{cnc}(v)$ to one vector $^{dat}\mathbf{p}^{cog}(q)$ by the assignment function $w(v) = q$.

Therefore, the function $\Phi(^A\mathbf{p}_1, {}^A\mathbf{p}_2, {}^A\mathbf{p}_3)$ is defined, that calculates a transformation matrix in a coordinate system defined by three vectors:

$$\Phi\left(^A\mathbf{p}_1, {}^A\mathbf{p}_2, {}^A\mathbf{p}_3\right) = \begin{pmatrix} (^A\mathbf{e}_x)^T & 0 \\ (^A\mathbf{e}_y)^T & 0 \\ (^A\mathbf{e}_z)^T & 0 \\ 0 \quad 0 \quad 0 & 1 \end{pmatrix} \cdot \begin{pmatrix} 1 & 0 & 0 & \\ 0 & 1 & 0 & -^A\mathbf{p}_1 \\ 0 & 0 & 1 & \\ 0 & 0 & 0 & 1 \end{pmatrix} \tag{8}$$

with

$$^A\mathbf{e}_x = \frac{\left(^A\mathbf{p}_2 - {}^A\mathbf{p}_1\right)}{\left\|\left(^A\mathbf{p}_2 - {}^A\mathbf{p}_1\right)\right\|}, \quad ^A\mathbf{e}_z = \frac{\left(^A\mathbf{p}_3 - {}^A\mathbf{p}_1\right) \times {}^A\mathbf{e}_x}{\left\|\left(^A\mathbf{p}_3 - {}^A\mathbf{p}_1\right) \times {}^A\mathbf{e}_x\right\|}, \quad ^A\mathbf{e}_y = {}^A\mathbf{e}_z \times {}^A\mathbf{e}_x \tag{9}$$

The correlation is performed by calculating coordinate systems for all triples of vectors $^{pin}\mathbf{p}^{cnc}(v)$ and $^{dat}\mathbf{p}^{cog}(q)$ and transforming all remaining vectors in these coordinate systems. If four vectors $^{dat}\mathbf{p}^{cog}(q_n)$, $n = [1..4]$ are the projections of four real markers $^{pin}\mathbf{p}^{cnc}(v_m)$, $m = [1..4]$ in the frame, the position of one vector transformed in the coordinate system that is defined by the three others must be equal:

$$^{q_1,q_2,q_3}\mathbf{T}_{dat} \cdot {}^{dat}\mathbf{p}^{cog}(q_4) = {}^{v_1,v_2,v_3}\mathbf{T}_{pin} \cdot {}^{pin}\mathbf{p}^{cnc}(v_4) \tag{10}$$

with

$$^{q_1,q_2,q_3}\mathbf{T}_{dat} = \Phi\left(^{dat}\mathbf{p}^{cog}(q_1) \quad {}^{dat}\mathbf{p}^{cog}(q_2) \quad {}^{dat}\mathbf{p}^{cog}(q_3)\right) \tag{11}$$

$$^{v_1,v_2,v_3}\mathbf{T}_{pin} = \Phi\left(^{pin}\mathbf{p}^{cnc}(v_1) \quad {}^{pin}\mathbf{p}^{cnc}(v_2) \quad {}^{pin}\mathbf{p}^{cnc}(v_3)\right) \tag{12}$$

For the quantity of v_{max} original vectors $^{pin}\mathbf{p}^{cnc}(v)$, the coordinate systems for all triple combinations are constructed. For each of these coordinate systems, $(v_{max} - 3)$ remaining vectors are examined.

The comparison with the vectors of the centers of gravity of the voxel groups is done by building the coordinate systems of all triple permutations of the vectors $^{dat}\mathbf{p}^{cog}(q)$. This is for considering the order of vectors in equ. (11). The total number of transformations for the original vectors n^{cnc} and for the vectors of found groups n^{cog} are:

$$n^{cnc} = \binom{v_{max}}{3} \cdot (v_{max} - 3) \quad \text{and} \quad n^{cog} = \binom{q_{max}}{4} \cdot 4! \tag{13}$$

For each $^{dat}\mathbf{p}^{cog}(q)$, a vector $\mathbf{c}^{cog}(q) = [c_1^q, c_{v\,max}^q]$ with v_{max} consistency values is defined. The consistency value c_{va}^{qa} shows the probability that the vector $^{dat}\mathbf{p}^{cog}(q_a)$ is the projection of the marker at the position $^{pin}\mathbf{p}^{cnc}(v_a)$. Each vector of the n^{cog} transformations is now compared with the n^{cnc} vectors of the original data. The consistency values are incremented, if the length of the difference between the vectors is below the maximum deviation ε_{dist}:

$$\underbrace{\left\| ^{q1,q2,q3}\mathbf{T}_{dat} \cdot {}^{dat}\mathbf{p}^{cog}(q_4) - {}^{v1,v2,v3}\mathbf{T}_{pin} \cdot {}^{pin}\mathbf{p}^{cnc}(v_4) \right\| < \varepsilon_{dist}}_{\downarrow} \tag{14}$$

$$c_{v1}^{q1} = c_{v1}^{q1} + 1,\ c_{v2}^{q2} = c_{v2}^{q2} + 1,\ c_{v3}^{q3} = c_{v3}^{q3} + 1,\ c_{v4}^{q4} = c_{v4}^{q4} + 1$$

The assignment between an original marker v_i and the group q' is done, if this group has the maximum consistency value c_{vi}^q of all groups for this marker and the consistency value is greater or equal the number of transformations that are performed for one original marker:

$$w(v_i) = \begin{cases} q' & \text{if}\ \ c_{vi}^{q'} = \max_q\left(c_{vi}^q\right) \wedge c_{vi}^{q'} \geq n^{cnc} \cdot \left(1 - \dfrac{n^{cnc} - 4}{n^{cnc}}\right) \\ 0 & \text{else} \end{cases} \tag{15}$$

If a minimum of four groups has been assigned, their geometry is verified again to avoid random hits by other groups. The remaining markers can be reconstructed by the known geometry of the original markers and the geometry of the identified and verified groups.

5. Experiments

In an experimental study, the medical data of n=45 patients has been tested with the algorithm, whereas 25 patients were edentulous. All patients had a reference frame in the mouth during the scan. The frame has 6 titanium cylinders with a diameter of 1.5mm and a length of 5 mm. The minimum distance between the two cylinders is 9 mm, the maximum distance is 50 mm. The data from the original structure is calculated with the CAD Software ProEngineer (PTC, Waltham, USA). The frame is manufactured on a high precision computer driven milling machine based on the CAD data with a tolerance below 0.05 mm.

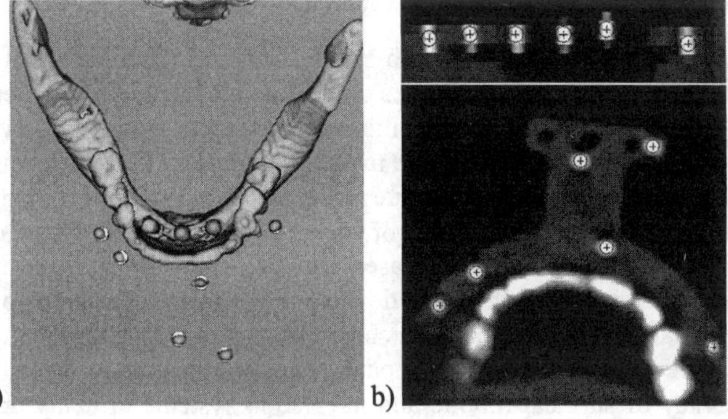

Fig. 2   a) 3D- and b) 2D visualization of detected marker structure of 6 titanium cylinders in a reference frame (© RoboDent GmbH 2001)

The patients were scanned using the imaging devices Somatom Plus 4, Somatom Plus 4 Volume Zoom (both Siemens, Munich, Germany), Picker 3000 (Marconi, London, GB), DVT9000 (Newtom AG, Munich, Germany) and a Tomoscan M (Philips, Netherlands). Slice thicknesses of the data sets range from 0.5 mm to 2 mm with field of views in the imaging data between approx. 130 mm and 300 mm. No filters were used for the 3D reconstruction of the data.

The data is stored in DICOM-3 Format and transferred to the System on a CD. The marker detection is integrated in the planning software of the navigation system for dental implantology RoboDent in the Version 1.0.25. Calculation is carried out on a Standard PC with a Pentium III on 1 GHz with 512 MB memory.

In the experiment, the time and the success of the marker detection are measured. To measure the success of the marker detection, the found markers were visually integrated in the two dimensional views of the medical imaging data and in the three dimensional surface model of the data. Markers were drawn as white spheres in the 3D-view and dark circles in 2D views (Fig. 2).

6. Results/Conclusion

The automatic registration succeeded to find the structure in the reference frame in 93 % of the study cases. No identification of wrong structures occurred. The time for the successful search was between 1 and 15 sec. with a mean of 3.02 sec. and a standard deviation of 2.34 sec. The maximum time for a successful search is 15 seconds. The failed detections were on studies with strong artifacts caused by crowns, bridges or fillings.

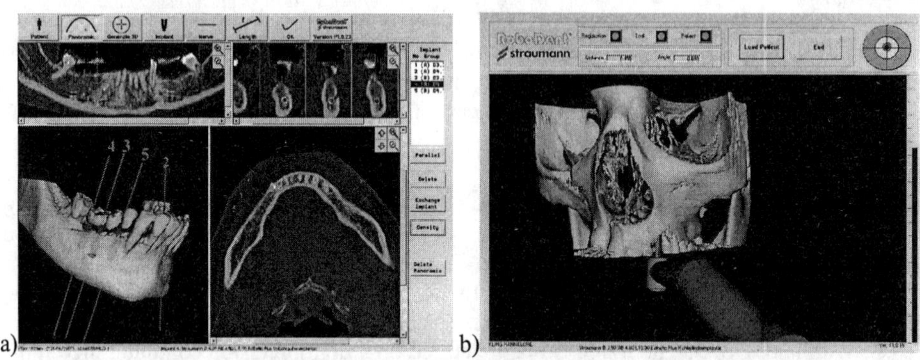

Fig. 3   a) Planning software and b) treatment software of the navigation system RoboDent for oral implantology (© RoboDent GmbH 2001).

A new method has been presented, which has the capability to register patients without any interaction with the user. The method relies on the knowledge of the geometry of the devices that are integrated during the image acquisition and during the surgical intervention.

The algorithm that is used to identify the marker structure in the data volume is robust, fast and secure and succeeds to find the structure in the patient data. Even if many artifacts caused by fillings, crowns or prosthetics occurred or when parts of the frame where out of the volume the algorithm kept the reliability in most cases. However, in some cases, strong artifacts cover too many of the markers, so that the identification fails. In this case, the algorithm detects that it fails and does not deliver wrong data which would cause a wrong treatment of the patient.

The authors believe, that this new method for patient registration has the potential to increase the accuracy of surgical robotic and navigation systems in many applications. However, it can only be used, if the area that is to be navigated is directly accessible during the image acquisition.

The new method has been integrated in the navigation system RoboDent (RoboDent, Berlin, Germany) for oral implantology (Fig. 3). More than 50 patients have been treated successfully by using the automatic patient registration.

Acknowledgment

This research work has been performed at the Department for Maxillofacial Surgery, Prof. Dr. Dr. Juergen Bier, within the Surgical Robotics Lab, Prof. Dr. Tim C. Lueth, Medical Faculty Charité, Humboldt-University Berlin. The work has been supported by the Deutsche Forschungsgemeinschaft with the Graduiertenkolleg 331 – Temperaturabhängige Effekte (granted to Prof. Dr. Dr.h.c. R. Felix, PD Dr. N. Hosten) and by the Real-Time Control Group, Prof. Dr.-Ing. Guenter Hommel, of the Technical University Berlin. Parts of the research have been supported financially by the Deutsche Krebshilfe (granted to Prof. Dr. Dr. J. Bier, PD Dr. P. Wust) and the Berliner Sparkassenstiftung Medizin (granted to Prof. Dr. T. Lueth, Dr. Dr. Ernst Heissler, Prof. Dr. Dr. Berthold Hell). Special thanks to the companies NDI, Rohwedder Visotech, Elekta, Metalor and Philips for their support of the project. We would like also to thank Thomas Hölper, Edgar Schüle, Dr.-Ing. Armin Freybott, and W. Scholz. Their personal engagement was the basis for this challenging research.

References

[1]   Birkenfellner W. et. al. (1999): Computer - Aided Implant Dentistry -An early Report-. MICCAI99, Cambridge, pp. 883-891.
[2]   Brief, J., S. Hassfeld, U. Sonenfeld, N. Persky, R. Krempien, M. Treiber, J. Mühling (2001): Navigated Insertion of Dental Implants. ISRACAS Fourth Israeli Symposium on Computer-Aided Surgery, Medical Robotics and Medical Imaging, Tel-Aviv, Israel, May 17, 2001.
[3]   Haßfeld, S. , J. Brief, R. Krempien, J. Raczkowsky, J. Münchenberg, H. Giess, H.P. Meinzer, U. Mende, H.Wörn, J. Mühling (2000): Computergestützte Mund-, Kiefer- und Gesichtschirurgie. Der Radiologe, 40, pp. 218 - 226.
[4]   Hein, A.; M. Klein, T. C. Lueth, J. Queck, M. Stien, O. Schermeier, J. Bier: Integration and Clinical Evaluation of an Interactive Controllable Robotic System for Anaplastology. MICCAI 2001, Utrecht, Netherland, 14.-17. Oct., 2001, in print.
[5]   Lavallee, S.: Registration for Computer-Integrated Surgery: Methodology, State of the Art. In Taylor, R. H., S. Lavallee, G. C. Burdea, R. Mösges (Ed.), Computer-Integrated Surgery, Technology and clinical Applications, MIT Press, 1996, pp. 77-98.
[6]   Khadem, R., C.C. Yeh, M. Sadeghi-Tehrani, M.R. Bax, J.A. Johnson, J. Nerney Welch, E. P. Wikinson, R.Shahidi (2000): Comparative Tracking Error Analysis of Five Different Optical Tracking Systems. Computer Aided Surgery, 5, pp. 98-107.
[7]   Marmulla, R., M. Hilbert, H. Niederdellmann (1998): Intraoperative Präzision mechanischer, elektromagnetischer, infrarot- und lasergeführter Navigationssysteme in der computergestützten Chirurgie. Mund Kiefer GesichtsChir, 2, pp. 145-148.
[8]   Queck, J. (2001): Ein navigierter mobiler Computertomograph für medizinische Anwendungen. Dissertation an der TU Berlin, in print.
[9]   Schermeier, O., D. Hildebrand, T. C. Lueth, D. Szymanski, J. Bier: Accuracy of an Image Guided System for Oral Implantology. Computer Assisted Radiology and Surgery (CARS), Berlin, Germany, June, 2001.
[10] Schermeier, O., R. Tita, J. Glagau, D. Hildebrand, M. Klein, J. Bier, T. Lüth (2001): Navigierte Insertion von Dentalimplantaten mit dem Behandlungssystem RoboDent. Automed2001, Bochum, Germany, Sep. 17., 18.
[11] Stien, M., T. Schubert, D. Szymanski, T. C. Lueth (2000): A System for Monitoring Robot-Assisted Surgical Interventions. Advanced Robotics and its Applications, Shanghai, China, 5./6. 10., pp. 6.

Medicine Meets Virtual Reality 02/10
J.D. Westwood et al. (Eds.)
IOS Press, 2002

Exploratory Design and Evaluation of a User Interface for Virtual Reality Exposure Therapy

Martijn J. Schuemie MSc.[1], Charles A.P.G. van der Mast Ph.D.[1], Merel Krijn MA.[2],
Paul M.G. Emmelkamp Ph.D.[2]
*[1] Department of Mediamatics, Delft University of Technology, Mekelweg 4, 2628 CD,
Delft, the Netherlands*
*[2] Department of Clinical Psychology, University of Amsterdam, Roetersstraat 15,
1018 WB, Amsterdam, the Netherlands*

Abstract. Virtual reality exposure therapy is slowly becoming a viable option for therapists. For virtual reality systems to be used in the daily practice of therapists, their usability needs to be taken into consideration. This paper describes the current state-of-the-art in interfaces for these systems, and describes several proposals for improving the design of these systems. An exploratory evaluation is performed to assess the merits of aspects of the proposed user interface.

1. Introduction

Already a great number of studies have shown virtual reality to be effective in the treatment of phobias such as acrophobia [1][2][3][4], claustrophobia [5], arachnophobia [6], agoraphobia [7] and fear of flying [8][9]. Slowly, Virtual Reality Exposure Therapy (VRET) is becoming a viable and acceptable option for therapists. When compared to current standard in vivo therapy, VRET can be less expensive, less intimidating for the patient and can provide the therapist with greater control of the stimuli with which the patient is confronted.

Currently, most research has been focused on proving the effectiveness of VRET. However, for VRET to become accepted in the daily practice of the therapist, the system should be easy to use for both therapist and patient. Our research is focused on improving the usability of VRET. For this, we have looked at the user interfaces of current VRET systems, and have made an analysis of the user interaction during virtual reality therapy sessions to identify possibilities for enhancing the user interface. This article describes our exploratory research into options for improving the user interface design of such systems.

2. Current VRET systems

An investigation into the user interfaces of existing systems for VRET, based on a web-based questionnaire and personal inquiry at the several suppliers of these systems, shows that these interfaces are quite similar and of a simple design. Table 1 shows an overview of the systems included in this research.

Without exception, these systems use a Head Mounted Display (HMD) to immerse the patient in the Virtual Environment (VE). The exact same view that is provided for the patient is also shown on a standard monitor for the therapist. In five of the seven systems, the therapist could alter certain elements of the VE during the exposure by keystrokes on the keyboard. In three systems, the therapist could also control the viewpoint of the patient, often by use of a joystick or similar input device.

The patient could look around in the world by use of a tracking device attached to the HMD. In case the VE consisted of a driving simulation, the patient was provided with appropriate steering controls. In some cases, the user was provided with a tracked device to interact with objects in the VE.

Table 1: Overview of commercially available systems for treatment of phobias

Name System	*URL website*	*Phobias (other disorders)*	
Hanyang University	bme.hanyang.ac.kr/vr	Acrophobia Fear of driving	Fear of speaking Agoraphobia
Virtually Better	www.virtuallybetter.com	Acrophobia Fear of flying Fear of speaking Agoraphobia	Fear of thunderstorms (Post traumatic stress disorder for Vietnam veterans)
VRHealth	www.vrhealth.com	Claustrophobia (Panic disorders)	(Eating disorders)
Previ	www.previsl.com	Fear of Flying Claustrophobia	(Eating disorders)
DriVR	www.driVR.com	Fear of Driving	
VRT-2002	science.kennesaw.edu/ ~mnorth/vrt1/vrt1.html	Acrophobia Fear of flying Agoraphobia	(Obsessive Compulsive disorders) (Attention Deficit Disorders)
CYBERmed	www.insight.co.at	Fear of flying	

To investigate the usability of these systems in more detail we created a virtual reality testbed configuration [10] with which different types of user interfaces can be tested. The testbed was configured to offer a user interface similar to the interfaces found in the systems described above. A usability study and a task analysis were made based on the observations of several therapists using this system in treatment of acrophobia [11].

The task analysis showed that by far the most frequent activity during VRET is determining the fear level of the patient by the therapist. Further usability analysis also showed that therapists have to memorize several arbitrary keyboard commands to control the VE, thus increasing the memory load and training time for the therapist on each VE. Another problem was that the therapist's view of the VE was restricted to the view of the patient, which was determined by the looking direction of the patient. Combined with the fact that the patient could also move him/herself within a limited range in the VE through use of the headtracking this made navigating the patient through the VE sometimes difficult for the therapist.

3. Proposed user interface

Research has indicated that interaction can increase the sense of presence [12]. Presence is seen by some as a key element in VRET. To enhance the sense of presence, patients are provided with a means to navigate themselves through the VE. For this, we used a technique based on the position of the HMD. If the patient stepped out of the middle of his or her moving space, (s)he would automatically start to move in that direction in the VE with a constant velocity. This motion would stop either when the patient stepped back, or when the patient collided with an obstacle (e.g. a wall) in the VE.

In the reviewed systems there was no specific screen for the therapist. Because the same image was projected both in the HMD and on the monitor, extra information for the therapist could not be included because this would also show in the HMD. Using our testbed we created a separate screen for the therapist by including a second computer that could communicate over the network with the virtual reality station generating the stereoscopic images for the HMD.

Based on the findings of our aforementioned study, we designed a user interface specifically for the therapist. Figure 1 shows an overview of the screen presented to the therapist. Through use of the familiar Window Icon Mouse Pointer (WIMP) metaphor the therapist could control the various parts of the graphical user interface. The two three-dimensional views in the middle of the screen displayed the VE from the viewpoint of the patient (top) and from a second, external viewpoint (bottom). Furthermore, patient name and session-number could be stored with additional treatment data and a clock was provided to keep track of session time.

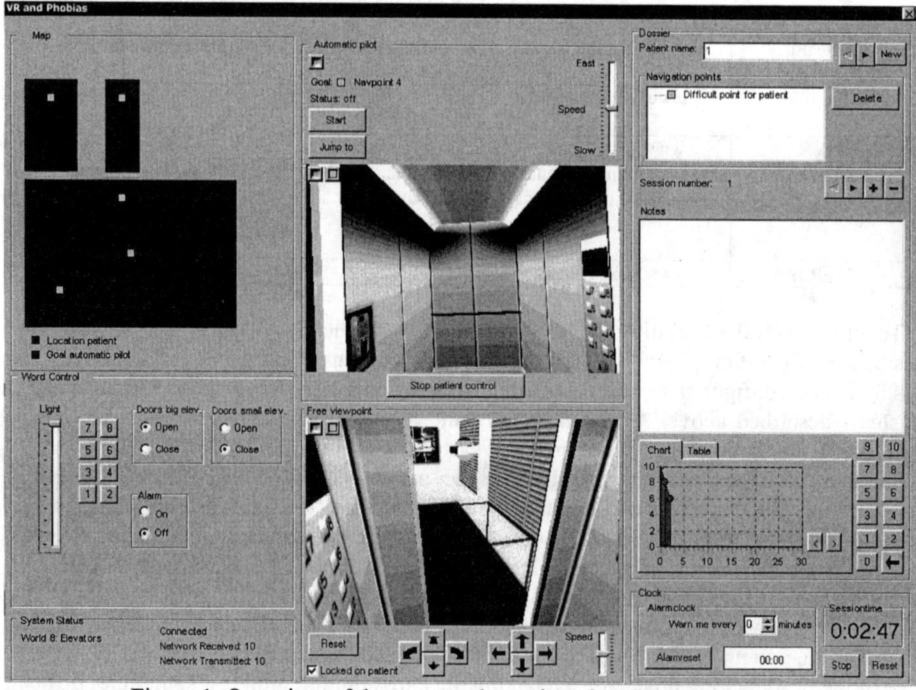

Figure 1: Overview of the proposed user interface for the therapist

3.1 SUDs recording

During therapy, patients are often asked to report their current level of anxiety on a scale from zero to ten, where zero means not anxious at all and ten indicates the highest level of fear the patient can imagine. Such Subjective Units of Discomfort (SUDs) are used by therapist to determine amongst others whether the fear has diminished during the exposure treatment.

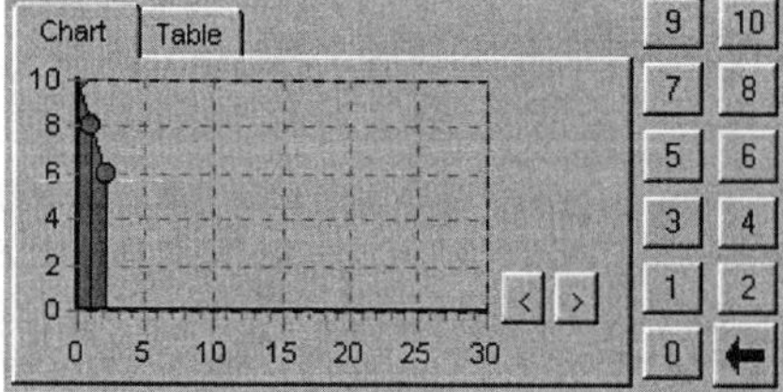

Figure 2: Tool for keeping track of SUDs

Figure 2 show the tool designed to keep track of these SUDs. By clicking on one of the numbers the SUD as well as the time is recorded and displayed either on a chart or in the form of a table. The back arrow could be clicked to erase the last SUD notation.

3.2 Automatic pilot

Even though the patient could also move him/herself through the VE, the therapist was also provided with several controls to manipulate the patient's location. One way was through use of the automatic pilot that could be programmed by dropping a token ▢ representing a location in the VE on the widget ◩ of the autopilot panel displayed in figure 3. By pressing the 'start' button the patient would gradually be moved to the location at the speed set with the speed control. By pressing 'jump to' the patient would immediately be teleported to that location. The location tokens could be picked up from the two-dimensional map of the VE and could be stored and retrieved from the patient dossier so the therapist could later return with a patient to a specific situation.

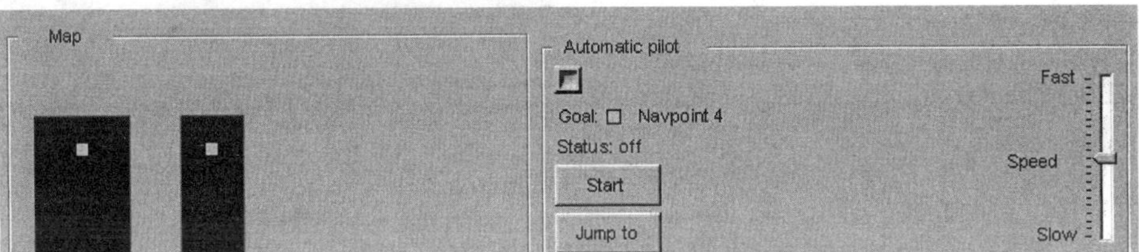

Figure 3: A part of the two-dimension map (left) and the control for the automatic pilot (right)

3.3 Free viewpoint

To solve the navigation problems experienced by some therapists, an external viewpoint was provided as shown in figure 4. This viewpoint was by default locked on the patient, showing the viewpoint of the patient in the shape of a head wearing an HMD.

In reality a railing surrounded the patient, and this railing was also represented in the external view. This not only enabled the therapist to determine where the patient was standing within the railing without looking up, but it also made it possible for the therapist to determine when a virtual railing corresponded to the real railing, thus creating the illusion that the patient could physically touch the virtual railing.

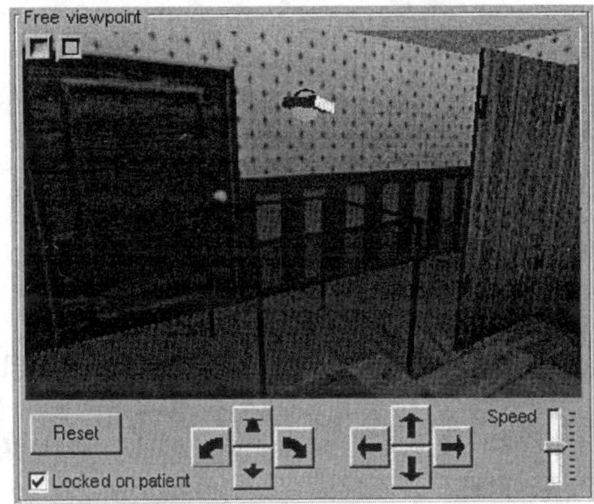

Figure 4: Extra viewpoint displaying the VE as well as a representation of the HMD and the railing surrounding the patient in reality

Controls to alter the viewing direction were also provided, configured according to guidelines set for these types of interfaces [13].

4. Method

A user interface was designed to represent the current state-of-the-art as described in section 2. This user interface (UI1) and the proposed new design (UI2) were used for exposure therapy on 27 students diagnosed as having a reasonable amount of acrophobia or claustrophobia. The therapy was performed by six students of the clinical psychology department trained in phobia treatment. For acrophobia treatment our VEs of a construction site, firestairs and rooftop terrace were used in combination with UI1. For claustrophobia treatment a virtual elevator, closet and narrow hallway were used in combination with UI2.

Questionnaires for both 'patients' and 'therapists' were used to acquire insight into the overall system usability and the usability of specific elements of the user interface. The patients were also required to fill in the Igroup Presence Questionnaire [14]. Additionally, the therapists were interviewed based on videorecordings of the treatment sessions.

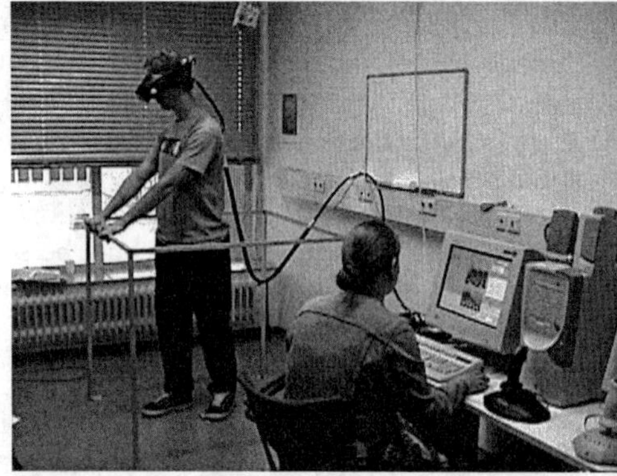

Figure 5: The test environment with a patient standing in the railing wearing the HMD, and a therapist behind the controls.

5. Results

In all, 3 students performing the therapy were interviewed. Two of these preferred UI2 to UI1. The other student indicated that her preference for UI1 was primarily based on the fact that the acrophobia worlds provided better possibilities for the exposure therapy; it was possible to increase the fear for the patient more gradually and to a higher extent. Interestingly, this student did rate UI2 much higher on our questionnaire with questions regarding sense of control during the session, ease of use of the system and whether it was subjectively pleasing to use the system. The other students rated both user interfaces equally.

Analysis of the questionnaires and interviews indicated that several elements of the proposed design were found helpful in the therapy. The SUDs registration tool was most popular, receiving 5 out of 5 points both for being used frequently and for easy of use.

The students indicated that the automatic pilot was hardly used at all. This was because the patient could navigate him/herself through the virtual environment. The students reported the autopilot to be moderately easy to use, and that they could achieve their goals with the automatic pilot. Storing certain locations for later use with that patient was never used because patients were never exposed to the same VE twice.

The external viewpoint was considered useful (average 4 out of 5 points). Users commented that the viewpoint increased their overview of the situation, reduced the need to look at the patient directly and facilitated moving the patients in tight spots. However, none of the students ever used the controls to change the viewpoint. The main reason given for this was that the controls were too complicated.

The fact that the patients could navigate themselves in UI2 was evaluated positively by the therapists (average 4 out of 5 points). Due to an error in filling in the questionnaires, only 4 of the patients treated with UI1 actually filled in the usability questionnaire, compared to 14 using UI2. Nevertheless, a one-way-ANOVA showed scores to be significantly lower (p=.008) for UI2 in response to the question whether the interventions of the therapists in the controls were considered to be annoying. Also interesting is that subjects using UI2 scored almost significantly higher on questions regarding how much they looked around in the VE (p=.058) and the ease with which they could do this (p=.087).

The presence experienced by the patients, as measured with the IPQ, did not differ significantly between conditions.

6. Conclusions

The fact that the different types of user interfaces were used for treatment of different phobias made comparison between the systems difficult. As expected, responses showed usability to be not only a function of the type of user interface but also of the design of the VE itself. However, qualitative insight was gained into the contribution of several user interface design elements to system usability. The tool for recording SUDs as well as the external viewpoint were evaluated positively in terms of their usability. It is also clear that the controls for changing the external viewpoints need to be simplified before therapists will use them.

The patient's navigation control was considered to enhance usability, both for therapists and patients. However, this type of interaction had no measurable effect on the sense of presence that the patients experienced.

The study reported here is, of course, only of an exploratory nature. Future experiments are planned to provide more quantitative insight in the way in which the usability of VRET systems can be improved.

References

[1] B.O. Rothbaum, L.F. Hodges, R. Kooper, D. Opdyke, J. Williford, M.M. North, Effectiveness of computer-generated (virtual reality) graded exposure in the treatment of acrophobia, *American Journal of Psychiatry* 152,4, pp.626-628, 1995

[2] M.J. Schuemie, M. Bruynzeel, L. Drost, M. Brinckman, G. de Haan, P.M.G. Emmelkamp, C.A.P.G van der Mast, Treatment of Acrophobia in Virtual Reality: a Pilot Study, F. Broeckx and L. Pauwels (Eds.) *Proceedings of the Euromedia 2000 Conference*, May 8-10, Antwerp Belgium, pp.271-275, 2000

[3] P.M.G. Emmelkamp, M. Bruynzeel, L. Drost, C.A.P.G. van der Mast, Virtual Reality Treatment in Acrophobia: A Comparison with Exposure in Vivo, *Cyberpsychology and Behavior*, Vol.4, No.3, pp.335-341, June 2001

[4] P.M.G.Emmelkamp, M. Krijn, L. Hulsbosch, S. de Vries, M.J. Schuemie, C.A.P.G. van der Mast, Virtual Reality Treatment versus exposure in vivo: A Comparative Evaluation in Acrophobia, *Behaviour Research & Therapy* (in press)

[5] M. Alcaniz, R.M. Banos, C. Botella, C. Perpina, A. Rey, H. Villa, Virtual Reality Treatment of Claustropobia, *Behaviour Research & Therapy*, Vol.36, No.2, pp.239-246, Februari 1998

[6] A.S. Carlin, H.G. Hoffman, S. Weghorst, Virtual Reality and Tactile Augmentation in the Treatment of Spider Phobia: A Case Study, *Behaviour Research and Therapy*, Februari 1997

[7] J.R. Coble, M.M. North, S.M. North, Effectiveness of virtual reality environment desensitization in the treatment of agoraphobia, *International Journal of Virtual Reality*, Vol.1, No.2, pp.25-34, 1995

[8] D.N. Chorofas , L.F. Hodges, G.D. Kessler, D. Opdyke, B.A. Watson, Virtual Reality exposure therapy in the treatment of fear of flying: a case report, *Behaviour Research & Therapy*, Vol.34, 1996

[9] B.O. Rothbaum, L.F. Hodges, S. Smith, J.H. Lee, A Controlled Study of Virtual Reality Exposure Therapy for the Fear of Flying, Journal of Consulting and Clinical Psychology, Vol.68, No.6, pp.1020-1026, 2000

[10] M.J. Schuemie, C.A.P.G. van der Mast, 2001, VR Testbed Configuration for Phobia Treatment Research, in: M.E. Domingo, J.C.G. Cebollada & C.P. Salvador (Eds.), *Proceedings of the Euromedia 2001 Conference*, April 18-20, Valencia, Spain, pp.200-204, 2001

[11] M.J. Schuemie, Design of Virtual Reality Exposure Therapy Systems - Task Analysis, *CHI 2000 Extended Abstracts*, ACM press, 2000, pp. 354-346, 2000

[12] M.J. Schuemie, P. van der Straaten, M. Krijn. C.A.P.G. van der Mast, Research on Presence in VR: a Survey, *Cyberpsychology and Behavior*, Vol.4, No.2, April 2001, pp.183-202

[13] H.M. Sayers, S. Wilson, W. Myles, M.D.J. McNeil, Navigation in Non-Immersive Virtual Environments, Proceedings of the 7th UK VRSIG Conference, pp.43-53, University of Strathclyde, Glasgow, Scotland, 2000

[14] T.W. Schubert, F. Friedman, H.T. Regenbrecht, Decomposing the sense of presence: Factor analytic insights, *Presented at the second international workshop on presence*, University of Essex, UK, 6-7 april 1999

Medicine Meets Virtual Reality 02/10
J.D. Westwood et al. (Eds.)
IOS Press, 2002

Limits of Human Perception of Haptic Information in Minimally Invasive Surgery Tools for Use in Simulation

A. Seehusen and A. Harrison
University of Bristol
Department of Mechanical Engineering
Queen's Building, University Walk
Bristol, UK BS2 8EW

Abstract. This research looks at the human ability to perceive haptic information when using Minimally Invasive Surgery (MIS) tools. In the simulation of MIS it is important to understand what haptic information can be perceived by a user. Understanding what can be felt allows the force feedback system of the simulator to be optimized.

1. Introduction

Haptic force feedback systems are important to the realism of surgical simulators as they increase a user's ability to become immersed in a virtual surgical environment. [1-3] In addition, finding the limits of human haptic perception helps to determine the limits of haptic reproduction that are necessary in a simulator. The human hand is not capable of feeling every aspect of the haptic information present at the handle of a MIS tool. The sensors located in the skin limit human sensing. The sensors have limits on frequency, amplitude, spatial and relative nature of the stimuli that they can detect. [4-7] These limits were explored in this research, and the ability to detect small changes in frequency and amplitude of a repeating signal at various frequencies was determined. Also, the ability to discriminate between two closely spaced impulses and to distinguish between waveforms was determined. Knowledge of human haptic perception will allow the force feedback system of a MIS simulator to be optimized and will prevent over design.

2. Methods

A testing rig was constructed using a MIS tool cut in the middle and attached to a linear actuator (Linear Drives, Ltd Thrust Tube 2504). The linear actuator controls the scissor action of the tool handle.

For the frequency and amplitude tests the rig generated sets of sinusoidal pulses. Each set of pulses was two seconds in duration and was separated from the next set by a pause, also of two seconds. For each pair of sets the frequency or force amplitude of the second set was either increased or decreased by a specific percentage. This was done over a range of frequencies and at different force amplitudes. It was then determined whether a test subject could feel the changes in frequency and amplitude.

For the impulse test, a test subject was sent sets of two sharp pulses which were separated by a steadily increasing delay. The test subject determined whether two signals could be felt instead of one.

The waveform test sent different waveforms to the test subjects to see if one could be distinguished from another. These waveforms were created using sine waves plus increasing odd harmonics waves. During each test the subject was asked to distinguish between two waveforms at several different frequencies.

3. Results

For both the frequency and amplitude tests, perception of change was poor at 1Hz, but rose at 2Hz and then dropped off again after 8Hz. A 12% change in frequency was generally detectable over 2-8 Hz, however, there was a large rise in confidence of perception at percentages of 16% and 20%. An 8% change in amplitude was not always felt, but a change of 11% was consistently perceived. It was also determined for both frequency and amplitude tests that perception rises slightly with an increase in force amplitude from 4-10N.

The impulse test showed that when the delay between the pulses exceeded 0.02s, two pulses could be felt. From this information, human perception can be modeled using a second order critically damped system with the time constant of 0.085 seconds.

For the waveform test, it was believed that harmonics present in the waveforms would stop being perceived at certain underlying sine wave frequencies. However, this was not proved to be true so alternative methods of analysis were considered. It was then found that the difference in rate of force change for each waveform determined whether or not two waves could be distinguished. The difference required to be felt increased as the base frequency of the waveforms increased.

4. Conclusions

Together these haptic data begin to indicate what humans can and cannot feel when manipulating Minimally Invasive Surgery tools. They will allow the demand on haptic systems to be minimized and system designs to be optimized.

References

[1] Barfield, W. & Hendrix, C. 1995, "Factors affecting presence and performance in virtual environments," in *Interactive Technology and the New Paradigm for Healthcare*, K. Morgan & R. M. Satava, eds., IOS Press and Ohmsha, Amsterdam, pp. 21-28.

[2] Cotin, S., Delingette, H., & et al. 1996, "Geometric and physical representations for a simulator of hepatic surgery," in *Health Care in the Information Age*, H. Sieburg, S. Weghorst, & et al., eds., IOS Press and Ohmsha, Amsterdam, pp. 139-151.

[3] Rosenberg, L. 1995, "Human interface hardware for virtual laparoscopic surgery," in *Interactive Technology and the New Paradigm for Healthcare*, K. Morgan, R. M. Satava, & et al., eds., IOS Press and Ohmsha, Amsterdam, pp. 322-325.

[4] Johansson, R. 1976, "Skin Mechanoreceptors in the human hand: receptive field characteristics," in *Sensory functions of the skin in primates with special reference to man*, vol. 27 Y. Zotterman, ed., Pergamon Press, Oxford, pp. 159-170

[5] Stone, R. 1997, *A distributive tactile sensing technique for soft deformable contact*, Ph.D., University of Bristol.

[6]. Sinclair, D. 1981, *Mechanisms of cutaneous sensation*, 2 edn, Oxford University Press, Oxford.

[7] Vallbo, A. & Johansson, R. 1978, "The tactile sensory innervation of the glabrous skin of the human hand," in *Active Touch*, C. Gordon, ed., Pergamon Press, Oxford, pp. 29-51.

Medicine Meets Virtual Reality 02/10
J.D. Westwood et al. (Eds.)
IOS Press, 2002

The DextroBeam:
a stereoscopic presentation system
for volumetric medical data

Luis Serra[1], Ralf Kockro[1,2], Goh Lin Chia[1], Ng Hern[1] and Eugene Chee Keong Lee[1]

1. Volume Interactions Pte Ltd, 5 Shenton Way #37-04, Singapore 068808
2. Department of Neurosurgery, National Neuroscience Institute, Singapore 308433

Abstract. This paper describes an interaction system called the DextroBeam designed for manipulating objects in 3D space while looking at a 3D stereoscopic display located in front of the user. Three-dimensional interaction is two-handed and is achieved by means of a stylus with a single button or switch. We have been planning several neurosurgical cases with the DextroBeam, including the separation of Nepalese Siamese twins in April 2001, and have conducted a course on surgery of the Temporal Bone (as part of the 9th ASEAN ORL Head and Neck Congress in Singapore, March 2001).

1.   Motivation

Over the past years we have been using the VR environment of the Dextroscope to plan neurosurgery with patient specific 3D reconstructions of fused MR and CT data [4][7]. The Dextroscope is a personal workstation that presents stereoscopic 3D data via a mirror reflection in a virtual workspace, which allows precise and hand-eye co-located manipulation in real-time, by reaching into the 3D data with both hands. This interface offers a suitable discussion platform for of up to three people, beyond which the display becomes too small for comfortable work.

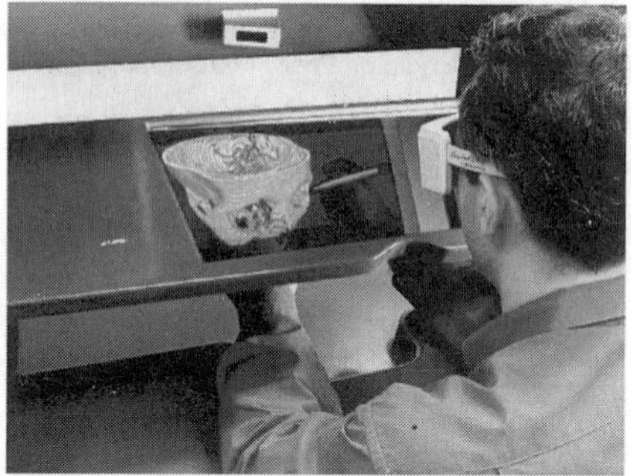

Figure 1.   The Dextroscope: the user looks into a mirror and sees the virtual object floating in front

There has been increasing interest among clinicians to extend the collaborative discussions with 3D patient data to more than three people, in particular for radiological discussions. Since the set-up of the Dextroscope is inadequate for this purpose, the first work around to this limitation was to project the graphics onto a large projection screen, while keeping the Dextroscope as the interactive console. The result was awkward, since the person interacting was detached from the group of clinicians viewing the projection screen, and thus could not react to their input.

We were thus confronted with the question of how to provide a way for 3D collaborative discussion while maintaining the benefits of 3D paradigm of interaction provided by the Dextroscope? Our solution was the DextroBeam.

2.　The DextroBeam

The DextroBeam replaces the monitor and mirror set-up of the Dextroscope with a screen projection system positioned in front of the user. Instead of looking where the hands are as in the Dextroscope, the user looks ahead at large stereoscopic screen projections while working with the virtual data as though it was in reach of the hands. The DextroBeam provides support for the user's arms to facilitate interactions in the 3D space. It also provides a surface required for the control of 2D widgets in a similar way to [8]. This design is a compromise that ensures comfortable interactions in 3D space and efficient and unambiguous operation of 2D widgets while addressing a large audience. This is done at the expense of hand-eye co-location.

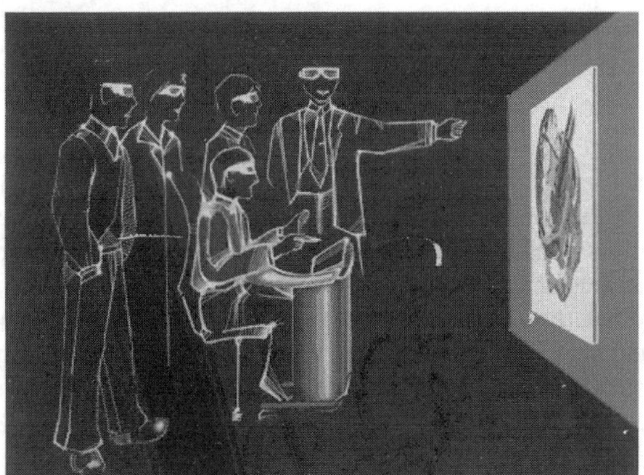

Figure 2.　　A typical scenario of interaction using the DextroBeam

3.　Background

This approach was chosen against the exisiting variety of interaction devices and methods in the literature because of its superior comfort and efficiency of interaction. It combines interaction with 3D objects by using simple hand-held 3D pointers and comfortable arms-rest, with widget control by means of a surface that provides mouse-like interactions.

Glove-based systems were found uncomfortable and cumbersome to wear in comparison to hand-held pointers [6]. Another device, the Cubic Mouse, although allowing freedom of movement, is bulky, needs to be held with both hands and also requires the user to learn multiple controls [1]. Another method to overcome the problems of interacting with controls in free space is the hand-held pen and tablet, the tablet providing the necessary passive haptic feedback in operating buttons [9]. The shortcoming, however, is having to devote one hand to holding the tablet.

In the case of 3D pointer-based systems, the issue is how to control the application widgets. If one uses a physical button on the 3D input device itself, activating the virtual button tends to lead d to errors in selection since the physical pressure on the button tends to shift the device and its pointed target. This is typically the case with the "virtual ray" approach [for example [3]]. Without the aid of anything to steady the hands, it is difficult to make precise movements, such as hitting a button or worse, dragging a slider to a specific point. The user has to hold the input devices while trying to perform intricate operations, which can be difficult to do, tiring and hard to sustain for long periods.

4.   Operation of the DextroBeam

The entire space of interaction is divided by the software into 3D space and 2D space as shown below.

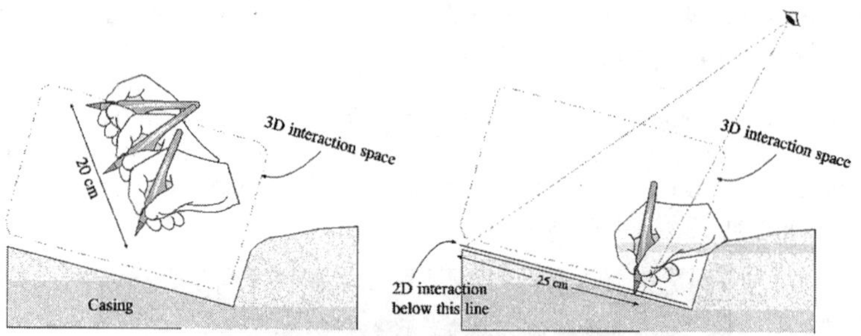

Figure 3.   Division of interaction space

As in the Dextroscope, the user interacts with the 3D objects using both hands, one holding a single-button stylus held in the hand and the other a 3D joystick. With the lower arms supported and the hands pivoted at the wrists, the user can reach a sufficiently large volume comfortably and naturally. When access to the application controls is required, the user touches the surface of the control panel with the tip of the stylus, triggering the display of the 2D panel. When the 2D panel with the widgets is not active it is not visible, to speed up performance and also to avoid confusion caused by cluttering the screen with too many objects. The physical surfaces provide a hard medium against which the buttons can be pushed unequivocally.

In the DextroBeam, unlike in the Dextroscope, the user sees the virtual objects floating, but sees the stylus moving in synchronism with the hand in a hand-eye coordinated manner, but not co-located. When touching the bottom surface, the user sees a virtual representation of the 2D interface plane, and interacts with the buttons and sliders there using the stylus.

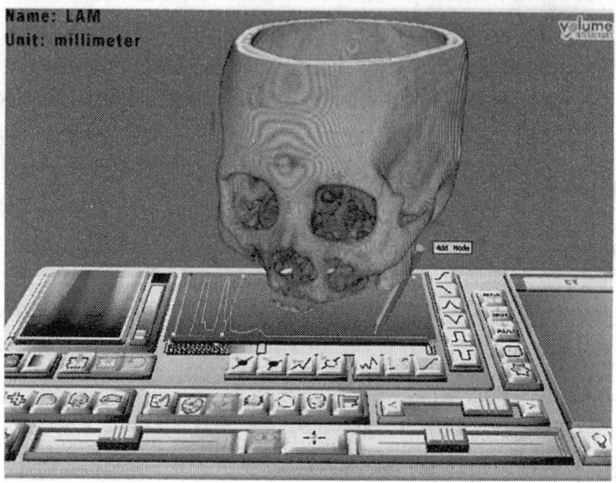

Figure 4.   The DextroBeam. What the user sees.

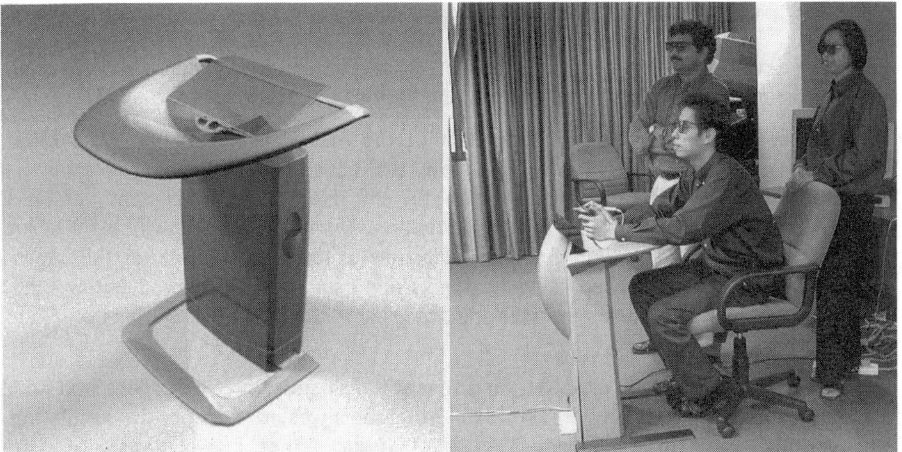

Figure 5.　　The DextroBeam: Left: The console. Right: Users in action.

5.　　Planning the separation of the Nepalese Craniopagus Twins

We are using the DextroBeam as a collaborative environment to allow a group of specialists to discuss, plan or train certain surgical procedures. The necessary segmentation procedures, either centred on patient-specific data or models (like in the case of the virtual temporal bone), are usually carried out beforehand in the Dextroscope, since it allows superior hand-eye coordination.

In the case of the planning of surgical separation of the conjoined craniopagus Nepalese twins in Singapore in April 2001 [2], we used the segmentation tools of the Dextroscope to segment the four brain hemispheres, the brain stems, and cerebella. Once this segmentation was done, the neurosurgical team in charge of the operation met around the DextroBeam to discuss the case. The 3D segmentation and measurement tools as well as the large stereoscopic working environment revealed to be crucial for the planning, since the pathological complexity of the case significantly challenged the spatial comprehension of radiologists and surgeons.

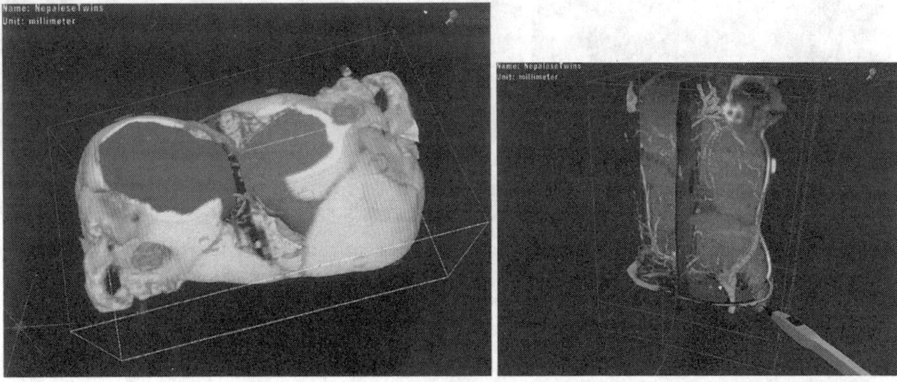

Figure 6.　　The Craniopagus Twins. Left: CT and MRA with segmented brain hemispheres obtained from MRI. Right: MRI (in triplanar mode) and volume rendered MRA displayed together.

6.   The Virtual Temporal Bone

We have developed a detailed model of the Virtual Temporal Bone and cerebello-pontine angle for the purpose of simulation and training various skull base approaches [5].

The model is based on the imaging data of the male Visible Human Data (VHD). Volumetric rendering of the CT generated the virtual bone. Using segmentation tools in the Dextroscope and the VHD photographic data, the soft tissue of the brain stem, vessels and cranial nerves were modelled as polygonal structures. Minute structures, which were hardly visible in the imaging data like the complete course of the 7th cranial nerve, the labyrinth and the ossicles were modelled using textbooks and cadaver dissections. Lesions such as acoustic schwannomas of different sizes and shapes or petroclival meningiomas were added to provide a training scenario.

The DextroBeam was then used to train different trans petrosal, retro-sigmoid, and middle fossa approaches to the CP angle. A suite of virtual tools was provided for the simulation of bone drilling with different drill sizes, soft tissue removal, adjustment of virtual microscopic viewpoints and measuring.

A course was conducted by the team of the National Neuroscience Institute of Singapore on surgery of the Temporal Bone (as part of the 9th ASEAN ORL Head and Neck Congress in Singapore, March 2001). Groups of 10 to 12 surgeons were trained on surgical procedures by employing virtual tools for bone drilling, soft tissue removal and microscopic viewing. It was found to provide a unique way to view and discuss the complexity of anatomical and pathological spatial relationships in relation to different surgical corridors. The integration of the system in a temporal bone and skull base workshop has shown, that it offers a valuable supplementation to cadaver dissections.

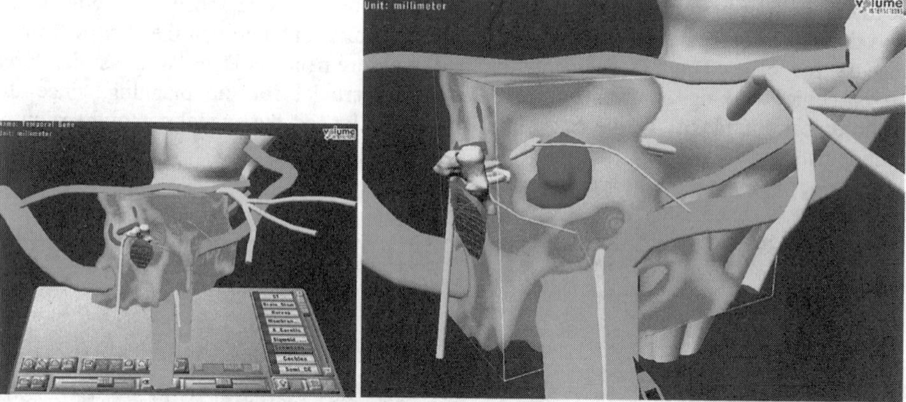

Figure 7.   Model of the Virtual Temporal Bone. Left: The bone in the centre, the conjunct venous sinuses, the course of the carotid artery, the brain stem and cranial nerves. Right: magnified view of the middle and inner ear showing the ossicles (left) and the cochlea (centre).

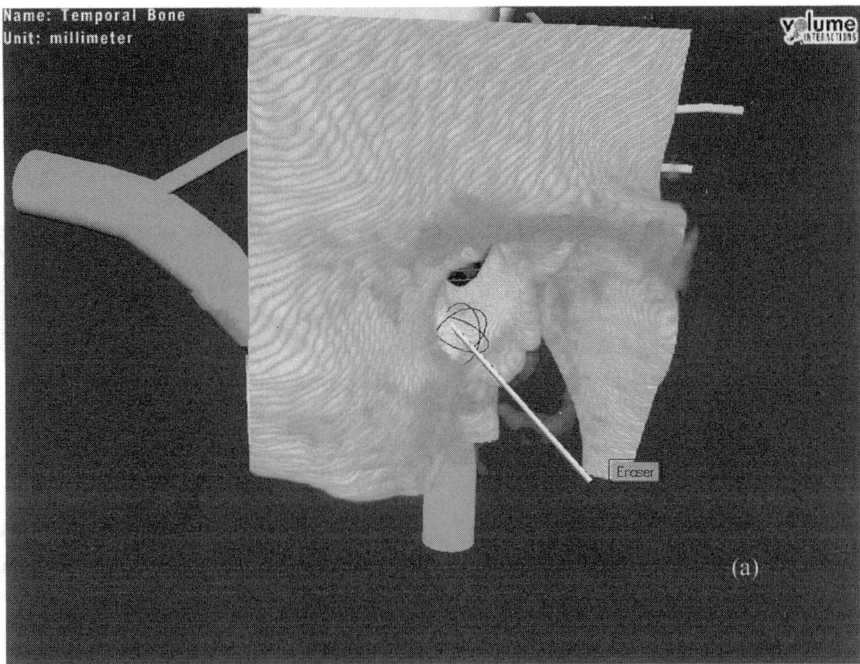

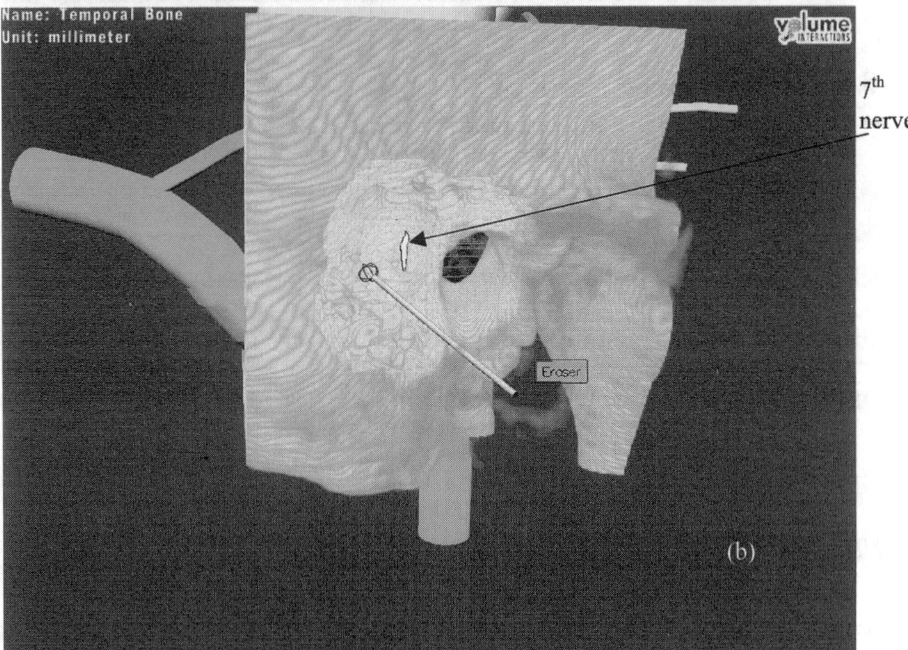

Figure 8. Drilling into the Virtual Temporal Bone. (a) Bone drilling starts behind the ear. (b) Exposure of the 7th cranial nerve (pointed by arrow).

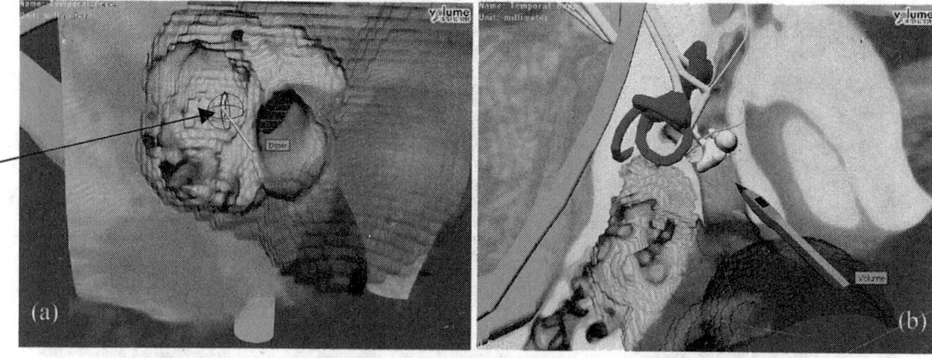

Figure 9.		Drilling into the Virtual Temporal Bone. (a) Magnified view of Figure 8b.
(b) Superior view revealing the inner ear structures to check on the progress of the simulation.
The craniotomy is extending towards the semicircular canals.

7.   Conclusion

We have designed an interactive console called the DextroBeam intended to reach a large audience while maintaining the 3D interactivity of the Dextroscope. This design ensures precise and comfortable interactions in 3D space, as well as efficient and unambiguous operation of 2D widgets.

The DextroBeam is installed at the National Neuroscience Institute of Singapore where it is used to hold radiological conferences. We are currently evaluating its clinical impact.

8.   References

[1] Fröhlich B, Plate J, Wind J, Wesche G, Göbel M, Cubic-Mouse-Based Interaction in Virtual Environments, IEEE Computer Graphics and Applications, July/August 2000, Vol. 20, No. 4.

[2] Goh KYC, Kockro RA, Serra L, Rajendra T and Chan C, Virtual Reality Simulation and Intra-operative Neuronavigation in the Surgical Separation of Craniopagus Twins. Medical Imaging and Augmented Reality MIAR 2001, Hong Kong, June 2001.

[3] Green M and Liang K JDCAD: A Highly Interactive 3D Modeling System, Computers and Graphics, 18(4), 1994, 499-506.

[4] Kockro RA, Serra L, YeoTT, Sitoh YY, Chua GG, Ng H, Lee E, Lee YH, Nowinski W: Planning and Simulation of Neurosurgery in a Virtual Reality Environment, Neurosurgery, Vol. 46, No. 1, pp. 118-137.

[5] Kockro RA, Yeo SB, Hwang P, Yeo TT, Goh C, Serra L, The Virtual Temporal Bone: Training of Skull Base Surgery in Virtual Reality Environment, In Proceedings of the conference World Federation of Neurological Surgeons, 2001, Sydney, Australia.

[6] Hinckley K, Pausch R, Goble C J, Kassel NF: A Survey of Design Issues in Spatial Input, Proceedings of ACM UIST'94 Symposium on User Interface Software & Technology, pp. 213-222.

[7] Serra L, Kockro RA, Chua GG, Ng H, Lee E, Lee YH, Chan C and Nowinski, WL, 1998, Multimodal Volume-based Tumor Neurosurgery Planning in the Virtual Workbench. MICCAI 98, Cambridge MA, USA, October 11-13, 1998, pp 1007-1016.

[8] Serra L, Ng H, Chua GG, Lee CK, Lee YH, Yeo TT, Chan C, and Kockro RA, An Interface For Precise And Comfortable 3D Work With Volumetric Medical Datasets, in Medicine Meets Virtual Reality: 7, January 20-23, 1999 - San Francisco, pp. 328-334.

[9] Sowizral H.A., (1994) Interacting with virtual environments using augmented virtual tools, In Proc. Stereoscopic Displays and Virtual Reality Systems 94, SPIE, 2177, pp. 409-416.

Medicine Meets Virtual Reality 02/10
J.D. Westwood et al. (Eds.)
IOS Press, 2002

Interactive Visualization of Four-Dimensional Ultrasound Data

Raj Shekhar and Vladimir Zagrodsky
Department of Biomedical Engineering, The Cleveland Clinic Foundation
Cleveland, Ohio 44195

Abstract. We present a hardware-accelerated method using three-dimensional (3D) textures to visualize four-dimensional (4D) images of the heart. Novel data subdivision and caching ideas enable interactive performance even though 4D data exceed the size of 3D texture memory. The capability to visualize 4D images is critical to continued evolution and clinical acceptance of 4D imaging.

1. Introduction

Acquisition of 4D ultrasound, especially of the heart, is gaining popularity. 4D acquisition is powerful in that it reveals the complex 3D geometry and motion of the heart. Historically, 4D images have been assembled by retrospectively gating planar images taken at multiple locations over multiple heart cycles. Such a gated 4D acquisition is slow and prone to distortions. Real-time 3D acquisition, a faster, more accurate and more convenient alternative, was recently introduced and is an area of active research and development.

Irrespective of the acquisition mechanism, challenges for 4D visualization remain the same. Methods to visualize 4D data must handle large data size (100-300 MB) and maintain a frame rate (20-30 Hz) so as not to alter the underlying heart motion. Important diagnostic cues are derived from the heart motion; maintaining the original heart motion is, therefore, critical to making accurate diagnoses. Additionally, many applications require visualizing two 4D images, either side-by-side or overlaid, simultaneously, thus doubling the data size requirement.

The use of 3D texture mapping hardware for accelerating volume rendering is well reported in the literature [1-2]. Many volume rendering libraries, such as Volumizer by Silicon Graphics, have been built upon this technology. The work reported so far, however, has focused mostly on 3D data. We report here the use of 3D texture mapping hardware as a means to achieve the desired frame rate in 4D visualization. The rendering speed of 3D texture mapping hardware is near instantaneous as long as the image data fit in the accelerated texture memory. The above condition is, however, seldom met when using 4D data. We describe here our novel use of data subdivision and caching schemes to meet challenges unique to 4D visualization. As for terminology, the term "texture memory" will imply "accelerated 3D texture memory" in the remainder of this article.

2. Data Subdivision

A 4D image (>100 MB) is typically larger than the size of the texture memory (32-64 MB) available even on most high-end graphics boards. Therefore, to still be able to use the limited texture memory, we "brick" the 4D data by dividing up each 3D image (or frame) of the sequence into 3D subblocks of identical size. An array of 3D texture objects equal in size to a 3D subblock are created in the texture memory. The required data subblocks are copied to the existing texture objects before and/or during rendering.

Not all data contribute to a visualization task. Data subdivision provides the "granularity" to pick the subblocks that contribute to visualization and discard the ones that do not, thus reducing data requirement. The discarded subblocks are the subblocks either away from the cutting plane in multi-planar reformatting (MPR) (Figure 1) or containing transparent voxels in volume rendering. The size of the subblocks plays a key role in determining the amount of reduced data. In general, smaller-sized subblocks lead to more specific data selection, but they also cause a greater percentage of data duplication because neighboring subblocks must overlap by a single layer of voxels. Computation costs also rise with decreasing subblock size.

3. Caching

The data required for visualization, even after data reduction, may still exceed the available texture memory. In such situations, some data subblocks must be brought into the texture memory, overwriting preexisting ones during rendering. In this sense, the texture memory also functions like a cache if data overflow occurs. Initialization of this cache and the associated cache replacement rules influence the frame rate that can be achieved. There are two features that make the current caching task unique. First of all, unlike most caching applications, the cache items (data subblocks) here are identical in size. Furthermore, due to the periodic (looping) nature of 4D visualization, cache items have identical lag time between their successive usages, i.e., subblocks to render the first frame will be required as frequently as those to render the second frame. The familiar Least-Recently Used and Least-Frequently Used cache replacement rules, which assume disproportionate usage, therefore, offer the worst performance in our case. Our caching strategy is explained below.

We first explain caching for the steady-state or no-interaction case. We treat all but one texture object as residing in the "long-term" cache, whereas the remaining texture object is used for short-term caching. Given a visualization task and its viewing parameters, the subblocks needed per frame for all the frames are determined. The long-term cache is then populated with as many selected subblocks as possible. During rendering, a subblock is first searched in the long-term cache; if unavailable, it is brought into the short-term cache to complete the rendering. We use the term "cache initialization" to refer to the initialization of the long-term cache and "leftover" subblocks to refer to subblocks that are left out of the long-term cache. Cache initialization ensures that the number of leftover subblocks per frame is roughly equal and hence the time spent in short-term caching is equally distributed between frames. If a certain subblock is used more than once per frame, it is given priority in the long-term cache.

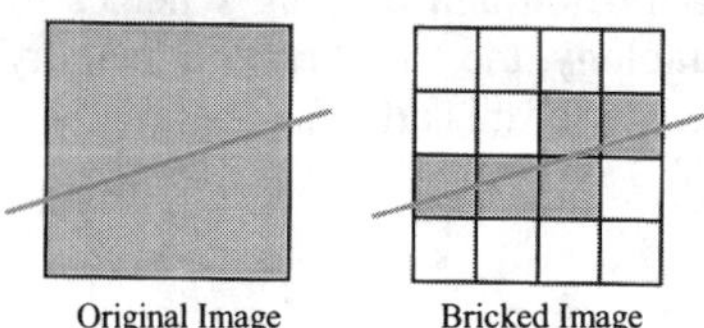

Figure 1 The oblique line shows the plane of MPR. Without data subdivision, the entire data must be copied to the texture memory; only shaded subblocks need to reside in the texture memory following data subdivision.

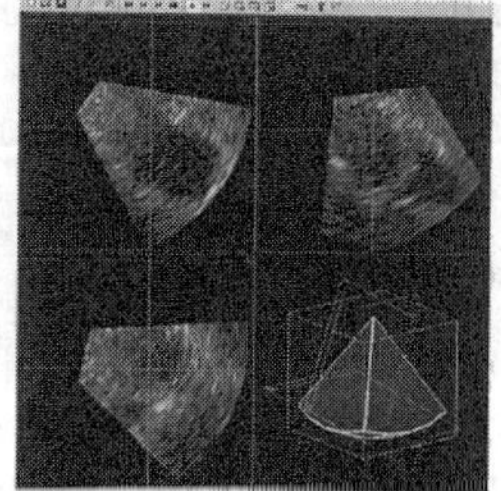

Figure 2 A snapshot of an interactive cine MPR session.

As long as the viewing parameters are unchanged, the contents of the long-term cache stays intact. However, the subblock requirement changes once interaction begins. Although many existing subblocks continue to be needed, a subset of new subblocks emerges and also a subset of existing subblocks is no longer needed. We, therefore, constantly compare the contents of the long-term cache with the continuously changing subblock requirement and update the long-term cache entries such that they are optimal for rendering a few upcoming frames in the current orientation but not the entire sequence. These incremental changes are made in such a way that when the interaction stops, the contents of the long-term cache are restored optimally upon one loop through the sequence.

4. Results

A snapshot of an interactive cine MPR session is shown in Figure 2 ("cine" refers to the looping feature). A reference schematic shows the orientation of the three reformatted planes inside the ultrasound acquisition pyramid and its bounding box. The 4D data set used for the cine MPR demonstration was a sequence of twenty 128 x 128 x 512 3D images. The data size was thus 160 MB. A typical frame rate achieved in conjunction with 3DLabs Wildcat 4210 graphics accelerator board with effectively 64 MB of texture memory for byte data was 30 Hz when all three planes were animated simultaneously. This rate was higher than the desired frame rate of 25 Hz (equal to the acquisition frame rate). The subblock size was 16 x 16 x 32 and each viewport was sized 360 x 360 pixels.

5. Discussion and Conclusions

4D visualization algorithms need to be developed as 4D data acquisition techniques emerge and gain clinical acceptance. 4D visualization is unique in that even in the steady-state, when no user interaction takes place, the rendered views must be animated at the original acquisition frame rate to prevent any motion distortion. The data subdivision and caching schemes presented here provide a general framework to visualize 4D data using the 3D texture mapping hardware. We have used this framework to perform cine MPR of three perpendicular cross-sections through a 4D cardiac data set, as well as other tasks. We have further shown that we can achieve the necessary frame rate in cine MPR visualization. The visualization framework we present offers many advantages: (1) hardware acceleration, (2) handling of one or more 4D data sets at one time, (3) usability across many visualization tasks, (4) capability to use any-sized 4D data on any-sized texture memory, and (5) achievement of higher frame rates. The highest frame rate that can be achieved in a given visualization task depends on a number of factors, namely, the amount of data, the amount of texture memory, the data transfer rate between the system and the texture memories, and the size and number of viewports on the screen. Although the hardware acceleration of texture mapping together with our solutions maximizes the frame rate, limited resources, especially limited texture memory, may not permit achievement of the desired frame rates. Fortunately, texture memory is becoming inexpensive, which is an encouraging trend for continued development of interactive 4D visualization algorithms and techniques.

References

[1] B. Cabral, N. Cam and J. Foran, Accelerated volume rendering of tomographic reconstruction using texture mapping hardware, In: Workshop on Volume Visualization, Washington, DC, 1994, pp. 91-98.
[2] A. Van Gelder and K. Kim, Direct volume rendering with shading via three-dimensional textures, In: *Proc. Symp. Vol. Visual.*, 1996, pp. 23-30.

Medicine Meets Virtual Reality 02/10
J.D. Westwood et al. (Eds.)
IOS Press, 2002

Reshaping Medical Volumetric Data for Enhanced Visualization

D. Silver
Department of Electrical and Computer Engineering
Rutgers, The State University of New Jersey
Piscataway, NJ 08855
silver@caip.rutgers.edu

N. Gagvani
Sarnoff Corporation
201 Washington Road, Princeton, NJ 08540
gagvani@caip.rutgers.edu

Abstract. Three dimensional volume datasets are now commonly produced in the medical sciences. These datasets are generated by observational equipment such as CT, MRI, and ultrasound. There is a significant amount of research in techniques to render these datasets quickly and more realistically. However, there is little or no work on intuitive methods to manipulate volume datasets and volume models. For example, one may want to view a colon stretched out or unraveled. While techniques exist to transform polygonal models, similar techniques are not available for volumetric data. In this work, we describe our methodology to "reshape volumes" and remap existing volumetric datasets using volumetric skeletons. We demonstrate our results by unraveling a 3D colon dataset and discuss the many potential uses of this new visualization methodology.

1. Introduction

Three dimensional volume datasets are commonly produced in the medical and scientific domains. These datasets are generated by observational equipment such as CT, MRI, and ultrasound or are the result of mathematical simulations, such as computational fluid dynamics. There is a significant amount of research in techniques to render these datasets quickly and more realistically. Volume rendering API's are available for many different software packages and there is even special purpose volume rendering hardware [18].

However, there is little or no work on intuitive methods to manipulate volume datasets and volume models. Note that the term *volume dataset* refers to a cubic dataset with *NxMxP* voxels and scalar values at each voxel. An MRI dataset of 512^3 resolution, is one example. The term *volumetric model* or *volume model* refers to a part of the dataset representing a segmented region or model which is of interest. In the literature, the terms volumetric and volume are used interchangeably as adjectives. Furthermore, "volume" refers to both binary and sampled volume datasets. In this document, we generally use the term volume except when it would be ambiguous. The manipulation of volume models includes deformation, animation, smoothing, reshaping and moving/removing parts of volumes for scientific (analysis) and non-scientific (computer graphics) applications. It is hard to pick regions, cull occluding regions, and it is impossible to reshape or rearrange part of a volume dataset. These are tasks that are potentially important for diagnostics and research.

The work on volume modeling and/or volume animation for scientific and non-scientific applications is sparse. The most common solution is to convert a volume models to a polygonal model, then perform the deformations and animations in the polygonal domain. The interior of a model and the intensity values at voxels are lost during this conversion. Other approaches in volume modeling/deformation involve applying a transformation to every voxel in the object such as spring-like models and continuum models [9], finite element methods [19] and landmark deformations [3]. Other approaches include deforming the rendering rays [12] and flat mapping [14]. A more complete review can be found in [5]. However, these methods are not intuitive and most do not give the type of fine user control permitted by the method described in this paper.

2. Methodology

"Volumetric skeletons" are used as the basis of our methodology. The skeleton[1] acts as a ubiquitous abstraction for volume models and allows us to manipulate them in a much more intuitive and general manner. The skeleton is computed from the actual volume using a reversible thinning procedure based upon the distance transform [6]. Polygons are never computed, and the entire process remains in the volume domain. The skeletal points are connected and arranged in a skeleton-tree structure. The key to the deformation process is the reconstruction phase which re-grows the volume model from the skeleton-tree. If the skeleton-tree is deformed, then the corresponding voxels also deform and remap to a new location, thus creating a deformed volume model [7].

The basic steps in this methodology include:
1. *Volume Segmentation:* The first step is to identify the volumetric model which is to be deformed by segmenting the voxels which are part of the model from the background. This creates a binary volume which is the input for thinning. However, the original sampled volume must be maintained for reconstruction. Various segmentation techniques are available for medical images; examples are provided in [16].
2. *Volume thinning*: This process is used to thin the volume model into a smaller set of "representative voxels". The thinned volume retains the essential shape of the original model, and is centered within it. A *parameter-based thinning algorithm* is used to determine the thinned voxels. A distance field is computed over the volumetric model with a 3D Distance Transform [15]. The distance field at a voxel represents the minimum distance from a boundary voxel; therefore a sphere centered at a voxel with a radius equal to its distance field, will touch at least one boundary voxel. A set of voxels, the union of whose spheres touch every boundary voxel, can be used to accurately reconstruct the object. Such a set of thinned voxels and their distance field

---

[1] The term skeleton has many different meanings in different contexts. The volumetric skeleton refers to a thinned version of the original volume and is unconnected. A connected skeleton, or skeleton-tree refers to a connected set of skeleton nodes. An IK-skeleton or a skeleton used for animation is a graph which has joint nodes identified. None of these are the same as the musculo-skeletal structure.

values can be used to compactly represent the object. The number of voxels in the thinned subset determines how accurately the volume can be reconstructed. The thinness of the volumetric skeleton can be controlled by a parameter called the *Thinness Parameter (TP)*. Once the distance field has been computed, the voxels in the volumetric skeleton are identified using the thinness condition, as described in [6].

3. *Connecting the Thinned Voxels*: The set of voxels from the thinning algorithm are unconnected. To perform most manipulations, these voxels must be connected. A number of different algorithms can be employed to get the best connectivity, including minimum spanning tree and clustering, or for more control, manual selection [1,7].

4. *Skeleton Deformation:* Once a connected skeleton results, it can be manipulated and deformed interactively. There are many computer graphics packages which allow the user to manipulate skeletons (examples include popular animation software such as Maya or 3D Studio Max). Furthermore, automatic graph matching or graph relaxing programs can also be used on these skeletons.

5. *Reconstruction*: This step involves retrieving back the deformed volume which is reconstructed from the deformed skeleton. Reconstruction is the inverse of thinning. Since the distance field value at every voxel in the volumetric skeleton is saved along with the voxel position, the volume model can be reconstructed by scan-filling all of the spheres (with radius equal to the distance field) centered at skeletal voxels. The quality of reconstruction depends on the number of voxels in the volumetric skeleton. Better reconstruction is achieved by using a lower thinness parameter during the volume thinning step, giving a thicker skeleton. Sample values are recovered at voxel locations while scan-filling. This is done via an inverse transformation and lookup into the original sampled volume model. When spheres are reconstructed around these transformed skeletal voxels, the model is re-generated in its deformed pose.

6. *Rendering:* Rendering the volume model is the last step. Since the reconstructed model is a volume, any type of volume rendering algorithm can be used, including ray casting, shear-warp, texture mapping, etc.

3. Results

An example of this process to perform "colon unwinding" is shown in Figure 1. In this example, an original colon MRI dataset at resolution 212x150x260 is "unwound" or straightened into a new dataset with a resolution of 991x90x94. In Figure 1a, the original 3D dataset is shown. Figure 1b contains the connected skeleton computed by first thinning the volume and then connecting the resulting thinned voxels. The skeleton is color coded to show which parts of the original volume map to each of the different skeletal segments. The number of skeletal segments can be controlled by the user. Figure 1c shows the coiled skeleton stretched into a line. The deformed volume is then regrown about this line. Two images of the new volume are shown in Figure 1C and 1D. This dataset can be sliced in half, thereby presenting a snapshot encompassing the entire interior of the colon in one image (as opposed to a virtual navigation [10] of the interior which must be stored as a movie). *(The colon dataset is courtesy of R. Robb, Mayo Clinic.)*

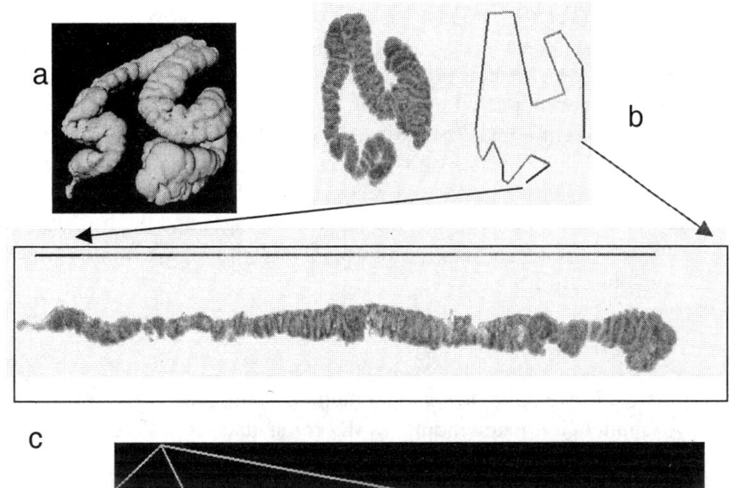

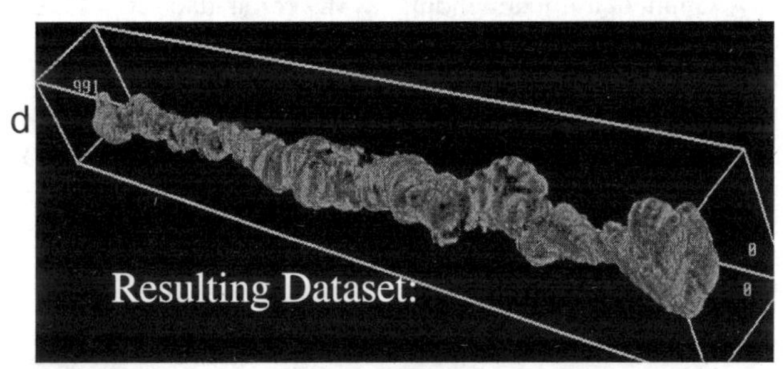

Figure 1. Unwinding the colon. The original colon dataset (a) is 212x150x160. A skeleton was computed (b) and color coded to show the segments of the colon which correspond to the joints in the skeleton. A stretched out colon is shown in (c) and (d). The resulting 3D dataset results is 991x90x94 voxels.

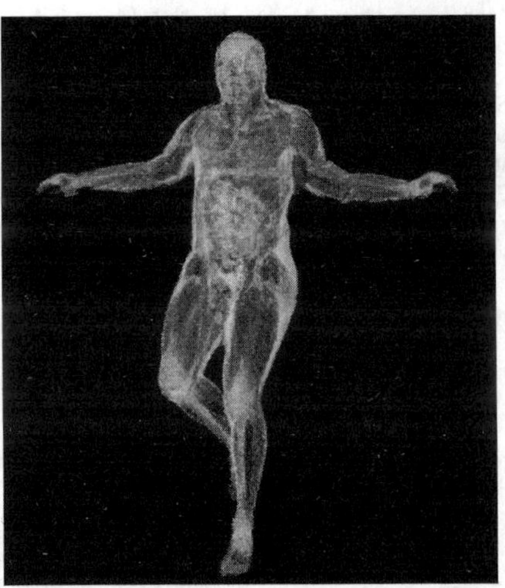

Figure 2. A frame from an animation of the visible human dataset using the methodology described here. The full animation can be seen at
http://www.caip.rutgers.edu/vizlab.html

The skeleton can also be used to remap the voxels to create an animation. This is shown in Figure 2 and described in [5]. In this example, the 3D Visible Human Dataset [17] is used. A skeleton is computed from the volume using the thinning process. This skeleton is then imported into a computer graphics animation package (Character Studio) and motion data is used to animate the skeleton. Figure 2 contains one frame from the animation which consists of a jumping rope sequence. Each frame represents a new 3D visible man dataset which was reconstructed from the animated skeletal poses and then volume rendered to create the movie Other images and the full animations can be seen on the web site: http://www.caip.rutgers.edu/vizlab.html. A full description of the algorithms can be found in [5].

4. Conclusion

In this work, we have presented a method to unravel and deform 3D volume models and have applied it to unwinding a 3D colon dataset. This methodology is based upon computing a reversible volume-based skeleton. The volume-based skeleton and skeleton-tree are powerful and versatile tools which can be used for reshaping or remapping volumes as well as for many other visualization tasks such as collision detection [8], volume morphing, shape matching, virtual navigation and virtual colonoscopy [10], and volume registration [13].

References:
1. A. Bhattacharya, An Interactive Volume Animation Toolkit, MS. Thesis, Rutgers, The State University of New Jersey, October 2001.
2. Character Studio, 3DS MAX, Discreet, Inc. http://www.discreet.com
3. Y. Chen, Q. Zhu, and A. Kaufman, Physically-based Animation of Volumetric Objects. Technical Report TR-CVC-980209, SUNY Stony Brook, February 1998.
4. S. Fang, R. Srinivasan, R. Raghavan, and J. Richtsmeier, Volume Morphing and Rendering -- An Integrated Approach. Computer Aided Geometric Design, 17(1):59--81 January 2000.
5. N. Gagvani and D. Silver, Animating Volumetric Models, Graphical Models, in press, March 2002.
6. N. Gagvani and D. Silver, Parameter Controlled Volume Thinning, Graphical Models and Image Processing, 61(3):149--164, May 1999.
7. N. Gagvani, D. Kenchammana-Hosekote, and D. Silver, Volume Animation Using The Skeleton Tree. Proceedings of IEEE Volume Visualization Symposium, October 1998.
8. N. Gagvani and D. Silver, Shape-based Volumetric Collision Detection. In Proc. IEEE Volume Visualization Symposium, pages 57--61, October 2000.
9. S.F. Gibson and B. Mirtich, A Survey of Deformable Modeling in Computer Graphic Technical Report TR97-19, MERL, November 1997. http://www.merl.com/reports/TR97-19/TR97-19.ps.gz.
10. T. He, S. Wang, and A. Kaufman, Wavelet-Based Volume Morphing, in Proc. Visualization 94, pages 85--92, October 1994.
11. L. Hong, A. Kaufman, Y-C. Wei , A. Viswambharan, M. Wax and Z. Liang, 3D Virtual Colonoscopy, IEEE Symposium on Frontiers in Biomedical Visualization, 1995.
12. Y. Kurzion and R. Yagel, Space Deformation Using Ray Deflectors, 6th Eurographics Workshop on Rendering, 1995, pp. 21-23.
13. A. Liu, S. Pizer, D. Eberly, B. B. Morse, J. Rosenman, E. Chaney, E. Bullitt, and V. Carrasco, Volume Registration using the 3D Core. Visualization in Biomedical Computing, SPIE 2659, pages 217--226, 1994.
14. C. Rezk-Salama, M. Scheuering, G. Soza, and G. Greiner, Fast volumetric Deformation On General Purpose Hardware, in Proc. Eurographics SIGGRAPH Workshop on Graphics Hardware, Los Angeles, August 2001.
15. T. Saito and J. Toriwaki, New Algorithms for Euclidean Distance Transformation of an n-Dimensional Digitized Picture with Applications, Pattern Recognition, volume 27, pages 1551-1565, 1994.

16. A. Singh, D. Goldgof and D Terzopoulos, Deformable Models in Medical Image Analysis, IEEE Computer Society, 1998.
17. The Visible Human Project, National Library of Medicine, http://www.nlm.nih.gov.
18. VolumePro Board, RTVis, www.rtvis.com, 1998.
19. W. Zhongke and E.C. Prakash. Visible Human Walk: Bringing Life Back to the Dead Body, in Proc. International Workshop on Volume Graphics, March 1999.

Medicine Meets Virtual Reality 02/10
J.D. Westwood et al. (Eds.)
IOS Press, 2002

Visualization of conserved structures by fusing highly variable datasets

Jonathan C. Silverstein, Ankur Chhadia, and Fred Dech
University of Chicago, Center for Clinical Information
Room A-105, MC 6051, 5841 S. Maryland Avenue
Chicago, IL 60637-1470
jcs@uchicago.edu, fdech@uchicago.edu, achhad1@uic.edu

Introduction: Skill, effort, and time are required to identify and visualize anatomic structures in three-dimensions from radiological data. Fundamentally, automating these processes requires a technique that uses symbolic information not in the dynamic range of the voxel data. We were developing such a technique based on mutual information for automatic multi-modality image fusion (MIAMI Fuse, University of Michigan). This system previously demonstrated facility at fusing one voxel dataset with integrated symbolic structure information to a CT dataset (different scale and resolution) from the same person. The next step of development of our technique was aimed at accommodating the variability of anatomy from patient to patient by using warping to fuse our standard dataset to arbitrary patient CT datasets.

Methods: A standard symbolic information dataset was created from the full color Visible Human Female by segmenting the liver parenchyma, portal veins, and hepatic veins and overwriting each set of voxels with a fixed color. Two arbitrarily selected patient CT scans of the abdomen were used for reference datasets. We used the warping functions in MIAMI Fuse to align the standard structure data to each patient scan. The key to successful fusion was the focused use of multiple warping control points that place themselves around the structure of interest automatically. The user assigns only a few initial control points to align the scans. Fusion 1 and 2 transformed the atlas with 27 points around the liver to CT1 and CT2 respectively. Fusion 3 transformed the atlas with 45 control points around the liver to CT1 and Fusion 4 transformed the atlas with 5 control points around the portal vein. The CT dataset is augmented with the transformed standard structure dataset, such that the warped structure masks are visualized in combination with the original patient dataset. This combined volume visualization is then rendered interactively in stereo on the ImmersaDesk in an immersive Virtual Reality (VR) environment.

Results: The accuracy of the fusions was determined qualitatively by comparing the transformed atlas overlaid on the appropriate CT. It was examined for where the transformed structure atlas was incorrectly overlaid (false positive) and where it was incorrectly not overlaid (false negative). According to this method, fusions 1 and 2 were correct roughly 50-75% of the time, while fusions 3 and 4 were correct roughly 75-100%. The CT dataset augmented with transformed dataset was viewed arbitrarily in user-centered perspective stereo taking advantage of features such as scaling, windowing and volumetric region of interest selection.

Conclusions: This process of auto-coloring conserved structures in variable datasets is a step toward the goal of a broader, standardized automatic structure visualization method for radiological data. If successful it would permit identification, visualization or deletion of structures in radiological data by semi-automatically applying canonical structure information to the radiological data (not just processing and visualization of the data's intrinsic dynamic range). More sophisticated selection of control points and patterns of warping may allow for more accurate transforms, and thus advances in visualization, simulation, education, diagnostics, and treatment planning.

1. Introduction

Skill, effort, and time are required to identify and visualize anatomic structures in three-dimensions from radiological data. A series of axial two-dimensional CT slices are examined one by one, as the viewer attempts to follow anatomic structures of interest from slice to slice and create a three-dimensional understanding of these structures and their relationships. The ability to identify the structure is dependent on the particular structure, its relative location, its anatomic variability, and the modality and resolution of the imaging as well as a priori structure knowledge. It can be challenging to distinguish the hepatic vein and the portal vein from each other within the substance of the liver if the contrast is not ideal. Though these are conserved structures, they are highly variable in their precise three-dimensional description from person to person. The ability to visualize the structure is dependent on knowing symbolic information about the generic structure, its relative location, and its specific geometry. It is even more challenging to determine the course and finer branches of the hepatic vein and portal vein from slice to slice and visualize its three-dimensional anatomy.

Fundamentally, automating these processes requires a technique that uses symbolic information not in the dynamic range of the voxel (CT) data. Others have done this with variable success. The voxel data consists of three coordinate values and one intensity value. These four data values give the viewer two pieces of information: location and shade. The viewer then determines which anatomic structure that voxel belongs to based on these two pieces of information. The difficulty lies in that the absolute and relative location of conserved structures can be variable from person to person. Furthermore the shading of a structure can be indistinguishable from a neighboring structure making it difficult to identify the border or it can be indistinguishable from a geometrically similar nearby structure making it difficult to identify which is which.

Automatic identification of a structure requires a technique to add a fifth data value representing a symbol or structure to groups of voxels (they may also overlap). Three-dimensional visualization of a structure requires rendering these stacks of voxels selected for the structures of interest based on symbolic value. We have previously developed such a technique [1] based on mutual information for automatic multi-modality image fusion (MIAMI Fuse) [2]. MIAMI Fuse is a fusion algorithm capable of accurately fusing two datasets of different modalities at high fidelity. We have been able to create a standard dataset with known structure location, fuse this to a CT dataset of different scale and resolution from the same person, and thus know the structure location in the CT dataset. We have further been able to render this modified CT dataset in a virtual 3D environment and select for structures based on the symbolic information added by the fusion. MIAMI Fuse has also been used by its principal creator to fuse multiple studies of different patients with warping to generate a probabilistic atlas of the abdomen (personal communication). This next step of development of our technique was aimed at accommodating the variability of anatomy from patient to patient by using warping to import structures from our standard dataset into arbitrary patient CT datasets.

2. Methods

A standard symbolic information dataset (NTSC atlas) was created from the full color Visible Human Female [3] by segmenting the liver parenchyma, portal veins (including the spleen), and hepatic veins (including the IVC) and overwriting each set of voxels with a fixed color (red, green, and blue respectively). The original 32-bit dataset was converted to an 8-bit dataset using the NTSC standard formula (0.299 R + 0.587 G + 0.114 B). Eight bit data is required for the MIAMI Fuse program. Two standard structure datasets were created from the NTSC atlas. A liver atlas was created by turning all the liver voxels white and everything else black. Similarly, a portal vein atlas was created by cropping the portal vein segmentation to remove the spleen, and turning all the portal vein voxels white and everything else black.

Two arbitrarily selected patient CT scans of the abdomen were used for reference datasets. CT1 was an abdominal CT with out contrast that extended from the lower lung fields to just below the level of the kidneys. There was an intrahepatic mass identified in this dataset. CT2 was an abdominal/pelvic CT with out contrast that extended from the middle of the liver to below the pelvic bones. Both CT dataset were quite variable from the NTSC atlas (Figure 1). The 12-bit DICOM format CT datasets were converted to 8-bit using a linear contrast function with an input range of negative 200 to positive 2000 Hounsfield Units.

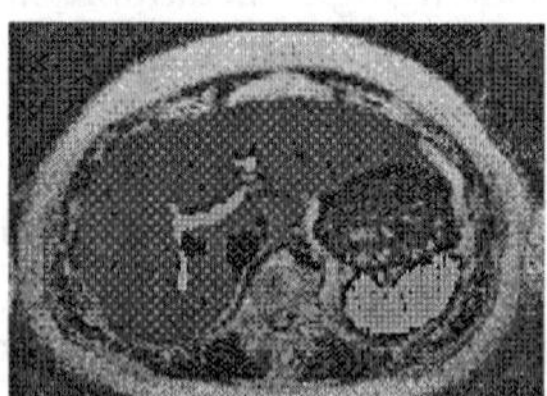 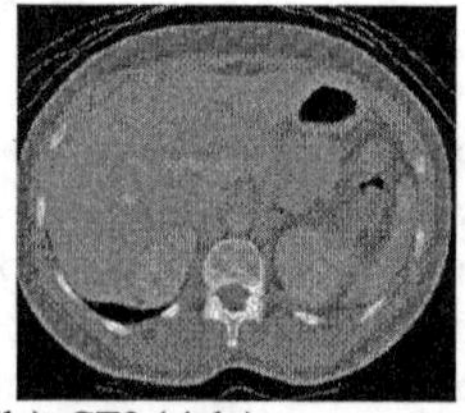 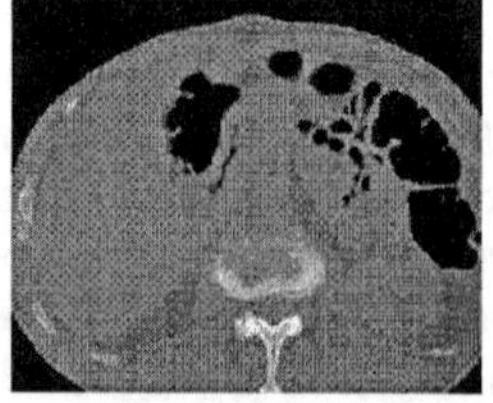

Figure 1: NTSC Atlas (left), CT1 (middle), CT2 (right)

MIAMI Fuse was used to perform 4 different fusions of a standard dataset to a CT dataset. This program optimizes the mutual information between the reference dataset and the transform iteration of the standard dataset. Larger structures, such as the liver will have more influence in determining the mutual information and thus the transform. Various combinations of control points and parameters were selected when running MIAMI Fuse. The control points are important in guiding the fusion in terms of accuracy and time. More control points tend to result in more accuracy but increased processing time. Control points in a concentrated area tend to focus the accuracy to that area. The parameters are important in determining the transform function and final scaling desired. Initially, the transform is set to rotate, translate, and scale to align and scale the two datasets. Next, the transform is set to warp to accurately fuse the desired structures.

Fusion 1 was of the NTSC atlas to CT1. Initially, 4 control points that would be automatically preselected around the border of the liver (1 each at the superior, inferior, and lateral tip of the right lobe and 1 at the superior-lateral tip of the left lobe) were selected on the atlas. Points that anatomically corresponded to these on the CT were selected by the user. These 4 points were used to rotate, translate, and scale the atlas to the CT. Next 27 control points uniformly dispersed around the border of the liver that would be automatically preselected on the atlas were selected. The program selected the corresponding points in the CT based on the initial rotate, translate, and scale transform and then went on to optimize a warp function based on these points. It took approximately 4 hours of processing time on Onyx2 Deskside to perform the transform. The liver atlas was then transformed based on this optimization to create liver1, which should correspond to the liver in CT1.

Fusion 2 was performed the same way as Fusion 1 except CT1 was replaced with CT2. The same control points that were preselected in the atlas in the Fusion 1, were used here. The user was only required to select the initial 4 points that anatomically corresponded to those preselected in the atlas. It also took approximately 4 hours of processing time to perform the transform. The liver atlas was then transformed based on this optimization to create liver2, which should correspond to the liver in CT2.

Fusion 3 was performed the same way as Fusion 1 except 45 control points instead of 27 uniformly dispersed around the border of the liver that would be preselected on the atlas were selected for the warping transform. It took approximately 7 hours of processing time to perform the transform. The liver atlas was then transformed based on this optimization to create liver1-45, which should correspond to the liver in CT1.

Fusion 4 was of the portal vein atlas to CT1. 5 control points that would be preselected around the bifurcation of the portal vein into right and left main branches on the atlas were selected. Points that anatomically corresponded to these on the CT were selected by the user. A warping transform fusion was performed based on these 5 points alone with out pre-optimization of rotation, translate, and scale. It took approximately 1 hour of processing time to perform the transform. The portal vein atlas was then transformed based on this optimization to create PV1, which should correspond to the portal vein in CT1.

Completed atlas transformations were parsed and each image data slice was extracted and expanded from 8bits to 12bits. The resultant raw data files were converted to Dicom MONOCHROME2 format using the rawtodc utility from David Clunie's Dicom3 toolkit [4]. Both the CT Dicom dataset and the transformed atlas Dicom series were loaded into the VR application [5] and rendered together back-to-front with respect to the view-point. The fused portion of the resulting image shows up as white due to the fact that it is more or less monochromatic with a level close to that of bone.

3. Results

The goal at this stage of development was to approach an accurate fusion of conserved structures of interest in variable datasets. The accuracy of the fusions was determined qualitatively by comparing the transformed atlas overlaid on the appropriate CT. It was determined where the transformed structure atlas was incorrectly overlaid (false positive) and where it was incorrectly not overlaid (false negative). This was limited to the external borders of the liver for fusions 1, 2, and 3 and the portal vein for fusion 4. The internal borders between the liver and intrahepatic venous systems were not evaluated due to difficulty delineating them by eye.

According to this method, fusions 1 and 2 were correct roughly 50-75% of the time. These transforms were inadequate most probably due to insufficient number of control points placed on the standard dataset for the warping transform. Fusions 3 and 4 had an accuracy of approximately 75-100% for individual slices (Figure 2). The internal borders were difficult to evaluate based on poor contrast between the liver and intrahepatic venous systems. In fusion 4, the atlas portal vein was mapped correctly onto the CT portal vein. However, only the main portal vein and its right and left main branches were transformed, while the smaller distal branches were not successfully warped.

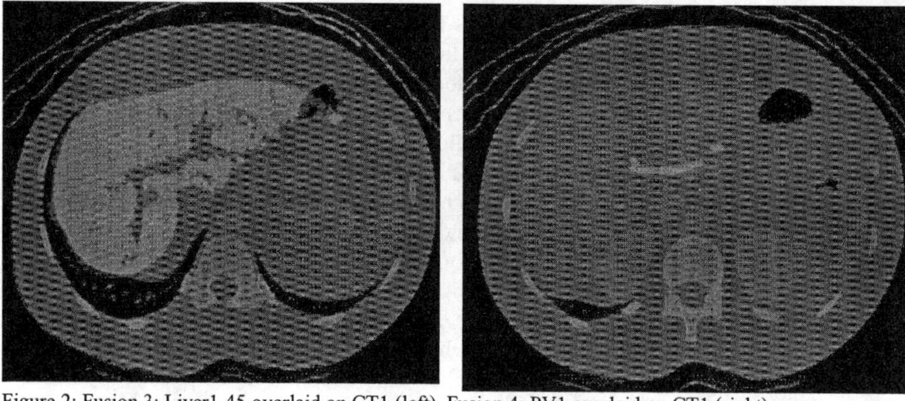

Figure 2: Fusion 3: Liver1-45 overlaid on CT1 (left), Fusion 4: PV1 overlaid on CT1 (right)

The rendered datasets can be arbitrarily viewed from a user-selected perspective in a windowed, clipped, and shaded display. Transformed structure atlases can be selected and added, removed, or colored within the CT dataset based on this transformation of symbolic structure information added to the CT dataset (figure 3).

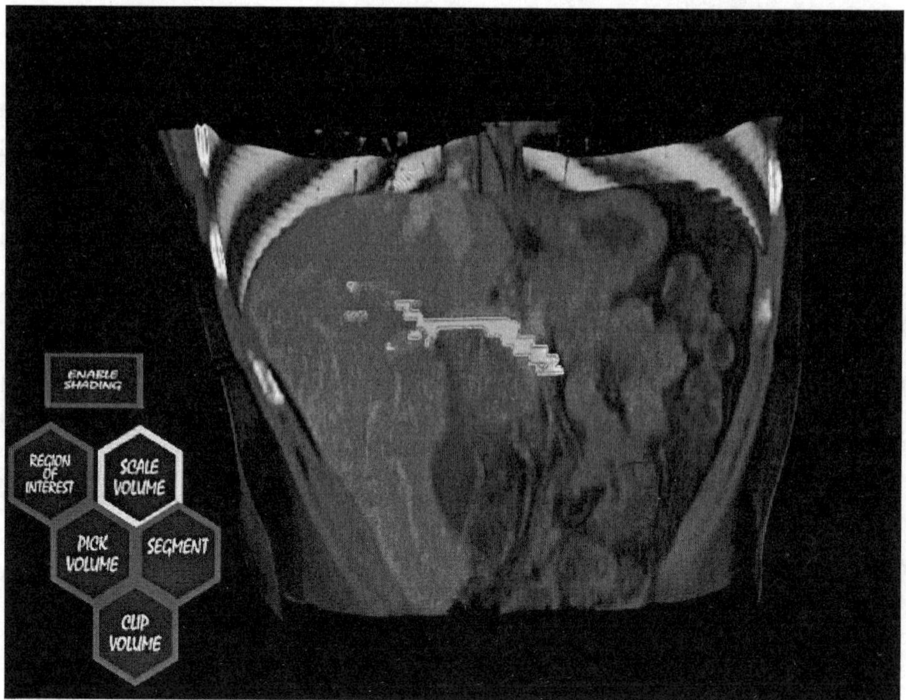

Figure 3: Fusion 4, PV1 overlaid on CT1 and arbitrarily clipped in volumetric display

4. Discussion

This work involves fusing data from two different humans into single dataset for visualization. The symbolic information for identification and visualization of structures is derived from the mutual information between the datasets. MIAMI Fuse is a fusion algorithm capable of accurately fusing two datasets of different modalities at high fidelity. Charles Meyer, its principal creator, has demonstrated that multiple studies of different patients can be fused with warping to generate a probabilistic atlas of the abdomen [6]. We used the warping functions in MIAMI Fuse in a similar fashion to align standard structure data to each patient scan by maximizing the mutual information between them and calculating the three-dimensional transformation required to move from standard to reference data. Therefore, the patient (reference) CT data remains unchanged while it is augmented by the standard anatomic segmentations warped to fit. The reference dataset is augmented with the transformed standard structure dataset one structure at a time by warping (with MIAMI Fuse) the voxels that represent the segmented symbolic structure mask into the CT data space. Then the warped structure masks are visualized in combination with the original patient dataset. Where the mask overlaps with the patient data, voxels are blended. Where there is no overlap, the original patient data is retained. This combined volume visualization is then rendered interactively in stereo on the ImmersaDesk in an immersive Virtual Reality (VR) environment. This augmented data can then be viewed arbitrarily in user-centered perspective taking advantage of features such as scaling, windowing in stereo and volumetric region of interest selection.

There was significant variability in the liver morphology between the standard dataset and each of the reference datasets. This increased variability required more robust parameters (significantly more control points) and more time when running the fusions. The key to successful fusion was the focused use of multiple warping control points that place themselves around the structure of interest automatically. The user assigns only a few initial control points to align the scans. We have transformed the liver and portal veins from a standard dataset to a variable arbitrary CT dataset. The accuracy of warping is a function of the number and location of control points. The more control points used in the standard dataset when warping the structures of interest, the more accurate the transform. This is at the expense of processing time. The more control points concentrated in a *specific area* of the dataset, the more accurate that *area* will be transformed. Notably, in this method, while adding more points to the standard dataset will result in better accuracy with increased processing time, *the user intervention would remain the same*. An objective measurement of accuracy was not used at this stage of the development. The augmented patient scans were simply viewed in the VR environment at interactive speeds.

Our goal at this stage was to be able to fuse conserved structures between highly variable datasets to add symbolic information to the CT datasets in attempts to improve the visualization and understanding of the anatomic relationships. Useful three-dimensional visualization and communication of these relationships ultimately requires rendering these stacks of voxels by selecting or deleting the structures of interest based on symbolic value ("Show me just the right hepatic arterial arcade"). Structures in these CT datasets that have been augmented with transformed standard dataset information (or that have symbolic structure information added) would be selected, colored, isolated, or combined with other combinations of augmented structures, or removed based on the symbolic information.

This augmentation and 3D visualization technique is a step closer to our long-term goal of a broader, standardized automatic structure colorization method for radiological data. More sophisticated selection of control points and patterns of warping will allow for more accurate transforms. This may ultimately provide a foundation for advances in visualization, simulation, education, diagnostics, and treatment planning.

5. Acknowledgments

This project has been funded in whole or in part with Federal funds from the National Library of Medicine, National Institutes of Health under Grant No. R01-LM-06756-01.

References

[1] Chhadia A, Dech F, Ai Z, Silverstein JC   Autocolorization of Three-Dimensional Radiological Data. Stud Health Technol Inform 2001;81:90-96.

[2] C.R. Meyer, J.L. Boes, B. Kim, P. Bland, K.R. Zasadny, P.V. Kison, K. Koral, K.A. Frey, and R.L. Whal. Demonstration of accuracy and clinical versatility of mutual information for automatic multimodality image fusion using affine and thin plate spline warped geometric deformations. Medical Image Analysis 1997, 3, 195-206.

[3] http://www.nlm.nih.gov/research/visible/visible_human.html

[4] http://idt.net/~dclunie/dicom3tools.html

[5] Dech F, Ai Z, Silverstein JC. Manipulation of Volumetric Patient Data in a Distributed Virtual Reality Environment. Stud Health Technol Inform 2001;81:119-25.

[6] Personal Communication - Charles Meyer

Medicine Meets Virtual Reality 02/10
J.D. Westwood et al. (Eds.)
IOS Press, 2002

A system for simulation and monitoring of robot-assisted and navigation-assisted surgical interventions (Part 1)

Malte Stien, Andreas Hein, Daniel Szymanski, Tim Lueth
Berlin Center for Mechatronic Medical Devices
Fraunhofer IPK – Charité • Campus Virchow, Clinic for Maxillofacial Surgery
Augustenburger Platz 1, 13353 Berlin/Germany
stien@ieee.org

Abstract. Location monitoring systems for surgical applications are getting more and more common in clinical daily life. Navigation treatment systems are also a form of a location monitoring system. These systems always consist of an optical, US-, electromagnetic or mechanical navigation system. If two or more navigation systems are combined or one navigations system is combined with a robot system the kinematic model of the entire system consists of closed kinematic loops. In this paper, an approach is presented to gain more information from the closed kinematic chains instead of breaking the kinematic loops.

1.   Introduction and Problem Description

Location monitoring systems for surgical and other applications capture the location information concerning one or more geometrical objects. The information is gained by one or more navigation systems. These navigation systems can be either optical, ultra-sonic, electromagnetical or mechanical systems. Even a robot system can be regarded as a navigation system since the location of the tool center point can be computed from the joint angles of the kinematic structure. If two or more navigation systems are combined, like it is done in many surgical robot systems, the monitoring model of the entire system consists of closed kinematic chains. In this paper, a mechanism will be described to handle closed kinematic chains consisting of redundant location information [1].

2.   State of the Art

Navigation treatment systems [2] do not combine location information from two or more navigation systems. They just visualize the location data of a single navigation system. In some robot-assisted surgery systems, a combination of a navigation system and a robot system is made. Thus, a redundant information concerning the location of the tool is the consequence. Today, in these cases a simple solution is to chose one of both location information to determine the location of the surgical tool. Using this method, the kinematic transformation from the measured object to the non-used navigation system is calculated from the used navigation system, although there is an information from the non-used navigation system that is ignored. This method makes no use of the multiple location information available from the combination of several navigation systems. Today, methods are known to combine a number of location information with different characteristics such as high noise (optical navigation system) or a given medium error (mechanical robot system) to an enhanced location information.

3.   Methods

The monitoring functionality of the system described in this contribution is based on a monitoring model. This model consists of some geometrical objects each containing a name n_i, a base coordinate system B_i and various mount coordinate systems $\mathbf{M_i}$. The geometry g_i of the object is stored in the base coordinate system of the object. The mount coordinate systems are dedicated for indicating locations where other objects can connect to.

$$O_i = \left(n_i, g_i, B_i, \mathbf{M_i}\right) \tag{1}$$

A mount coordinate system consists of a name n_i, a geometry object o_i it belongs to, a type t_i and a gender g_i. Mount coordinate systems can only be linked with mount coordinate systems of other geometry objects.

$$M_i = \left(n_i, o_i, t_i, g_i\right) \tag{2}$$

The link can only be established if the type of both mount coordinate systems are equal and the gender of both mount coordinate systems correspond to each other. The gender can be either neutral, male or female. For linking two coordinate systems both of them has to be neutral or one of them has to be male and the other has to be female.

$$g \in \left\{\mathbf{n}, \mathbf{m}, \mathbf{f}\right\} \tag{3}$$

$$\exists t_i \in M_i, \exists t_j \in M_j \big\|\left(t_i = t_j\right) \tag{4}$$

$$\exists g_i \in M_i, \exists g_j \in M_j \big\|\left[\left(g_i = g_j = \mathbf{n}\right) \vee \left(g_i = \mathbf{m} \wedge g_j = \mathbf{f}\right) \vee \left(g_i = \mathbf{f} \wedge g_j = \mathbf{m}\right)\right] \tag{5}$$

Example: A robot flange has one base coordinate system and four mount coordinate systems. One coordinate system is for mounting the robot flange to the robot body. The second mount coordinate system is for mounting a tool to the flange. Two optical localizers can be mounted to the mount coordinate systems left. This is only possible because the type of the mount coordinate system on the flange and that one on the localizer are identical. The gender of the localizer mount system is female while the one of the flange is male.

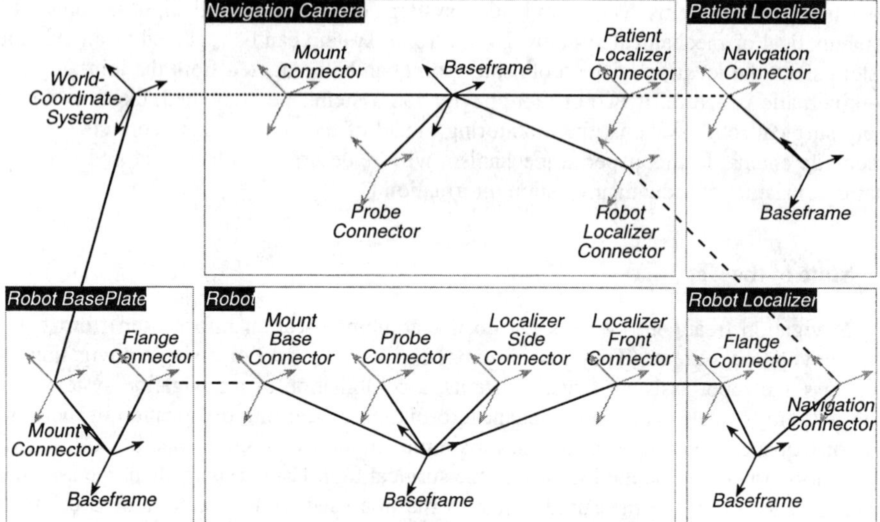

Fig. 1.:   An example for a monitoring model. The dashed lines represent flexible connections while the solid lines represent rigid connections and dotted lines represent snap connections.

The coordinate systems are linked together with kinematic connections. Each connection can implement a different behavior. Regarding reality, one can notice, that many different types of kinematic relations between objects exist. Some objects seem to be independent of each other (represented by a flexible connection), other objects are connected rigidly (rigid connection) to each other. In some cases two objects are in a constant but unknown relation to each other (snap connection). A kinematic connection consists of two coordinate systems K_{si} and K_{ei} the connection is established between. Each connection has a type t_i determining the behavior of the connection. The core attribute of each kinematic connection is given by a transformation matrix $\mathbf{T_i}$ determining the transformation from K_{si} to K_{ei}. Additionally, each kinematic connection represents its quality by two parameters. The medium error μ_i and the standard deviation σ_i represent the reliability of the transformation matrix $\mathbf{T_i}$. Especially for connections that represent values measure by a position measurement device these features are of great importance. In Tab. 1 a survey about three different kinds of kinematic connections is given.

$$C_i = \left(K_{si}, K_{ei}, t_i, \mu_i, \sigma_i, \mathbf{T_i}, \Pi_{im}, \Pi_{ii}\right) \tag{6}$$

Tab 1:   Survey on three different types of kinematic connections and their parameters

	μ_i	σ_i	$\mathbf{T_i}$	Example
rigid	variable, mostly 0	constant 0	constant	The connection between a robot flange and a mounted tool
flexible	variable	variable	depending on sensor data	The connection between a navigation camera and one of the navigation system's localizer
snap	constant 0	constant 0	depends on the transformation between adjoining objects	The navigation camera is located at a fixed location in the operation theatre but the location is unknown due to the possibility to move the navigation camera around.

4. Results and Conclusion

The system has been successfully tested in a clinical environment consisting of a patient model, a navigation system and a surgical robot. The presented modeling approach that has been presented in this paper leads to a more realistic model than traditional ones. In this contribution the basic model was described for the location propagation algorithm presented in the second part of this paper [4].

References

[1]   Stien, M (2002): Ein offenes System zur grafischen Überwachung und Simulation roboterunterstützter chirurgischer Eingriffe. PhD. Thesis in preparation., in preparation.

[2]   Schermeier, O.; T. Lueth, J. Glagau, D. Szymanski, R. Tita, D. Hildebrand, M. Klein, K. Nelson, J. Bier (2001): Automatic patient registration in computer assisted maxillofacial surgery. Medicine Meets Virtual Reality 2002, Newport Beach, California/USA, 23-26 January 2002.

[3]   Maybeck, Peter S. (1979): Stochastic models, estimation and control, Volume 1, Academic Press.

[4]   Stien, M.; A. Hein, D. Szymanski, T.C. Lueth (2002): A new approach for modelling kinematic dependencies for monitoring locations of objects in closed kinematic chains (Part 2). Medicine Meets Virtual Reality 2002, Newport Beach, California/USA.

Medicine Meets Virtual Reality 02/10
J.D. Westwood et al. (Eds.)
IOS Press, 2002

A new approach for modelling kinematic dependencies for monitoring locations of objects in closed kinematic chains (Part 2)

Malte Stien, Andreas Hein, Daniel Szymanski, Tim Lueth
Berlin Center for Mechatronic Medical Devices
Fraunhofer IPK – Charité • Campus Virchow, Clinic for Maxillofacial Surgery
Augustenburger Platz 1, 13353 Berlin/Germany
stien@ieee.org

Abstract. Location monitoring systems for surgical applications are getting more and more common in clinical daily life. Navigation treatment systems are also a form of a location monitoring system. These systems always consist of an optical, US-, electromagnetic or mechanical navigation system. If two or more navigation systems are combined or one navigations system is combined with a robot system the kinematic model of the entire system consists of closed kinematic loops. In this paper, an approach is presented to gain more information from the closed kinematic chains instead of breaking the kinematic loops. This is the second part of [1].

1. Methods

This is the second part of [1]. Thus, the paper immediately starts with the explanation of the methods. During operation of the monitoring system, the sensor data of the navigation system and the robot system is transmitted via a network connection to the monitoring system. In this paper, the algorithm for determining the locations of the geometry objects of the scene is described. The algorithm can be divided in five parts:

1. During the preparation of the first location propagation the coordinate systems initialize their data fields used for the location fusion algorithm (e.g. a Kalman filter). Additionally, the flexible connections are equipped with the appropriate sensor data. In this step, the transformation between the two adjoining coordinate systems is determined. The medium error and the standard deviation of this information are also determined. For example a software model representing the navigation camera can calculate these values based on an internal model of the accuracy of the system in a certain location. All snap connections inside the monitoring model disable themselves.

2. The first location propagation cycle is started. The algorithm starts with the world coordinate system which location can be expressed by the identity matrix. The medium error of this initial location information is 0 and the standard deviation is also 0.

$$L \equiv \left\{ {}^{\text{WCS}}\mathbf{T}, \mu, \sigma \right\} = \{\mathbf{I}, 0, 0\} \tag{1}$$

This location information is propagated through connection 1 (see numbers in Fig. 1) to the first coordinate system. From there it is distributed to all directly linked connections. See below for a further description of this step.

3. This step is called the second preparation phase. It is very similar to step 1. Additionally to step 1, in this step the location fusion algorithms determine the locations of all coordinate systems in the graph. The snap connections enable themselves. Afterwards,

the location fusion algorithm initializes again. The sensor data used for this step is the same as in step 1.

4. This step is identical to step 2.

5. In this step the location fusion algorithm determines the locations of all coordinate systems in the graph. Afterwards, the scene is visualized according to the new locations of the coordinate systems.

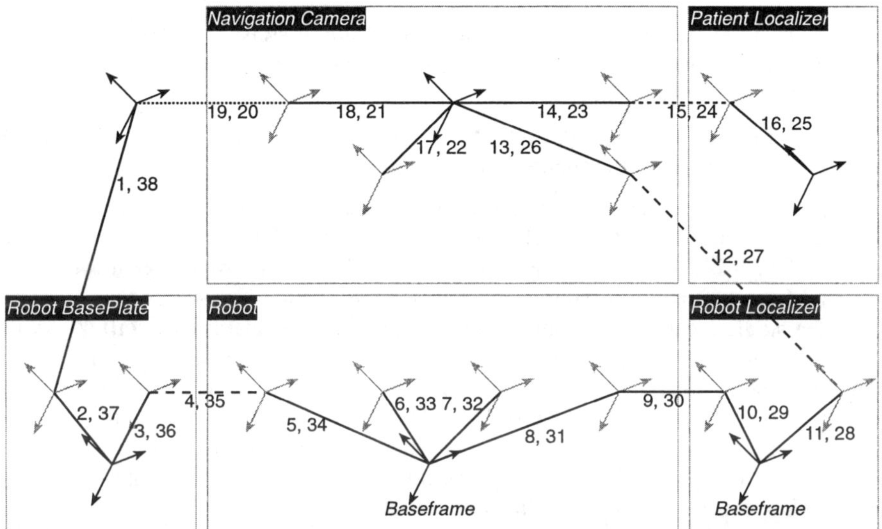

Fig. 1.: An example for a monitoring model. The dashed lines represent flexible connections while the solid lines represent rigid connections and dotted lines represent snap connections. The numbers represent one possible sequence or the location information propagated through the graph.

In the following section the location propagation phase (step 2 and 4) is explained more precisely. Every time a location information reaches a kinematic connection, it behaves as follows: Every kinematic connection calculates a new location information form the location information coming from one of the adjoining coordinate systems K_{from} and the internal location propagation consisting of $\mathbf{T}_{\text{internal}}$, μ_{internal} and σ_{internal}. The calculations for the rigid connection are described in (2) while these for the flexible connections are described in (3).

$$\mathbf{T}_{\text{result}} = \mathbf{T}_{\text{from}} \cdot \mathbf{T}_{\text{intern}}, \quad \mu_{\text{result}} = \mu_{\text{from}} \text{ and } \sigma_{\text{result}} = \sigma_{\text{from}} \tag{2}$$

$$\mathbf{T}_{\text{result}} = \mathbf{T}_{\text{from}} \cdot \mathbf{T}_{\text{intern}}, \quad \mu_{\text{result}} = \mu_{\text{from}} + \mu_{\text{intern}} \text{ and } \sigma_{\text{result}} = \sqrt{\sigma_{\text{from}}^2 + \sigma_{\text{intern}}^2} \tag{3}$$

The behavior of the snap connection is more complex. The snap connection investigates if the transformation between both of the adjoining coordinate systems stays under a given threshold without the influence of the snap connection. Thus, the snap connection disables itself during the first location propagation cycle (step 2). It does nothing during that step. During the second location propagation cycle (step 4) the connection is active again. It calculates the transformation between both coordinate systems based on the location of both systems determined in during the first location propagation cycle (step 2).

$$\mathbf{T}_{\text{difference}} = \left(\mathbf{T}_{\text{source}}\right)^{-1} \cdot \mathbf{T}_{\text{target}} \tag{4}$$

If the resulting transformation matrix stays under the given threshold, the connection gets rigid. In this case the movement of both coordinate systems relative to each other seems to be a result of noisy sensor data but not of a real relative movement of both objects. The internal transformation matrix $\mathbf{T}_{\text{intern}}$ of the snap connection is determined by averaging the transformations from the last n cycles ($n=30$ has been used). Based on $\mathbf{T}_{\text{intern}}$ the resulting transformation $\mathbf{T}_{\text{result}}$ is calculated.

$$\mathbf{T}_{\text{result}} = \mathbf{T}_{\text{from}} \cdot \mathbf{T}_{\text{intern}}, \ \mu_{\text{result}} = \mu_{\text{from}} \text{ and } \sigma_{\text{result}} = \sigma_{\text{from}} \tag{5}$$

If the resulting transformation value exceeds the threshold the snap connection simply stores $\mathbf{T}_{\text{difference}}$ for averaging and terminates. In this case no location information is propagated by the connection.

All kinematic connections propagate the location information $\mathbf{T}_{\text{result}}$ to the coordinate system on the other side or the connection.

Every time a location information reaches a base coordinate system or a mount coordinate system, it behaves as follows: The coordinate system analyses the location information gained in the current location propagation cycle (step 2 and 4 are two different cycles). The location information is combined to a new location information considering the characteristics of the single location information (medium error and standard deviation). A Kalman filter or a similar algorithm can be used for that task. If the quality of the new location information is better than the old one the location information is propagated to all adjoining kinematic connections without the one that delivered the location information to the coordinate system. If the quality of the location information is lower than the one already known by the coordinate system, the coordinate system does nothing but returning the control to the coordinate system that delivered the location information.

After step 5 has terminated for every geometry object in the kinematic graph (Fig 1.) witch is connected directly or indirectly to the world coordinate system an optimal and plausible location information is known. During the visualization these objects can be rendered in their correct position and orientation. Objects which location information has not been updated during the current location propagation cycle are rendered in wireframe mode.

2. Results and Conclusion

The system has been successfully tested in a clinical environment consisting of a patient model, a navigation system and a surgical robot. A network connection from the real robot and navigation system to a single monitoring system has been established. The visualization is performed in real-time according to the real process. The location data can be recorded on a harddisk and played back. A system has been presented that can be used for teaching the use of surgical robot's and navigation systems by watching the monitored interventions of professionals. The data stream that is transmitted from the real robot system to the monitoring client can be used for documentation. The monitoring system stores the stream to a persistent storage media that can be archived. The presented modeling approach that has been presented in this paper leads to a more realistic model than traditional ones.

References

[1]   Stien, M.; A. Hein, D. Szymanski, T. Lueth (2002): A system for simulation and monitoring of robot-assisted and navigation-assisted surgical interventions (Part 1). Medicine Meets Virtual Reality 2002, Newport Beach, California/USA.

TEMPORAL BONE DISSECTION SIMULATION – AN UPDATE

D Stredney,[1] Gregory J Wiet, M.D.[2,4], J Bryan[1], D Sessanna[1], Jim Murakami, M.D.[3],
P Schmalbrock Ph.D.[5], Kimerly Powell, Ph.D[6]. and B Welling, M.D.[2]

[1]*Ohio Supercomputer Center (OSC), Columbus, OH*
[2]*Department of Otolaryngology, Children's Hospital, Columbus, OH*
[3]*Department of Radiology, Children's Hospital, Columbus, OH*
[4]*Department of Otolaryngology, The Ohio State University, Columbus, OH*
[5]*Department of Radiology, The Ohio State University, Columbus, OH*
[6]*Bimedical Engineering, Cleveland Clinic Foundation, Cleveland, OH*

ABSTRACT We report on our continued development of a virtual simulation for temporal bone dissection that provides stereoscopic display, haptic feedback, and aural simulation into a straightforward, comprehensive learning environment. The multimodal interface provides a seamless simulation for non-deterministic drilling and cutting of bone in the surgical context, as well as an intuitive interface for the intelligent tutor for learning regional anatomy. We present novel methodologies for integrating multimodal and multiresolution data sets, including extension to functional and structural segmentation. We will present our initial efforts to validate this environment. Through continued iterations, it is our hope that the system will provide a valuable tool for training future otologic surgeons as well as an environment for the quantitative evaluation of surgical skill.

1. INTRODUCTION

We have previously reported on our justification, initial techniques, and development of a seamless, multimodal   environment for simulating temporal bone dissection [1,2,3]. The overall goal of this effort has been the emulation of otologic techniques that are traditionally learned in temporal bone dissection laboratories using cadaveric specimens. While our previous reports discuss the initial designs and integration of patient specific data within the system, this report focuses on our efforts to acquire and integrate multimodal and multiresolution data into the simulator, thus providing a rich and varied environment for learning temporal bone anatomy and surgical techniques. We have also extended portions of the system for a more user-friendly method to functionally and structurally segment data. Additional improvements include the integration of an intelligent tutor. Through further development we intend to increase the realism and utility of the system, and to conduct multi-institutional studies that validate the efficacy of the system as a training tool.

2. BACKGROUND/PURPOSE

Successful otologic surgeries are based on fundamental understanding of the regional anatomy and the application of this knowledge to patient variance through demonstration of proficiency in subtle microsurgical technique. Traditional methods including text and atlases [4,5,6,7], CDROM's [8,10], and physical models [11,12]. These various levels of schema provide limited and determined approaches for understanding the complex regional anatomy. By using cadaver dissections which more closely emulate surgical techniques, a period of four to five years is still required to develop a comprehensive understanding of the subtle spatial relationships, anatomical variances presented by pathologies, and permutations of surgical technique [4]. However, the physical limitation of the material, associated risks, and decreased availability make this method increasingly   problematic.

Harada first introduced the concept of exploiting 3D volumetric reconstructions for emulating the drilling of bone and exposing the intricate regional anatomy of the temporal bone [13]. However, because of the computational overhead of volumetric representation at the time, surface-based approaches have been predominantly employed for model simulation. [14,15,16,17]. Recently, development of volumetric, physically based simulations has been proposed, emphasizing the need for secondary characteristics seen during surgery [18]. Albeit important to the eventual simulation of the surgeries themselves, we do not feel that these attributes are essential for initial training, where context and procedure is key. In fact, these attributes may lead to confusion for the novice [19]. We have pursued a volumetric approach to rendering the structural model of the regional anatomy and because of recent developments in commodity computing hardware, a more realistic and robust system is emerging. This approach allows us to more directly integrate anatomical variance with little or no preprocessing. Through evaluative trials, we believe we have reached a level of realism for the system to be useful in resident training as an adjuvant to temporal bone dissection with cadaveric temporal bones.

3. METHODS
3.1 Data Acquisition
Our initial development data was with a dry skull specimen and was accomplished on a spiral CT and resulted in a 64MB isotropic volume with a voxel resolution of 0.35mm inplane resolution and a 1mm slice thickness. To obtain multimodal data sets, our second acquisition was from a fresh cadaver, (72 year old male < 24hrs following death) and was obtained through the Body Donation Program of the Department of Biomedical Informatics at The Ohio State University. Intact imaging was provided to preserve the relationships with soft and hard tissue. Magnetic Resonance imaging (1.5Tesla) was conducted at the magnetic resonance Facility at OSU. Clinical Computed Tomography (CT) was conducted at Children's Hospital, Columbus. Subsequently, bilateral excision of the temporal bone was performed and the specimens were trimmed to contain the middle ear laterally, and the otic capsule and internal acoustic canal medially (See Figure 1). Additional 1.5 T and 8T acquisitions were acquired at OSU, and microCT was conducted by the Biomedical Engineering Center at the Cleveland Clinic Foundation. CT images were acquired with a single-detector row CT scanner (CTi; GE Medical Systems, Milwaukee, Wis.). The cadaver was scanned and reconstructed using the following parameters: section thickness of 1.0 mm using a helical acquisition with a pitch of 1.0, gantry rotation time of 1 second, x-ray tube voltage of 120 kV, x-ray tube current of 200 mA, an imaging field-of-view of 10 cm, images reconstructed every 0.5 mm (50% overlap between adjacent sections). The imaging protocol yielded 1.0 mm thick axial images of the temporal bone with a 512 x 512 image matrix. Image resolution was therefore 0.19 x 0.19 x 1.0 mm.

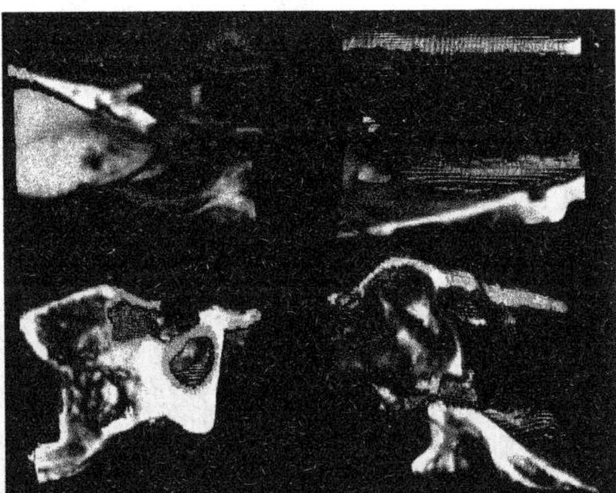

Figure 1: Section of trimmed temporal bone reconstructed from CT. Functional segmentation appears tinted. Upper: Left = Anterior, Right = Posterior, Lower: Left = Lateral, Right = Medial

Micro-computed tomography images of the excised temporal bone were obtained using a dedicated microradiography system consisting of a microfocal x-ray source (Phoenix X/ray, Wunstorf Germany) a 7-axis micro-positioning system and a high resolution X-ray image intensifier coupled to a scientific CCD camera (Thomson Tubes Electroniques, Cedex France) (See Figure 2). In order to safely expose the specimens to air, a 70% ethanol solution was used to exchange the formalin initially used to fix the specimens. Three hundred and sixty 2048 x 2048 12-bit projection radiographs were collected in a circle at 1degree intervals around the entire specimen. The projection radiographs were collected at 40 kV and 200 microA with the II operating in 7-inch mode. The images were subsampled by a factor of four (spatial resolution = 200 micrometers), background corrected, and the gray level intensities were scaled relative to that of air. A 512 x 512 x 512 volume was reconstructed using a modified Feldkamp cone-beam reconstruction algorithm [20].

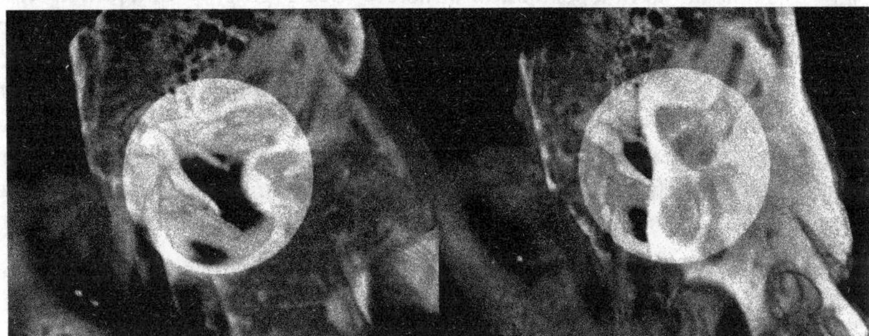

Figure 2: MicroCT of otic capsule. Left: Relationships of ossicles are highlighted. Right: Section through cochlea and semicircular canals

The MRI data for the excised temporal bone were acquired on a GE 1.5 Tesla employing 3D fast-spin echo sequence with a TR of 2000ms TE 80ms using custom 1inch RF receive coil. The data was reconstructed to an isotropic voxel resolution of .3 mm. 8T images were acquired a small single strut TEM RF coil. A set of localizer images was acquired to determine specimen orientation. High resolution images were obtained in 2hrs with a 3D spin echo sequence using TR 300ms, TE16.6ms FOV 5.5x5.5cm and a 5cm slab, matrix 256x256x128 with a final pixel resolution of 214x214x390μm. Gradient echo images were acquired in 20 minutes with identical resolution using TR=50ms, TE=5.3ms and about 90 degree flip angle. The 2nd specimen was acquired with 256x128x128 matrix, final pixel size 214x428x390μm)

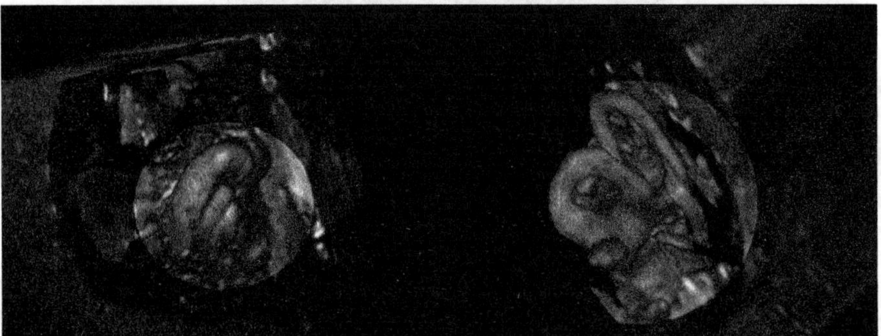

Figure 3: Left = Cochlea highlighted Note: Vestibulocochlear nerve to the immediate left. Right = Semicircular canals highlighted

3.2 Segmentation

We have integrated the physical interface of the simulator system into the segmenting system, to facilitate the segmentation process The segmentation software allows one to segment structures within the volume rather than image by image. The system allows the user to view the structures in stereo, and to use the haptic device to validate location of a tool to mark (3D paint) the actual structure, with a single voxel of precision if required. These masks "tag" volume elements with structural or functional information, i.e., information that is surgically relevant but is independent of structure (See Figure 4). In addition, the system allows for arbitrary sectioning of the data (See Figure 1). Thus segmentation can occur not only on surface structures, but on internal structures as well. This provides an extremely intuitive environment for segmentation, allowing the user to "paint and feel" in real-time the curves of the semicircular canals as they are delineated. In addition, the system allows for several user-imposed constraints, including the option to write over or preclude write over of existing segments, or to effect only structures within a certain threshold value. In addition, a revert function allows the user to correct any mistakes.

3.3 Integration

To create the most accurate and useful volumetric reconstruction of the regional anatomy, the acquired and multiscale data must be combined, or merged, into a single dataset. To help manage this process, we are developing a novel application that allows experts to interactively control the entire merging procedure. First, an appropriate mapping between datasets must be determined. This is accomplished by visualizing at least two datasets simultaneously, and interactively manipulating a set of control points to place one dataset in the correct location with respect to another. The user can manipulate clipping planes, zoom, rotate, and alter the opacity of each dataset to help verify the mapping. This process is repeated for all datasets until their common space is well defined. That is, given any dataset, the transformation mapping it to every other dataset has been user defined. Once the final mapping between each dataset is obtained, the destination dataset must be defined. The destination dataset is first defined by choosing a region-of-interest within the common space. Next, a resolution or the final dataset is chosen, for example 256x256x256. Finally, the sampling rules are defined. These rules allow the user to customize how different data are copied and blended with one another. Once the final dataset has been parameterized, the application creates the final dataset by sampling the source datasets using the appropriate mapping, and combining the samples according to the set of rules.

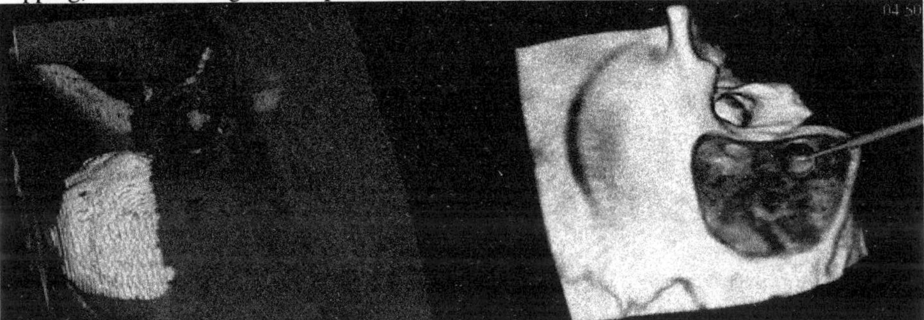

Figure 4: Left - Segments tinted on left temporal bone. Right - View from surgical simulation with burr after mastodiectomy performed on right temporal bone.

4. RESULTS

The system has been integrated with both left and right temporal bones from the two acquisitions. Current efforts include the segmentation and registration of soft-tissue structures derived from MRI acquisitions. The system defaults to the surgical context for a series of expose and identify procedures. At any time, the use may select interaction with a spaceball to arbitrarily orient the data. Also, burr size and type is readily changed. The phantom interface serves to deliver haptic feedback during palpation and drilling as well as a control for menu selection.

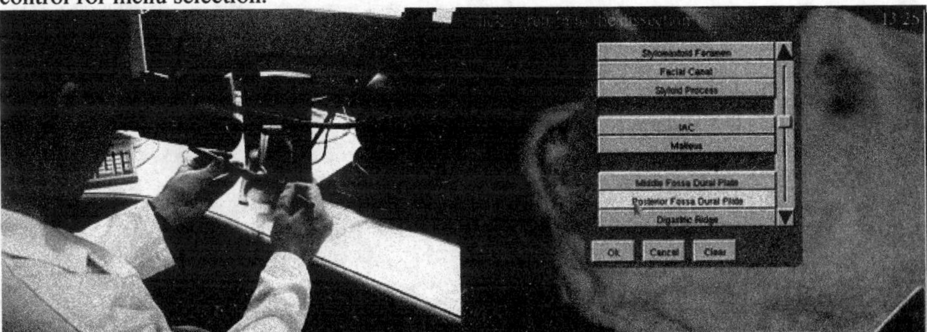

Figure 5: Left: Current System configuration. Right: View of menu for selecting structures

If requested, the user can select the menu of either ID or ED mode. The ED is an expert demo, where a previously captured session by an expert s is reconstructed. This is fully simulated in real-time, and through the use of the space ball, the user can arbitrarily change the viewing parameters for the expert session. In ID mode, the user may ask "What" is the structure, and by using the haptic device, the system will spawn prerecorded voice files identifying the structure chosen. Or the user may select "Where" is the structure, where a menu of segmented structures appears, and the user can select one or more structures to be highlighted. The session reduces the opacity of the bone and allows the user to arbitrarily view the highlighted structure(s). Upon request to return, the system returns to the surgical context. We have presented the simulator at the American Academy of Otolaryngology-Head and Neck Surgery Foundation (AAO-HNSF)(in Denver, September 9-12, 2001, as well as conducting evaluation sessions at the Department of Otolaryngology at The Ohio State University Medical Center , October 1 –5, 2001 (See Figure 6).

5. Discussion

We have presented an integrated simulation environment for learning the regional anatomy and procedures involved in otological surgeries. Preliminary results from our efficacy study indicate the simulator has immediate potential for improving anatomical training in a temporal bone curriculum. Respondants also gave high marks for the overall utility of the system. As expected, user feedback indicates that both visual quality and haptic fidelity requires further improvement. These issues will be addressed in subsequent iterations of the development cycle.

6. Acknowledgements

We would like to acknowledge the continuing support of the Dr. David Schuller, Dr. Iain Grant, and the Department of Otolaryngology at OSU, Al Stutz at OSC, and Dr. Joel Saltz and the Department of Biomedical Informatics, and honorable mention to Edward Auyang for the assistance with the data acquisition. Additional thanks go to Sensable Technologies, Virtual Research, Inc., Silicon Graphics, Inc., Nvidia and Medtronic Xomed. This work is funded by the National Institute for Deafness and Communicative Disorders, I-R21 DC04515-01.

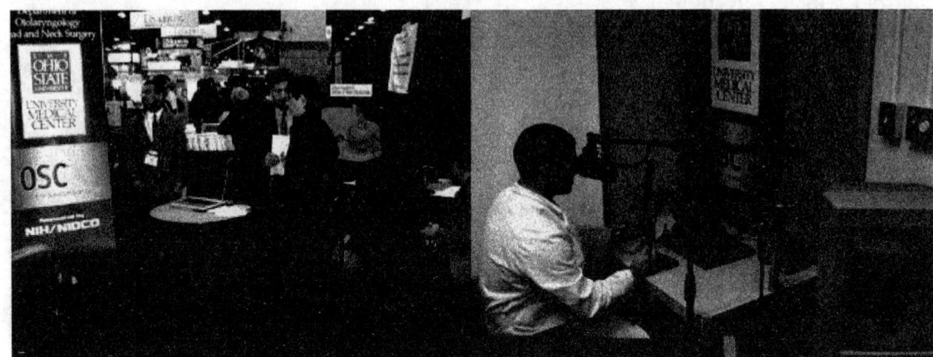

Figure 6: Left: Simulation at AAO-HNSF conference Right: System under evaluation in Dept. of Otolaryngology, The Ohio State University

REFERENCES

[1] Wiet GJ, Bryan J, Dodson E, Sessanna D, Stredney D, Schmalbrock P and B Welling, *"Virtual Temporal Bone Dissection*, Proceedings of MMVR8, 2000,Westwood et. al., (Eds). IOS Press Amsterdam: 378-384

[2] Wiet, G.J., D. Stredney, D. Sessanna, J. Bryan. *Volume-based Temporal Bone Dissection Simulator*, AAO-HNSF/ARO Research Forum, 2001 Annual Meeting of the American Academy of Otolaryngology-Head and Neck Surgery Foundation, Denver, Colorado, September 9-12, 2001

[3] Bryan J, Stredney D, Sessanna D, Wiet GJ, *Virtual Temporal Bone Dissection: A Case Study*", Proc. of IEEE Visualization 2001, San Diego, CA, 2001:497-500.

[4] Nelson RA, Temporal Bone Surgical Dissection Manual, 2nd Edition, House Ear Institute, Los Angeles, 1991.

[5] Schuknecht HF and AJ Gulya, Anatomy of the Temporal Bone with Surgical Implications, Lea & Febiger, Philadelphia, 1986.

[6] Glasscock, ME and GE Shambaugh, "Surgery of the Ear", Fourth Edition, WB Saunders Company, Philedelphia, 1990.

[7] Donaldson JA, Surgical Anatomy of the Temporal Bone"Fourth Ed. Raven Press, New York, 1992

[8] Swartz JD and HR Harnsberger, "Imaging the Temporal Bone". Third Edition, Thieme, New York. 1998,

[9] Brodie, H and T Singh, "Interactive Temporal Bone Anatomy" University of California Davis Medical School, October 13, 1997.

[10] Blevins NH, Jackler RK and C Gralapp, "Temporal Bone Dissector: The Interactive Otology Reference, Mosby -year Book, Inc. 1998.

[11] Golding-Wood DG, "Temporal bone dissection for display" Journal of Laryngology and Otology, January 1994, pgs-3-8.

[12] www.temporal-bone.com/plastic.htm

[13] Harada T, Ishii S, and N Tayama, "Three-dimensional Reconstruction of the Temporal Bone From Histological Sections," Arch Otolaryngol Head Neck Surg,1988;114:1139-1142.

[14] Takagi A, and I Sando, "Computer-aided three-dimensional reconstruction and measurements of the vestibular end-organs, Otolaryngology – Head and Neck Surgery, (98) 3:1988, 195-202.

[15] Green JD Jr, Marion MS, Erikson BJ, Robb RA, and R Hinojosa, "Three-Dimensional Reconstruction of the Temporal Bone" Laryngoscope100, January 1990:1-4.

[16] Kuppersmith RB, Johnston R, Moreau D, Loftin RB, and H Henkins, "Building a Virtual Reality Temporal Bone Dissection Simulator", Proc. of Medicine Meets Virtual Reality, K.S. Morgan et al. (Eds.) IOS Press Amsterdam, 1997:180-186.

[17] Mason TP, Applebaum EL, Rasmussen M, Millman A, Evenhouse R, and W Panko, "The Virtual Temporal Bone", Proc. of Medicine Meets Virtual Reality, J.D Westwood et al., (Eds.) IOS Press Amsterdamn 1998:346-352.

[18] John N, et al, "An Integrated Simulator for Surgery of the   Petrous Bone" Proc. MMVR9,2001:218-224.

[19] Lintern "Back-to-Basics Training", Tech. Rev, 80(October) 1992.

[20] Grass M, Kohler Th, Proksa R. 3D cone-beam CT reconstruction for circular trajectories. Phys Med Biol 2000, 45:329-347.

Medicine Meets Virtual Reality 02/10
J.D. Westwood et al. (Eds.)
IOS Press, 2002

Measurement of *In-vivo* Force Response of Intra-abdominal Soft Tissues for Surgical Simulation

B.K. Tay[1], N. Stylopoulos[2], S. De[1], D.W. Rattner[3], M.A. Srinivasan[1]

[1] Laboratory for Human and Machine Haptics,
Massachusetts Institute of Technology, Cambridge, MA 02139

[2] Department of Surgery,
Massachusetts General Hospital, Boston, MA 02114

[3] Division of General and Gastrointestinal Surgery,
Massachusetts General Hospital, Boston, MA 02114

Abstract. The lack of data on *in-vivo* material properties of soft tissues has been a significant impediment in the development of virtual reality based surgical simulators that can provide the user with realistic visual and haptic feedback. As a first step towards characterizing the mechanical behavior of organs, this work presents *in-vivo* force response of the liver and lower esophagus of pigs when subjected to ramp and hold, and sinusoidal indentations delivered using a haptic feedback device, Phantom, employed as a mechanical stimulator. The results show that pulse significantly affects the reaction forces and that the lower esophagus is 2 to 2.5 times stiffer than the liver.

1. Introduction

Laparoscopic surgery is being employed for an increasing variety of procedures, spawning a crucial need for tools to train surgeons for surgeries. A surgical simulator is one such tool that involves an immersive virtual environment where the human user interacts with virtual organs using his/her sense of vision and touch. For the virtual environment to be realistic and result in positive training transfer, it is generally expected that physically based models of organs and tissues must be used. Computation of realistic surgical tool-tissue interaction forces and organ deformations requires elucidation of physical laws governing the behavior of soft tissues [1]. To compute these deformations and reaction forces, apart from the consideration of force equilibrium and boundary conditions, *in-vivo* material properties of the soft tissues are required. *Ex-vivo* data [2] is not suitable since the material properties vary considerably from *in-vivo* data due to a variety of factors such as loss of blood pressure and degeneration of tissues.

Determination of *in-vivo* properties of soft tissues is a difficult problem. Efforts have been made to measure *in-vivo* intra-abdominal tissues [3, 4]. Attempts have also been made to measure *in-vivo* intra-abdominal tissue properties using specially designed instruments [4-6]. However, the measurements made until now are not suitable for our application, because of the limitations on the range, resolution or frequency bandwidth of the measurements as well as the particular organs that were tested. We are interested in the linear as well as the nonlinear response of the soft tissues and their viscoelastic properties under compressive and shear loading. For realistic simulation of laparoscopic procedures we require a systematic study of the mechanical behavior of organs and data suitable for the development of the simulator.

In this paper, we present the *in-vivo* force response of the liver and lower esophagus of pigs subjected to ramp and hold stimuli as well as low frequency vibration stimuli delivered using the Phantom haptic interface device.

In the next section, we briefly describe the setup for the experiment, including the equipment used, the type of stimuli applied and the experimental procedure and in section 3, we present some of our experimental results.

2. Methods

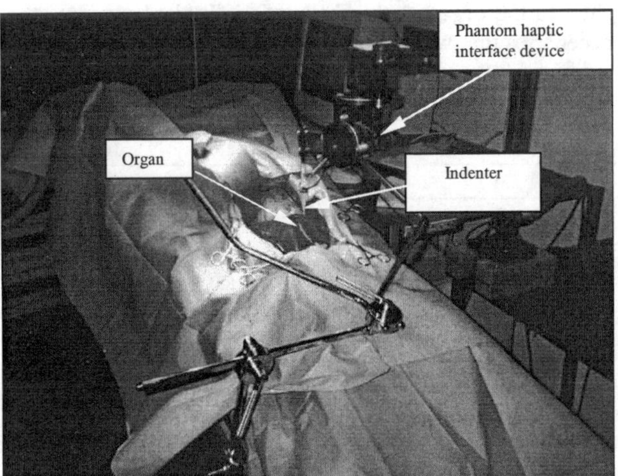

Figure 1: Experimental setup for tissue property measurement.

a) Setup

In-vivo force response of the intra-abdominal organs of pigs was obtained by applying indentation stimuli to the organs and measuring the corresponding reaction forces. The indenter used was a 2mm diameter flat-tipped cylindrical probe. The stimuli were delivered using a force feedback haptic device, Phantom Premium-T 1.0 (SensAble Technologies) that was programmed to perform as a mechanical stimulator. The Phantom has a nominal position resolution of 30μm and a frequency bandwidth that exceeds stimulus frequencies employed here.

A six-axis force sensor from ATI Industrial Automation, Nano 17, was used for measuring the reaction forces. The Nano 17 has a force resolution of 0.781mN along each of the three orthogonal axes when attached to a 16-bit A/D converter. The indenter was fixed to the tip of the Phantom with a force sensor in-between to accurately sense the reaction forces. Using position control, the Phantom was programmed to indent the organ to different depths at different ramp velocities. Force measurement was sampled at 200Hz using custom software. An 850MHz Pentium III PC was used for both position control and data acquisition.

b) Indentation Stimuli

Indentation stimuli included both ramp and hold in the three orthogonal directions as well as sinusoidal indentations. Ramp and hold indentations explore the force response of the organs to different displacements and the effect of ramp velocities on the response. These indentations reveal the viscoelastic nature as well as non-linear steady state force-displacement relationship of the soft tissues. Indentations up to 8mm from the resting surface of the organs and ramp velocities up to 8mm/s were applied.

Effects of anisotropy may be studied by comparing the force-displacement relationships of the organ in the three orthogonal directions. Ramp and hold indentation stimuli in the normal (Z) direction were applied by ramping the indenter to the prescribed depth in one second. The indenter was then held in place for 20 seconds. Force response was recorded for the entire period. For the indentation stimuli in the other two orthogonal directions, a preindentation of 4 – 6mm was applied to the organ in the Z direction. Table 1 presents the different ramp and hold indentation scenarios that were used.

Displacements (mm)	Ramp Velocity (mm/s)	Direction
1.0	1.0	Z, X, Y
2.0	2.0	Z, X, Y
4.0	4.0	Z, X, Y
6.0	6.0	Z
8.0	8.0	Z

Table I. Ramp and hold indentation conditions applied to the organs.

Sinusoidal indentations reveal the frequency dependency of the organ response. Low frequency sinusoidal indentations (0.5, 1.0, 2.0 and 3 Hz) were applied to the organs in only the Z-direction. The amplitude of the sinusoids was 1.5mm superimposed over a pre-indentation of 4mm. This ensured that the indenter stayed in contact with the organ over the entire course of stimulation.

c) Experimental Procedure

The pig was first put under general anesthesia and placed on the surgical table (see Figure 1). A midline incision was made at its abdominal region and dissection carried out on the anatomical structures to expose the organs. The tip of the Phantom, with the indenter attached, was then lowered into the abdominal region. Preliminary experiments revealed that breathing caused motion and forces that exceeded the stimulus ranges employed here. Only during the stimulus application periods was the respirator turned off and breathing of the pig held, so that the force response of the organ was unaffected by breathing cycles.

3. Results

Force response from indentation stimuli performed on the liver and the lower esophagus of pigs is presented in this section. These indentation stimuli were delivered to three female pigs that weighed about 32kgs to 65kgs. Typical results are presented below.

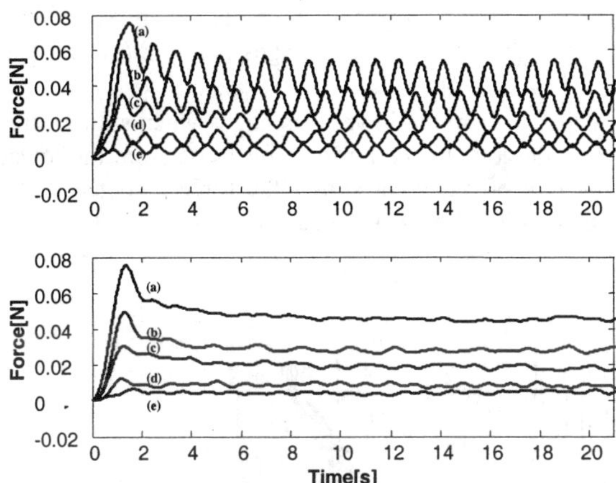

Figure 2.   *In-vivo* force response from the liver to ramp and hold stimuli under displacement control. (a) velocity of indentation=8mm/s, depth of indentation=8mm; (b) velocity of indentation=6mm/s, depth of indentation=6mm; (c) velocity of indentation=4mm/s, depth of indentation=4mm; (d) velocity of indentation=2mm/s, depth of indentation=2mm; (e) velocity of indentation=1mm/s, depth of indentation=1mm. Raw data is shown in the top panel and data with the effect of pulse on force response removed is shown in the bottom panel.

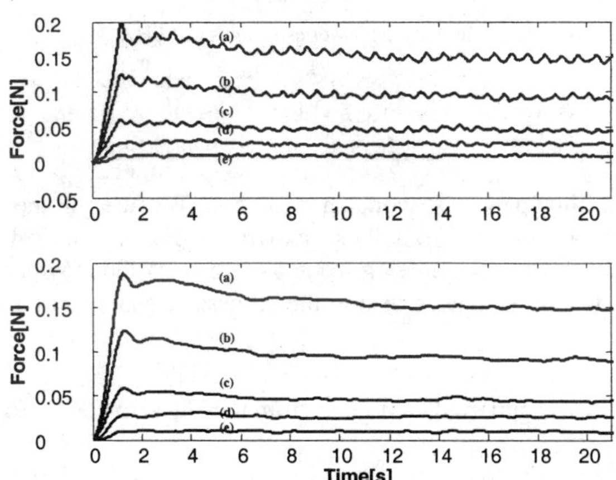

Figure 3.   *In-vivo* force response from the lower esophagus to ramp and hold stimuli under displacement control. Same format as Figure 2.

Figures 2 and 3 above show some typical force response as a function of time of the liver and the lower esophagus subjected to ramp and hold indentations in the Z-direction. Various velocities and depths of indentation were delivered as shown in the figures. The approximately sinusoidal variations in the force response in the upper panels of the figures indicate the forces generated due to the pulse of the pig. These forces are superimposed on the inherent force responses of the organs as the indenter is held in place at the required depth.

To observe the force response of the organs to the ramp and hold indentations without the influence of the pulse, a low pass digital filter was designed with a cutoff frequency just below the frequency of the pulse rate to generate the plots in the lower panels of the figures. These plots show the relaxation behavior of the organs as well as steady state force response. Comparing Figures 2 and 3, we see that the lower esophagus is 2 to 2.5 times stiffer than the liver.

Figure 4 shows the force response from the lower esophagus when subjected to sinusoidal indentation at 1.0Hz. The plot on the left shows the force response from the lower esophagus as a function of time while the plot on the right shows the force response as a function of displacement. The nonzero area of the loop indicates viscous energy dissipation.

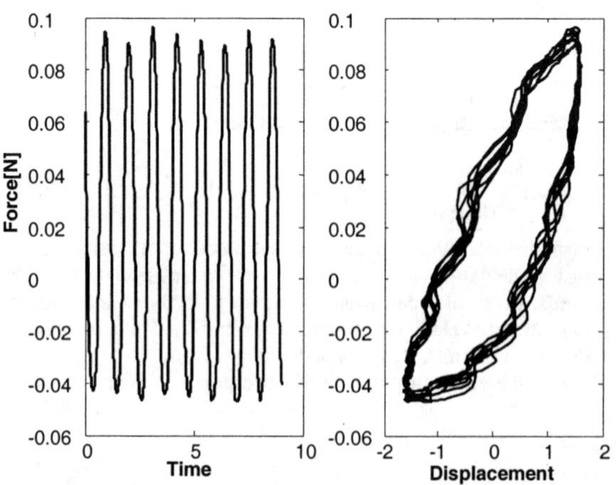

Figure 4. *In-vivo* sinusoidal force response from the lower esophagus at 1.0Hz.

4. Concluding remarks

What we have presented in this paper is work in progress. We are in the process of incorporating the material response data from these experiments in a surgical trainer for laparoscopic Heller myotomy [7]. Efforts are being made to determine the effects of boundary conditions on the organ force response. We are also in the process of quantifying the effects of anisotropy on tissue response.

Acknowledgment: This work was supported by a grant from the Harvard Center for Minimally Invasive Surgery.

References

[1] S. De, J.K., M.A. Srinivasan, A Meshless Numerical Technique for Physically Based Real Time Medical Simulations, *Proceedings of MMVR Conference* (2001) 113-118.

[2] Y. C. Fung, Biomechanics: mechanical properties of living tissues, Springer-Verlag, New York (1993).

[3] Inman Brouwer, J.U., Loren Bentley, Alana Sherman, Neel Dhruv, Frank Tendick, Measuring In Vivo Animal Soft Tissue Properties for Haptic Modelling in Surgical Simulation, *Proceedings of MMVR Conference* (2001) 69-74.

[4] F. J. Carter, T.G.F., P. J. Davies, D. McLean, A. Cuschieri, Biomechanical Testing of Intra-abdominal Soft Tissues, *Medical Image Analysis* (2000).

[5] Mark P. Ottensmeyer, E.B.-U., J. Kenneth Salisbury, Input and Output for Surgical Simulation: Devices to Measure Tissue Properties *in vivo* and a Haptic Interface for Laparoscopy Simulators, *Proceedings of MMVR Conference* (2000) 236-241.

[6] Blake Hannaford, J.T., Mika Sinanan, Manuel Moreya, Jacob Rosen, Jeff Brown, Rainer Leuschke, Mark MacFarlane, Computerized Endoscopic Surgical Grasper, *Proceedings of MMVR Conference* (1998) 265-271.

[7] S. De , M. Manivannan, J. Kim, M. A. Srinivasan, D. Rattner, Medical Simulation of Laparoscopic Heller Myotomy using a Meshless Technique, *Proceedings of MMVR 2002 Conference* (2002).

Medicine Meets Virtual Reality 02/10
J.D. Westwood et al. (Eds.)
IOS Press, 2002

Estimation of Soft-Tissue Model Parameters Using Registered Pre- and Postoperative Facial Surface Scans

Matthias Teschner
National Biocomputation Center
Stanford University, USA

Sabine Girod
National Biocomputation Center
Stanford University, USA

Abstract

Computer–based techniques for the simulation of craniofacial surgical procedures and for the prediction of the surgical outcome have been shown to be very useful. However, the assessment of the accuracy of the simulated surgical outcome is difficult. In this paper, a technique is described which allows to compare the simulated surgical outcome and the actual surgical result. The simulated postoperative patient's appearance is compared to a second surface scan which is obtained postoperatively. The pre- and postoperative surface scans, which are different due to the surgery, are registered employing a robust registration method which minimizes distances of corresponding points. Parameters of the soft–tissue model can be adapted with respect to minimized differences of corresponding points of the simulated postoperative and the actual postoperative surface of a patient's face.

1 Introduction

Simulation methods are used to support osteotomy planning and to predict the patient's postoperative appearance preoperatively. These techniques support the surgical planning process and enable an efficient, economical, and save study of craniofacial surgery methods [1], [2], [3], [4]. Based on a CT scan of a patient's head and a photorealistic surface scan of a patient's face, a craniofacial surgery simulation system is used to simulate surgical procedures [5]. Soft tissue is represented by mass points with nonlinear forces between adjacent mass points. In order to predict soft–tissue deformation due to simulated surgical procedures, an optimization approach is employed.

2 Deformable Soft–Tissue Model

Soft tissue is represented using a nonlinear mass–spring model. Mass points and springs are classified with respect to certain characteristics. The model considers the layered structure of soft tissue, the skin turgor, gravity, and nonlinear elasto–mechanical properties of soft tissue.

The computation of soft–tissue deformation due to bone realignment or external forces is based on the optimization of a nonlinear cost function. The cost function considers the sum of magnitudes of resulting forces at all mass points. The cost function is parametrized by the positions of all mass points.

The technique for soft-tissue deformation is integrated in a system for craniofacial surgery simulation. The system handles patient-individual data sets. It is capable of simulating bone cutting and bone realignment with integrated interactive collision detection. Soft–tissue deformation due to simulated surgical procedures can be computed. The system can be used to predict the postoperative patient's appearance preoperatively [5].

3   Framework for Estimating Model Parameters

In order to assess the precision of the simulated surgical outcome, the simulated postoperative patient's appearance has to be compared with the actual postoperative appearance. Therefore, a pre– and a postoperative photorealistic surface scan of a patient's face are obtained. In order to enable the comparison, the pre– and postoperative surface scan have to be registered. Registration is required due to the fact, that the pre– and the postoperative scan are most probably obtained with different positions of the patient's head relative to the scanner.

In contrast to the well–known Iterative Closest Point algorithm (ICP) [6], which minimizes the mean of the Euclidean distances between corresponding points, a robust registration method is employed, which minimizes the median of the Euclidean distances of corresponding points [7]. This is due to the fact, that the pre– and the postoperative facial scan differ in certain areas, i.e., corresponding points in these areas will still have comparative large Euclidean distances. In case of minimizing the median error instead of the mean error these points do not falsify the transformation computed by the registration process. If both scans are registered, the surgery simulation is performed using the preoperative scan of the patient's face and the simulation result is compared to the actual postoperative appearance by assessing the differences of corresponding points.

Parameters of the soft–tissue model, such as number of soft–tissue layers or spring constants, are adapted with respect to minimized differences of corresponding points of the simulated and the actual surface of a patient's face.

4   Results

A mass–spring model has been developed that enables the representation of realistic non-linear elasto–mechanical properties of multi–layer soft tissue. An integrated system for craniofacial surgery simulation has been developed. The system handles patient-individual data sets. It is capable of simulating bone cutting and realignment with integrated inter-active collision detection. Soft–tissue deformation due to simulated surgical procedures can be computed. Various surgical procedures have been simulated using six patient-individual data sets.

Registration of pre– and postoperative surface scans provides the opportunity to assess the accuracy of the simulation result by comparing the simulated and the actual postoperative patient's appearance. Differences between both scans can be minimized by the adaption of model parameters. Fig. 1 shows a pre– and postoperative surface scan of a patient's face. Both scans are registered and the registration error is visualized in the right–hand image. Dark colors represent large errors (Hausdorff distances up to $6mm$). Areas influenced by the surgery show large registration errors. However, these areas do not falsify the registration of the entire scan. The second group of images shows two scans with and without swelling. This swelling can be seen in the right–hand image which visualizes the registration error of these two scans. It can be seen that the registration approach is not influenced by areas which are different in both scans.

The registration shown in Fig. 1 can be used to compare the simulated postoperative patient's appearance and his actual postoperative appearance. The registration can also be employed to objectively assess the swelling, e. g. by measuring the volume of the swelling.

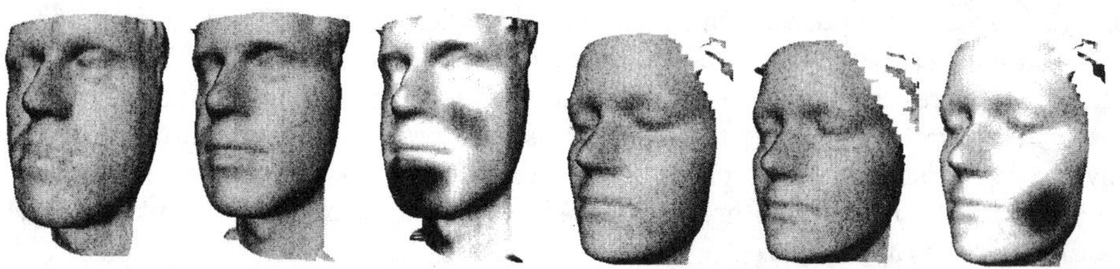

Figure 1: Two patient data sets. Left: Praeoperative surface scan. Middle: Postoperative surface scan. Right: Registration error mapped onto the postoperative surface scan. Dark areas represent a large Hausdorff–distance up to $6mm$. Bright areas are regions with no significant registration error.

References

[1] R. Kikinis, H. Cline, D. Altobelli, M. Halle, W. Lorensen, F. Jolesz. "Interactive Visualization and Manipulation of 3D Reconstructions for the Planning of Surgical Procedures". In *Proc VBC '92*, pages 559–563, 1992.

[2] R. M. Koch, M. H. Gross, D. F. Bueren, G. Frankhauser, Y. Parish, F. R. Carls. "Simulating Facial Surgery Using Finite Element Models". *SIGGRAPH '96, ACM Computer Graphics*, 30, August 1996.

[3] M. Bro-Nielsen. "Finite Element Modeling in Surgery Simulation". *Proc of the IEEE: Special Issue on Virtual & Augmented Reality in Medicine*, 86(3):524–530, Mar 1998.

[4] H. Delingette, S. Cotin, N. Ayache, "A Hybrid Elastic Model Allowing Real–Time Cutting, Deformations and Force–Feedback for Surgery Training and Simulation," *Proc Computer Animation 1999*, IEEE Comput. Soc. Los Alamitos, CA, USA, pp. 70–81, 1999.

[5] M. Teschner, S. Girod, B. Girod, "Surgical Planning," *Principles of 3D Image Analysis and Synthesis*, Girod, Greiner, Niemann (ed.), Kluwer Academic Publishers, Boston, 2000.

[6] B. K. P. Horn, "Closed Form Solution of Absolute Orientation using Unit Quaternions," *Journal of the Optical Society A*, vol. 4, no. 4, pp. 629–642, April 1987.

[7] P. J. Rousseeuw, A. M. Leroy, *Robust Regression and Outlier Detection*, ISBN 0471852333, John Wiley and Sons Inc., New York, 1987.

Medicine Meets Virtual Reality 02/10
J.D. Westwood et al. (Eds.)
IOS Press, 2002

Virtual Endoscopy using Spherical QuickTime-VR Panorama Views

Ulf Tiede[1], Norman von Sternberg-Gospos[1], Paul Steiner[2], Karl Heinz Höhne[1]

[1]*Institute of Mathematics and Computer Science in Medicine (IMDM),*
[2]*Dept. of Radiology*
University Hospital Hamburg-Eppendorf, Germany

Abstract. Virtual endoscopy needs some precomputation of the data (segmentation, path finding) before the diagnostic process can take place. We propose a method that precomputes multinode spherical panorama movies using Quick-Time VR. This technique allows almost the same navigation and visualization capabilities as a real endoscopic procedure, a significant reduction of interaction input is achieved and the movie represents a document of the procedure.

1 Introduction

Virtual endoscopy (VE) and especially virtual colonoscopy (VC) have gained much attention in diagnostic radiology recently. After acquisition of a MRI or CT volume data set the procedure involves the following computation steps:

- segmentation of the colon
- determination of the (typically central) path through the colon
- navigation through the colon and visualisation of the colon wall
- documentation of the flight through the colon as a movie
- transfer of the document together with the report to the referring physician
- in a modern environment: archiving and communication of the document in a PACS

In clinical practice it has turned out to be advantageous to do the segmentation in advance and also to compute a path before viewing, because otherwise the navigation is extremely tedious and time consuming and needs a complex user interface. In ideal cases segmentation can be done automatically [1], however, in some cases manual control is required due to noise in the data or motion artefacts. A common approach for path computation is skeletonization [2]. For noisy data and due to wrickles in the colon highly sophisticated heuristics are needed to remove dead ends and loops, to end up with a smooth path. Another way to support navigation is described in [3]. Here a potential field is calculated, which is used to compute a force that pushes the virtual viewer back onto the central path. The strength of the force depends on the distance of the current view point to the path. At the colon wall the force is infinite thus inhibiting the user to pass through the wall. Other approaches unfold the inner colon surface to a 2D image map [4]. However, clinicians are unfamiliar with these images in addition to geometric distortion problems.

The visualization of the colon wall requires a conversion of the colon surface to polygonal meshes in order to utilize standard computer graphics hardware and software, which allow to compute 3D views at near real-time speed for modest size datasets. Available voxel-based accelerators (e.g. Mitsubishi VolumePro) cannot perform perspective transformations directly which are a essential for calculating endoscopic views [5].

Outgoing from the fact, that navigation is complex (even when a central path is already defined) and real-time visualization for high quality rendering cannot be achieved on standard PCs, we investigated an approach that also precomputes a large part of the visualization. Expected advantages are that visualization is restricted to "meaningful" images and interaction becomes easier.

2   Method and material

If we would try to include any possible view in a precomputed movie, the amount of data would be huge and navigation would not be simple at all. If we use only a fixed field of view and a constant viewing direction while moving through the colon along the central path one might miss important details which are outside the selected field of view (e.g. behind wrinkles). A well-known technique from classical photography is the use of wide angle ("fish-eye") lenses, but these yield strong geometric distortions. Another approach that we propose here is the generation of panorama images where a number of overlapping photographs are taken while the camera is rotated around the vertical axis. The single photographs are then connected to form a cylindrical image also known as a panorama view. While this technique needs some effort in photography it can easily be simulated in computer graphics. However, cylindrical projections do not allow straight views up and down, i.e. 90° upwards or downwards from the horizon due to geometric distortions that become apparent at viewing angles larger than 45°. A generalization of cylindrical panoramas are spherical panoramas, which allow viewing in all directions. Recently Apple Computer, Inc. has incorporated spherical panoramas into their QuickTime-VR technology. They provide a data structure where six images corresponding to the six faces of a cube are interpreted as a spherical panorama [6]. The QuickTime player has a build-in distortion correction method for viewing these *cubic panoramas* as spherical scenes. In contrast to other precomputed movies, the amount of data is thus decisively reduced. In addition the interaction with QTVR movies is very simple.

Cubic panoramas are computed as follows: From a given viewpoint we compute six 3D projections, which correspond to the six faces of a cube. The viewpoint is assumed to be located at the center of the cube, i.e. the first projection looks into the direction along the central path, then we turn 90° to the right, compute the 2nd image. Turn again 90° to the right, now we are looking back into the direction we came from, turn again and finally we compute the images when looking 90° upwards and downwards. As can easily be seen the six projections must be calculated with a field of view of exactly 90° so that the images fit nicely together and form the faces of a cube (Fig. 1). The images are stored as a sequence of frames together with additional information that allows QuickTime to recognize the images to be a cubic panorama. The QuickTime player then allows continuous navigation across the entire panorama in real-time using the two degrees of freedom of the mouse.

For a continuous motion through the colon we compute such cubic panoramas along the central path every few millimeters with a high resolution rendering algorithm described in [7]. The single panoramas, which are called nodes in QuickTime terminology, must then be connected to enable the player to "jump" from one node to the next. This is accomplished using so called hot spots, which are just an additional image layer, where the pixel values correspond to the node number the player may move to. These hot spot images are very simple and can be calculated automatically for colonoscopy, because there are no bifurcations. Thus if we are at node n the pixel value of the hot spot for all possible forward-looking directions, i.e. 180° field of view from the initial viewing direction, is n+1, and the value for all backward-looking directions is n-1. The result is a multi-node cubic panorama movie.

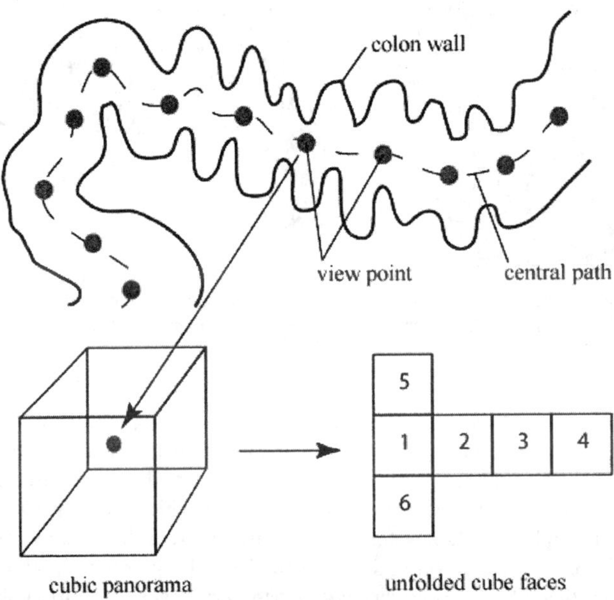

Fig. 1: Cubic panorama generation. At any viewing position 6 projections corresponding to the 6 faces of a cube are computed with a field of view of 90°.

As each panorama node has its own initial viewing parameters, i.e. pan and tilt angles and field of view, it is important for a smooth transition from one node to the next not to use these initial values to preserve and transfer the parameters of the current node. We modified the behaviour of the player to handle this requirement, so that it become possible to move through the colon while inspecting the colon wall laterally.

For diagnostic purposes it is not sufficient to provide endoscopic views only. For the radiologist, who is familiar with interpreting CT and MR images, it is a necessity to have access to the original data at any stage of the viewing process. Therefore we do not only store the panorama images but the corresponding z-buffers and the related viewing transformation matrices as well (Fig. 2). With this additional information available we can easily get back from any surface location into the original gray scale volume. Furthermore this allows the simultaneous display of different views such as 3D outside views, in which the current virtual camera position and orientation can be marked to facilitate orientation.

3   Results

We applied the described method to about 20 contrast enhanced MRI datasets of the colon. The datasets were segmented by thresholding and the central path as well as up to 200

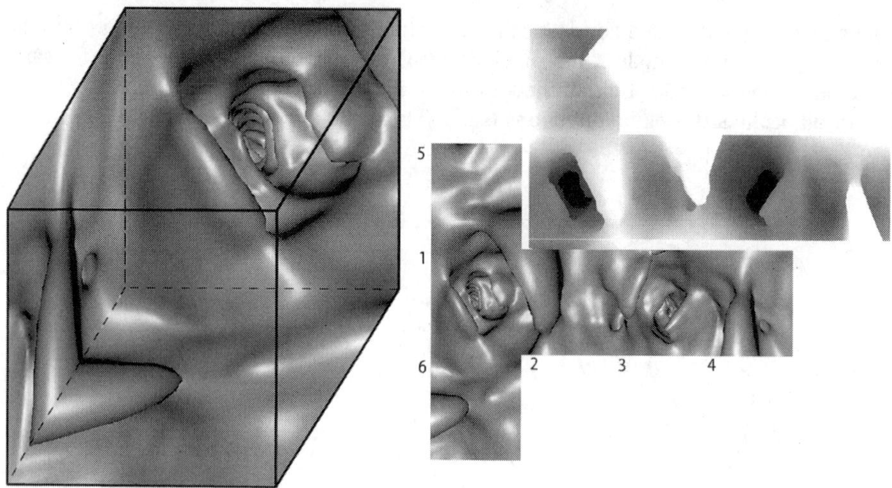

Fig. 2: Left: Cubic panorama projections. Right: Image map of the 6 unfolded cube faces (front) and their corresponding z-buffers (rear). The distortion correction for viewing a panorama is performed automatically by the QuickTime player

high resolution cubic panoramas together with their corresponding z-buffers were computed and stored in the QuickTime VR movie format. Additionally a matrix of 3D overview images that show the colon from outside were created to facilitate orientation. These images are stored as a QuickTime VR object movie which is very similar to panorama movies. The radiologist can then access the final movie over the intranet on his desktop PC. He can "move" through the colon in real-time while looking around in all directions searching for abnormalities. On the 3D overview he can verify were the virtual endoscope is currently located. Also, just by clicking on the colon surface at any location, the corresponding position is marked on three orthogonal cross-sections showing the original MR values. This helps the radiologist who is familiar with 2D cross-sections in the assessment of suspected lesions. Fig. 3 shows the simple graphical interface we have developed for virtual colonoscopy. Our radiologists feel comfortable with the user interface. The entire procedure takes a couple of minutes for establishing a diagnosis.

4   Conclusion

Using precomputed spherical panorama images for virtual endoscopy allows quasi real-time viewing and easy navigation on a standard PC. Especially the very simple user interface has proved helpful for the acceptance of the procedure. The method can also be applied to structures with bifurcations like blood vessels or the bronchi. Fig. 4 shows as an example the bifurcation of the bronchi computed from the Visible Human data set [8]. As a decisive advantage the panorama movie represents a document similar to classical video recordings of real endoscopic examinations with additional functionality that can be viewed with standard software at any PC or with browser technology in an Intranet. Due to the fact that computation time is not an issue, also more sophisticated rendering methods like automatic color labeling of suspicious regions can easily be incorporated. If connected to a knowledge base [9] additional features like symbolic descriptions and manipulation capabilities become possible, which allow to generate even more comprehensive teaching and learning material [10].

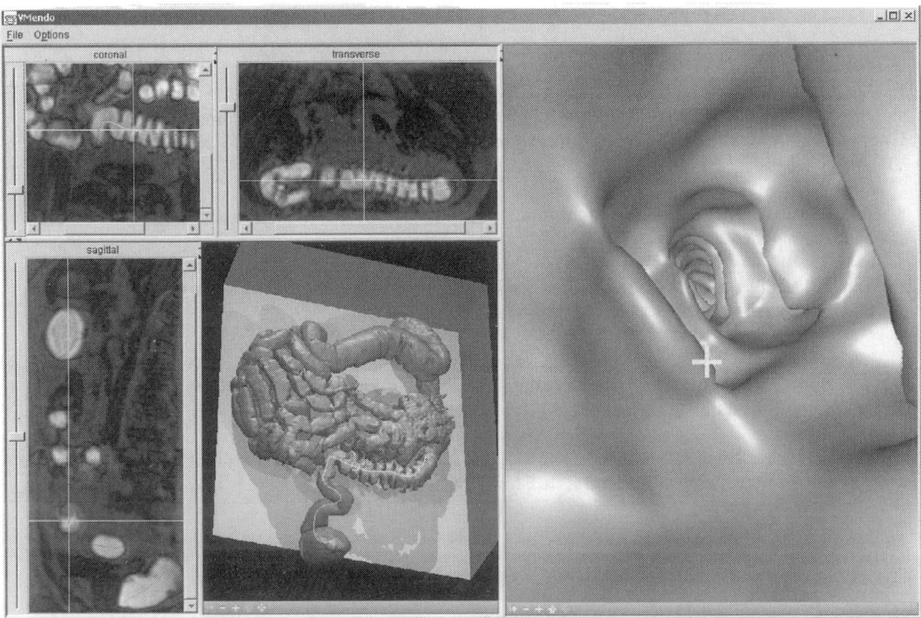

Fig. 3: User interface showing an endoscopic view (right), a 3D overview image (middle bottom) and three orthogonal MR cross-sections. The marked position on the colon wall (white cross) corresponds to the positions on the cross-sections and in the overview.

Currently the number of panoramas in a single QuickTime VR movie is limited to 255 which is not a real restriction for the application shown here. Further research should also take stereoscopic viewing into account.

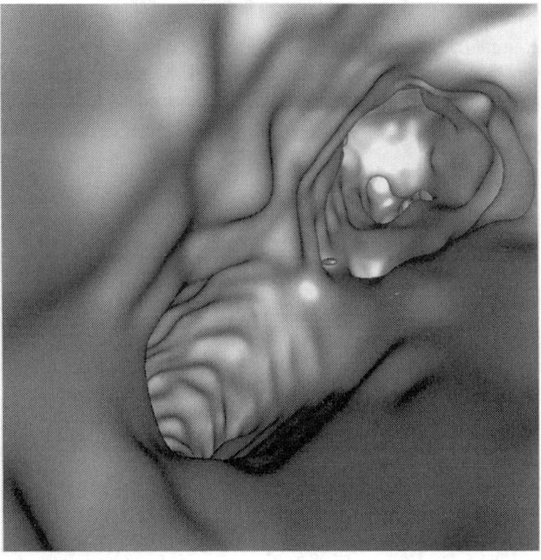

Fig. 4: Panorama view of the main bifurcation of the bronchi computed from the Visible Human Dataset.

5   References

[1] M. Sato, S. Lakare, M. Wan, A. Kaufman, Z. Liang, and M. Wax, An automatic colon segmentation for 3D virtual colonoscopy, IEICE Trans. Information and Systems, Vol. E84-D, No. 1, January 2001, pp. 201-208.

[2] Y. Zhou, A. W. Toga, Efficient Skeletonization of Volumetric Objects, IEEE Transactions on Visualization and Computer Graphics, vol. 5 (3), 1999, pp. 196-209.

[3] M. Wan, F. Dachille, and A. Kaufman, Distance-Field Based Skeletons for Virtual Navigation, Visualization 2001, San Diego, CA, October 2001, in press

[4] A. V. Bartroli, R. Wegenkittl, A. König, E. Gröller, Virtual Colon Unfolding, Technical Report TR-186-2-01-08, April 2001: Institute of Computer Graphics and Algorithms, Visualization and Animation Group, Vienna University of Technology.

[5] M. Wan, W. Li, K. Kreeger, I. Bitter, A. Kaufman, Z. Liang, D. Chen and M. Wax, 3D Virtual Colonoscopy with Real-time Volume Rendering, In: Chin-Tu Chen, Anne V. Clough (eds.) Proc. SPIE Medical Imaging 2000, San Diego, CA., Feb. 2000, Vol. 3978, pp. 165-171

[6] Interactive Movies: QuickTime VR, Apple Computer, Inc., 2001
http://developer.apple.com/techpubs/quicktime/qtdevdocs/PDF/insideqt_qtvr.pdf

[7] U. Tiede, T. Schiemann, K.H. Hoehne, High Quality Rendering of Attributed Volume Data, In: David Ebert et al. (eds.): Proc. IEEE Visualization '98, IEEE Computer Society Press, Los Alamitos, CA, 1998, 225-262.

[8] A. Pommert, K.H. Höhne, B. Pflesser, E. Richter, M. Riemer, T. Schiemann, R. Schubert, U. Schumacher, U. Tiede: Creating a high-resolution spatial/symbolic model of the inner organs based on the Visible Human. *Med. Image Anal. 5*, 3 (2001), 221-228.

[9] R. Schubert, B. Pflesser, A. Pommert, K. Priesmeyer, M. Riemer, T. Schiemann, et al., Interactive volume visualization using 'intelligent movies', In: Westwood JD et al., editors. MMVR 99. Proceedings of the Confenrence Medicine Meets Virtual Reality; 1999 Jan 20–23; San Francisco, CA. Amsterdam: IOS Press 1999. Studies in Health Technology and Informatics 62. p. 321-327.

[10] K.H. Höhne, B. Pflesser, A. Pommert, K. Priesmeyer, M. Riemer, T. Schiemann, R. Schubert, U. Tiede, H.-C. Frederking, S. Gehrmann, S. Noster, U. Schumacher, VOXEL-MAN 3D-Navigator: Inner Organs. Regional, Systemic and Radiological Anatomy, Springer-Verlag Electronic Media, Heidelberg, 2000. (3 CD-ROMs, ISBN 3-540-14759-4).

Medicine Meets Virtual Reality 02/10
J.D. Westwood et al. (Eds.)
IOS Press, 2002

Integration of intraoperative radiotherapy (IORT) dose distribution into the postoperative CT-based external beam radiotherapy (EBRT) treatment planing

*Martina Treiber, **S. Daeuber, * R. Krempien, **H. Hoppe, *FW. Hensley, *J. Brief, **H. Woern, ***T. Lehnert, ***M. Buechler, *M. Wannenmacher

* *University of Heidelberg, Department of Clinical Radiology, Germany*
** *University of Karlsruhe (TH), Institute for Process Control and Robotics, Germany*
*** *University of Heidelberg, Dept. of Surgery, Germany*

Abstract:

In the treatment of malignant disease external beam radiation therapy (EBRT) is often combined with surgery. Intraoperative radiotherapy (IORT) improves the local control by dose escalation. For reasons of recording, improvement and security of the intervention, it would be necessary to merge the IORT-dose distribution with the postoperative CT-based EBRT-planing. The aim of this work was to develop a method to reconstruct the IORT field and register it with the postoperative planing CT. This enables the reconstruction of the IORT dose distribution and merge it with the CT-based EBRT planing data. We use a surface scanner to receive a large amount of surface points which enables us reconstruct the IORT-field and to register it with the CT-based EBRT planning data. Scanning and calculation time is not over 2 seconds, depending mainly on the CPU power. The error of a single point is below 1 mm. The density of the point cloud is approx. 4 per mm^2. In this paper we give an overview of our experimental setup and the accuracy of the method.

1. Background/Problem

In the treatment of malignant disease external beam radiation therapy (EBRT) is often combined with surgery [Gunderson]. EBRT dose is limited due to radiosensitive surrounding tissue. Intraoperative radiotherapy (IORT) improves the local control by dose escalation (direct access; adjacent risk organs can be removed from the IORT field) [Eble1, Lehnert]. For reasons of recording, improvement and security of the intervention, it would be necessary to merge the IORT-Dose distribution with the postoperative CT-based EBRT-planing.

2. Method and Tools Used

The aim of this work was to develop a method to reconstruct the IORT field and register it with the postoperative planing CT. This enables the reconstruction of the IORT dose distribution and merge it with the CT-based EBRT planing data. Unfortunately the dose distribution can not be reconstructed post-operatively [Eble2]. Missing essential parameters are the exact position and angle of the IORT beam relative to the patient and the topology of the exposed area.

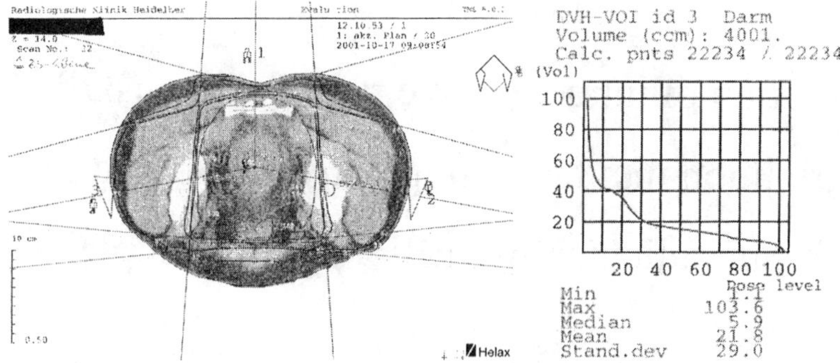

Fig. 1: EBRT-planing of rectal carcinoma. Left: Dose distribution over the planing target volume. Dose limitations of due to risk organs in the clinical target volume. Right: Due to the close anatomic relations, part of small bowel receives 100% of the planed dose (Dose volume histogram DVH). Due to the organ tolerance of the small bowel the max. EBRT dose is 45 Gy, which often is not sufficient for tumor control.

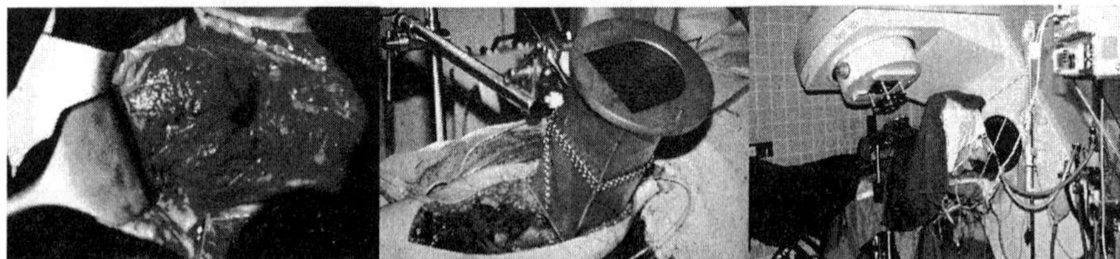

Fig. 2: IORT-procedure. Irradiation of the tumor bed i.e. the area of highest risk for local recurrence. In the IORT-procedure risk-organs can be removed from the target volume. Due to the IORT-dose to the tumor bed a dose escalation with higher local control rates without increase of side effects can be achieved.

The latter one affects the dose distribution by attenuation and scattering of the (electron) beam. We scan the IORT-field surface using a coded light projection [Gaertner, Tang]. In addition with fiducials to mark of the field we get both the exact position of the beam and the topology.

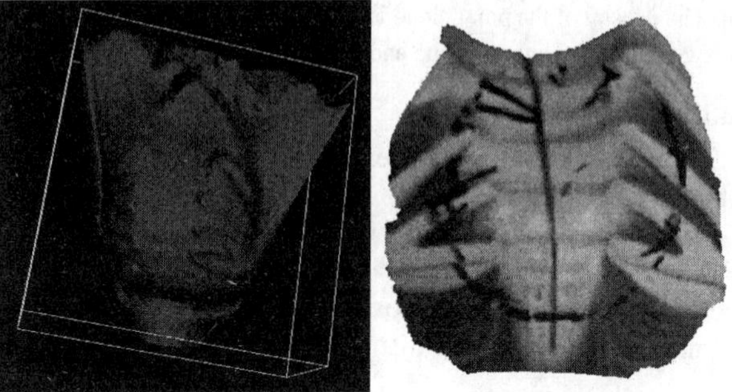

Fig. 3: Surface reconstruction of the tumor bed using a IORT-phantom. Left. Surface reconstruction using a laser scanner. Right: the blue circle represents the IORT-field. After registration with the EBRT planing-CT a reconstruction of the dose-distribution ca be performed in the EBRT planing CT data.

The scanning hardware consists of a conventional video projector, two CCD-cameras and a state-of-the-art PC (800 MHz CPU, 256 Mbytes RAM). The system generates a set of three-dimensional coordinates, i.e. points, which all are located on the surface of the IORT-field. After reconstructing the IORT-field the afore mentioned fiducials remain in the patient and are used to register the IORT-field reconstruction with a postoperative CT. The transfer to postoperative CT is a standard task (rigid registration).

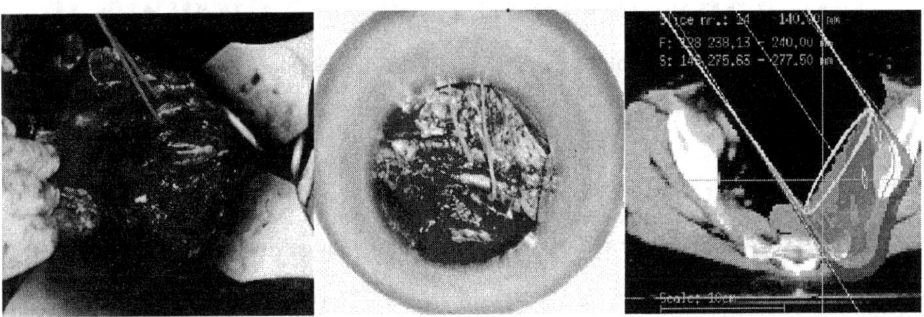

Fig. 4: IORT-field and reconstruction of dose distribution in the EBRT planing CT. Left: Tumor bed with risk structure (ureter). Middle: IORT-field through electron tube. Risk structure can be removed from IORT-field. Right: After surface reconstruction a reconstruction of the IORT dose distribution can be simulated in the EBRT planing CT.

3. Results, Conclusions

We have tested the approach using a pelvis model for intraoperative simulation of an IORT field to rectal carcinomas. As mentioned above the IORT-field was clipmarked and then a surface image of the IORT-field was acquired using the light projection. It was important to visualize the fiducials in the surface image. After this procedure a planning CT for EBRT planning in RT-position was obtained. The surface image of the IORT-field then was registered within the CT scan using the fiducials.

Scanning and calculation time is not over 2 seconds, depending mainly on the CPU power. The error of a single point is below 1 mm. The density of the point cloud is approx. 4 per mm^2.

4. Conclusions

Structured light is a global measurement technique, particularly useful where the behavior of an entire surface is of interest. It's use in the definition of the IORT field and the registration of the field and the field shape to a planning CT in order to incorporate the IORT dose in the EBRT planing is a possible solution. In this paper we give an overview of our experimental setup and the accuracy of the method.

5. References

S. Tang, C. Kwoh, M. Teo, N. W. Sing, and K. Ling, "Augmented Reality Systems for Medical Applications", IEEE Engineering in Medicine and Biology (May/June 1998), pp. 49-58, 1998.

H. Gaertner, "Quantitative ∫3D-Vermessung mit codierter Beleuchtung", Institut für Technische Optik, Universität Stuttgart, 1998.

Eble M.J., M. Treiber, Th. Lehnert, Ch. Herfarth, M. Wannenmacher IORT for recurrent rectal carcinoma. Font-Radiat-Ther-Oncol 1997 31:229-33

Eble MJ., Hensley F, Wannenmacher M Dosimetra of IORT fieldsin the pelvic cavity International Society of Intraoperative Radiation Therapy (ISIORT) 1998

Lehnert T, Treiber M, Tiefenbacher U, Wannenmacher M Intraoperative radiotherapy for carcinoma of the gastrointestinal tract Seminars in Surg. Oncol. In press

Gunderson LL, Willett CG, Harrison LB, Petersen IA, Haddoch MG Intraoperative irradiation: current and future status. Semin Oncol. 1997 Dec;24(6):715-31.

Medicine Meets Virtual Reality 02/10
J.D. Westwood et al. (Eds.)
IOS Press, 2002

The application of eyeglass displays in changing the perception of pain

Mimi M. Y. Tse[1], Jacobus K.F. Ng[2], Joanne W.Y. Chung[1] and Thomas K.S. Wong[1]

*Department of Nursing & Health Sciences, The Hong Kong Polytechnic University, Hung Hom,
Kowloon, Hong Kong [1]*
Department of Anaesthesiology, Faculty of Medicine, The University of Hong Kong [2]

E-mail: hsmtse@inet.polyu.edu.hk
Tel: 852 2766 6541
Fax: 852 2364 9663

Abstract. We have been examining the potential value of visual stimulation via the eyeglass displays in changing the perception of pain. In this randomized, controlled, cross-over study, 72 healthy university student volunteers were asked to wear a light-weighted eyeglass projecting a feeling of watching a fifty-two-inch television screen in a close distance while pain was produced by a modified tourniquet technique. There is a significant increase of pain threshold and pain tolerance with the effect of visual stimulation. These findings having implications of using visual stimulation as positive adjunct to other methods of pain relief and to different pain conditions in clinical areas.

1. Introduction

For many people, the experience of hospitalization is anxiety and pain (1). Fifty percent of patients regarded their pain relief as inadequate despite the use of pharmacological and non-pharmacological techniques to relieve pain (2). Unfamiliar hospital settings, various diagnostic and therapeutic procedures, and the sight and sounds of medical procedures exacerbate pain and anxiety in the hospital environment.

To block off the anxiety-induced sights and sounds of the hospital surroundings and create a pleasing environment, the use of light-weighted eyeglass displays might be able to change the sensation and perception of pain.

2. Research Method

It was a randomized, controlled, crossover study. An eyeglass was used and was connected to a VCD player (picture 1). The eyeglass only weights 120g, and could easily slip onto the user's face as a pair of spectacles (picture 2). Wearing the eyeglass displays gives the feeling of watching a fifty-two-inch television screen from only six and a half feet away.

Picture 1　An eyeglass was connected to a VCD

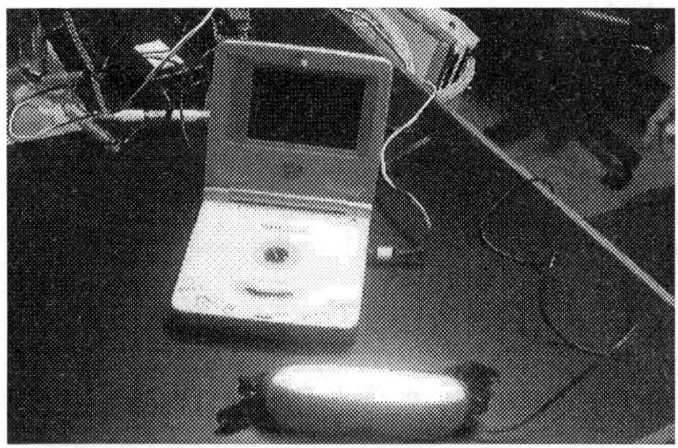

Picture 2　Wearing the eyeglass

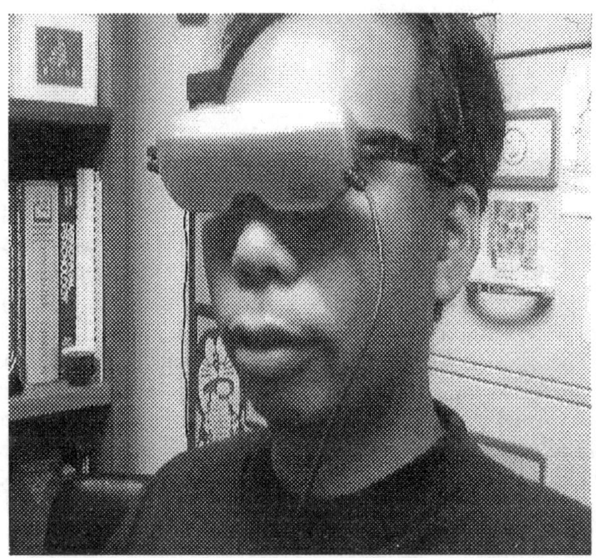

The sensation of pain was produced by a modified tourniquet technique (3). Subjects were randomly allocated into two groups (Group V and Group B) with subsequent cross-over. For those in Group V, subjects were instructed to wear the eyeglass and watch the soundless displays of natural scenery during the inflation. Whereas in Group B, the eyeglass they worn would project a static blank screen.

Pain threshold was defined as the time when subjects reported the first detectable pain, whereas pain tolerance was the time pain was reported to be intolerable and deflation of the tourniquet was requested. Level of anxiety, extent of simulation sickness and the degree immersion (getting into the visual stimulated world) were measured using a ten point numeric scale.

3. Results

There were seventy-two subjects participated in the study. (36 female, 36 male, age 20.97±1.97).   With visual stimulation generated by wearing the eyeglass displays, there was a significant increased in pain threshold (t=5.647, d.f. =71, p=0.000); with mean tourniquet time increased from 123 seconds to 187 seconds. Likewise, pain tolerance was significantly increased (t=7.088, d.f.=71, p=0.000), with mean tourniquet time increased from 271 seconds to 380 seconds.

It was a gender difference in pain threshold (p<0.01) when participants watching the static blank screen. Yet, both genders had an increased in pain threshold and pain tolerance after using the eyeglass displays. The degree of immersion was positively correlated with the improvement in pain threshold, whereas anxiety level was negatively correlated with the improvement in pain threshold. Only 4 out of 72 participants reported to have a slight degree motion sickness.

4. Conclusions and future work

The findings from this study highlighted the therapeutic potential of using eyeglass displays visual stimulation as positive adjunct to pain control. The gate control theory of pain supports the use of cognitive processes such as distraction to alter pain perception (4). The results of our study support the theory. Indeed the impact of visual stimulation on pain threshold and pain tolerance has been examined in voluntary subjects (5).   A convenience sample of forty-six (32 female and 14 male, age 21.7±1.58) university-age Chinese students was recruited. Watching videotapes via a 29-inch television generated visual stimuli. There was a 33% increased in pain threshold and 27% increased in pain tolerance as compared to the control group. In the present study, wearing an eyeglass displays generated visual stimuli. There was a 52% increased in pain threshold and 40% increased in pain tolerance. It is found that the use of eyeglass displays might be more effective in blocking off the unpleasant sights of the immediate environment, and creating a pleasing environment by the video world.

It is found that only 4 out of 72 participants reported to have a slight degree of motion sickness. Thus, visual stimuli provided via the eyeglass displays are unlikely to create many undesirable effects such as motion sickness or other discomfort. Anxiety is known to increase subjective complaints of pain (6). In the present study, the advantage in watching videotapes via the eyeglass displays might be more effective in less anxious individuals in enhancing their pain perception. Visual stimulation is acting at least partially as a distraction for pain relief. The more immersed the subjects perceived themselves in the video stimulated world, the more distraction they were engaged and the awareness of pain might be decreased.

Likewise, providing visual stimuli to patients requires no prescription by the physician, and is convenient to use and acceptable to patients, making the use of various visual stimuli an appealing non-pharmacological intervention for pain relief. Nurses and other health care professionals are encouraged to use these interventions when performing painful procedures to patients.

The content of the visual displays could be tailored made to create a more immerse environment; and alleviate anxiety might be useful to enhance a better pain control when using the eyeglass displays device. The present study takes the first step towards establishing an innovative pain control technique, which may be practically applied in the clinical areas. There has not been any research and application of visual stimulation via the eyeglass displays in the local Chinese community as an adjunct to pain relief. Our study will add knowledge to the existing pain relief methods.

References

(1) Solomon, L. Film offers hospitals a kid-friendly makeover. WebMD Health Atlanta. (2000) On-line. Available: http://atlanta.webmd.com:80/content/article/2789.172

(2) McCaffrey, M. (1999). Pain management: problems and progress. In: McCaffrey M, Pasero C (eds.) *Pain: Clinical Manual.* (2nd. ed.). St. Louis, MO: Mosby.

(3) Janal, M.N., Glusman, M., Kuhl, J.P. & Clark, W.C (1994). On the absence of correlation between responses to noxious heat, cold, electrical and ischemic stimulation. *Pain* 58, 403-411.

(4) Sparks, L. (2001). Taking the "Ouch" out of injections for children: using distraction to decrease pain. *The American Journal of Maternal/Child Nursing* 26 (2), 72-78.

(5) Tse, M.M.Y., Yang, J.C.S., Chung, J.W.Y., & Wong, T.K.S. (2000). "The effect of visual stimuli on pain threshold and tolerance." Second International Health Care Conference, South Africa, 14-17 August, South Africa, pp.126 (manuscript in press)

(6) National Institutes of Health (1996). Integration of Behavioral and Relaxation Approaches into the Treatment of Chronic Pain and Insomnia. *JAMA*, 276 (4), 313-318.

Medicine Meets Virtual Reality 02/10
J.D. Westwood et al. (Eds.)
IOS Press, 2002

Evaluation of Visualization Techniques for Image-guided Navigation in Liver Surgery

Marcus VETTER[1], Peter HASSENPFLUG[1], Matthias THORN[1], Carlos CÁRDENAS[1],
Götz Martin RICHTER[3], Wolfram LAMADÉ[2], Christian HERFARTH[2],
Hans-Peter MEINZER[1]

*[1]Deutsches Krebsforschungszentrum, Div. Medical and Biological Informatics,
Im Neuenheimer Feld 280, 69120 Heidelberg, Germany*

*[2]Div. of Surgery, University of Heidelberg, Im Neuenheimer Feld 110,
69120 Heidelberg, Germany*

*[3]Div. of Radiology, University of Heidelberg, Im Neuenheimer Feld 110,
69120 Heidelberg, Germany*

Abstract. A substantial component of an image-guided surgery system (IGSS) is the kind of three-dimensional (3D) presentation to the surgeon because the visual depth perception of the complex anatomy is of significant relevance for orientation. Therefore, we examined in this contribution four different visualization techniques, which were evaluated by eight surgeons. The IGSS developed by our group supports the intraoperative orientation of the surgeon by depicting a visualization of the spatially tracked surgical instruments with respect to intrahepatic vessels that have to be conserved vitally, the tumor, and preoperatively calculated resection planes. In the prelimenary trial presented here we examined the human ability to percept an intraoperative virtual scene and to solve given navigation tasks. The focus of the experiments was to measure the ability of eight surgeons to orientate intrahepaticaly and to transfer the percepted spatial relation to movements in real space. An auto-stereoscopic visualization with a prism-based display yielded that the navigation can be performed faster and more accurately than with the other visualization techniques.

1. Introduction

Within the scope of this project we examine the human ability to orientate in a virtual environment by the means of different visualization techniques and to transfer the perceptions from the virtual world to the real anatomy of the patient. A good depth perception is especially important for the application of virtual environments within image-guided navigation in interventional medicine. An accurate spatial tracking of the surgical instruments is required during the intervention. Therefore, next to 3D visualizations on conventional displays quasi holographic visualizations on autostereoscopic displays come in question.

The surgeons expect an improved orientation during the invervention by the three-dimensional visualization of the complex structure and context of the organ's anatomy. A typical task of an IGSS is the virtual depiction of the surgical instruments in spatial relation to the individual anatomy

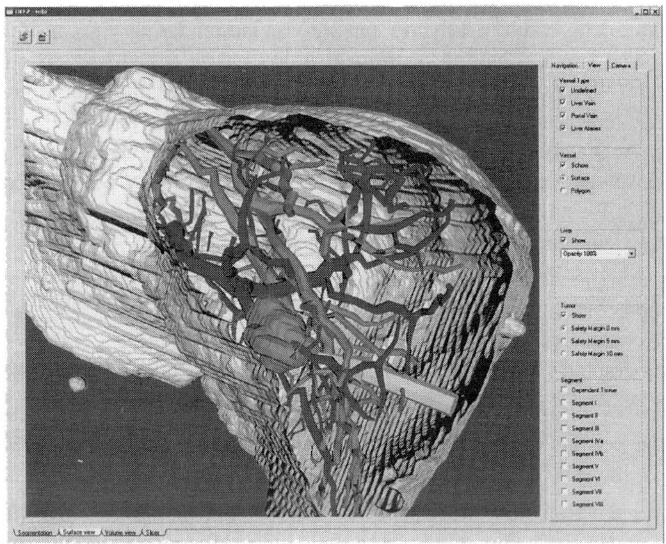

Figure 1: Screenshot of the devoloped application with view on a surface visualization of a clipped liver with intrahepatic vessels, tumor, and a depiction of the virtual instrument

of the patient [1]. Therefore, preoperative CT- and MRI data are preprocessed and enhanced with data from interventional planning [2]. These data are then registered with the current situs during the intervention and readapted to the current deformation of the organ. In many cases the mutual depiction of pre- and intrainterventional data is required that permits the specific selection of the kind of data which are currently adequate during the intervention. The depiction of the surgical instrument in relation to chosen data from planning and anatomy is important for the ability of the surgeon to orientate by the means of the virtual visualizations.

We are developing a prototype of an IGSS for the application in oncological liver surgery. This IGSS will enable the surgeon to see her/his instrument in relation to important structures inside the liver. For the successful resection of tumors in oncological liver surgery (R0 resection) the exact knowledge of the localization of the tumorous tissue and the surrounding security margin is necessary [3,4,5]. The transfer of the preoperatively planned resection margins to the current situs is of interest: The complex run of the intrahepatic vessels like the liver veins and the portal veins assist the surgeon to orientate inside the liver. A life-threatening injury of vessels that have to preserved essentially is a major intraoperative risk. The transfer of the preoperative anatomy and planning results to the intraoperative situs involves intraoperative image acquisition, registration with the preoperative data, deformation tracking and modeling, and the adequate presentation to the surgeon. Therefore, an adequate interface of the IGSS to the surgeon is an important component for a successful application of the system.

2. Methods

We developed a prototype of an image-guided navigation system for liver surgery, which allows a comparison of the different visualization techniques. For this purpose, intrahepatic vessels and tumors are visualized in real-time by surface rendering (VTK) and also with volume-rendering via the Volume Pro hardware board. For depicting the instrument together with the volume data, combined hybrid surface-volume-rendering via z-buffer merging was implemented. The surgical cutting instrument is tracked in 6 DOF by an electro-magnetic tracking system (NDI Aurora). As displays were used: a conventional computer screen with and without shutter-glasses and an auto-stereoscopic display (Dresden 3D) with and without head-tracking. A Diamond Fire GL3 graphics card is used to control the auto-stereoscopic display. The developed applications runs on a 1.7 GHz Pentium IV personal computer. Eight surgeons had to solve navigation tasks for a preliminary evaluation.

Four different visualization techniques were presented:

1. non-stereoscopic visualization on a conventional monitor
2. stereoscopic visualization with shutter glasses
3. auto-stereoscopic visualization on a prism-based display
4. quasi-holographic visualization on a prism-based display with additional head-tracking

The realization of 3. and 4. was performed using a new prism-based auto-stereoscopic display [6] that permits the perception of a stereoscopic 3D impression without the use of additional aids like HMDs, shutter glasses, red-green glasses or see-through displays.

We measured the trajectory and the orientation of the instrument in virtual space, the required time under given constraints from the surgical planning: The instrument had to be moved within given corridors.

2.1 Experimental setup

The examination was performed as a preliminary study with eight surgeons. Every subject got a training period of ten minutes for each visualization technique. Type and difficulty of the training tasks was comparable to those of the following measurements.

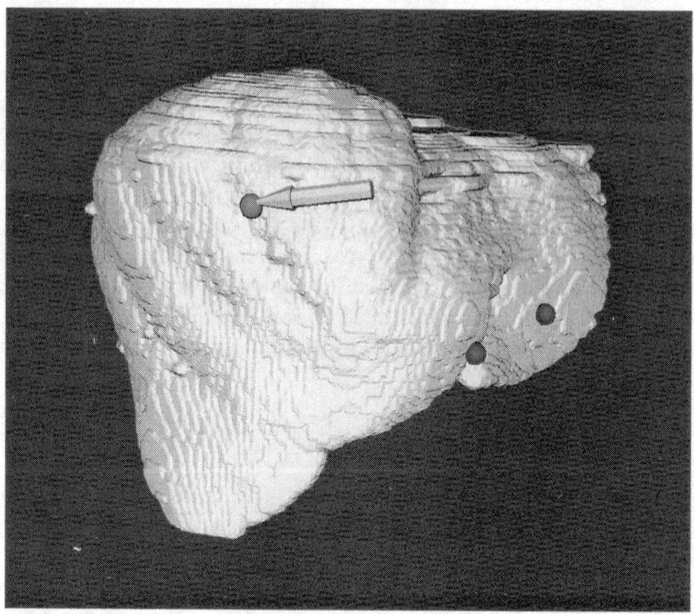

Figure 2: Surface visualization of the liver with three spheres as marks for experiment 1 and a depiction of the virtual instrument

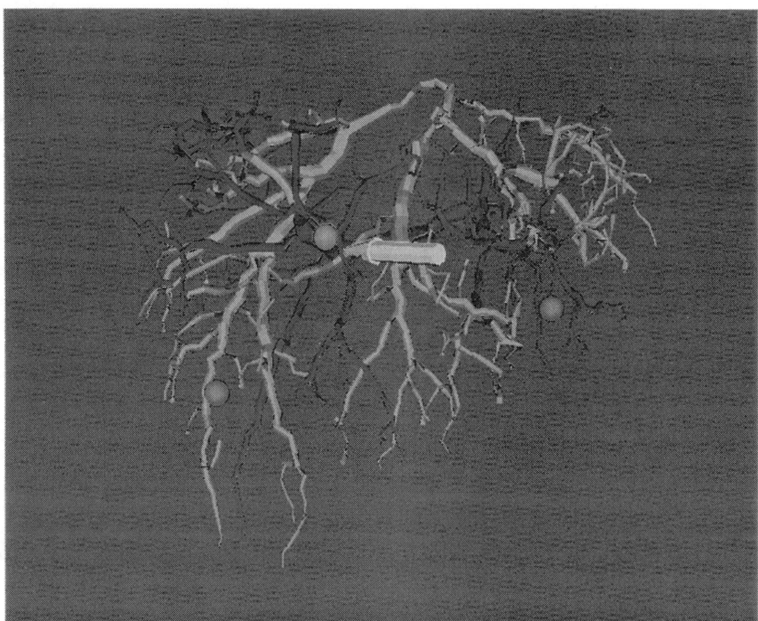

Figure 3: Surface visualization for experiment 2 depicting two intrahepatic vessel trees (blue: portal tree, turquoise: liver veins) , the virtual instrument and three destination spheres in the depth of the liver

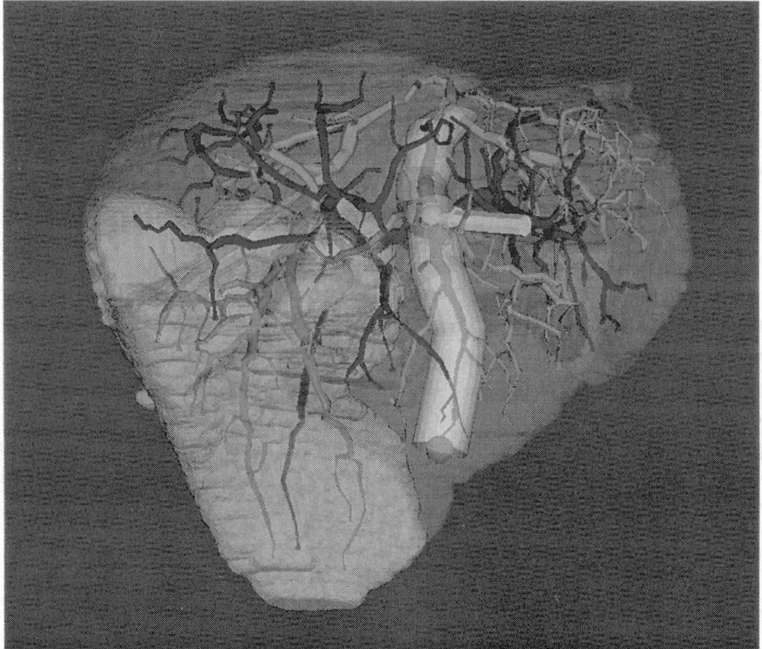

Figure 4: Surface visualization of the transparent liver with tumor, proposed resection region, intrahepatic vessles, the corridor with the three spheres, and the depiction of the virtual instrument (experiment 3)

For the second task the three spheres had to be reached at intrahepatic locations. Therefore, the destinations points were positioned at different depth between the intrahepatic vessels. The time required by the physician to reach every sphere was measured.

The first task consits of positioning an instrument at an exact position onto the surface of the organ. In this experiment only the surface of the liver and no intrahepatic structures were depicted. The time and trajectory from the defined starting position to the final destination was measured for each subject.

The third task consists of positioning the tip of the virtual instrument at three spheres staying inside a given intrahepatic corridor around the run of a vessel. The time of the instrument's tip inside and outside the corridor was measured and the number of corridor violations was counted.

3. Results

The non-stereoscopic display does not provide the surgeon with a sufficient depth perception because occlusion of objects is an insufficient depth cue. Nevertheless, the first task was solved fastest with this visualization technique with a mean time of 16 seconds. The evaluation of the trajectory yielded, that the users moved intuitively along the viewing ray in direction towards to object. The information about the occlusion of the instrument and the destination object is enough to determine the direction along the viewing ray.

The second task, finding objects in the inside of the organ, was solved worst with a mean time of 26 seconds. The task to stay inside a corridor could be solved with a mean 1.75 corridor violations worse than with shutter-glasses or the auto-stereoscopic display. Though the shutter-glasses yield good results with respect to intraheptic orientation they imply several disadvantages, which make them intraoperatively unacceptable for the surgeon. Reasons for this are tiresome flickering, significant light absorption and the limited field of view.

The stereoscopic visualization with the prism-based display yielded that the navigation can be performed faster and more accurately than with the other visualization techniques. The two first tasks were solved with a mean time of 18 and 22 seconds respectively. Particularly, the adherence to the corridor with an average of 1.13 corridor violations was significantly improved. Also, the relation of the surgical instrument with respect to interesting target structures is subjectively judged better by the surgeons.

For the quasi-holographic visualization it is necessary to additionally track the position of the observer's eyes to adaptively adjust the position of the virtual camera. This results in a improvement of orientation in the case of multiple occluding structures, e.g. vessel trees. The observer can look intuitionally and naturally around objects. For the corridor task the ideal path near the V. porta hepatica was partially occluded by another vessel. The observer could look around the viewing obstacle by intuitionally moving his/her had. This led to a significant reduction of corridor violations in this region.

4. Discussion and Conclusion

We developed a prototype for an image-guided navigation system for liver surgery. The evaluation of four different visualization techniques yielded significant improvements of orientation in the depth of the organ with respect to speed and accuracy in case of stereoscopic visualization techniques.

The stereoscopic visualization requires higher concentration by the observer. Its higher computational costs on current state of the art PCs yield a perceptible inferior response time in contrast to the 3D visualization on a conventional display. This drawback becomes especially perceivable during fast movements of the instrument. By the usage of next generation graphic cards this drawback will lose its importance.

The convenient auto-stereoscopic display is accepted best by the surgeons. Therefore, the prism-based visualization technique is a major step forward to intraoperativ stereoscopic visualization and orientation, respectively.

Acknowledgements

This work is being funded by the "Bundesministerium für Bildung und Forschung (BMBF)" grant 01EZ0008 within the scope of the "Innovationswettbewerb Medizintechnik".

References

[1] R. L. Galloway, R. J. Maciunas and C. A. Edwards, Interactive, image-guided neurosurgery. *IEEE Trans Biomed Eng* **39** (1992) 1226-1231.

[2] G. Glombitza, W. Lamadé, A. M. Demiris, M. R. Göpfert, A. Mayer, M. L. Bahner, H.-P. Meinzer, G. Richter, T. Lehnert and C. Herfarth, Virtual planning of liver resections: image processing, visualization and volumetric evaluation. *Int J Med Inf* **53**(2-3) (1999) 225-37.

[3] P. Hassenpflug, M. Vetter, M. Thorn, C. Cárdenas, G. Glombitza, W. Lamadé, G. M. Richter and H.-P. Meinzer: Navigation in liver surgery - requirement analysis and possible solutions. In: M. H. Kim and H.-P. Meinzer (eds), Proceedings of the Fifth Korea-Germany Joint Workshop on Advanced Medical Image Processing, Ewha Womans University, Seoul, Korea, May 15th/16th, 2001.

[4] P. Hassenpflug, M. Vetter, C. Cárdenas, M. Thorn and H.-P. Meinzer, Navigation in liver surgery - results of a requirement analysis. In: H. U. Lemke, M. W. Vannier,K. Inamura, A. G. Farman and K. Doi (eds), Computer Assisted Radiology and Surgery, CARS 2001 - Proceedings of the 15th International Congress and Exhibition, Berlin, June 27 - 30,, Elsevier, Amsterdam, vol. **ICS 1230** (2001) 1162.

[5] M. Vetter, P. Hassenpflug, M. Thorn, C. Cárdenas, G. Glombitza, W. Lamadé, G. M. Richter and H.-P. Meinzer, Navigation in der Leberchirurgie - Anforderungen und Lösungsansatz. In: Wörn H, Mühling J, Vahl C, Meinzer HP (eds), Rechner- und sensorgestützte Chirurgie, SFB 414, Lecture Notes in Informatics (LNI) - Proceedings, Gesellschaft für Informatik, Bonn, vol **P-4** (2001) 92-102.

[6] A. Schwerdtner and H. Heidrich, Dresden 3D Display: A Flat Autostereoscopic Display, Electronic Imaging / Photonics West 1998, San Jose Convention Center, San Jose, California, 1998.

Medicine Meets Virtual Reality 02/10
J.D. Westwood et al. (Eds.)
IOS Press, 2002

Enhanced stereographic x-ray images

Warren J Viant and James W Ward

Department of Computer Science, University of Hull, Hull, UK

Abstract. This project extends previous work on stereographic projection of 2D x-ray images and aims to overcome a number of problems, namely: confusing stereo cues; distortion between stereo pairs; and increased radiation exposure from additional x-ray images. Images are distortion corrected and a polygonal representation of a bone fitted to the x-ray image, to approximate the bone surface. The polygonal representation is rendered and blended with the x-ray image to add surface detail, without obscuring salient features within the original x-ray. A reduction in x-ray exposure by using a stereo pair of computer-generated polygonal bone images blended with a mono x-ray image is investigated. An experiment provides evidence that depth perception is increased with the inclusion of bone surface rendering, and is achievable with a mono x-ray image.

1   Introduction

X-ray images, generated from either fluoroscopic C-arm or plate film devices, are projections of the 3D world onto a 2D plane. The intensity of each pixel on the image is a function of the number of x-rays that penetrate the target medium and strike the receptor. The attenuation of the x-rays is due to the absorption and scattering effects of the material. Thus an x-ray image portrays information about the internal structure of an object rather than surface properties.

Clinicians perceive a patient as a complex 3D body, but rely heavily on only 2D x-ray images. Previous projects [2] have investigated the effects of translating these 2D x-ray images into stereographic projections, but with limited success.

This project extends previous work on stereographic projection of 2D x-ray images and aims to overcome a number of problems, namely:

- Confusing stereo cues,
- Distortion between stereo pairs,
- Increased radiation exposure from additional x-ray images.

Human perception of stereo relies on cues [4], such as parallax, occlusion, surface shading, etc. A number of significant cues are not present within x-ray images i.e. surface shading, as the x-ray image is a projection of the volume rather than the surface. Occlusion cues can be contradictory as x-ray images show objects intersecting other objects. Image distortion between stereo pairs can also provide disparities in stereo cues.

2   Method

This project approaches the problem in three stages. Initially all x-ray images are undistorted using an accurate distortion correction technique [1]. A polygonal representation of a bone is fitted to the x-ray image, to approximate the bone surface. The polygonal representation is rendered and mixed with the x-ray image to add surface detail, without obscuring salient features. The procedure is repeated for the second x-ray image in the stereo pair. The third stage aims to reduce x-ray exposure by using a stereo pair of computer-generated polygonal bone images blended with a mono x-ray image. By merging the computer-generated and mono x-ray images it is possible to trick the viewer into perceiving stereo, when only one x-ray image is available. This removes the need for increased radiation exposure. Various projection techniques including toed, parallel and non-symmetric viewing frustums and eye separation have also been investigated for increased stereo perception.

2.1   X-ray distortion correction

The fluoroscopic C-arm image intensifier (FII) was designed as a qualitative device for the surgeon, not as a quantitative vision system compatible with high accuracy image analysis. Poor image integrity, often described as image distortion, results from three factors, namely:

- Internal anomalies in the FII's internal structure e.g. irregularities in the focusing of the photoelectrons onto the CCD or the geometry of the receptor plate.
- Flexion of the FII's structure i.e. change of orientation from the vertical to horizontal causes a change in the relative position of the x-ray source to the receptor screen
- External magnetic fields i.e. affect the image intensification process within the 20-30 keV field.

This project uses a calibration process to reduce the problems of the FII's poor image integrity. A mapping for distortion correction is created through computer analysis of an image of a calibration phantom (i.e. a grid of spherical markers) representing a *virtual screen* against which all subsequent image measurements are referenced. This mapping defines the distortion correction required for each pixel on subsequent images.

2.2   Polygonal model

In order to mix the x-ray image with a surface rendered polygonal model, it is first necessary to align and fit the model to the available images. This was achieved through a combination of scale, translation, rotation and FFD (Free Form Deformation) operators.

The scale and rigid body transformations allowed for a good initial alignment of the model to be achieved, while the FFD allowed small-scale deformation of the model. This was needed to account for minor differences in shape between the generic polygonal model and the actual bone.

In the first instance, the images were prepared manually, so that a variety of techniques could be investigated. The trial images were produced and rendered using 3D Studio MAX (Discreet). In the longer term, software will be developed to simplify this process. The fitting technique is illustrated below in Figure 1. Note that the x-ray image is undistorted prior to the fitting.

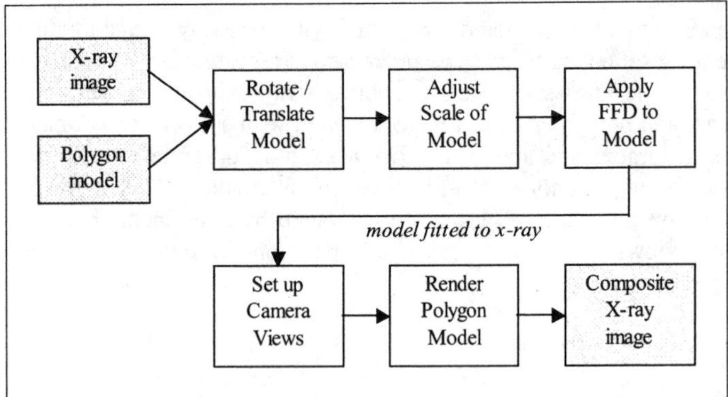

Figure 1. Block diagram of fitting process

The fitting process for the left and right eye views was identical:

1. The x-ray image was applied as a texture map to a square (planar quadrilateral), to represent the screen of the fluoroscopic C-arm.
2. A synthetic camera was created with adjustable viewing distance, field of view and aspect ratio. These parameters were chosen to produce the desired stereo projection, and vary for each image pair.
3. The polygon model was placed between the screen and camera, and manually fitted to the x-ray image. The process is illustrated in Figure 1.

Having fitted the model, the left and right views were rendered. Each view was rendered into two separate images; one containing only the rendered polygon model, and one containing the texture mapped screen. These images were then merged to form the final joint stereo image. Several different methods can be used to combine these images, including:

1. Multiplicative blending: the intensity of the x-ray image is modulated by the intensity of the rendered polygon model. This has the effect of applying the shading information from the surface rendered model to the x-ray.

2. Additive blending: the two source images are scaled and summed, to form a linear blend between the x-ray and rendered polygon model. For example, this method is appropriate for adding surface highlights to an x-ray.

The multiply operator appears to produce the best results, although care is needed to ensure that detail is not lost from the x-ray image. The two blending operations are described below.

Multiplicative Blending

For each pixel, the intensity I_d in the destination image is the product of the intensities in the two source images (I_{s1}, I_{s2}). The contribution of each image can be controlled by first scaling the source images by constants (k_1, k_2) as shown here:

$$I_d = k_1 I_{s1} . k_2 I_{s2}$$

When blending the images, a mask was used to ensure that the images were only multiplied in the areas corresponding to the polygonal bone model. This was necessary to prevent the background areas of the x-ray image from being darkened. The final contrast and brightness of the output image can also be adjusted if required, to ensure that a reasonable contrast range is preserved.

Additive Blending

The intensity I_d in the destination image is the sum of the intensities in the two source images (I_{s1}, I_{s2}). Again, the images are first scaled by constants (k_1, k_2) to control the relative contribution to the result:

$$I_d = k_1 I_{s1} + k_2 I_{s2}$$

With additive blending, it is not necessary to use a mask image since the areas that do not correspond to the polygonal bone model will be black, and therefore do not contribute to the result. Additive blending is useful for adding shading highlights to the image, but is less suitable for reproducing the shading of the rendered polygon model. For this reason, the multiplicative blending approach was found to give more useful results.

Images for Comparison

For comparison purposes, an original x-ray image and a blended image are illustrated below in Figure 2 and Figure 3. The blended image combines a distortion corrected x-ray with a rendered surface model, using multiplicative blending with a mask image. Much of the detail of the image is preserved, for example there are folds of fabric visible in the top left hand corner of the image, and the intra medullary cavity is preserved.

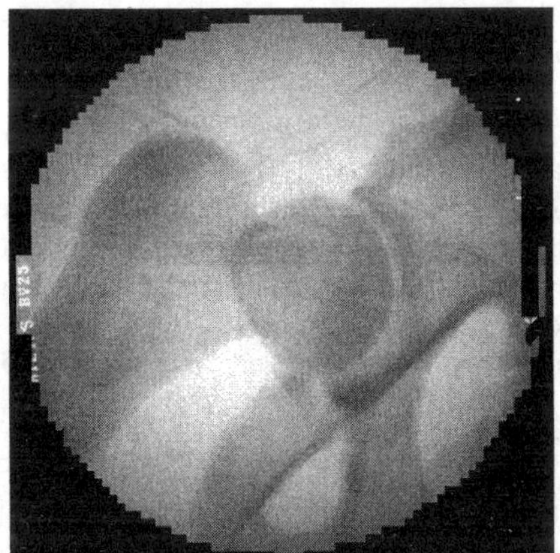

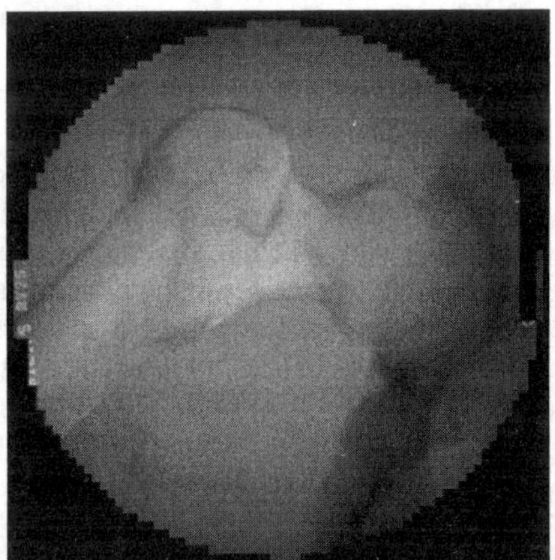

Figure 2. Distortion corrected x-ray image   **Figure 3. Distortion corrected x-ray image with bone surface rendering**

2.3 Stereo pairs

Two different projection methods were used for generating stereo images: *parallel projection* and *toed projection*, as illustrated below in Figure 4. The camera distance, screen size and field of view were matched to that of the FII, while the separation between the cameras (or angle in case of toed projection) varies for each image.

The camera distance is typically 960mm, with 290mm screen size. For toed projection, the angular offset ranges from 5 to 10 degrees. For parallel projection, the camera separation is typically between 0 and 100mm. The separation or angular offset is specified with each image.

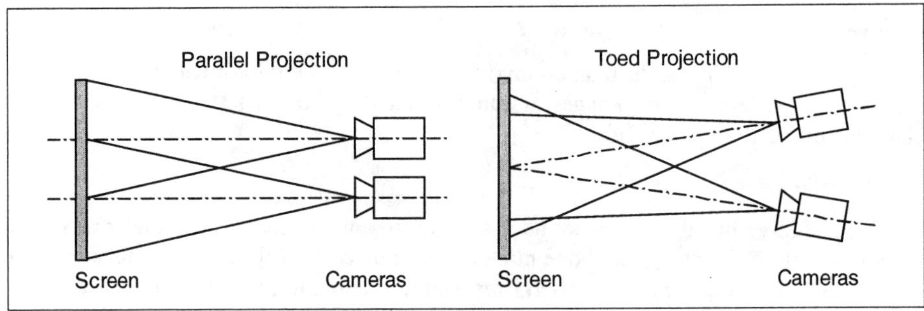

Figure 4. Parallel versus Toed Projection

3   Experiment

The aim of the experiment was to determine which stereographic x-ray technique provides the viewer with a balance of depth perception with ease of accommodation.

The experimental setup consisted of a 1.4Ghz Athlon PC with NVidia GeForce3 graphics processor. The images were viewed using StereoGraphics CrystalEyes glasses. The subjects were chosen at random from a selection of computer literate postgraduates and staff. Only 3 out of the 12 subjects had any recent experience in stereo viewing.

The subjects were first exposed to stereo viewing with a set of ten sample stereo photographs of natural scenes. The actual experiment was conducted using two sets of five stereo pairs. The first set comprised of contrast and colour variations. The second set comprised of surface properties and viewing frustum variations. The subjects were asked to rate the ease with which they were able to accommodate each stereo pair. The subjects were required to order each set of five stereo pairs by perceived depth. The five images within each set were randomly shuffled to avoid issues of prior history.

All the x-ray images were captured with a FII and have undergone image distortion correction.

Image 1: Stereo pair of raw x-ray images captured with a 5 degree angular offset.

Image 2: Single mono x-ray image mixed with a stereo pair of polygonal bone models (femur only), using parallel projection. There is a 10mm translational offset between the two computer-generated images.

Image 3: As image 2, except with higher contrast of superimposed bone model.

Image 4: As image 2, except with blue shading on superimposed bone model, applied using a mask image.

Image 5: As image 2, except blue shading on superimposed bone model and red shading on original x-ray image.

Image 6: Stereo pair of raw x-ray images captured with a 10 degree angular offset.

Image 7: Single mono x-ray image mixed with a stereo pair of polygonal bone models (femur only), using toed projection. There is an 8 degree angular offset between the two computer-generated images.

Image 8: Stereo pair of x-ray images mixed with a stereo pair of polygonal bone models (femur only), using toed projection. There is an 8 degree angular offset between the two computer-generated images.

4   Results

The results for the experiments 1 and 2 are given in Figure 5 and Figure 6, respectively. The experiment demonstrates that ease of accommodation is improved when toed projection is used, as opposed to parallel projection. Addition of surface rendering, colour and mono x-ray images does not adversely affect accommodation. Experiment 1 suggests that a viewer can be deceived into perceiving stereo by the use of higher contrast or coloured images. This supports the evidence by Rydmark, who suggests that colour and texture are important in the perception of a 3D object [3]. Experiment 2 suggests that the addition of bone surface rendering enhances the perception of depth. Stereo bone surface rendering blended with a stereo x-ray image provided the best perception of depth. The most significant result was that stereo bone surface rendering blended with a mono x-ray image provided a better perception of depth than a stereo-pair of raw x-ray images with no bone surface rendering.

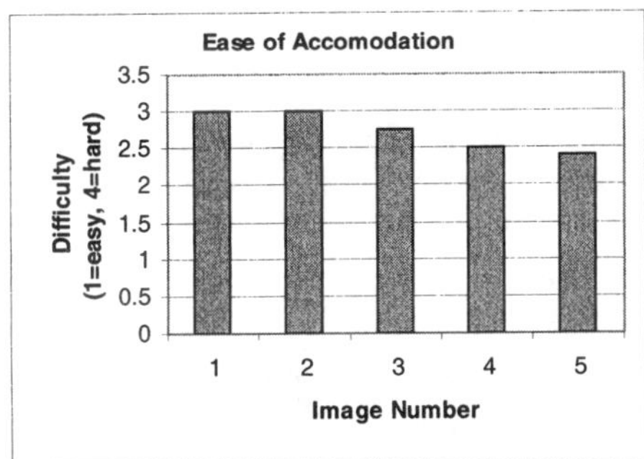
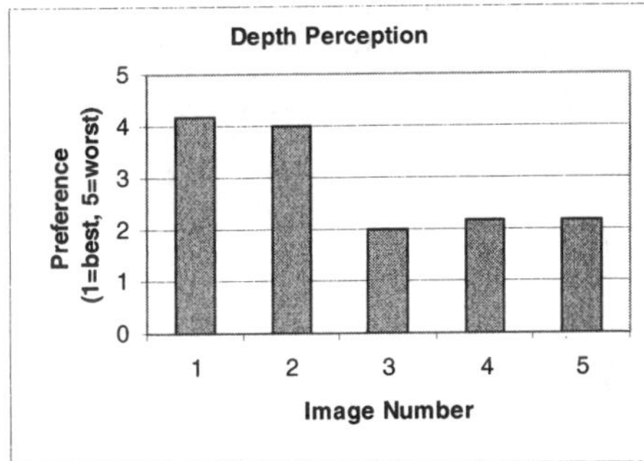

Figure 5. First experiment: Ease of accommodation, and depth perception.

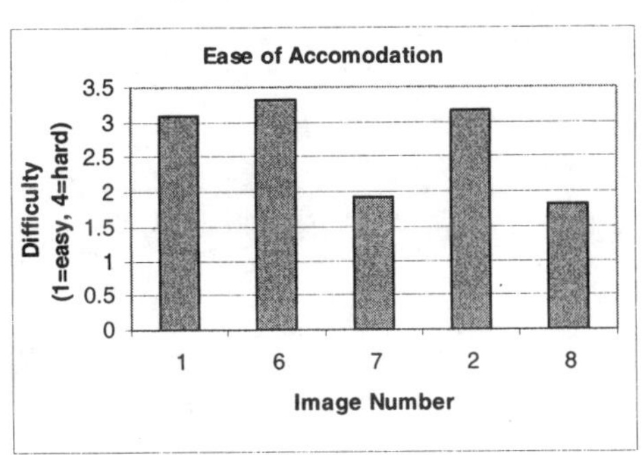
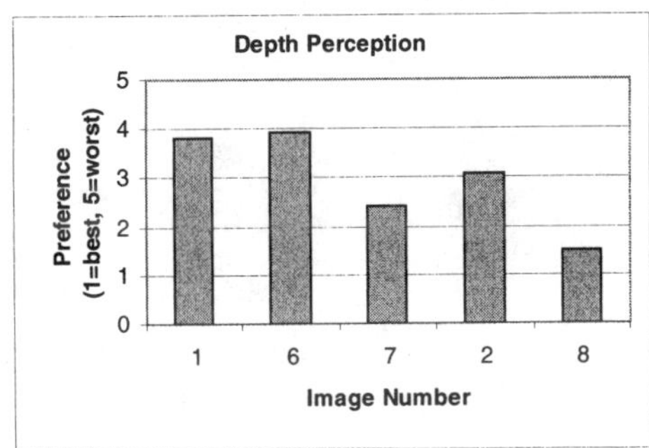

Figure 6. Second experiment: Ease of accommodation and depth perception.

5   Discussion

The experimental results indicate that it is possible to achieve a perception of stereo with a pair of standard x-ray images. Stereo perception is enhanced by inclusion of a bone surface rendering. Careful blending of the images is required to avoid removing salient features within the x-ray image and a number of candidate techniques were investigated.

The use of a mono x-ray image also results in stereo perception, but with a reduced stereo depth.

The novelty of this project is the combination of distortion correction, and surface model fusion, with single 2D images to achieve a perceived stereo result.

6   References

[1]   Viant WJ, Phillips, R, Bielby MS, Zhu Y, Griffiths JG, Mohsen AMMA, Sherman KP, "A technique for a very high accuracy image intensifier calibration", Proceedings of Medicine Meets Virtual Reality 1999, ISBN 9051994451, pp.379-380.

[2]   Berestov A, "Stereoscopic x-ray image processing", Proceedings of Medicine Meets Virtual Reality 2001, ISBN 1586031430, pp. 53-59.

[3]   Rydmark M, "3D Visualisation and Stereographic Techniques for Medical Research and Education", Proceedings of Medicine Meets Virtual Reality 2001, ISBN 1586031430, pp. 434-439.

[4]   Hsuy, Ke Sheny, Frank B. Venezia Jr.y, David M. Chelbergy, Leslie A. Geddesz. Application of Stereo Techniques to Angiography: Qualitative and Quantitative Approaches

The Communication Between Therapist and Patient in Virtual Reality: The Role of Mediation Played by Computer Technology

Francesco VINCELLI [1-3], Enrico MOLINARI [1-3], Giuseppe RIVA [2-3]

[1] *Laboratorio Sperimentale di Psicologia, Istituto Auxologico Italiano, Verbania, Italy*
[2] *Applied Technology for Neuro-Psychology Lab., Istituto Auxologico Italiano, Verbania, Italy*
[3] *Department of Psychology, Catholic University, Milan, Italy*

Abstract: Even if the number of reported application is constantly increasing, understanding how to use immersive virtual reality (VR) to support clinical practice presents a substantial challenge for the designers and users of this emerging technology. These opposite faces are resulting from the peculiar characteristics of VR. In fact, VR is not simply a particular collection of technological hardware, but can be considered as a new *medium* defined in terms of its effect on both basic and major psychological processes. In particular, the essence of VR is the inclusive relationship between the participant and the virtual environment, where direct experience of the immersive environment constitutes communication. Starting from this vision, the chapter tries to outline a theoretical framework for supporting the development and tuning of clinical oriented VR systems.

1. Introduction

Even if the number of reported application is constantly increasing, as reported by the contents of this special issue, understanding how to use immersive virtual reality (VR) to support clinical practice presents a substantial challenge for the designers and users of this emerging technology [1]. As noted by Banos and colleagues [2] VR has two opposite faces. On one side it can be used by clinicians as a "setting lab where to study anomalous behaviors, emotions and beliefs" (p.284). On the other side, "VR can be also seen as a creator of psychopathology" (p. 288) for its potential of inducing reality judgments and identity problems. Moreover, it is well known that this tool can induce important side effects such as cybersickness and aftereffects [3], forcing the clinician to a clear planning of his approach to lessen the probability of inducing harmful consequences for the patients. These opposite faces are resulting from the peculiar characteristics of VR. In fact, VR is not simply a particular collection of technological hardware, but can be considered as a new *medium* defined in terms of its effect on both basic and major psychological processes [4-6]. According to Bricken [7] the essence of VR is the inclusive relationship between the participant and the virtual environment, where direct experience of the immersive environment constitutes communication.

Biocca & Delaney [8] defined a communication interface as "the interaction of the physical media, codes and information with the sensorimotor channels of the user" (p. 59). Designers play a key role in defining the characteristics of this advanced communication interface.

Following this approach, it is also possible to define VR in terms of human experience [9]: "a real or simulated environment in which a perceiver experiences telepresence," where telepresence can be described as the "experience of presence in an environment by means of a communication medium" (pp.78-80).

Starting from these definitions, in the next paragraphs we will try to outline a theoretical framework for supporting the development and tuning of clinical oriented VR systems.

2. The patient-therapist dialogue

The research aimed at increasing psychotherapy effectiveness is quite active and its priority target is to find the application limits of the different treatments. Specialized literature clearly reports that virtual experience makes it possible to overcome some of these limits with regard to an ever increasing amount of different types of psychopathological disorders.

To better explain the advantages offered by this technology, let us examine, for instance, the so-called "Graded Exposure". One of the essential components of cognitive-behavioral therapies is the exposure of the subject to the stimuli causing his disorder. Virtual reality allows making this stage of the treatment easier. VR software makes it possible to re-create, together with the subject under treatment, a hierarchy of reality-matching situations, which the subject will experience in a real way thanks to the involvement of all sensory and motor channels. The realistic reproduction of virtual environments enables the interacting individual to immerse himself in a condition of real presence.

Another factor, which plays a major role in the psychotherapeutic treatments connected with the different schools of psychology, is the elicitation of antagonist responses rather than of maladjusted ones. The development of the ability to induce a condition of psychophysical relaxation is one of the goals aimed at by any psychotherapist anxious to limit the negative effects involved by psychophysiological arousal. In all cases in which dysfunctional thoughts and maladjusted behaviors are combined with the manifestation of the disorder through the hyperactivation of the psychophysiological parameters, some training to control one's own psychosomatic responses in a more adaptive way becomes essential.

But the effectiveness of this technique largely depends on the ability shown by the subject for whom the therapy has been designed, to produce the images, which are generally suggested by the therapist. The more these images will become vivid and realistic in the subject's fancy the more it will be easy to obtain a relaxation response [10].

The opportunities offered by virtual technology in this field are manifold and quite favorable. The guided administration by the VR therapist of scenes helping to induce a relaxation response has been fairly successful [11]. This is mainly due to the intrinsic effects of the VR instrument. The feeling of being really present as provided by the realistic representation of the cybernetic environments and by the involvement of all sensory and motor channels enables the subject under treatment to live the virtual experience more vividly and realistically than he would do through his own imagination [12].

Virtual Reality is a highly flexible instrument allowing to program manifold ways of managing psychological troubles. The opportunity to structure a large number of controlled stimuli and at the same time to monitor any response aroused by the program user allows to increase the chance of therapeutic success as compared to traditional procedures. The potential offered by this technology mainly comes from the central role played in psychotherapy by imagination and by memory. The limits of these two factors, which are essential in the life of all of us, are either absolute or connected with individual potentials. Thanks to virtual experience some of these limits can be overcome. Re-created world can sometimes be more vivid and real than the world that a large number of subjects can describe through their own imagination and through their own memory.

This innovative instrument brings about a change in comparison with the traditional relationship between patient and therapist [1]. The new pattern of this relationship is based of the awareness of being more capable to manage in the difficult operation of recovering past experience and of predicting future experience. The therapist who knows and is aware that he can make use of and derive benefit from this effective instrument in his own therapeutic practice feels more efficient and capable to act in a more incisive way on the course of the disorder suffered by his patient. At the same time, the subject under treatment perceives the advantage of being able to re-create and make use of a real experimental world within the walls of his own therapist's surgery.

3. Conclusion

Virtual Reality Assisted Therapy gives therefore a substantial impulse to the development of new opportunities for the prevention and treatment of psychological health. On the other hand, research-connected factors deal with the difficult cooperation between the community of experts concerned with Virtual Reality and the community of experts who establish the official standards for mental health investigations.

Quite often the results achieved by VR are not taken into consideration by experts who carry out their researching activity within some particular nosological environments, since this method of study is not included in the guidelines of traditional research. Although their attitude is rather common in our culture, being consistent with the difficulties shown by each of us in accepting innovations and differences, this limit can be overcome only through the establishment of specific standards to be applied to the guidelines for Virtual Reality research.

Acknowledgment

The present work was supported by the Commission of the European Communities (CEC), through the VEPSY UPDATED (IST-2000-25323) research project (http://www.psicologia.net).

References

[1]   G. Riva, Design of clinically oriented virtual environments: A communicative approach, *CyberPsychology & Behavior* **3** (2000) 351-358.

[2]   R. M. Banos, C. Botella, and P. C., Virtual Reality and Psychopathology, *CyberPsychology & Behavior* **2** (1999) 283-292.

[3]   A. Rizzo, M. Wiederhold, and J. G. Buckwalter, Basic issues in the use of virtual environments for mental health applications, in *Virtual environments in clinical psychology and neuroscience: Methods and techniques in advanced patient-therapist interaction*, G. Riva, B. Wiederhold, and E. Molinari, Eds. Amsterdam: IOS Press, 1998, pp. 21-42.

[4]   N. I. Durlach and A. S. E. Mavor, *Virtual reality: scientific and technological challenges*. Washington, D.C.: National Academy Press, 1995.

[5]   G. Riva, From technology to communication: Psycho-social issues in developing virtual environments, *Journal of Visual Languages and Computing* **10** (1999) 87-97.

[6]   G. Riva, Virtual Reality as a communication tool: a socio-cognitive analysis, *Presence, Teleoperators, and Virtual Environments* **8** (1999) 460-466.

[7]   W. Bricken, Virtual reality: Directions of growth, University of Washington, Seattle, WA HITL Technical Report R-90-1, 1990.

[8]   F. Biocca and B. Delaney, Immersive virtual reality technology, in *Communication in the age of virtual reality*, F. Biocca and M. R. Levy, Eds. Hillsdale, NJ: Lawrence Erlbaum Associates, 1995, pp. 57-124.

[9]   J. S. Steuer, Defining virtual reality: Dimensions determining telepresence, *Journal of Communication* **42** (1992) 73-93.

[10]   F. Vincelli, Y. H. Choi, E. Molinari, B. K. Wiederhold, and G. Riva, Experiential cognitive therapy for the treatment of panic disorders with agoraphobia: Definition of a clinical protocol, *CyberPsychology & Behavior* **3** (2000) 375-386.

[11]   G. Riva, M. Bacchetta, M. Baruffi, S. Rinaldi, F. Vincelli, and E. Molinari, Virtual reality based Experiential Cognitive Treatment of obesity and binge-eating disorders, *Clinical Psychology and Psychotherapy* **7** (2000) 209-219.

[12]   F. Vincelli and E. Molinari, Virtual reality and imaginative techniques in clinical psychology, in *Virtual environments in clinical psychology and neuroscience: Methods and techniques in advanced patient-therapist interaction*, G. Riva, B. Wiederhold, and E. Molinari, Eds. Amsterdam: IOS Press, 1998, pp. 67-72.

Medicine Meets Virtual Reality 02/10
J.D. Westwood et al. (Eds.)
IOS Press, 2002

Virtual Reality Assisted Cognitive Behavioral Therapy for the Treatment of Panic Disorders with Agoraphobia

F. Vincelli [1-2], H. Choi [3], E. Molinari [2], B.K. Wiederhold [4], S. Bouchard[5], G. Riva [1-2]

[1]*Laboratorio Sperimentale di Psicologia, ATN-P Lab, Istituto Auxologico Italiano, Verbania, Italy*
[2]*Department of Psychology, Università Cattolica, Milan, Italy*
[3]*Seoul Paik Hospital, Inje University, Seoul, South Korea*
[4]*Center for Advanced Multimedia Psychotherapy, CSPP Research and Service Foundation, San Diego, California*
[5]*Department of Psychology, Université du Québéc à Hull, Canada*

Abstract: The chapter describes the characteristics of the Experiential-Cognitive Therapy (ECT) protocol for Panic Disorder and Agoraphobia. The goal of ECT is to decondition fear reactions, to modify misinterpretational cognition related to panic symptoms and to reduce anxiety symptoms. This is possible in an average of eight sessions of treatment plus an assessment phase and booster sessions, through the integration of Virtual Experience and traditional cognitive-behavioral techniques. We decided to employ the techniques included in the cognitive-behavioral approach because they showed high levels of efficacy. Through virtual environments we can gradually expose the patient to feared situation: virtual reality consent to re-create in our clinical office a real experiential world. The patient faces the feared stimuli in a context that is nearer to reality than imagination.

For ECT we developed the Virtual Environments for Panic Disorders - VEPD - virtual reality system. VEPD is a 4-zone virtual environment developed using the Superscape VRT 5.6 toolkit. The four zones reproduce different potentially fearful situations - an elevator, a supermarket, a subway ride, and large square. In each zone the characteristics of the anxiety-related experience are defined by the therapist through a setup menu.

1. Introduction

A review of epidemiological studies suggests that in different geographic, cultural and racial groups approximately 5% of the population will have agoraphobia and 3.5% will have panic disorder at some time in their life [1].

Within the Diagnostic and Statistical Manual of Mental Disorders (DSM-IV) framework, the essential feature of panic disorder (PD) is the occurrence of panic attacks. A panic attack is a sudden onset period of intense fear or discomfort associated with a cluster of physical and cognitive symptoms, which occurs unexpectedly and recurrently, such as pervasive apprehension about panic attacks, persistent worry about future attacks, worry about the perceived physical, social or mental consequences of attacks, or major changes in behavior in response to attacks. The disorder is often associated with circumscribed phobic disorders such as specific phobias, social phobias, and especially with agoraphobia [2,3]. Indeed, avoidance of public places in order to reduce fear or panic becomes the main cause of incapacity in patients, who, in more serious cases, are confined to their homes patterns [6-9].

Evidence collected over the past 20 years has consistently shown the effectiveness of a multicomponent cognitive-behavioral strategy in the treatment of panic disorder with agoraphobia . The treatment package includes exposure to the feared situation, interoceptive exposure, cognitive restructuring, breathing retraining, and applied relaxation. On an average the duration of the protocol is twelve-fifteen sessions. The protocol involves a mixture of cognitive and behavioral techniques, which are intended to help patients identify and modify their dysfunctional anxiety-related thoughts, beliefs and behavior. Emphasis is placed on reversing the maintaining factors identified in the cognitive and behavioral patterns [10-14].

2.   Traditional versus Virtual Reality Therapy

One of the fundamental parameters in assessing the effectiveness of therapies is the ratio existing between the "cost" of administration of the therapeutic procedure and the resulting "benefits" [15]. By cost it is meant the expenditure not only in terms of money and time, but also in terms of emotional involvement by the person to whom the therapy is directed. The benefits regard the effectiveness of the treatment, i.e., the achievement of the target set, in the shortest time possible. Exposure therapy traditionally is carried out "in imagination" or *"in vivo"*. In the first case, the subject is trained to produce the anxiety-provoking stimuli through mental images; in the second case, the subject actually experiences these stimuli in semi-structured situations. Both of these methods present advantages and limitations as regards the cost-benefit ratio. In the first case, the prevalent difficulty is represented by teaching the subject to produce the images that regard experiences associated with anxiety: the majority of failures linked to this therapy are those subjects who present particular difficulties in visualizing scenes of real life. The cost of the application, however, is minimal, because the therapy is administered in the physician's office, thus avoiding situations that might be embarrassing for the patient and safeguarding his privacy. In the second case, the difficulty lies in structuring, in reality, experiences regarding the hierarchically ordered anxiety-provoking stimuli, with the result that the cost in terms of time, money and emotions is high. At the same time, the advantage of contending with real contexts increases the likelihood of effectiveness of the *"in vivo"* procedure [16,17,18].

Using VR software, it is possible to re-create, together with the subject undergoing treatment, a hierarchy of situations corresponding to reality, which he may experience in an authentic way thanks to the involvement of all his sensorimotor channels. The realistic reproduction of virtual environments enables the interacting individual to immerse himself in a dimension of real presence. This makes it possible to limit the costs as compared to traditional procedures of treatment, as pointed out above, and to consolidate the effectiveness of the treatment thanks to the possibility of re-creating a "three-dimensional world" within the walls of the clinical office [18].

Through the analysis of the current applications of VRT (Virtual Reality Therapy) some conclusions can be drawn as to the effectiveness of virtual experience.
First of all, individuals subjected to virtual environments have experienced the feeling of being present like real experience even when the virtual environment did not faithfully match the real world situations. This statement was confirmed by the evidence that the reactions and emotions originating from virtual experience were equal to those experienced by subjects involved in real experience. Another rather frequent conclusion in the analyzed studies concerns the fact that the concentration on a task shown by subjects engaged in

virtual experience significantly increases if compared to the control groups treated "in vivo". In addition, perceptions and behaviors connected with real world can be changed thanks to experience into virtual experience. This last datum confirms that it is possible to extend the results obtained by "in vitro" treatments, which make use of VR, to "in vivo" situations too.

3.   The Experiential-Cognitive Therapy Protocol

At the beginning the Experiential-Cognitive Therapy (ECT) protocol for Panic Disorder and Agoraphobia was developed at the Applied Technology for Neuro-Psychology Lab of Istituto Auxologico Italiano, Verbania, Italy, in cooperation with the Department of Psychology at the Catholic University of Milan, Italy [19]. The actual version included the efforts of researchers from the Center for Advanced Multimedia Psychotherapy, California School of Professional Psychology, San Diego (CA), USA, from the Department of Psychology, Universite du Quebec a Hull, Canada, and from the Seoul Paik Hospital, Inje University, Seoul, Korea [20]. The goal of ECT is to decondition fear reactions, to modify misinterpretational cognition related to panic symptoms and to reduce anxiety symptoms. This is possible in an average of eight sessions of treatment plus an assessment phase and booster sessions, through the integration of Virtual Experience and traditional techniques of CBT. We decided to employ the techniques included in the cognitive-behavioral approach because they showed high levels of efficacy. Through virtual environments we can gradually expose the patient to feared situation: virtual reality consent to re-create in our clinical office a real experiential world. The patient faces the feared stimuli in a context that is nearer to reality than imagination.

For ECT we developed the Virtual Environments for Panic Disorders - VEPD - virtual reality system. VEPD is a 4-zone virtual environment developed using the Superscape VRT 5.6 toolkit. The four zones reproduce different potentially fearful situations - an elevator, a supermarket, a subway ride, and large square. In each zone the characteristics of the anxiety-related experience are defined by the therapist through a setup menu. In particular the therapist can define the length of the virtual experience, its end and the number of virtual subjects (from none to a crowd) to be included in the zone.

Zone 1: In this zone, an elevator in which the subject has to enter, the subject becomes acquainted with the appropriate control device, the head mounted display and the recognition of collisions.

Zone 2: this zone show a supermarket in which the patient can go for shopping. The subject can pick up objects and pay for them at the cash-register.

Zone 3: this zone reproduces a subway ride. The subject is located in the train which moves between different stations.

Zone 4: the last zone is a large square in which are located a medieval church, different buildings, and a pub.

Subjects. Subjects will be consecutive patients seeking treatment who met will DSM IV criteria for panic disorders and agoraphobia for a minimum of 6 months as determined by an independent clinician on clinical interview. Individuals will be excluded if they were acutely suicidal, medically ill or pregnant, had abused alcohol or drugs within the last year or had evidence of cardiac conduction disease. Before starting the trial, the nature of the treatment will be explained to the patients and their written informed consent will obtained.

3.1   Assessment.

Subjects will be assessed by independent assessment clinicians who will not involved in the direct clinical care of any subject. They will be MA-level chartered psychologists or PhD-level chartered psychotherapist. For the clinical interview they will use a semi-structured interview with the aim of identifying relevant DSM IV diagnostic criteria in the subjects. All the subject will be assessed at pre treatment, upon completion of the clinical trial and after a 1-month, 3-month, 6-month, 12-month and 24-month follow-up period. The following psychometric tests will be administered at each assessment point:
1. **BDI-II** - Beck Depression Inventory [21];
2. **STAI** - State-Trait Anxiety Inventory [22];
3. **ACQ** - Agoraphobic Cognitions Questionnaire [23];
4. **FQ** - Fear Questionnaire [24];
During the assessment will be also used:
- Subjective measurements (self reports, diaries)
- Subjective Units of Distress (SUDs) during exposure to virtual environments. In particular SUDs will be taken at baseline, after 10 minutes and after 20 minutes

3.2   Treatment

The overall treatment is composed by 8 sessions and by different booster sessions for six months after the therapy (see Table 1).

The first goal of session 1 is to discuss with our patient the etiologic model of Panic Disorder and Agoraphobia and to describe the program of Experiential-Cognitive Therapy. The description is necessary to obtain an active role of the patient in the therapy.

Then we introduce our patient to Virtual Reality through the use of head mounted display and joystick. The innovative principle of ECT is to integrate cognitive and behavioral techniques with the experiential possibilities offered by Virtual Reality. Then the next step of the first session is to structure the Graded Exposure procedure to virtual environments: the patient is exposed to each of the four virtual environments, with the minimum level of difficulty (small number of subjects present in the environments, ready access to the exits, plenty of room in the elevator,...), and is asked to evaluate the experience on a SUD's scale. In this way we will obtain a hierarchy of virtual environments, from the least anxiety-provoking to the most, that will be used along the treatment.

After a hierarchy of administration between the environments has been established, it is necessary, in order to guarantee gradualism of exposure, to establish a hierarchy of stimuli within each environment. The virtual environments in our treatment program are designed to reach this goal. In the supermarket and on the underground, the increase in difficulty may be obtained by increasing the number of persons present in the environment and by moving away from the exits of the respective environments. In the square it is possible to increase the number of people present and to approach narrower spaces that offer fewer ways out. In the lift, it is possible to arrange for the presence of other people and to enlarge or restrict the space inside the lift.

The second step is to show the patient the role of avoidance as the main source of agoraphobic and panic behaviors. The therapist underlines the importance of regular exposure to feared situation and structures with his patient a self-exposure schedule. In vivo graded self-exposure as homeworks, initially with the co-therapist (when it is possible), is very important to empower the efficacy of the therapy. This step can be more easily approached by graded exposure to virtual reality and produce important advantages for the patient: reducing the number of sessions, reducing dependency on the therapist and helping to maintain therapeutic achievements.

Each session starts with the review of the homeworks, to verify the difficulties that have emerged during self-exposure and to reinforce the patient for the tasks that have been carried out. After the graded exposure procedure, session three is based on Cognitive Restructuring. In panic disorder cognitive treatment focuses upon correcting misappraisals of bodily sensations as threatening. The cognitive strategies reduce attentional vigilance for symptoms of arousal, level of chronic arousal, and anticipation of the recurrence of panic. Cognitive treatment starts by reviewing with the patient a recent panic attack and identifying the main negative thoughts associated with the panic sensations. Once patient and therapist agree that the panic attacks involve an interaction between bodily sensations and negative thoughts about the sensations, a variety of procedures are used to help patients challenge their misinterpretations of the symptoms.

Session 1
- Description of the etiologic model of PDA according cognitive behavioral approach.
- Connection between the model and a recent PDA of the patient.
- Introduction to Virtual Environments.
- Graded exposure to virtual environments and set a hierarchy of the virtual stimulus.
- Homework: diary of panic attacks.

Session 2
- Homework's review
- Cognitive assessment assisted through graded exposure to virtual environments
- Introduction and scheduling of in vivo Self-Exposure
- Homework: diary of panic attacks, in vivo Self-Exposure.

Session 3
- Homework's Review.
- Cognitive Restructuring assisted through Graded Exposure to virtual environments.
- Homework: diary of panic attacks, in vivo Self-Exposure.

Session 4
- Homework's Review
- Graded exposure to virtual environments
- Cognitive Restructuring face to face
- Homework: panic attacks diary, in vivo Self-Exposure

Session 5
- Homework's Review
- Interoceptive Exposure
- Interoceptive Exposure assisted through Graded Exposure to virtual environments
- Homework: in vivo interoceptive exposure, panic attacks diary.

Session 6
- Homework's Review
- Interoceptive exposure assisted through graded exposure to virtual environments
- Cognitive Restructuring face to face
- Homework: in vivo interoceptive exposure, diary of panic attacks.

Session 7
- Homework's Review
- Interoceptive Exposure assisted through Graded Exposure to virtual environments.
- Cognitive Restructuring face to face.
- Homework: in vivo interoceptive exposure, diary of panic attacks.

Session 8
- Homework's review
- Cognitive restructuring and prevention relapse
- Follow-up session schedule
- Retest

Booster sessions
- Follow-up after 1 month, 3 months and 6 months
- Review and Reinforcement of patient's tasks
- Management and Prevention of future relapse

Table 1: The Experiential-Cognitive Therapy Protocol for the treatment of Panic Disorder with Agoraphobia

A lot of patients interpret the unexpected nature of their panic attacks as an indication that they are suffering from some physical abnormality. In these cases a psycho-education program presenting the nature of anxiety can be helpful, especially if it is tailored to patients' idiosyncratic concerns. One of the prevalent errors in cognitions is *overestimation*. The panickers are inclined to jump to negative conclusions and to treat negative events as probable when in fact they are unlikely to occur. Another type of cognitive error is misinterpreting events as *catastrophic*. Decatastrophizing means to realize that the occurrences are not as "catastrophic" as stated, which is achieved by considering how negative events are managed versus how "bad" they are. This is best done in a Socratic style so that clients examine the content of their statements and reach alternatives. The cognitive strategies are conducted in conjunction with behavioral technique of graded exposure in virtual reality. The schedule of session four is similar to the one of session three. The first part is dedicated to graded exposure. The second part is dedicated to the careful inquiry of cognitive distortions and their modification.

The key feature of session five, six and seven is Interoceptive Exposure [6,9]. The theoretical basis for interoceptive exposure is one of fear extinction, given the conceptualization of panic attacks as "conditioned" alarm reactions to particular bodily cues. Since according to the cognitive model panic disorder is considered as a *"phobia of internal bodily cues"*, the purpose is to modify associations between specific bodily sensations and panic reactions. This technique is also used during the exposure to the virtual environments.

After cognitive restructuring, prevention relapse is an important step of the last session. In this session we have to schedule the self-exposure homeworks, the Booster sessions and to reinforce the patient for the tasks that have been carried out and for the future tasks. The number of booster sessions can be scheduled according to the results of our patients. In our experience three sessions after 1, 3 and 6 months is an appropriate number to improve the overall efficacy of the therapy. The objective of booster sessions is to verify the difficulties that have emerged and to reinforce the patient for the tasks that have been carried out. During this phase it is possible to repeat some steps of the therapeutic techniques to improve or to stabilize the results of treatment [19,20].

4.   Conclusion

The feeling of actual presence offered by the realistic reproduction of cybernetic environments and by the involvement of all the sensorimotor channels, enables the subject undergoing treatment to live the virtual experience in a more vivid and realistic manner than he could through his own imagination. VR constitutes a highly flexible tool, which makes it possible to programme an enormous variety of procedures of intervention on psychological distress. The possibility of structuring a large amount of controlled stimuli and, at the same time, of monitoring the possible responses generated by the user of the programme offers a considerable increase in the likelihood of therapeutic effectiveness, as compared to traditional procedures.

In the proposed method, we decided to integrate the experience of the virtual environments with the techniques included in the cognitive-behavioral approach because they showed high levels of efficacy. Through virtual environments we can gradually expose the patient to feared situation: virtual reality consent to re-create in our clinical office a real experiential world. The patient faces the feared stimuli in a context that is nearer to reality than imagination. Other significant advantages are the supervised exposure to agoraphobic situations and the possible boost to the effectiveness of cognitive restructuring by practicing it in anxiety inducing situations.

Acknowledgment

The present work was partially supported by the Commission of the European Communities (CEC), specifically by the IST programme through the VEPSY UPDATED (IST-2000-25323) research project (http://www.psicologia.net).

References

[1]   H.U. Wittchen & C.A. Essau, The epidemiology of Panic Attacks, Panic Disorder and Agoraphobia, in *Panic Disorder and Agoraphobia,* J.R. Walker, G.R. Norton & C.A. Ross, Eds. Pacific Grove: Brooks/Cole Publishing Company, 1991, pp. 103-149.

[2]   APA (1994). *Diagnostic and statistical manual of mental disorders,* 4th edition (DSM-IV). Washington, DC: American Psychiatric Press.

[3]   Goisman, R. M., Warshaw, M. G., Peterson, L. G., Rogers, M. P., Cuneo, P, Hunt, M. F., Tomlin-Albanese, J. M., Kazim, A., Gollan, J. K., Epstein-Kaye, T., Reich, J. H., & Keller, M. B. (1994). Panic, agoraphobia, and panic disorder with agoraphobia: Data from a multicenter anxiety disorders study. *Journal of Nervous and Mental Disease, 182(2),* 72-79.

[4]   Barlow, D. H., & Mavissakalian, M. (1981). Directions in the assessment and treatment of phobia: The next decade. In M. Mavissakallan & D. H. Barlow (Eds.), *Phobia:Psychological and pharmacological treatment.* New York: Gullford Press.

[5]   Chambless, D. L., & Goldstein, A. J. (1983). *Agoraphobia: Multiple perspectives on theory and treatment.* New York. Wiley.

[6]   Barlow, D. H. (1988). *Anxiety and its disorders: Tbe nature and treatment of anxiety and panic.* New York: Guilford Press.

[7]   Telch, M. J., Lucas, J. A., & Nelson, P. (1989). Nonclinical panic in college students: An investigation of prevalence and symptomatology. *Journal of Abnormal Psychology, 98, 300-306.*

[8]   Barlow, D. H., & Craske, M. G. (1994). *Mastery of your anxiety and panic II.* San Antonio, TX: Harcourt Brace & Co.

[9]   Clark, D. M., Salkovskis, P., Gelder, M., Koehler, C., Martin, M., Anastasiades, P., Hackmann, A., Middleton, H., & Jeavons, A. (1988). Tests of a cognitive theory of panic. In I. Hand & H. Wittchen (Eds.), *Panic and phobias II.* Berlin: Springer-Verlag.

[10]   R.M. Rapee & D.H. Barlow, The cognitive-behavioral treatment of panic attacks and agoraphobic avoidance, in *Panic Disorder and Agoraphobia,* J.R. Walker, G.R. Norton & C.A. Ross, Eds. Pacific Grove: Brooks/Cole Publishing Company, 1991, pp. 103-149.

[11]   Clark, D., Salkovskis, P., & Chalkley, A. (1985). Respiratory control as a treatment for panic attacks. *Journal of Behavior Therapy and Experimental Psychiatry, 16,* 23-30.

[12]   Clark, D. M., Salkovskis, P., Hackmann, A., Middleton, H., Anastasiades, P., & Gelder, M. (1994). A comparison of cognitive therapy, applied relaxation, and imipramine in the treatment of panic disorder. *British Journal of Clinical Psychology, 164,* 759-769.

[13]   Gitlin, B., Martin, M., Shear, K., Frances, A., Ball, G., & Josephson, S. (1985). Behavior therapy for panic disorder. *Journal of Nervous and Mental Disease, 173,* 742-743.

[14]   Shear, M. K., Ball, G., Fitzpatrick, M., Josephson, S., Klosko, J., & Francis, A. (1991). Cognitive-behavioral therapy for panic: An open study. *Journal of Nervous and Mental Disease, 179,* 467-471.

[15]   Vincelli F. (1999). From imagination to virtual reality: the future of Clinical Psychology. *CyberPsychology & Behavior. 2; 3; 241-248.*

[16]   Rothbaum BO, Hodges L, Kooper R. (1997) Virtual reality exposure therapy. *J Psychother Pract Res*;6:219-226.

[17]   Riva G, Galimberti C. (1997) The psychology of cyberspace: a socio-cognitive framework to computer mediated communication. *New Ideas in Psychology*;15:141-158.

[18]   Vincelli F., Molinari E., (1998). Virtual reality and imaginative techniques in Clinical Psychology. In Riva G., Wiederhold B K , Molinari E. (Eds.) *Virtual environments in Clinical Psychology and Neuroscience.* IOS Press Amsterdam.

[19]	Vincelli F., Riva G. (2000) Experiential Cognitive Therapy for the treatment of panic disorders with agoraphobia. *MMVR 2000, Medicine Meets Virtual Reality Conference.* January 27-30.

[20]	Vincelli F., Choi Y.H., Molinari E., Wiederhold B., Riva G. (2000). Experiential Cognitive Therapy for Treatment of Panic Disorder with Agoraphobia: definition of a clinical protocol. *CyberPsychology & Behavior. 3; 3; 375-385.*

[21]	Beck A.T., Ward C.H., Mendelson M., Mock J. & Erbaugh J. (1961) An inventory for measuring depression. *Archives of General Psychiatry, 4, 561-571.*

[22]	Spielberger C.D., Gorsuch R.L., Lushene R., Vagg P.R. & Jacobs G.A. (1983) *Manual for the Stait.Trait Anxiety Inventory.* Palo Alto,CA, Consulting Psychology Press.

[23]	Chambless D.L., Caputo G.S., BrightP. & GallagherR. (1984) Assessment of fear of fear on agoraphobics. The Bodily Sensation Questionnaire and the Agoraphobic Cognitions Questionnaire. *Journal of Consulting and Clinical Psychology, 52, 1090-1097.*

[24]	Marks I.M. & Mathews A.M. (1979) Brief standard self-rating for phobic patients. *Behavior Research and Therapy, 17, 263-267.*

Medicine Meets Virtual Reality 02/10
J.D. Westwood et al. (Eds.)
IOS Press, 2002

Dextrous and Shared Interaction with Medical Data: stereoscopic vision is more important than hand-image collocation

John A. WATERWORTH
Interactive Institute - Tools for Creativity Studio
Tvistevägen 47, P O Box 7964, 907 19 Umeå, Sweden.

Abstract. The current experiment was carried out to extend our knowledge about the relative importance of stereoscopic display and hand-image collocation for dextrous interaction. We devised a new task, the Volumetric Dexterity Test (VDT), which quite accurately duplicates the way professional personnel such as surgeons and radiologists interact with detailed medical data in a VR environment. Our results were surprising. Stereo vision was very important to both accuracy and speed of task completion, as we found previously. But the presence of hand-image collocation did not improve accuracy, despite the fact that this was a truly three-dimensional task. If this finding is borne out it has important implications for the volumetric presentation of medical data to individual practitioners and in group settings.

1. Introduction

Dextrous interaction refers to the use of non-immersive virtual reality to explore detailed medical (or other) data for diagnostic, surgery planning and educational purposes [1]. It typically uses a mirror to produce a virtual work volume into which the user can reach. Our earlier research [2] tested the importance of stereoscopic vision and hand-image collocation for a task requiring dextrous interaction with a virtual display [3]. The task - the Dexterity Game [1] - consists of a virtual version of the familiar "pass the loop over the wire without touching it" game. The player manipulates a tool, which corresponds to the "loop and handle" with his or her dominant hand. The task is to traverse from one end of a virtual wire to the other while "touching" the wire as little as possible. The non-dominant hand holds another tool, which allows the player to adjust the overall position of the wire and frame. When a virtual touch is detected, a sound is heard and the wire changes colour. There is no haptic feedback when the wire is touched.

In that earlier study [2] we compared performance on a trial task in a virtual environment, with and without stereoscopic display, and with and without hand-image collocation. Although both factors affected speed and accuracy of task completion, adding stereoscopy to desktop VR gave significantly greater benefits than adding hand-image collocation. Surprisingly, there was no additional benefit from combining the two.

The Dexterity Game is not a truly volumetric task, and there may be no deviation of the virtual wire in the third dimension (depth, in the z-plane) if the participant does not adjust the orientation of the virtual wire frame with the non-dominant hand. Even so, observing participants attempt this task brought home to us how difficult it is to work dextrously in three dimensions. Even when both cues are present the game is not easy. Another weakness of the earlier study was that we collected no data from the non-dominant hand, and so we could not tell, for example, if people moved the task object more often in the no stereo viewing conditions.

The current experiment was carried out to rectify these weaknesses, and extend our knowledge about the relative importance of stereoscopic display and hand-image collocation for dextrous interaction. We devised a new task, the Volumetric Dexterity Test (VDT), which quite accurately duplicates the way professional personnel such as surgeons and radiologists interact with detailed medical data. The VDT comprises a complex, three-dimensional structure composed of magenta voxels (see Figure 1 below). A thread, composed of blue voxels, winds in and around this structure. The task is to remove the blue thread while damaging the magenta structure as little as possible.

2. The Experiment

There were three completely different work-settings. The first offered hand-eye-collocation to the user (see Figure 2). The second used a standard monitor with no mirror and no hand-image collocation (Figure 3), while the third was similar to the second but used a large projector-screen (Figure 4). Our interest in the projected display stemmed from the fact that medical users frequently want to examine visualised data in a teaching or other group setting.

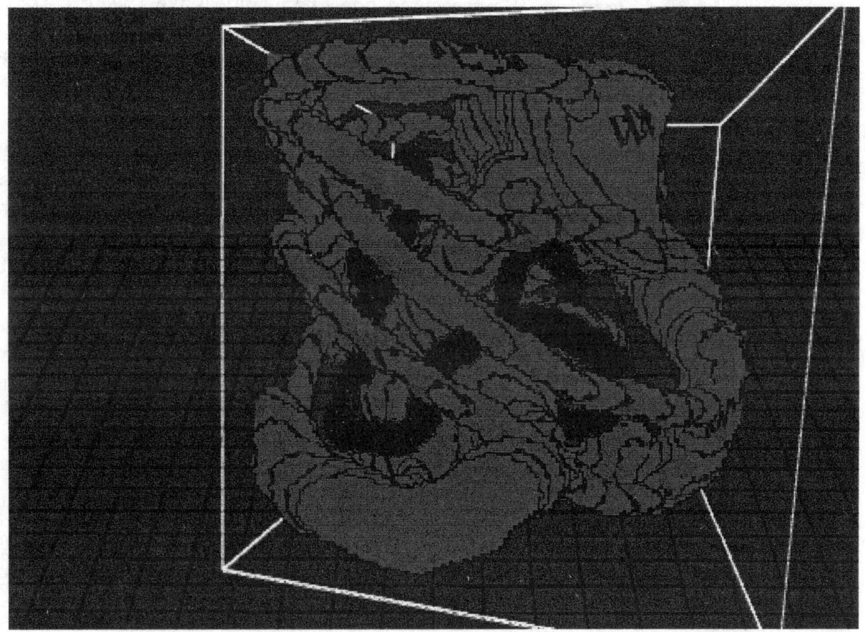

Figure 1 – The Voxel Dexterity Test

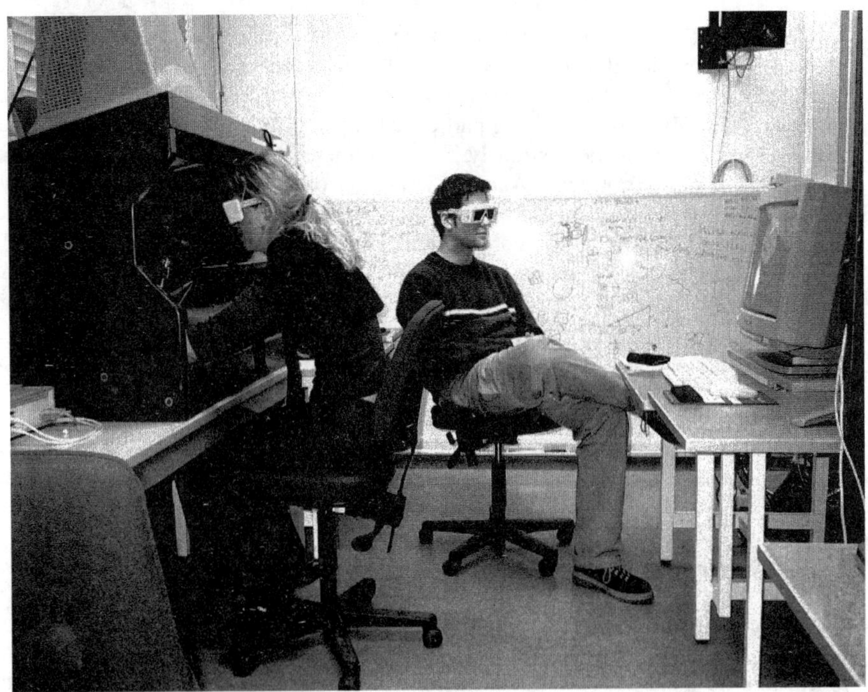

Figure 2 – The experimental set-up with hand-eye collocation

We compared performance on the VDT in each of these conditions, with and without stereoscopic viewing. We measured how many blue voxels were correctly removed, how many magenta voxels were erroneously removed, how long the task took to complete, and how often the non-dominant hand was used to manipulate the work volume.

We used equipment provided by the VRLab located at Umeå University in Northern Sweden for this study, consisting of an SGI Onyx-2 with a 21-inch colour monitor, screen resolution 1280 X 1024 pixels (1026 X 768 pixels in stereo conditions). Hand-image collocation was provided by the Dextroscope™ (formerly known as the Virtual Workbench) from Volume Interactions Pte. Ltd. of Singapore. A Polhemus FasTrack™ with pen-like receiver (held in the dominant hand) was used by participants for precise work, and a simple button and position sensor (held in the other hand) for moving the virtual object of interest. CrystalEyes™ time-multiplexed LCD shutter glasses were used to provide stereo capability. Participants viewed both stereo and monoscopic displays through the glasses, with zero disparity in the latter case. The refresh rate was 96Hz (48Hz per eye) in all conditions.

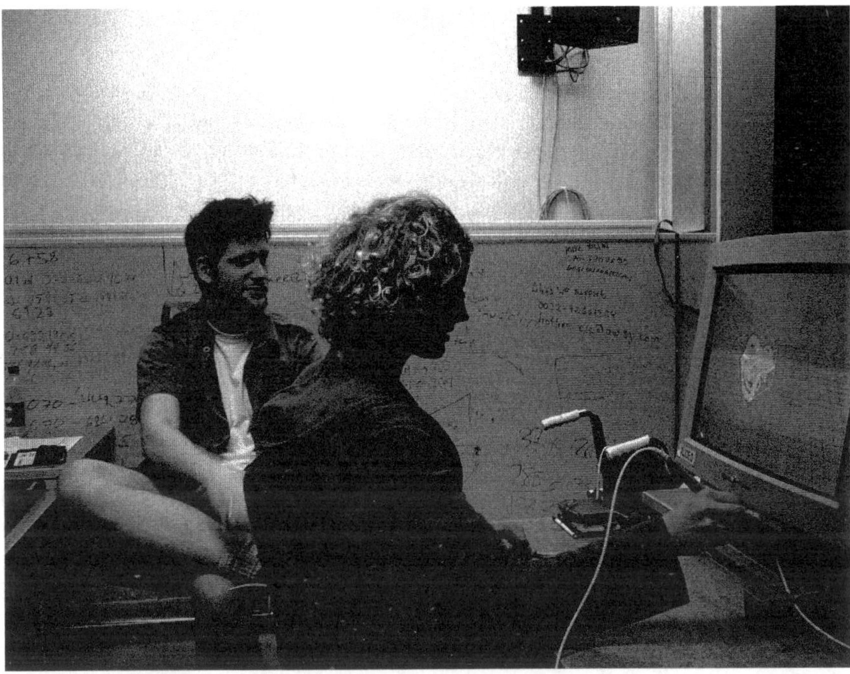

Figure 3 – The experimental set-up without hand-image collocation

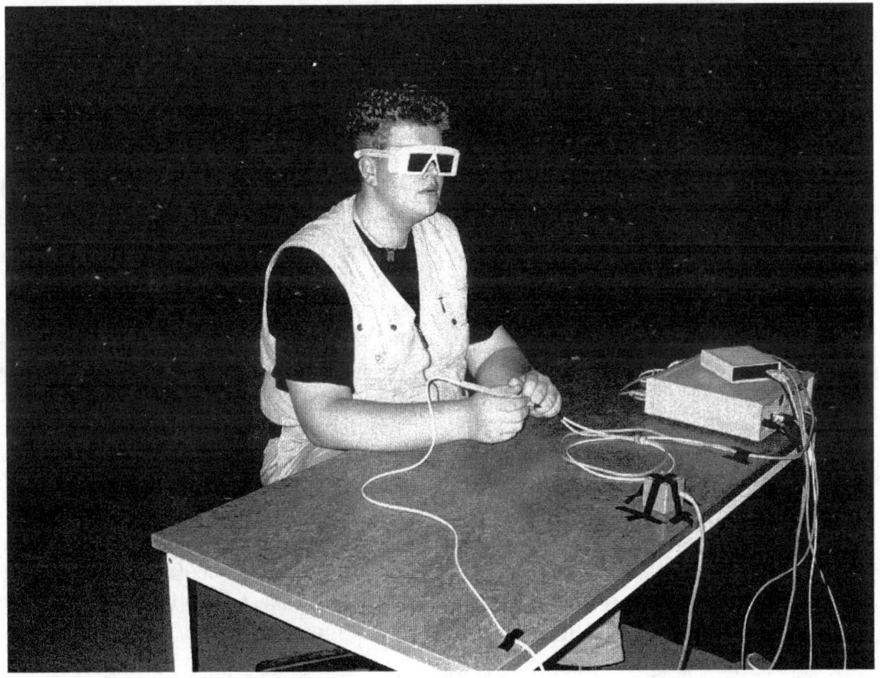

Figure 4 – The experimental set-up with projected image

3. Results

We recorded the numbers of blue and magenta voxels removed, and the time taken for each task, as well as the number of left hand button presses and holding times. The basic data obtained will be described first. In the following, PROJ refers to the condition with no hand-image collocation and projected display. HIC refers to the condition with hand-image collocation, and NHIC refers to the condition with a standard monitor position and without hand-image collocation.

Table 1 – Number of blue voxels correctly removed

	PROJ	HIC	NHIC	Means
Stereo	3340,30	1949,95	1553,15	2281,133
No-stereo	6512,95	3097,80	3078,40	4229,717
Means	4926,625	2523,875	2315,775	3255,425

From Table 1 it can be seen that performance was much better with stereo than with no-stereo. ANOVA confirmed that this was a highly significant difference ($p<.0002$).

Performance was much worse with the projector than with the two proximal conditions (HIC and NHIC). This was also a highly significant difference ($p<.0001$). Performance improved over the four trials ($p<.03$), but there were no interaction effects.

Table 2 - Magenta voxels erroneously removed

	PROJ	HIC	NHIC	Means
Stereo	8563,00	5680,75	3477,30	5907,017
No-stereo	42258,40	16982,30	17001,95	25414,217
Means	25410,700	11331,525	10239,625	15660,617

From Table 2 we can see that performance with stereo was again very much better than without ($p<.0001$) and that performance with the projected image was again much worse than both HIC and NHIC ($p<.0001$). There was also a highly significant learning effect across trials ($p<.0001$).

There were two interaction effects: a highly significant interaction between stereo/non-stereo and PROJ/HIC/NHIC ($p<.0001$), and a significant interaction between stereo/no-stereo and learning ($p<.05$). Inspection of Table 2 shows that the differences between stereo and no-stereo were greater for PROJ than for HIC or NHIC. The effect of learning was greater for stereo than for no-stereo.

Surprisingly, stereo performance was worse with HIC than with NHIC, whereas no-stereo performance was better with HIC than NHIC, although, as with blue voxels removed (where there was an apparent and similar benefit of NHIC over HIC for the stereo conditions) this difference was not statistically significant.

Table 3 reveals that stereo was faster than no-stereo ($p<.0001$) and that image location also had a significant effect ($p<.02$), mostly due to the fact that HIC was faster than PROJ and NHIC. The effect of learning was again highly significant ($p<.001$). There were no interaction effects.

Table 3 - Time to complete the task in seconds

	PROJ	HIC	NHIC	Means
Stereo	387,85	292,80	406,55	362,000
No-stereo	507,15	462,85	463,80	477,933
Means	447,50	377,825	435,175	420,167

Table 4 - Non-dominant hand button presses

	PROJ	HIC	NHIC	Means
Stereo	44,90	29,75	54,75	43,133
No-stereo	43,70	34,70	31,05	36,483
Means	44,30	32,225	42,90	39,808

In terms of non-dominant hand button presses, the only significant effect was the interaction between stereo/no-stereo and PROJ/HIC/NHIC ($p<.05$). This appears to reflect the tendency for HIC to result in considerably fewer button presses than NHIC with stereo, but in slightly more button presses than NHIC with non-stereo (Table 4).

Table 5 - Non-dominant hand button holding time

	PROJ	HIC	NHIC	Means
Stereo	119,55	99,60	158,6	125,917
No-stereo	86,50	114,60	57,20	86,100
Means	103,025	107,100	107,900	106,008

Stereo resulted in longer holding times than no-stereo ($p<.05$) and there was an interaction effect between stereo/no-stereo and PROJ/HIC/NHIC ($p<.05$). This appears to result from shorter holding times with HIC than NHIC for stereo conditions, but shorter holding times with NHIC than HIC for no-stereo conditions (Table 5).

4. Discussion

Performance with stereo was much better than performance without, in terms of blue voxels correctly removed, magenta voxels erroneously removed, and time taken to perform the task. This was true wherever the image was located. For magenta voxels, the effect of stereo versus non-stereo was greater with the projector than for the standardly-placed monitor or for the condition with hand-image collocation.

The effects of image location were less clear-cut. With the projector, accuracy was much worse than both the other conditions in terms of the number of both blue and magenta voxels removed. Users appeared to have some difficulty transposing dextrous manipulations to and from the wall projection. But hand-image collocation did not result in significantly better performance than the standardly-placed monitor in terms of these two measures (blue and magenta voxels removed). Completion was faster with hand-image collocation than with the other two conditions, although the difference was rather small.

The pattern of results is broadly compatible with those of our earlier study. In both experiments stereo was found to be more beneficial than hand-image collocation in improving performance. In both, hand-image collocation improved speed, but the benefit on performance was even smaller in the present study. As in the first experiment, there were few interaction effects. Hand-image collocation was not more beneficial when combined with stereo than without.

Learning effects were revealed in terms of blue voxels removed and, more dramatically, magenta voxels removed in error. In the latter case, there was an interaction effect between learning and stereo/no stereo indicating that there was more improvement for stereo than non-stereo.

There were complex interactions between stereo versus non-stereo, hand-image collocation and its absence, and work object movements with the non-dominant hand. Although it is not easy to interpret these results, it appears that users compensated for the absence of stereo in different ways in conditions with hand-image collocation than in those without, in terms of the number of times they moved the work object and the duration of each move.

5. Conclusions

Our results were surprising. Stereo vision was very important to both accuracy and speed of task completion, as we found previously. But the presence of hand-image collocation did not improve accuracy, despite the fact that this was a truly three-dimensional task. It may be that the ability to move the work object was much more important in this case than in the earlier study, and that object movement can adequately compensate for the absence of hand-image collocation.

If this finding is replicated by further studies, it has important implications for the volumetric presentation of medical data to individual practitioners and in group settings. For example, the complication and expense involved in using a "reach in" style of collocated hand and image display may not be justified. And in a group setting, it may be advantageous if the practitioner currently manipulating the volume of interest does not rely on the projected image. We have further experiments planned to test the effectiveness of different ways of displaying detailed medical data as collaborative tools.

Acknowledgements

The experiment was carried out by Daniel Bergh, using equipment and facilities provided by VRlab at Umeå University, Sweden. We thank our volunteers for their participation.

References

[1] Poston, T. and Serra, L. (1996). Dextrous Virtual Work. Communications of the ACM, 39, 5, 37-45, May 1996.

[2] Waterworth, J A (2000) Dextrous VR: the Importance of Stereoscopic Display and Hand-Image Collocation. In Mulder, J D and van Liere, R (eds.) Virtual Environments 2000: Proceedings of Eurographics Workshop in Amsterdam, June 2000. Vienna: Springer.

[3] Serra, L., Poston, T., Ng, H., Chua, B. C. and Waterworth, J. A. (1995). Interaction Techniques for a Virtual Workspace. Paper and video presented at the International Conference on Artificial Reality and Tele-Existence (ICAT)/Conference on Virtual Reality Software and Technology (VRST) '95, Maakuhari Messe, Japan, November 1995.

Usability Analysis
of VR Simulation Software[*]

Anna L. Weaver, Paul N. Kizakevich
Research Triangle Institute, Research Triangle Park, NC

Walt Stoy
Center for Emergency Medicine, Pittsburgh, PA

J. Harvey Magee
U.S. Army Medical Research and Materiel Command, Ft. Detrick, MD

William Ott, Kevin Wilson
Durham County EMS, Durham, NC

1. Background/Problem

Usability testing, commonly conducted for commercial software to ensure that it meets the needs of the end user, is likewise vital to creating effective training software employing VR technologies. However, developers often limit software testing to expert evaluation (by other developers or subject matter experts [SMEs]) to identify potential problems that might impede the usability or acceptability of the software. This paper describes a usability test—conducted with representatives of the end user—of VirtualEMS™, a VR software package designed to provide realistic practice for emergency medical technicians (EMTs) and paramedics. The purpose is to provide insight into the process of and value added by usability testing.

2. Test Design

Following Rubin's *Handbook of Usability Testing*[1], iterative usability testing of VirtualEMS was conducted with representatives of the end user: students and teachers in emergency medical services (EMS) programs and practicing EMTs and paramedics (referred to as firehouse users). Students and teachers were tested at the Center for Emergency Medicine of Western Pennsylvania (CEM) in Pittsburgh, PA, in mid-February 2001; testing with firehouse users took place at the Durham County EMS Base in Durham, NC, in late March 2001. Following CEM testing, preliminary recommendations were provided to developers; many of these recommendations were implemented prior to firehouse testing.

CEM and firehouse testing provided quantitative and qualitative information about software usability, including adequacy of the software's tutorial and help system, and provided preference information (e.g., Do these users enjoy working with VirtualEMS? Do they think it provides meaningful training and/or practice?).

Consistent with prior SME evaluations conducted on this software and concurrent with CEM testing, experts in emergency medicine evaluated the accuracy and realism of several aspects of VirtualEMS, including organization and completeness of tools and

---

[*] This software was supported in part by the U.S. Army Medical Research and Materiel Command under Contract No. DAMD17-99-2-9046. The contents of this software do not necessarily reflect the position or the policy of the government, and no official endorsement should be inferred.

several aspects of VirtualEMS, including organization and completeness of tools and devices; accuracy and realism of the visual representations of the patient, his injuries, and medical devices; and accuracy and realism of patient interactions and physiological responses represented in the software.

3. Method

Standard usability testing methods employed included scripted scenarios, pre- and post-test questionnaires, data logs, the think-aloud protocol, and test monitor observations[1]. The test monitor measured and recorded certain aspects of test participant performance, including observations and comments (test participant exhibits frustration or satisfaction or comments about the software positively or negatively); number of noncritical errors (an individual participant makes a mistake but is able to recover and complete the task); number of critical errors (an individual participant makes a mistake and is not able to recover and complete the task); time to complete tasks (when applicable); and number of times users accessed help screens and/or the user's guide. It is important to note that the test monitor did not offer participants assistance with the software or tasks.

SMEs were asked to self-record their evaluations, although an observer was occasionally present. In contrast to the test monitor role described above, the SME observer interacted freely with the SMEs, often providing explanations and assistance with software features.

4. Usability Results

Usability testing identified problems with and potential improvements to the tutorial, help system, and other elements of the interface (mouse commands, pop-up menus). Test participants also provided an overall rating for the software.

Tutorial

Perhaps the most important qualitative finding related to user immersion in the scenario and the importance that the software tutorial follow standard EMS procedures. Several users became frustrated when the tutorial, designed to teach users to operate the software, did not fully follow EMS procedures. Testing also revealed that users are quickly immersed in the simulation and that they have a strong desire to treat the patient correctly. Some were so distracted by this conflict that they strayed from the tutorial. Although it is encouraging to note that VirtualEMS engages its target users, users' ability to learn from the tutorial was often compromised.

Help System

The initial, web-based help system featured links from software elements (help buttons) to HTML pages offering helpful information. All users consulted help files when they could not figure out a software feature or became confused. If they did not find the answer immediately, they expected to be able to search the help files and indicated that searchable help was key to overall usability and user-friendliness. Although web-based help offered some of the desired functionality, users suggested that a Microsoft Windows®-compatible help system would be preferred.

Interface

Users indicated that they expect familiar Microsoft Windows® interface features (e.g., cursor displays as an hourglass when the program is busy). Problems and inconsistencies in the interface identified during testing included menus closing too quickly and message boxes sometimes obscuring text.

In addition, both CEM and firehouse users demonstrated significant problems with the "learn mode" (designed to provide users with a review of EMS assessment protocols), the software's simulation of scene assessment, and one of the primary navigational tools.

Overall Rating

On a scale from 1 (lowest or poorest) to 5 (highest or best), the average overall ratings given by students and firehouse users are indicated in Table 1.

Table 1. Average Evaluation Scores — Students and Firehouse Users

Test user	Overall usefulness	Meaningfulness for training/ practice	Likelihood of using outside classroom/ work environment	Likelihood of using if approved for continuing ed.
EMS students	3.4	4.0	3.7	**
Firehouse users	4.0	4.8	4.8	4.3

** Participant was not asked this question.

5. SME Results

SMEs identified several problems with accuracy and realism of the software. For example, visual representations of some wounds were determined to be unrealistic, and vital signs were determined to be "way too good" for the severity of injuries depicted in most scenarios. Accuracy, realism, and function of patient interactions and medical devices were deemed adequate for EMS training.

6. Conclusions

Usability testing identified markedly different problems than SME evaluations, thus proving that usability testing does add value to the software development effort. Problems with the interface that might have gone unnoticed in SME evaluations were identified and recorded through the testing, and their effect on overall user satisfaction was realized. Observing actual end users working with software can be key to developing training software that will be accepted by users and will, thus, achieve the intended training goal.

After the first round of tests (CEM), several recommended changes (e.g., to the tutorial and interface) were implemented. As shown in Table 1, subsequent firehouse testing revealed improvement in users' perception of the software's meaningfulness and overall usefulness, and an increase in the likelihood that users would use the software. (Because of the small sample size, formal hypothesis testing was not done). This would indicate that the changes recommended after initial usability testing increased user satisfaction with the software.

The usability testing methods applied in this study proved adequate for testing desktop-VR software like VirtualEMS™; however, other accepted usability evaluation methods might also be applicable, including heuristic evaluation (usability specialists judge whether a user interface follows established usability principles), cognitive walkthrough (expert evaluators construct task scenarios, then role play the part of a user working with that interface), and pluralistic walkthroughs (users, developers, and usability professionals step through a task scenario, discussing and evaluating each element of interaction)[2].

References

[1] Rubin, J. (1994). *Handbook of Usability Testing*. New York: John Wiley & Sons.

[2] Hom, J. (1996). *The Usability Methods Toolbox* [Online]. Available:
http://www.best.com/~jthom/usability/usable.htm

Medicine Meets Virtual Reality 02/10
J.D. Westwood et al. (Eds.)
IOS Press, 2002

Elastically Deformable 3D Organs for Haptic Surgical Simulation

Roger Webster, Ph.D.[1], Randy Haluck, M.D.[2], Rob Ravenscroft, Ph.D.[1]
Betty Mohler [1], Eric Crouthamel [1], Tyson Frack [1], Steve Terlecki [1], Jeremy Sheaffer [1]

*[1]Department of Computer Science School of Science and Mathematics H. Justin Roddy
Science and Technology Building Millersville University Millersville, PA. USA 17551
webster@cs.millersville.edu*

*[2] Department of Minimally Invasive Surgery Penn State University College of Medicine
Milton S. Hershey Medical Center Hershey, PA USA 17033*

Abstract. This paper describes a technique for incorporating real-time elastically deformable 3D organs in haptic surgical simulators. Our system is a physically based particle model utilizing a mass-springs-damper connectivity with an implicit predictor to speed up calculations during each time step. The solution involves repeated application of Newton's 2nd Law of motion: $F = ma$ using an implicit solver for numerically solving the differential equations.

1. Introduction

Surgical simulators are currently being developed by many research institutions and corporations to train medical students and surgeons in minimally invasive surgery. Among the primary research topics is the notion of deformable virtual organs and soft tissue for use in haptic surgical simulators. During the past decade many graphics researchers have contributed to the forefront of deformable 3D objects research, see D. Terzopoulos, et.al. in [1,2], and in cloth animation systems, Baraff and Witkin in [4], and N. Thalmann, et.al, in [5]. Haptic surgical simulators have primarily used either physically based models [6,7,8] or finite element models [9,10,11]. Although many techniques have been proposed for deformable object animation (see [12] for an overview), few can provide the performance necessary for real-time applications. The fundamental trade off therefore is accuracy vs interactivity. In haptic surgical simulation this problem is especially acute, as the user must feel contact forces (and see the graphical deformations) that are accurate yet computed in real time.

Our system is a physically based particle model utilizing a mass-springs-damper connectivity with an implicit predictor to speed up calculations during each time step. This system consists of a set of point masses (nodes) connected to each other with a network of springs and dampers. Each vertex in the organ geometry has a mass and is connected to every other vertex with springs and dampers. The solution involves repeated application of Newton's 2nd Law of motion: $F = ma$ using an implicit solver for numerically solving the differential equations. The dynamics equation for each mass point is $m_i x_i = -\gamma_i x_i + \Sigma g_{ij} + f_i$ where m_i is the mass at point $x_i \in R^3$, $-\gamma_i x_i$ is the damping force to prevent instabilities, g_{ij} is the linear Hookian force exerted on mass i by the spring between i and j, f_i is the sum of the external forces acting on mass i (gravity, pushing and probing the 3D organ). Combining the vectors of all mass points produces: $Mx + Dx + Kx = f$, where M is the mass matrix, D is the damping matrix, K is the stiffness matrix, and f is the aggregate force vector. As the system progresses through time dt, the first order differential equations are: $v = M^{-1} (-Dv - Kx + f)$, $x = v$, where v is the velocity vector. Baraff and Witkin [4] have used a similar technique effectively in modeling cloth systems for special effects in the motion picture industry. The fundamental problem with these implicit solvers is that they need to solve a linear system at each time step, which is not practical with today's computers. To get around this computational expense, we incorporate a technique, based upon the work of Desbrun et.al. [13], with an approximate solver that pre computes the solution to a linear system. In addition, we have written a pre-processor that builds the matrices for the predictor for each organ and writes them out to a file. The matrix generation process may take considerable time to calculate (several minutes). The surgical simulation application, however, can simply load a file with the prediction matrices pre-built.

Method and Tools

Our simulator uses the Sensable Technologies' PHANToM™ haptic device, the "Reachin Display"™ unit to provide the user with the ergonomic feel of actual surgery (see Figure 1). The Crystal Eyes™ stereo glasses are used to enhance the 3D effect. The graphics programming environment is EAI/Sense8's WorldToolkit™ API of OpenGL calls. The haptics programming environment is the Sensable Technologies' GHOST™ API calls. The control computer is a Pentium processor workstation running Windows2000™ with an Nvidia GeForce™ graphics OpenGl accelerator.

Our system has four basic forces. They are: (1) gravity, in which all masses are accelerated in the y-axis at 9.8 m/s/s. The collision forces (2) are calculated when the user pulls and probes the organs. All momentum being exerted is transferred back to the colliding mass points. The springs (3) are either stretched or compressed away from their initial resting length. Each spring is subject to the conventional Hooke's Law restoring force (F = -kx). To prevent numerical instabilities we use a damping coefficient (4) in which masses in motion will receive a small force opposite to their directional vector.

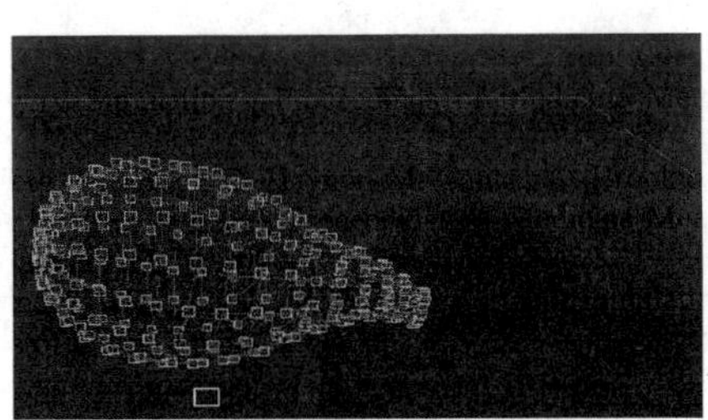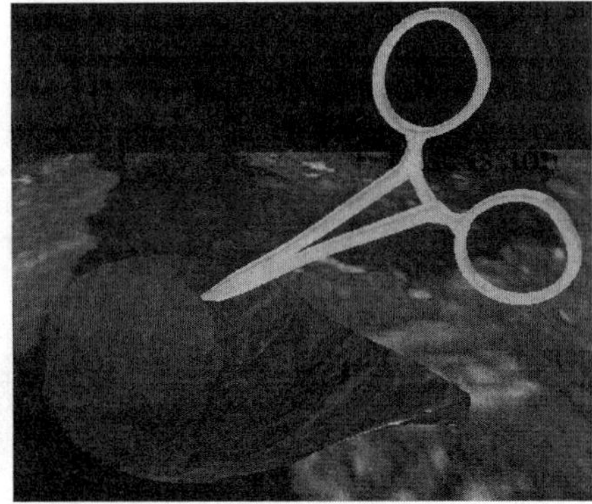

Figure 1. (a) Wire frame of gallbladder model showing mass points and (b) probing deformation.

Conclusions/Results

The goal of this project is to develop real-time elastically deformable 3D organs software for use in simulating a suite of surgical procedures. We have experimented using 3D organs with up to 1000 polygons with frame rates of 25 fps on a conventional intel 1.4 Ghz single processor PC with a GeForce OpenGL accelerator with no significant visual or haptic computational lag. The advantage of this technique is that the underlying physical model is simple, it uses well-understood dynamics, and interactive frame rates with modestly sized polygonal models are attainable. The downside is that the discretized mass-springs system is an approximation of the actual continuous real-world physics. In addition, proper values for the spring constants of non-isomorphic soft tissues are contrived and can cause instability problems as well as slow deformations. Further enhancements, testing and evaluation are in progress. See our web site http://cs.millersville.edu/~webster/haptics for updated information.

Acknowledgments

This project was funded, in part, by the National Science Foundation under grant numbers EIA-00116616, DUE-9950742 and DUE-965123. Additional funding provided by the Neimeyer-Hodgson Grants Program, and by the Noonan Endowment fund and the Faculty Grants Committee of Millersville University.

References

[1] D. Terzopoulos, J.C. Platt, H. Barr, K. Fleischer, "*Elastically Deformable Models*", Proceedings of the Annual ACM SIGGRAPH '87 Conference, ACM Press, Vol. 21. pp. 205-214, July 1987.

[2] D. Terzopoulos, K. Fleischer, "*Modeling InElastic Deformation: Vicoelasticity, Plasticity, Fracture*", Proceedings of the Annual ACM SIGGRAPH '88, ACM Press, Vol. 22. pp. 269-278, August 1988.

[3] D. Metaxas, D. Terzopoulos, "*Dynamic Deformation of Solid Primitives with Constraints*", Proceedings of the Annual ACM SIGGRAPH '92, ACM Press, Vol. 26. pp. 309-312, July 1992.

[4] D. Baraff and A. Witkin, "*Large Steps in Cloth Animation*", Proceedings of the Annual ACM SIGGRAPH '98 Conference, ACM Press, Vol. 33, pps. 43-54, July 1998.

[5] Nadia Thalmann, "*Cloth Animation*", Proceedings of the Annual ACM SIGGRAPH '98 Conference, ACM Press, Vol. 33, pps. 43-54, July 1998.

[6] Suvranu De, M. Srinivasan, "*Thin Walled Models for Haptic and Graphical Rendering of Soft Tissues in Surgical Simulations*", Proceedings of Medicine Meets Virtual Reality (MMVR '99), IOS Press, San Francisco, CA. January 1999, pps. 94-99.

[7] C. Basdogan, M. Srinivasan, S. Small, S. Dawson, "*Force Interactions in Laparoscopic Simulations: Haptic Rendering of Soft Tissues*", Proceedings of Medicine Meets Virtual Reality (MMVR 6), IOS Press, San Diego, CA. January 1996, pps. 19-22.

[8] D. James and D. Pai, "*ArtDefo Accurate Real Time Deformable Objects*", Proceedings of the Annual ACM SIGGRAPH Conference, ACM Press, August 1999, pps. 65-72 (see also http://www.cs.ubc.ca/~djames/deformable/index.html).

[9] Morten Bro-Nielsen, "Fast Finite Elements For Surgery Simulation", Proceedings of Medicine Meets Virtual Reality 5 (MMVR '97), 1997, pps. 395-400.

[10] Jeffrey Berkley, P. Oppenheimer, S. Weghorst, D. Berg, G. Raugi, D. Haynor, M. Ganter, C. Brooking, G. Turkiyyah, "Creating Finite Element Models from Medical Images", Proceedings of Medicine Meets Virtual Reality (MMVR '2000), Newport Beach, CA. January 27-30, 2000, IOS Press, pps. 26-32.

[11] Morten Bro-Nielsen and S. Cotin, "Real-time Volumetric Deformable Models for Surgical Simulation Using Finite Elements and Condensation", Proceedings of EuroGraphics, 1996, pps. 21-30.

[12] Sarah Frisken and B. Mirtich, "*A Survery of Deformable Modeling in Computer Graphics*", MERL Technical Report TR-97-19, November 1997, http://www.merl.com/reports/TR-97-19/.

[13] Mathieu Desbrun, G. Debunne, A. Barr, M, Cani, "*Interative Multi-Resolution Animation of Deformable Models*", Proceedings of the Annual ACM SIGGRAPH Conference, pps. 82-89, ACM Press, August 1999.

[14] "General Haptic Open Software Toolkit GHOST Programmer's Guide", Sensable Technologies Inc., June 1999.

Medicine Meets Virtual Reality 02/10
J.D. Westwood et al. (Eds.)
IOS Press, 2002

A Generic Arthroscopy
Simulator Architecture

D P M Wills[1], E Abblard[1] and K P Sherman[2]

1. *Department of Computer Science, University of Hull, Hull, UK*
2. *Orthopaedic Department, Hull and East Yorkshire Hospitals NHS Trust, Hull, UK*

Abstract. Virtual Environments offer considerable potential to improve training for arthroscopic surgery. However, current systems are developed for individual joints, which requires healthcare providers to purchase and maintain multiple environments with differing interfaces and capabilities. This paper describes a generic arthroscopy system architecture that allows the fast development of training environments for any joint, each sharing a common user-interface. The use of the architecture in developing a simple ankle simulator is also described.

1 Introduction

The potential of Virtual Environment techniques to enhance the arthroscopic training of both surgical trainees and experienced surgeons has already been demonstrated [1,2], providing an environment for a safer, more effective and rapid training process. Further, such techniques can provide a method for the early selection of those surgical trainees who require more concentrated teaching in specific skills areas. The Royal College of Surgeons of England has explored the possibility of testing basic surgical skills as a requirement for the MRCS diploma and the possibility of assessing higher-level practical surgical skills is also being considered by the intercollegiate board for higher surgical training (FRCS) [3]. The costs involved in such methods of assessment are a major obstacle to their widespread acceptance.

However, current systems are developed for individual joints, which would require healthcare providers to purchase and maintain multiple systems with differing capabilities and interfaces. We believe that the area is now sufficiently mature that a generic system can be developed that will allow multiple joints to be simulated within a single system architecture, sharing common components in software, hardware and, at a higher level, trainee scoring and assessment. The development of such a system would benefit health care purchasers, trainees and experienced surgeons and, above all, patients.

In this paper we report our initial development of a Generic Arthroscopy Simulator Architecture (GASA), which provides a set of core components and infrastructure for developing arthroscopy training simulators. The development of a simple Virtual Ankle Arthroscopy Training Systems has been conducted within this architecture.

2 Method

Based upon our previous development of training systems for Knee Arthroscopy [4,5] and Vitreous Eye Surgery [6], a set of common components have been identified, which include visualization, collision detection, haptic feedback, kinematic joint representation, deformable objects and user-interface. An initial Object-Oriented design has been produced for the generic system and a number of software components developed in C++. OpenGL has been used for the visualization. Further, a scene configuration interface has been implemented that allows a user to quickly describe the internal anatomy, including kinematical linkages, of the joint for arthroscopic training.

2.1 The GASA Design

An arthroscopy simulator involves a simulation scene containing objects of various anatomical types and one or more surgical instruments. The position and orientation of the instruments are detected by a tracking system with the virtual arthroscope providing the main training visualization. The anatomical elements are organised as kinematic chains consisting of links articulated by joints. The top-level design of the generic architecture is summarised in Figure 1.

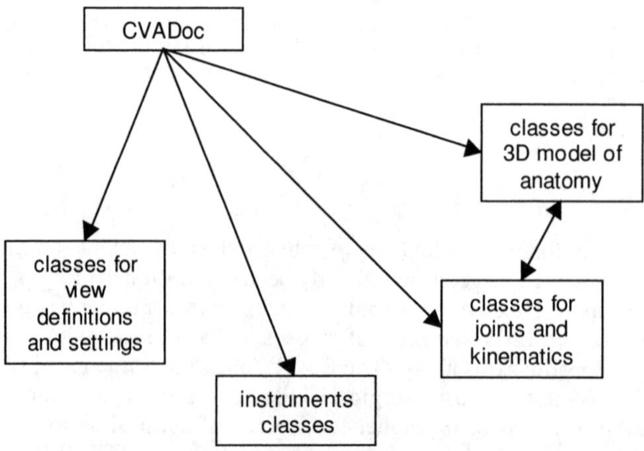

Figure 1 – General organisation of the program

The document class CVADoc stores the configuration data for the simulation. It contains pointers to the anatomical definition, which includes a list of anatomical elements and their types (bones, ligaments, etc.). It also contains a list of joints, pointers to the instruments (the arthroscope and possibly a second tool) and information about the current view and its settings. This configuration data is loaded from a file and can be modified within the system when a new joint simulation is being created. Methods are provided in CVADoc that allow for the addition and removal of anatomical objects, the setting of viewing parameters, and the loading and saving of the configuration data.

The main views currently supported within the system are the arthroscopic view and an anatomical overview. The parameters for the arthroscopic view are dependent on the arthroscope being modelled, the current point of view, and the position and type of the light source. The anatomical overview allows the trainee to have an external view of the joint, allowing for orientation and better anatomical understanding in the early stages of training. All aspects of these views are user-definable and can be customised for the type of scope and joint under consideration. Other views are provided that are used in the definition of a particular training system, for instance, allowing specific joint properties to be specified. They provide a visual representation of the current joint structure and the interactive definition of new linkages and related properties such as coordinates axis and centres of rotation.

Two kinds of anatomical objects are defined: the anatomical "structures" and the anatomical "elements" (Figure 2). The anatomical structures correspond to different biomechanical functions in the body, or, more simply, to different types of anatomical bodies. For instance, such a structure could group all the bones or all the ligaments. All objects within an anatomical structure will share a set of properties. The anatomical elements are the individual anatomical bodies. For instance, the tibia, the patella, the cruciate ligaments, could be described as anatomical elements within the knee.

Each element object depends on one structure object and the structure object is defined as containing element objects. Therefore, the anatomical element, amongst its attributes, has a reference to the structure object it belongs. The anatomical structure object maintains a list of the elements in the simulation scene that are relevant to its definition.

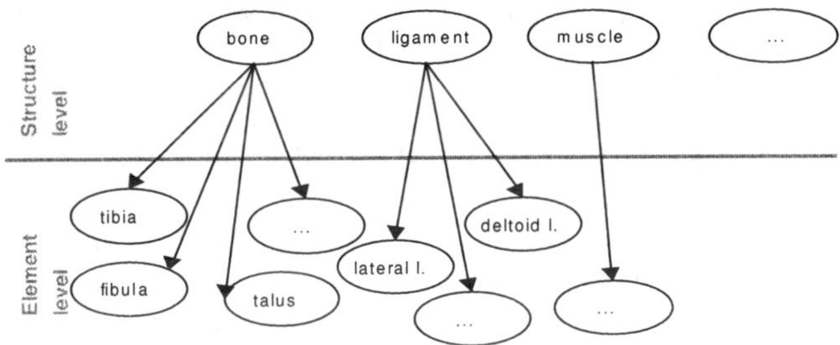

Figure 2 – two level design of anatomy

This approach has two advantages:
- properties can be defined at the structure level and refined at the element level
- methods can be applied either to individual elements, or to the group of elements defined in a structure.

A further breakdown (Figure 3) occurs for elements into rigid (CrigidElem) and non-rigid (CnonRigidElem) elements. Each element then has a pointer to a CGLObj object that defines the corresponding 3D computer model, currently a triangular mesh. Methods are provided that allow object loading, object drawing using OpenGL, ray intersection (for collision detection), low level access to the object geometry and bounding box.

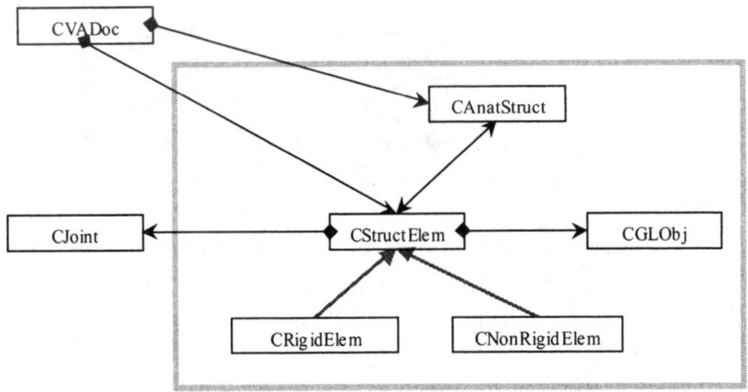

Figure 3 – Classes defining the anatomical elements

The document class also contains information about instruments (an arthroscope is always defined) and about the tracking system being used. It is in charge of updating the state of the instruments as often as required, based upon information provided by classes that provide an interface to the tracking hardware being used (Figure 4).

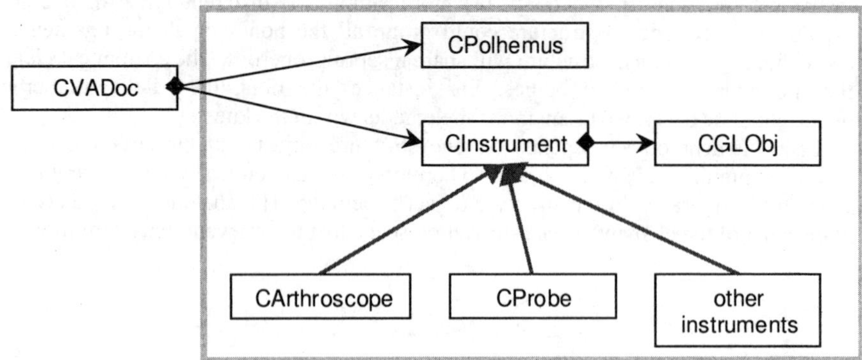

Figure 4 – Classes for the definition of the instruments

Animation of the anatomical object is provided for by the definition of a kinematic chain, that is an arrangement of joints and links. The type and structure of a joint dictates the range of motion of the links, defined as constraints, which are derived from the shape of the bones and the forces exerted by tissues such as muscles and ligaments. Links are typically bones and ligaments. Joints may have up to 6 degrees of freedom, modelled by elementary joints with a single degree of freedom. It was decided at an early stage that the user should not have to define joints at the elementary level and therefore methods are provided that will transform the high level information defining the joint into the appropriate set of elementary joints. The classes involved in the kinematic definition of joints are shown in Figure 5.

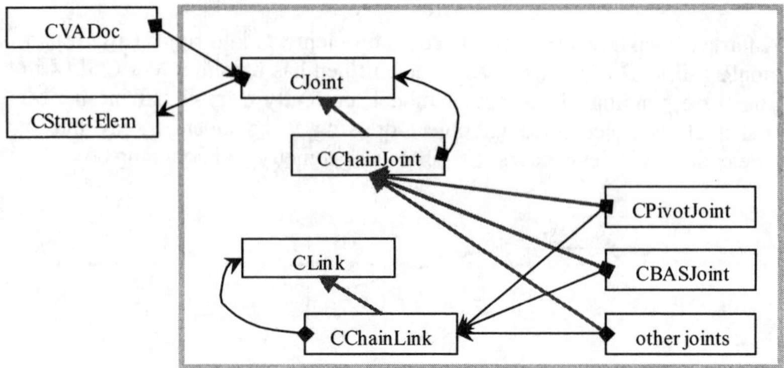

Figure 5 - Classes for the definition of the joints and kinematics

3   Results

Microsoft Visual C++ and Microsoft Foundation Classes were used to implement a subset of the GASA design with OpenGL being used for the visualization. Based upon this implementation, a simple ankle arthroscopy training system was constructed. Dialog boxes available from a menu (Figure 6) were used to first define the anatomical structures (bone, ligaments, etc) and then the individual elements within the structures (tibia fibula, talus etc). For each anatomical element, a name and valid file containing the 3D mesh was given. By default new elements are visible and fixed (not attached to any joint). Since the 3D meshes of the anatomy were not specifically created for use in the training system, provided tools were used to redefine the coordinate planes of the objects and to specify centres of rotation.

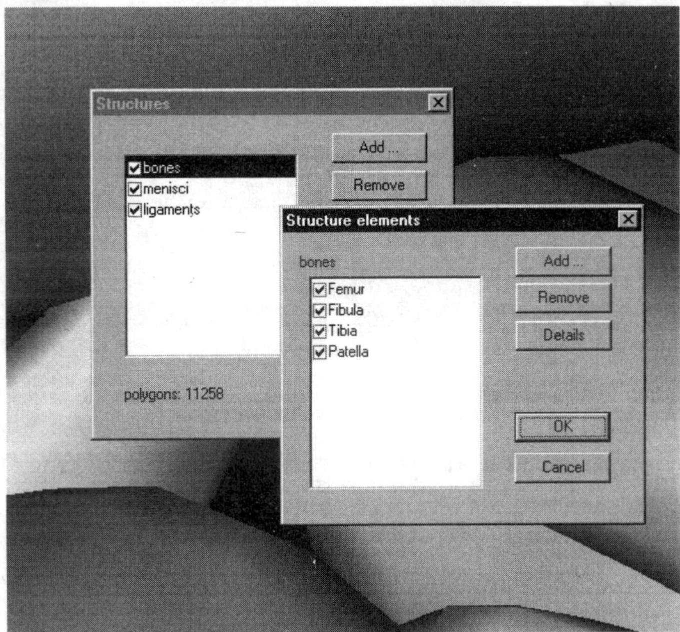

Figure 6 – Dialog boxes for the definition of the anatomical structures and elements. Here, three structures are defined: bones, ligaments and menisci. The elements defined as being bones are: the femur, the fibula, the tibia and the patella. By default, they are all visible as shown by the check boxes.

The joints were defined to form a kinematic chain, which is an alternation of joints and links between joints. At any time, the current joint list was available from a menu, which allowed the addition and deletion of joints, the setting of their properties and their articulation. When a joint was required, a dialog box was requested which allowed the specification of an appropriate mechanical model and position of the new joint within an existing chain (Figure 7). A number of default properties are given to new joints, which can then either be accepted or updated via a further dialog box. The placement of pivot points for joints was performed through the use of dialog boxes and a 3D graphical representation, increasing the intuitiveness of the system.

Since arthroscopes differ in size and other physical characteristics (such as angle and field of view), the arthroscope may not be the same for all training systems. Therefore the user is given the opportunity to accept a default arthroscope or to describe the properties of the arthroscope required. These properties include a named file containing the geometry of the scope, the angle of sight and an indication as to the accuracy required in detecting collisions between the scope and other object in the scene.

In a similar vein, further aspects of the training system were defined which included: the arthroscopic and anatomical view, collision detection methods and accuracy, selection of tracking system and calibration.

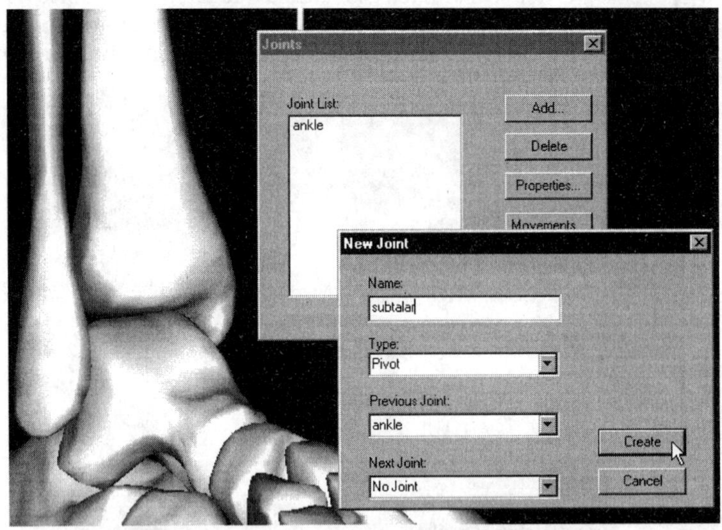

Figure 7 - Creation of a joint. Here, a joint named "subtalar" is created that is located after the joint "ankle" in the kinematic chain. The joint is of type "pivot".

4   Discussion

A generic arthroscopy simulator has been developed to provide a solution to arthroscopy training. The need for such a simulator comes from the difficulty of arthroscopic procedures and the weaknesses of traditional training methods, in terms of cost, risk, realism and efficiency. The provision of a generic training system will avoid the need to produce individual simulators for each joint that can be subject to arthroscopy.

One of the main tasks has been to produce an architecture that allows further developments with minimal changes in the overall design. Particular attention has been given to this issue.

An example implementation of the design has been programmed and this has been used to create a simple ankle training system that includes manipulation of the arthroscope, interaction between the user and the programme, and the detection of collisions between the arthroscope and other objects in the scene.

A major achievement of this project has been to include a generic model of a kinematic chain in order to articulate the model. During the production of the ankle training system it has become apparent that this area needs improvements in terms of both the level of realism available and the operation of the configuration interface.   However the main structure is complete and further developments can be built upon it. The use of mechanical models to model the joints is relevant to arthroscopy simulation, but does not necessarily require an accurate simulation of how the articulation takes place. Further, it has been shown to be easy to include this articulation in a generic simulator, as the initialisation of the joint requires only a few parameters. However, future research will investigate the feasibility of including classes to simplify the inclusion of accurate biomechanical models when required.

The interface of the application already allows simulation scenes to be built, including various kinds of elements, a description of the kinematics and the choice of an arthroscope. Further configuration tools should be designed for this purpose, including utilities to ensure the correct correspondence between the virtual model and the physical model. The design adopted for the management of anatomical bodies has allowed the easy implementation of some anatomy "browsing" facilities. The anatomical bodies of a joint can be hidden or shown individually or according to their type. This feature can be helpful at early stages of training, since the number of bodies overlapping other parts of the anatomy may confuse the trainees. At the first stage of the training, the trainee will also benefit from the opportunity to use an "overview", consisting of an external view of the joint where the arthroscope is illustrated.

5 References

[1] W. Muller and U. Bockholt, The Virtual Reality Arthroscopy Training Simulator, Medicine Meets Virtual Reality, *Technology & Informatics* **50** IOS Press and Ohmsha, (1998) 13-19.

[2] K. P. Sherman, The Specifications and Role of a Virtual Environment System for Knee Arthroscopy Training, PhD Thesis, University of Hull, UK, 2000.

[3] Discussion Document, Joint Committee Intercollegiate Examinations, Royal College of Surgeons, May 2001, UK.

[4] K. P. Sherman, J. W. Ward, D. P. M. Wills, A. M. M. A. Mohsen, A Portable Virtual Environment Knee Arthroscopy Training System with Objective Scoring, Studies. In: J. D. Westwood and H Hoffman *et al* (eds.), *Health Technology and Informatics* **62**, IOS Press and Ohmsha, 1999, pp. 335-336.

[5] J. Ward, K. Sherman, D. Wills, A. M. M. A. Mohsen, M. Crawshaw, The Acquisition of Force Feedback Data For a Virtual Environment Knee Arthroscopy Training System read at the 1999 Advanced Simulation Technologies Conference, San Diego, April 1999. Published in proceedings.

[6] D. Verma and D. P. M. Wills, A Virtual Reality Simulator for Vitreoretinal Surgery, BEAVRS, Cambridge, UK, 7-8 October 1999.

Medicine Meets Virtual Reality 02/10
J.D. Westwood et al. (Eds.)
IOS Press, 2002

Virtual Reality in 3D Echocardiography: Dynamic Visualization of Atrioventricular Annuli Surface Models and Volume Rendered Doppler-Ultrasound

Ivo WOLF[1], Raffaele DE SIMONE[2], Mark HASTENTEUFEL[1],
Tobias KUNERT[1], Sibylle LINK[2], Hans-Peter MEINZER[1]
[1]Deutsches Krebsforschungszentrum, Im Neuenheimer Feld 280,
69120 Heidelberg, Germany
[2]Div. of Cardiac Surgery, University of Heidelberg, Im Neuenheimer Feld 110,
69120 Heidelberg, Germany

Abstract. Knowledge about annuli shape and blood flow patterns, both optimally assessed by transesophageal 3D Doppler echocardiography, can be used in computer assisted surgical planning of heart valve reconstruction. Moreover, information about the individual shape of the annulus anatomy can guide the design of annular prostheses. The problem is that the annulus cannot be easily differentiated from the valve and the myocardium with standard visualization methods. We have developed a nearly automatic method for annulus segmentation. The algorithm provides the annulus shape in a symbolic description, which can be used for surface visualization. Best results to visualize the blood flow from the Doppler signal and the myocardial morphology are obtained by volume rendering. A hybrid visualization technique combining surface rendering and volume rendering enables to dynamically visualize the surface rendered annulus combined with a volume rendered 3D (plus time) reconstruction of either backscatter (morphology) and Doppler information (in original color coding), or together with backscatter only or Doppler only. Visualization of annuli structures combined with blood flow and general myocardial morphology provides a new tool to analyze heart diseases.

1. Introduction

The severity of heart valve insufficiencies (regurgitation) can be analyzed by studying the blood flow leaking through the defect valve. Different types of flow patterns can be linked to different heart valve diseases [1]. Regurgitation is not always caused by defects of the valve itself. Although the causes of regurgitation without valvular disease are still unclear, the condition is associated with changes in annular shape and dynamics [2]. The annulus is the ring where the valve is fixed at the myocardium. Annulus dilation, for example, may hinder the valve to close completely and therefore may cause regurgitation. Valvular disease and annular anomalies may also exist in combination. Moreover, knowledge about annuli form can be used in computer assisted operation planning of heart valve reconstructions and to design annuli prostheses guided by the individual anatomy. It is therefore desirable to visualize the annulus together with the regurgitant flow patterns, especially if the dynamics of the process can be displayed.

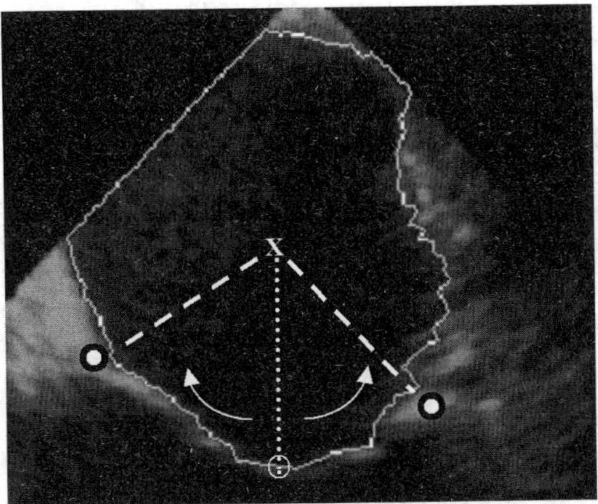

Figure 1. Annulus segmentation: First, the contour of the atrium is detected (solid line). Vertical below (dotted line) the centroid of the atrium (X) lies a point (circle) belonging to the valve, which is used as the start point for searching for wall thickness discontinuities. Dashed lines: Directions of detected discontinuities in wall thickness (filled circles).

Transesophageal three-dimensional Doppler echocardiography optimally assesses morphology, including the annulus, as well as blood flow patterns. The segmentation of the annulus is necessary to extract diagnostic valuable information. This is a very time-consuming step if performed manually. We have developed a nearly automatic method for annulus segmentation, reducing the time necessary for user interaction. The segmentation result is transformed in a surface representation of a tube and visualized together with the volume rendered morphology and/or blood flow.

The segmentation as well as hybrid visualization methods have been integrated in our EchoAnalyzer® software system, which is designed for three-dimensional echocardiographic visualization and quantification [3]. The software will be available for multi-center evaluation after successful completion of internal tests.

2. Methods

2.1 Echocardiographic Imaging

For data acquisition, we use a Sonos 2500DSR/Sonos 5500DSR ultrasound system (Philips Medical Systems, Andover, Mass, USA) with a transesophageal multiplane probe (5 MHz), which allows digital data storage. Four-dimensional data sets are acquired by the built-in rotational controller of the system triggered by ECG and respiratory gating. The backscatter and Doppler data are stored separately.

After acquisition, the data are either stored on a magneto-optical disc for transfer to the off-line processing system or transferred directly using the optional LAN interface from Agilent. The EchoAnalyzer® analysis software is developed in C++ using the GUI library Qt (Trolltech, Oslo, Norway) and runs on all 32-bit Windows systems and on all major Unix derivatives including Linux.

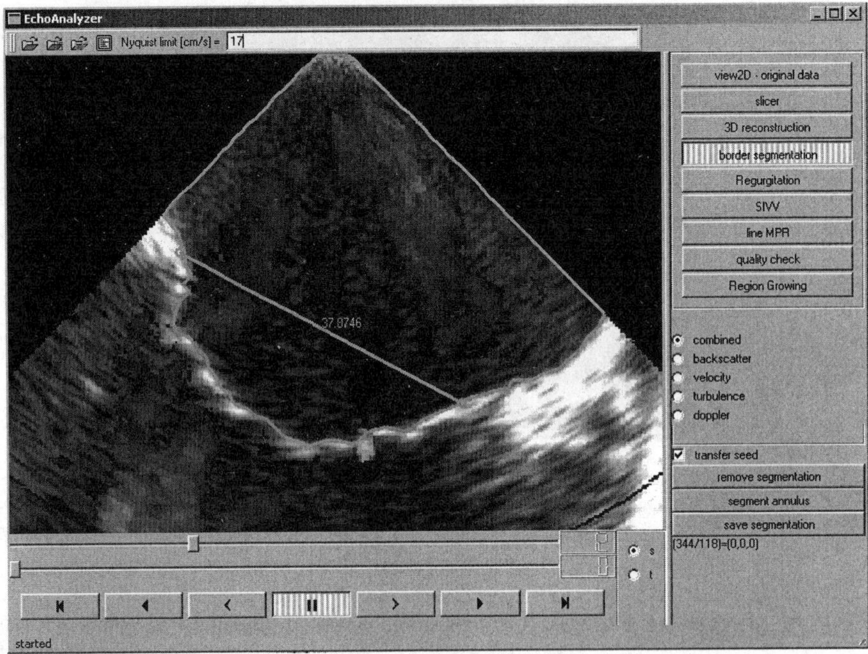

Figure 2. Segmentation module of the EchoAnalyzer® software: The contour of the automatically segmented atrium and the result of the annulus detection (line between the two intersections of the annulus with the slice) are shown.

2.2 Segmentation

The segmentation procedure for the detection of the annulus consists of two major steps [4]. First, one of the cavities adjacent to the annulus is segmented. Usually, we use the atrium for this purpose, because its contour is often better visible than the contour of the ventricle [5].

The second step, based on the result of the first step, is the actual annulus segmentation. The approach is based on the fact that the heart valve is much thinner than the myocardium. Thus, the valve can be detected as the part of the cavity's contour that is considerably thinner than the adjacent parts. The discontinuities in wall thickness along the contour of the cavity on either side of the valve are used to define the position of the annulus (see Figure 1).

2.3 Conversion of Segmentation Result in Surface Representation

The result of the segmentation process is an unstructured list of points in cylindrical co-ordinates. The unstructured list of points has to be transformed in a non-planar polygon in a Cartesian co-ordinate system for visualization. The center of mass $\bar{c}$ of the points and a least-squares-fit of a plane with normal $\bar{n}$ through the points are calculated. The unstructured list of points is sorted by calculating the angles φ of the points in the cylindrical co-ordinate system with $\bar{c}$ as a point on the cylinder axis and $\bar{n}$ as its direction (orientation of the plane $\varphi = 0$ arbitrarily chosen) and rearranging the points according to increasing φ. Additional points are added to the polygon by spline interpolation to achieve a smooth visualization.

The display of the annulus as a filled polygon can now be performed and is useful to determine in which part of the valve the defect is located, if visualized in combination with the blood flow.

The form of the annulus with respect to the morphology and the dynamics of its motion can be more easily appreciated if the annulus is displayed as a ring. The ring must have a

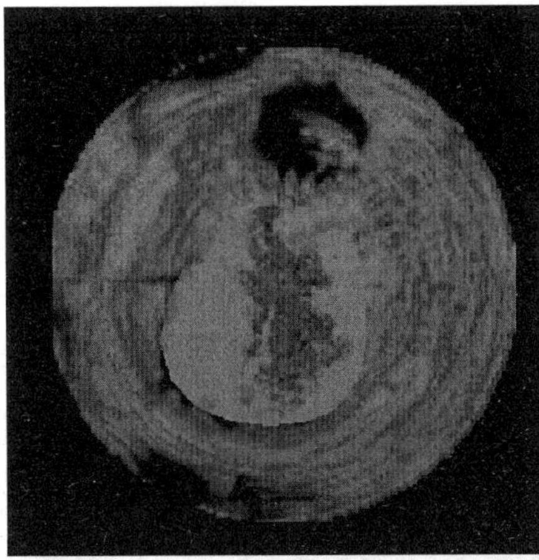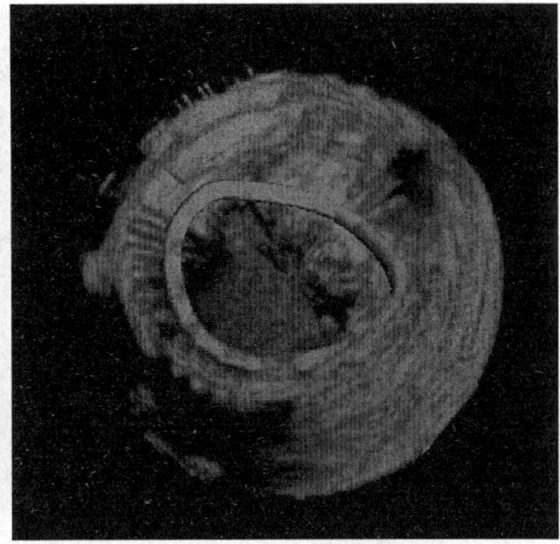

Figure 3. Visualizations of the annulus as a filled polygon (left) and a torus (right), combined with volume rendered morphology and blood flow.

sufficient thickness to be visible simultaneously with the volume rendered morphology and blood flow. Therefore, we have to construct a torus out of the polygon data. The construction of the torus is described in the following.

The torus is built of cylinders with slanted caps fitting to the following cylinder. Each cylinder consists of rectangular patches. Let r be the desired radius (thickness) of the torus, $\vec{p}_i$ the i-th point of the polygon and $\vec{s}^i_j$, $j=1..n$, the vectors defining the cap of the cylinder at point $\vec{p}_i$. The cap of the cylinder is a circle approximated by the points $\vec{p}_i + \vec{s}^i_j$, $j=1..n$. We define $\vec{s}^i_0 = r \cdot \vec{s}^{i*}_0 / \left| \vec{s}^{i*}_0 \right|$, $\vec{s}^{i*}_0 = \vec{v}_{i,-1} \times \vec{v}_{i,+1}$, $v_{i,w} = \vec{p}_i - \vec{p}_{i+w}$. If $\vec{v}_{i,-1}$ and $\vec{v}_{i,+1}$ are collinear, $\vec{p}_i$ is eliminated, thus it is always $\vec{s}^i_0 \neq 0$. $\vec{s}^i_0$ is rotated around the axis through $\vec{p}_i$ with the direction $\vec{a}_i = \vec{v}_{i,-1} / \left| \vec{v}_{i,-1} \right| - \vec{v}_{i,+1} / \left| \vec{v}_{i,+1} \right|$ to construct the remaining $\vec{s}^i_j$ (rotation angle $\alpha = 2\pi \cdot j / (n+1)$).

The next step is to connect the points of two caps to build the surface of the cylinder without causing an internal twisting of the torus. Therefore, $\vec{s}^i_0$ is connect with $\vec{s}^{i+1}_l$, where $l = \arg\max\{\vec{s}^i_0 \cdot \vec{s}^{i+1}_l, l=1..n\}$, then $\vec{s}^{i+1}_l$ with $\vec{s}^{i+1}_{l+1}$ and $\vec{s}^{i+1}_{l+1}$ with $\vec{s}^i_1$. The next patch starts with connecting $\vec{s}^i_1$ and $\vec{s}^{i+1}_{l+1}$, etc. Of cource, $i+1$ and $l+1$ is meant modulo the number of points in the polygon and the number of patchs (n), respectively.

3. Results

The segmentation module of the EchoAnalyzer® software is shown in Figure 2. The cavity segmentation is started by manually setting a seed point inside the cavity of interest, or, if "transfer seed" is activated, the centroid of the detected contour of the current slice (if available) is used for the next selected slice. The annulus segmentation is started by clicking the respective button. Less than a second is needed to segment the cavity and the annulus on a standard PC with 1 GHz processor. The segmentation result of both, the cavity segmentation as well as the annulus segmentation, can be interactively corrected.

Figure 3 shows the annulus displayed as a filled polygon (left) and as a torus (right), in both cases combined with the volume rendered morphology and the Doppler signal. A time series showing the dynamics of the annulus motion combined with the blood flow only is displayed in Figure 4. Notice how the annulus moves up and down during the heart cycle. A color version of the paper can be requested from the author.

 I. Wolf et al. / Virtual Reality in 3D Echocardiography

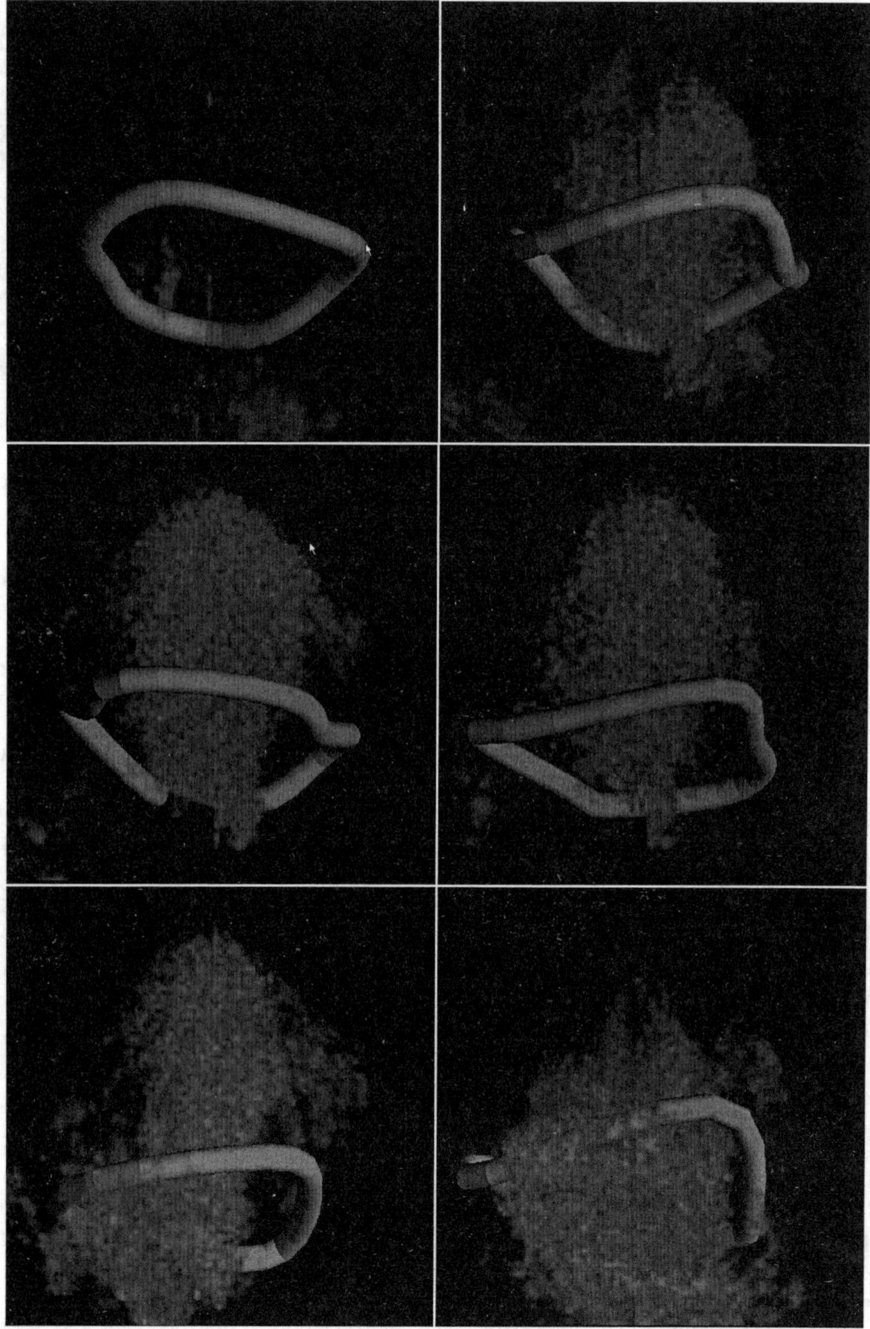

Figure 4. Annulus dynamics over a heart cycle displayed in combination with blood flow.

4. Discussion and Conclusion

The presented methods enable an enhanced visualization of three-dimensional echocardiographic data. The annulus, which normally can not easiliy be distinguished in volume (as well as surface) rendered views, is inserted in the volume rendered scene as a clearly visible overlay. The segmentation of the annulus necessary to construct the overlay is facilitated by a nearly automatic algorithm reducing the time necessary for user interaction. Both, segmentation and visualization methods have been integrated in our EchoAnalyzer® software package, which will be made available for multicenter evaluation in the future.

The combined visualization of the annulus with the morphology and/or the blood flow may help to elucidate the conditions of regurgitation in the absence of structural valvular abnormalities as well as how much the annulus is involved in regurgitation with valvular disease. Futhermore, it can be used for operation planning of heart valve reconstructions and to design annuli prostheses guided by the individual anatomy.

Acknowledgements

This work was supported by the Deutsche Forschungsgemeinschaft within the Special Research Area 414 "Information Technology in Medicine – Computer and Sensor Supported Surgery".

References

[1] R. De Simone, G. Glombitza, C.F. Vahl, H.P. Meinzer, S. Hagl, Three-dimensional color Doppler reconstruction of intracardiac blood flow in patients with different heart valve diseases, *Am J Cardiol* **86**(12) (2000):1343-8.

[2] S.R. Kaplan, G. Bashein, F.H. Sheehan, M.E. Legget, B. Munt, X.N. Li, M. Sivarajan, E.L. Bolson, M. Zeppa, R.W. Martin, Three-dimensional echocardiographic assessment of annular shape changes in the normal and regurgitant mitral valve, *Am Heart J* **139**(3) (2000):378-87.

[3] I. Wolf, R. De Simone, G. Glombitza, H.P. Meinzer, EchoAnalyzer – A system for three-dimensional echocardiographic visualization and quantification. In: H.U. Lemke, M.W. Vannier, K. Inamura, A.G. Farman, K. Doi (eds.), Proc. Computer Assisted Radiology and Surgery 2001. ISBN: 0 444 50866 X, Elsevier Science, Amsterdam, 2001, pp. 902-7.

[4] I. Wolf, M. Hastenteufel, R. De Simone, G. Glombitza, C.F. Vahl, S. Hagl, H.P. Meinzer. Three-Dimensional Annulus Segmentation and Hybrid Visualisation in Echocardiography. *IEEE Computers in Cardiology* (2001), in print.

[5] I. Wolf, R. De Simone, G. Glombitza, H.P. Meinzer, Automatic segmentation of heart cavities in multidimensional ultrasound images. In: Hanson KM (ed.), Proc. SPIE Medical Imaging 2000, Vol. 3979. Bellingham: SPIE, 2000, pp. 273-83.

Medicine Meets Virtual Reality 02/10
J.D. Westwood et al. (Eds.)
IOS Press, 2002

Engineering and Algorithm Design for an Image Processing API: A Technical Report on ITK - the Insight Toolkit

Terry S. Yoo[1], Michael J. Ackerman[1], William E. Lorensen[2], Will Schroeder[3], Vikram Chalana[4], Stephen Aylward[5], Dimitris Metaxas[6], Ross Whitaker[7]

[1]*National Library of Medicine, National Institutes of Health, Bethesda, MD 20894*
[2] *General Electric Corporate Research and Development, Niskayuna, NY 12309*
[3] *Kitware, Inc. Clifton Park, NY 12065*
[4] *Insightful, Inc, Seattle WA 98109*
[5] *Dept. of Radiology, Univ. of North Carolina at Chapel Hill, Chapel Hill, NC 27599*
[6] *Computer and Information Science Dept, Univ. of Pennsylvania, Philadelphia, PA 19104*
[7] *School of Computing, Univ. of Utah, Salt Lake City, UT 84112*

Abstract. We present the detailed planning and execution of the Insight Toolkit (ITK), an application programmers interface (API) for the segmentation and registration of medical image data. This public resource has been developed through the NLM Visible Human Project, and is in beta test as an open-source software offering under cost-free licensing. The toolkit concentrates on 3D medical data segmentation and registration algorithms, multimodal and multiresolution capabilities, and portable platform independent support for Windows, Linux/Unix systems. This toolkit was built using current practices in software engineering. Specifically, we embraced the concept of generic programming during the development of these tools, working extensively with C++ templates and the freedom and flexibility they allow. Software development tools for distributed consortium-based code development have been created and are also publicly available. We discuss our assumptions, design decisions, and some lessons learned.

1. Introduction

The National Library of Medicine (NLM), in partnership with the National Institute for Dental and Craniofacial Research (NIDCR), the National Eye Institute (NEI), the National Science Foundation (NSF), the National Institute for Neurological Disorders and Stroke (NINDS), the National Institute on Deafness and other Communication Disorders (NIDCD), and the National Cancer Institute (NCI), has founded the Insight Software Consortium to support the creation of a public resource in high-dimension data processing tools. The initial emphasis of this effort is to provide public software tools in 3D segmentation and deformable and rigid registration, capable of analyzing the head-and-neck anatomy of the Visible Human Project data. The eventual goal is for the consortium to provide the cornerstone of a self-sustaining software community in 3D, 4D and higher dimensional data analysis. The consortium is committed to open-source code, public software including open interfaces supporting connections to a broad range of visualization and graphic user interface platforms.

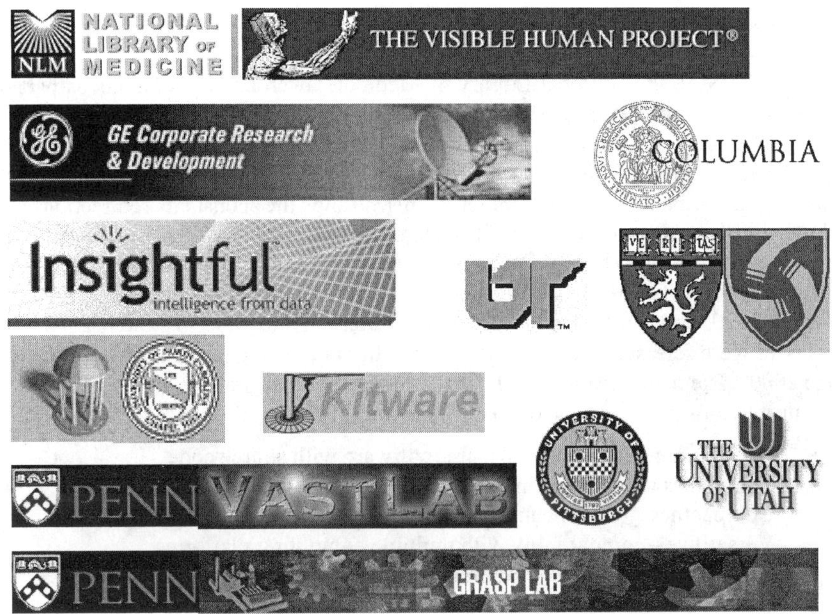

Figure 1. The Insight Software Consotium Members: The Office of High Performance Computing and Communications – NLM, General Electric Corporate R&D, Kitware, Inc., Insightful, Inc., the University of North Carolina at Chapel Hill, the University of Pennsylvania (the VAST Lab and the Department of Radiology), and the University of Tennessee, Harvard Brigham and Women's Hospital, U. Penn's GRASP Lab, the University of Pittsburgh, the University of Utah, and Columbia University.

The Insight Software Research Consortium including partners in academia and in industry has been formed to carry this work forward. The prime contractors are: General Electric Corporate R&D, Kitware, Inc., Insightful, Inc., the University of North Carolina at Chapel Hill, the University of Pennsylvania (the VAST Lab and the Department of Radiology), and the University of Tennessee. Subcontracts from the prime contractors have been extended to: Harvard Brigham and Women's Hospital, U. Penn's GRASP Lab, the University of Pittsburgh, the University of Utah, and Columbia University. The prime contractors and their subcontractors comprise the software research consortium with the principal investigators of the prime contractors serving as the governing board. Together with the NLM Office of High Performance Computing and Communications as the executive member, the Insight Software Consortium is working to deliver a software toolkit to improve and enable research in volume imaging for all areas of health care.

This work is a continuation of the successful Visible Human Project™. The original project was a far-reaching enterprise in human anatomy [3]. However, it fell short of the goal of creating a self-supported community of imaging research. The absence of inexpensive adequate imaging software tools eroded the momentum of the community. The current effort is one part of a multi-prong effort in anatomical and imaging research, the Visible Human Project™: From Data to Knowledge [1]. Two other efforts, one on advanced data acquisition and the other on distributed delivery of Visible Human Project™ content in the form of an online head and neck atlas are also in progress. Together, through these three works-in-progress as well as through three sponsored projects in Next Generation Internet distributed anatomical education and collaboration, we are attempting to stimulate the research community by providing new vehicles for the distribution of content, new data and data acquisition techniques, and new software image analysis tools.

2. Background

In the Fall of 1999, the National Library of Medicine awarded six contracts as part of an announced consortium effort called the Visible Human Project™ Image Processing Tools. The collective image processing contracts represent a 3-year, $7.5 million project in image analysis software tools. These contracts were organized through a flexible administrative mechanism of annual work assignments, permitting the constant redirection of the development of a software tool set as its design principles evolved. A first meeting of the software consortium was held in November 1999, and the initial vision for the software consortium was published at MMVR2000 [4]. A software architecture meeting was held in January 2000, and a meeting on algorithm validation was held in March 2000. Initial C++ classes were released at the second organizational meeting of the software consortium in June 2000. The name *Insight* was formally adopted at that time.

In our previous paper [4], we described our commitment to:

- Open Source Software – cost-free software with source code
- Toolkits as a Software Engineering Philosophy - APIs
- Compactness – not encumbering the software with multiple licenses
- Versatility – compatibility with multiple computing platforms
- Long Range Support – including distribution, education, and maintenance
- Validation – shared validation methods to promote algorithm development
- 3D – a strong preference for volume techniques and higher dimensions

The Insight Software Consortium has completed design and development of an initial version of a public medical image segmentation and registration toolkit known as the Insight ToolKit (ITK).

3. Architecture – Requirements

Beyond governing principles, the first task in formulating any software engineering task is to evaluate the user requirements as well as assess the available resources and current practices. We briefly cover the design decisions, the targeted user community, and the user requirements selected early in the evolution of ITK.

Primary users - We have selected application developers as the primary audience for ITK. Specifically, a clinician or other practitioner is not the first target user of the products of this work. The goal is to create an application programmer's interface (API) which can be used by developers in medical programs and software products wherever the problems of image or volume segmentation and registration exist. Unlike previous NIH imaging software development efforts, the goal is specifically NOT to create a single monolithic program. Rather, we are pursuing a software foundation from which a broad range of programs can be supported. The Insight mission is to provide: a software foundation for future research, an archival repository of image processing algorithms, a catalog of validation techniques, as well as a platform for advanced product development.

ITK supports native and generic data types (native: long, unsigned long, float, double, Char, Unsigned char, Int, unsigned int, shorts, unsigned shorts. Generic: u9, u16, etc.) as well as multi-component (intensity, intensity/α, RGB, RGB/α, vector or diffusion tensor data, etc.) and multidimensional data (x-y-z, x-y-z-time, x-y-z-scale, etc.). Insight has supported this notion of high dimensionality, both in independent and dependent variables, from its inception. N-dimensional datasets are explicitly support for specific operations, and where possible all pixel-wise operations support n-dimensions. These requirements lead to the widespread use of templates and generic types.

Processing requirements – ITK supports the processing of large datasets on modest processing platforms including multiprocessor systems. At the time of the design meeting (January 2000), the consortium selected mid-range desktop machines as the target (450 MHz CPU with a 0.5 GB of core memory). It was anticipated that mid-range desktops would track growing dataset sizes with a ratio of 10: 1 for dataset size to main-memory capacities. Current mid-range desktop computers (January 2002) can be found in the range of 1.25 GHz CPUs and main memory sizes of 2 GB are not uncommon. However, we continue to believe that our target of 10:1 dataset size to main memory is still valid as dataset sizes continue to increase. The increase in availability of multiprocessing shared-memory computers was also anticipated, and accommodations for pipelined and streaming software architectures were made early in the design.

Language and hardware support requirements – C++ was selected as the project programming language with the caveat that the library support multiple language bindings, permitting compilation and linking with a range of contemporary computer languages. Java provided better cross-hardware-platform portability, but it was deemed too young a language. Since part of the mission of Insight is to provide an archival mechanism for algorithms, C++ is adequate for programming a library. We observe that many of the software libraries in use today are written in C or even in Fortran. They serve the purposes of usable APIs and algorithm archives so long as they support multiple language bindings.

ITK is supported on multiple hardware systems. We specifically targeted Sun, SGI, Linux, and Windows/9x/NT/2000 as primary goals. Macintosh systems are not excluded, but were not specifically included in the original specifications. The advent of Mac OSX makes support for Apple systems more likely. By far, the greatest constraint on the platform support has been the adequate availability of compilers that correctly handle C++ templates. As mentioned before, the requirement for handling multi-dimensional images drives the use of generic types and a broad incorporation of templates in the ITK software.

Available resources and current practices – Engineering as an enterprise is always subject to the available resources and the current methods in use. Software engineering is no exception; the resources in question are measured in the expertise of your personnel, access to machines, and other intangible factors. The Insight Software Consortium is geographically widely distributed, so collaboration and communication have been limiting resources. Much of our software engineering has been in support of the distributed software development enterprise, including automated test and build procedures, online reporting of the state of the software, automated generation of documentation, and bug tracking. As a result, all software elements have been accompanied by inline documentation and built-in software regression tests.

As a rule, we adopted the most current software development practices in object oriented programming, while adhering to the principles of compactness and versatility. We selected the *vxl* numerical programming library from another open source initiative; vxl has no encumbering language preventing free development or distribution of derivative work. The consortium also incorporated the Standard Template Library (STL) as well as programmed through the creation of new templated classes. The compactness principle dictates that the toolkit shall not have any dependencies on specific visualization software; however it must have hooks and interfaces for interactive operations, callback, and event handlers for dynamic visualization.

4. Software Design and Project Execution

The user requirements and design goals of the Insight project directed the project along certain predictable lines. The memory and parallel processing requirements dictated a pipelined streaming software architecture. The distributed and sophisticated nature of the programming effort placed other, more novel concerns before the consortium, setting specific directions for the group. Nevertheless, knowing the direction of our code development and foreseeing the impact and breadth of the work being attempted are two different things. The Insight Consortium has broken new ground in collaborative software development and the use of generic programming in API development.

Extreme programming – The brevity of our development cycle and limited communications among the programming teams suggested a departure from the traditional government sponsored software development process of design specification followed by implementation, quality assurance, and testing. A continuously re-iterative design, implementation, and coding process, called *extreme programming* [2], has been adopted by the consortium. The ITK API has undergone continuous review and modification by the expert developers on the programming team. GE Corporate R&D along with Kitware, Inc. serve as the lead design groups, with GE CRD handling issues of testing and quality control during development and Kitware serving as system integrators for the project. Other teams from across the consortium are contributing new implementations of complex medical image processing algorithms, helping to refine the software architecture as the toolkit grows in complexity and mathematical sophistication. There are substantial costs to the constant redesign, but the reward is early implementation and rapid improvement through frequent revision.

Generic Programming – The Insight Software Consortium has undertaken an aggressive approach in the design and execution of ITK. Advanced programming concepts and techniques in object-oriented programming have been incorporated into the toolkit. C++ is the chosen language for the software development; however, it is the comprehensive use of programming templates and the adoption of generic programming practices which have driven this project to the edge-of-the-art in programming. These choices permit algorithm development without strong typing of the atomic image elements, providing for great flexibility in the toolkit. Color data, greyscale, floating point, and other image values are handled with equal facility. More importantly, the generic programming style permits rapid development of the toolkit by many team members simultaneously, allowing large changes to the software across all aspects of the toolkit with minimal disruption. The pervasive use of these methods makes ITK unique among software APIs.

CMake and CABLE - Early in the development process, we recognized the need for a comprehensive build and test environment. We were also aware of the need to support multiple languages, especially interpretive development languages for rapid application prototyping, including the Tool Control Language (TCL), Python, and Java. As part of our design process, we therefore included the creation of CMake, a cross platform build environment supporting Windows (Microsoft Visual C++), GNU C++, and SGI Irix C++. CMake prevents skew of our code by eliminating the need for simultaneous development f the software on multiple platforms. In addition to CMake, we included the development of CABLE, a generic code wrapping tool to provide multiple language bindings for languages such as TCL. These advanced software engineering concepts are applicable to a wide cross section of programming initiatives and are available in source code form as separate tools offered from the Insight Software Development Consortium Indeed, CMake has already been adopted internationally among software developers faced with writing code for Windows and Unix platforms.

Engineering a Collaboration: DART – an automated build and test environment – Finally, we have created a comprehensive test environment that supports build and regression testing. Continual and nightly builds of ITK Test results are posted on a web-accessible dashboard, providing immediate feedback for software developers as to the integrity of their modifications and their compatibility with all supported computing platforms. Coordination of a large software project, especially one with a geographically distributed team would be nearly impossible without this facility. Like CMake and CABLE, DART is available as a separate software engineering suite in source code form.

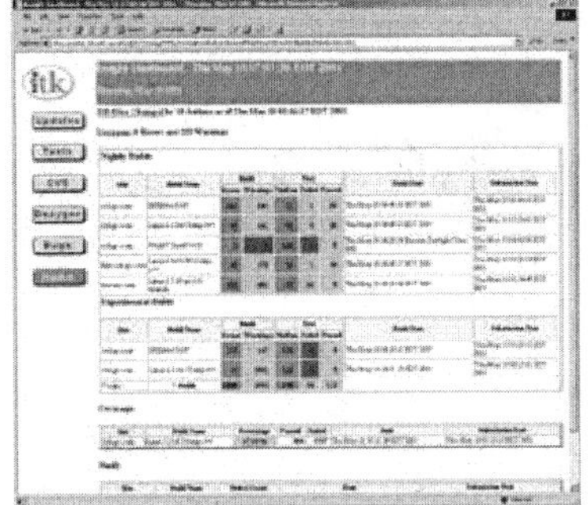

Figure 2. A DART Dashboard for ITK. This is a postage stamp view representing a full web page that reflects the state of the toolkit at any time. Nightly and continuous builds constantly update the online report showing failed tests and warnings on multiple platforms with multiple compilers. These builds are run at different locations in the consortium with the results displayed on a single portal. Recent changes to the source code can be tracked through the dashboard including the programmers responsible for changes that lead to build failures. Distributed development teams can be coordinated in multiple time zones using this facility. DART is a product of the Insight Software Consortium and is available as an open source product.

5. Algorithms, Examples and the ITK Beta Release: an invitation

The consortium members represent a broad cross-section of skills and backgrounds, each with considerable expertise in medical image analysis. The algorithm developers in the group have proposed and are contributing methods representing a comprehensive range of approaches for the filtering, processing, segmenting, and registering high-dimensional medical data. Watersheds, level set mathematics, geometric partial differential equations, finite element models, finite differencing engines, statistical pattern recognition techniques, and Voronoi spatial decomposition hybridized with deformable models for segmentation are among the many methods represented in ITK. Many of these methods are multithreaded and pipelined for maximum performance. Insight is dedicated to open-source code, so all of these methods are publicly available through the API source.

The Insight Software Consortium is beginning a public beta release of ITK. Interested programmers should search the following URL – http://www.itk.org. Additional documentation, examples, and a thorough review of the materials in this paper can be found at that site. The consortium is especially interested in feedback from application developers on the integration of ITK with existing visualization and interactive medical image analysis packages. Beta test results will be solicited in June 2002 with the goal of a full release of ITK by October 2002.

6. Conclusions

The Insight Software Consortium has developed a first version of the Insight ToolKit (ITK), an open source software API for medical image segmentation and registration. We have described the design criteria and user requirements that later led to our software engineering practices used throughout ITK. Chief among these practices are *generic programming* through extensive use of C++ templates and the rapid iterative development strategy of *extreme programming*. To support our distributed software development team, multiple programming platforms, and the need for multiple language bindings, the Insight Software Consortium has endorsed and created DART (for automated build and testing on multiple software and hardware architectures), CMake (a cross-platform make system), and CABLE (a language wrapping tool providing link capabilities in TCL, and soon for Python). ITK has an internal data-flow architecture supporting threading, streaming and pipelining for multiprocessor and large data support. ITK is currently publicly available.

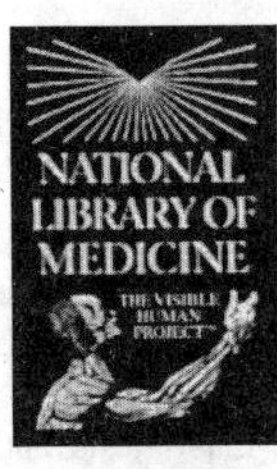
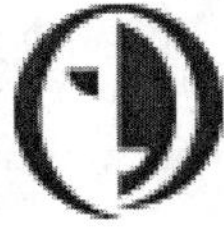
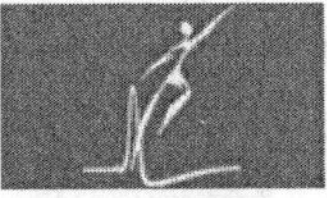

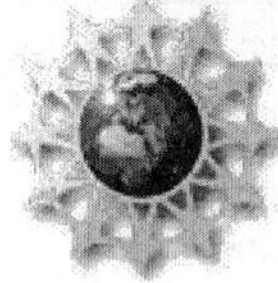
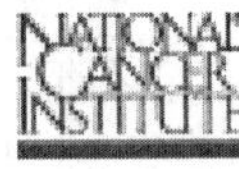
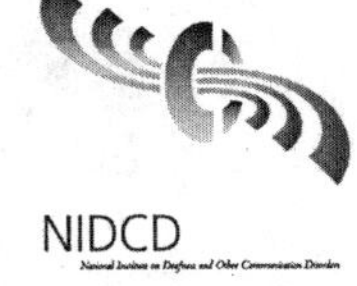

Figure 3. The sponsors of the Visible Human Project: From Data to Knowledge. This is a trans-NIH and inter-agency initiative in information technology for health care research.

7. Acknowledgements

The authors would like to thank the National Library of Medicine (NLM) and its Visible Human Project™ for its support for this project, along with its partners: the National Institute for Dental and Craniofacial Research (NIDCR), the National Eye Institute (NEI), the National Science Foundation (NSF), the National Institute for Neurological Disorders and Stroke (NINDS), the National Institute on Deafness and other Communication Disorders (NIDCD), and the National Cancer Institute (NCI). This project has been carried through the dedication of our research investigators, our subcontractors and their PIs, and our staff and student programmers. We would also like to thank our colleagues in the Insight Software Consortium, including (among many): Jim Miller (GE CRD), Peter Ratiu (Harvard BWH), Bill Hoffman, Ken Martin, and Brad King (Kitware), Lydia Ng (Insightful), Luis Ibanez and Julien Jormier (UNC-CH), George Stetten, and Aaron Cois (UPitt), Jim Gee, Jay Udupa and Ting Chen (UPenn), Celina Imielinska, Pat Moholt, and Hillary Schmidt (Columbia), and Josh Cates (Utah).

References

[1] Ackerman, M.J., T.S. Yoo, D. Jenkins. 2000. The visible human project: from data to knowledge. Computer Assisted Radiology and Surgery (Proceedings of CARS2000), H. U. Lemke, et al. eds., Elsevier Press, Amsterdam: 11-16.

[2] Beck, Kent. 1999. Embracing change with extreme programming. IEEE Computer, October 1999. 32(10). 70-77.

[3] V. Spitzer, M. J. Ackerman, A. L. Scherzinger, and D. Whitlock. 1996. The Visible Human Male: A Technical Report. J. of the Am. Medical Informatics Assoc. 3(2) 118-130.

[4] Yoo, T.S. and M.J. Ackerman, 2000, A new program in medical image data processing, Medicine Meets Virtual Reality 2000 (Proceedings of the 8th Annual Medicine Meets Virtual Reality Conference), James Westwood, et al. eds., IOS Press, Amsterdam. 385-391.

Finite Element (FE) Modeling of the Mandible: from Geometric Model to Tetrahedral Volumetric Mesh

Linping Zhao[1,2]   H. Han[2,3]   P. K. Patel[1,2,3]   G. E. O. Widera[1]   G. F. Harris[1,2]
[1]Marquette University, P.O. Box 1881, Milwaukee, WI 53201
[2]Shriners Hospital for Children, 2211 Oak Park Avenue, Chicago, IL 60707
[3]Northwestern University Medical School, Chicago, IL 60611

Abstract. This paper presents our experience in using FE modeling of clinically relevant cases specifically in mandibular surgery. A semi-automatic procedure integrated with a group of Virtual Basic-based codes has been developed to clean the geometric models. Consequently, the time required for generate the tetrahedral volumetric mesh of mandible from patient-specific CT data has been reduced to less than 40 hours. Pre- and post-operation FE meshes are shown to be consistent and can be used for further modeling and analysis.

1. Introduction

A critical step in a patient-specific FE modeling process is the generation of the geometrical model of bony components. Current approach for the creation of three-dimensional models of craniofacial anatomy is time-consuming and prone to errors [1, 2].

In our preliminary study [3], a different approach for the routine development of child-specific mandibular model was proposed. The basic idea of this consists of generating the geometric models using an available medical imaging visualization package (ANALYZE AVW, Biomedical Imaging Resource, Mayo Foundation, Rochester, MN), and then importing such geometric models into a FE analysis package (DEFORM 3D, Scientific Forming Technologies Corp., Columbus, OH) to generate the volumetric tetrahedral mesh. The time- and labor-intensive step in this approach is the editing, including cleaning, repairing and smoothing, of the geometric model.

This paper presents our recent progresses with regard to geometric model editing. A child with an isolated mandibular deformity is used to demonstrate our procedure. In particular, problems encountered during surface editing are investigated and a semi-automatic approach is developed.

2. Procedure

The procedure employed for generating a geometrical model of the mandible from patient-specific CT/MRI data is shown in Figure 1.

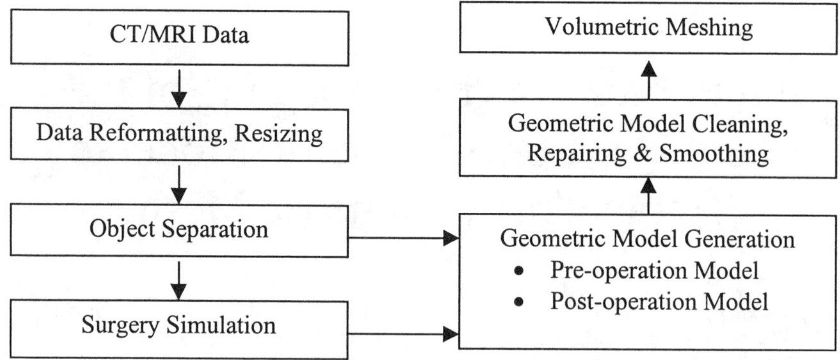

Figure 1. Procedure for geometrical model generation and meshing from patient-specific CT/MRI data.

3. Results

3.1. Identification and Removal of Geometric Discontinuities

In order to generate the mesh of the solid model successfully, the preprocessor of DEFORM 3D requires that the input geometry consist of only one unique surface topologically. However, the geometric model of the mandible generated by use of ANALYZE AVW does not fulfill this requirement since it includes some geometric discontinuities. The geometric discontinuities detected by the preprocessor include inner cavities, free edges, holes, and irregularities. Figure 2 shows two examples of the inner cavities in the geometric model of mandible.

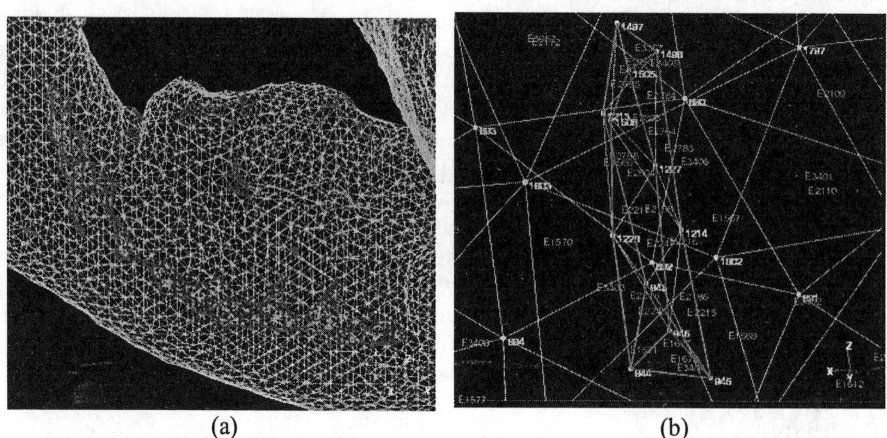

Figure 2. Inner cavities in the geometric models of mandible: (a) long pipe; (b) small inner cavity.

A group of Virtual-BASIC (VB) codes have been developed as additional macros of Microsoft Excel to remove the inner cavities. Several points representing the inner cavity and its dimensions were picked up visually. Using these data as input, the corresponding macros are then run to identify the points of the inner cavities. The surface elements or the connectivity representing the inner cavities were then separated from the element set of the entire surface. Using this semi-automatic approach, up to 80 to 90% of the inner cavities can be removed. The remaining free edges and holes, as shown in Figure 3, are relatively easy to remove manually.

Other surface irregularities often need to be removed by redefining those surface elements or the connectivity involved so as to smooth the surface. This was complemented manually in our study.

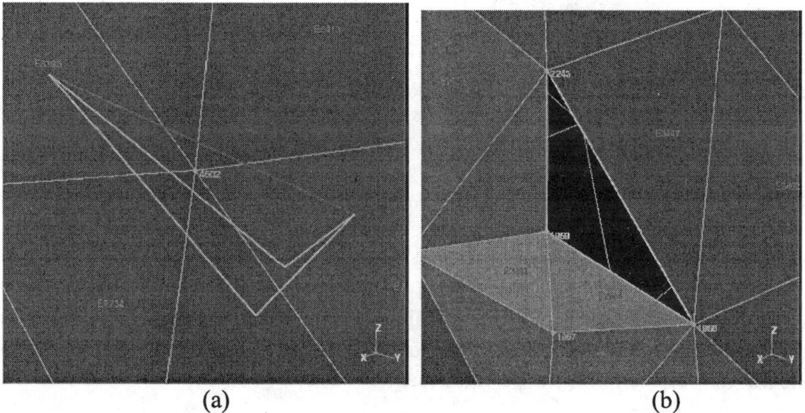

(a)   (b)

Figure 3. Discontinuities in the geometric model of mandible: (a) free edges; (b) hole on the surface.

3.2. Volumetric Mesh

After various discontinuities in the geometric models had been removed, volumetric tetrahedral meshes of both the pre- and post-operation mandible were generated, as shown in Figure 4. They are consistent visually and can be used for further modeling and analysis.

Using the above approach, the time required for the geometric model editing, including cleaning, repairing and smoothing, can be reduced to less than 30 hours for a single mandible model. For the same subject and the same model, more than 100 hours can be expended if the model is set up manually, based on our previous experience. Using our approach, the total modeling time required for a mandible from the patient–specific CT data to the volumetric tetrahedral mesh is less than 40 hours.

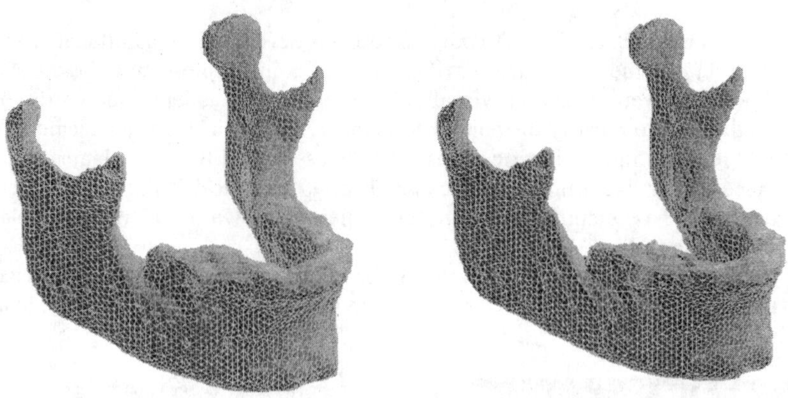

Figure 4. Finite element mesh of mandible subject to the mandible advancement: (a) pre-operation, (b) post-operation.

4. Summary

The procedure to rapidly generate a patient-specific volumetric model for FE analysis from CT scan data has been further developed. A semi-automatic approach to remove the inner cavities of the geometric model of mandible has been integrated into the procedure. With this approach, the time required for the development of a patient-specific solid model and tetrahedral mesh generation can be significantly reduced.

Acknowledgement

This research was supported by Shriners Hospital for Children and the Orthopaedic & Rehabilitation Engineering Center (OREC) jointly sponsored by Marquette University and the Medical College of Wisconsin.

References

[1] T.W.P. Korioth, A.,Verslius, Modeling the Mechanical Behavior of the Jaws and their Related Structures by Finite Element(FE) Analysis, *Crit Rev Oral Biol Med*, 8(1), pp.90-104, 1997.

[2] Linping Zhao, P. K. Patel, G. E. O. Widera, H. Han, G. F. Harris, Medical Imaging Genesis for Finite Element-Based Mandibular Surgical Planning in the Pediatric Subject, 23rd Annual International Conference of the IEEE Engineering in Medicine and Biology Society, Istanbul, Turkey, October 25-28, 2001.

[3] R. A. Robb, Biomedical Imaging, Visualization, and Analysis. Willey-Liss, pp. 237-272, 2000.

Author Index